Introduction to the
Neurophysiology of Movement

Introduction to the Neurophysiology of Movement

Andrew J. Fuglevand

University of Arizona, USA

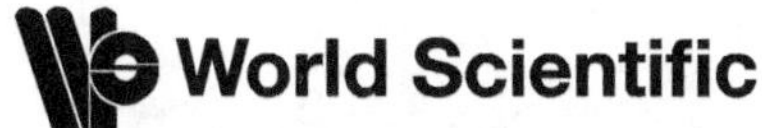

World Scientific

NEW JERSEY · LONDON · SINGAPORE · BEIJING · SHANGHAI · TAIPEI · CHENNAI

Published by

World Scientific Publishing Co. Pte. Ltd.

5 Toh Tuck Link, Singapore 596224

USA office: 27 Warren Street, Suite 401-402, Hackensack, NJ 07601

UK office: 57 Shelton Street, Covent Garden, London WC2H 9HE

British Library Cataloguing-in-Publication Data
A catalogue record for this book is available from the British Library.

INTRODUCTION TO THE NEUROPHYSIOLOGY OF MOVEMENT

ISBN 978-981-98-1352-0 (hardcover)
ISBN 978-981-98-1395-7 (paperback)
ISBN 978-981-98-1353-7 (ebook for institutions)
ISBN 978-981-98-1354-4 (ebook for individuals)

For any available supplementary material, please visit
https://www.worldscientific.com/worldscibooks/10.1142/14324#t=suppl

Typeset by Stallion Press
Email: enquiries@stallionpress.com

Dedication

This work is dedicated to my remarkable mentors: Drs. Ellen Krieghbaum, Doris Miller, David Winter, Roger Enoka, and Brenda Bigland-Ritchie.

Preface

This is an introductory textbook that examines how the brain and spinal cord control movement. It is primarily directed toward senior undergraduates and junior graduate students in the movement sciences (kinesiology, motor control, exercise sciences), physiology, applied physiology, biomedical engineering, and in early stages of clinical programs such as physical therapy, occupational therapy, rehabilitation sciences, and speech sciences. I have found that many students enrolled in such programs (and even some investigators who work in these areas) often have relatively poor understanding of basic principles of neurophysiology that are foundations of motor control. Therefore, this book begins with chapters outlining fundamentals of cellular neurophysiology. This information is not only useful for understanding the control of movement but also for understanding many aspects of nervous system function. As a consequence, this material should also provide a solid footing for students of these programs to exchange important ideas and collaborate with colleagues trained primarily in the neurosciences.

The playing of a musical instrument, the swinging of a tennis racquet, dancing, speaking, changing a light bulb, or simply walking down a street are all examples of exquisitely controlled behaviors enacted by our nervous system. Yet, these behaviors are not produced by a "motor system" in isolation. Indeed, virtually all motor behaviors critically depend on input from a variety of sensory systems. In particular, the somatosensory (literally "body sense") system is essential for producing controlled movements. As such, this book outlines the organization and operation of the somatosensory system—from sensory receptors in the periphery to high-level processing in the somatosensory cortex. Furthermore, the somatosensory system is reasonably comprehensible and enables understanding of general principles of sensory processing that are applicable to other sensory systems.

The "motor system" proper is also described by beginning in the periphery (with the motor unit) and working up to motor areas of the cerebral cortex. Other brain structures (cerebellum and basal ganglia), known to have important influences on motor function, are also described. The functions that these regions play are described in the context of three broad categories of movement: reflexes, rhythmical behaviors, and voluntary movements. Also, along the way, various disorders of the nervous system affecting movement are described, and some approaches applied to treat these disorders are outlined.

An extensive appendix providing a conceptual overview of electricity and electrical circuits is also included as part of this book. This appendix has been added because of the importance of electrical signaling within the nervous system. Indeed, students should have a solid understanding of electricity if they are to grasp how the brain processes information and produces behaviors. Yet, many students struggle with basic electrical concepts. Therefore, Appendix A is provided as a gentle but thorough (re-) introduction to principles of electrical circuits.

The study of how the nervous system controls movement is undergoing a renaissance. Remarkable genetic tools combined with advanced methods for quantifying behavior have enabled investigators to probe the function of individual neurons in the production of various types of movements. Furthermore, it is now possible to record the activities of hundreds of neurons simultaneously during the performance of motor acts in awake behaving animals. Such approaches have unveiled new and important insights (and many new questions) as to how the nervous system controls movement. Yet, many of the basic principles identified in over 125 years of careful investigation since the time of Cajal and Sherrington remain relevant today and are the building blocks for understanding motor control. This book focuses primarily on those building blocks, but some of the new ideas are also introduced.

Relatively few references are provided in this book. Much of the work described has been thoroughly established over many years of careful investigations by a host of researchers. As such, it did not seem necessary to reacknowledge all those important contributions. In some cases, however, where experimental studies are not yet part of the canon of motor control neurophysiology, citations are provided. Also, citations to particularly readable and seminal works are given. In addition, citations are provided for all figures used in the book.

It must also be acknowledged that my thinking about the topic of this book has been strongly shaped by a set of foundational textbooks and monographs. These include *Principles of Physiology—Electrophysiology* by the University of Washington group (Patton *et al.* 1989), *Neurobiology* (Shepherd 1994), *Corticospinal Function and Voluntary Movement* (Lemon & Porter 1995), *From Neuron to Brain* (Nicols *et al.* 2001), *The Neuron* (Kazmerick & Levitan 2001), *Principles of Neural Science* (Kandel *et al.* 2012), and *The Motoneurone and Its Muscle Fibres* (Kernell 2006). These works permeate this book. I have attempted to cite them where their influence is direct and obvious—but there are certainly many other instances where their influence was subconscious, and as such, may not have been cited.

All illustrations, unless otherwise indicated, were made by the author.

Contents

Part 1

Cellular Neurophysiology

Chapter 1
Introduction to Neurophysiology

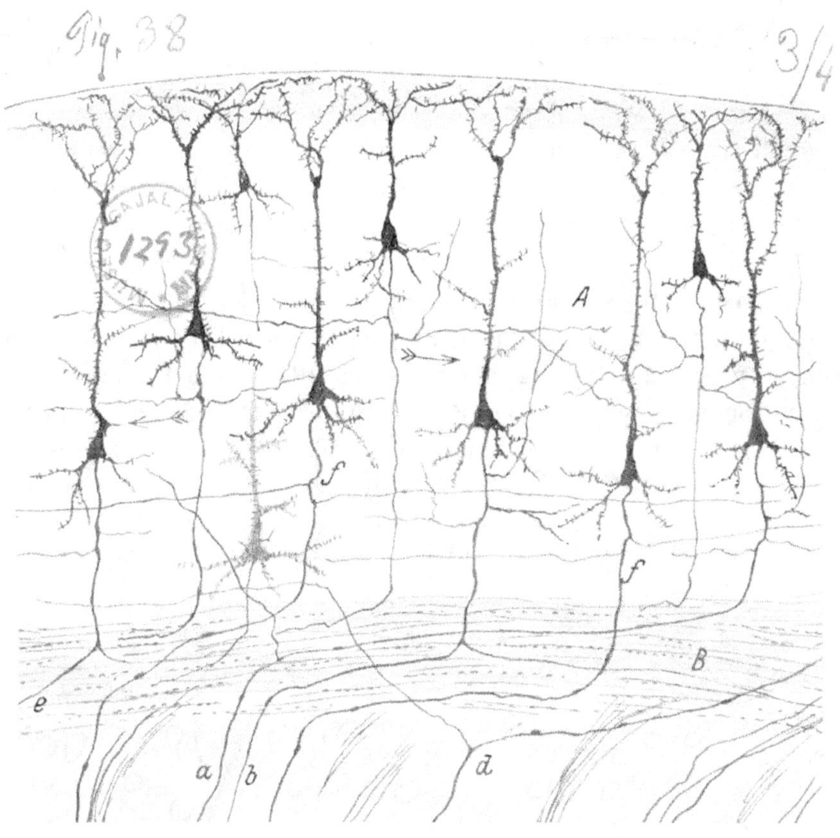

Pyramidal neurons of the cerebral cortex. Santiago Ramon y Cajal.

Overview

From the broadest perspective, the nervous system is a massive assembly of cells that continuously takes in information about the external environment through various sensory systems (Figure 1A), monitors the internal state of the organism via the autonomic nervous system (Figure 1B), and draws upon stored knowledge related to previous experiences using memory systems (Figure 1C). This array of converging information is processed and analyzed moment-by-moment and is used by the organism to make decisions about what it should do next. Such decisions involve selection and generation of a behavior from a repertoire of behaviors available to the organism through the motor system (Figure 1D). The outcome of the selected behavior is monitored and used as an additional source of information back to the nervous system (Figure 1E). Behavior itself is almost always expressed in some form of movement mediated by muscular activity—and it can be as subtle as the gentle contractions of facial muscles to produce a smile or as conspicuous as the powerful contractions of the leg, trunk, and arm muscles as an athlete sprints down a track.

These operations of taking in information, processing it, making decisions, and generating behaviors are accomplished by communication among an inconceivably large number of cells (the neurons). For example, the human brain is thought to possess on the order of 100 billion neurons. Fortunately, there are some simplifying features of the nervous system

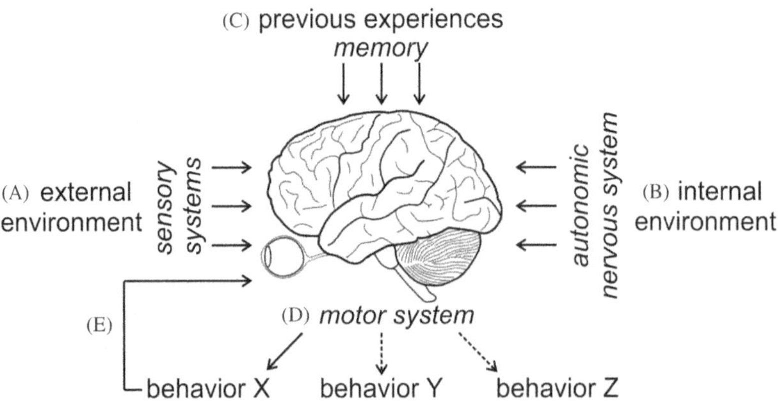

Figure 1.   Overview of the operations of the nervous system.

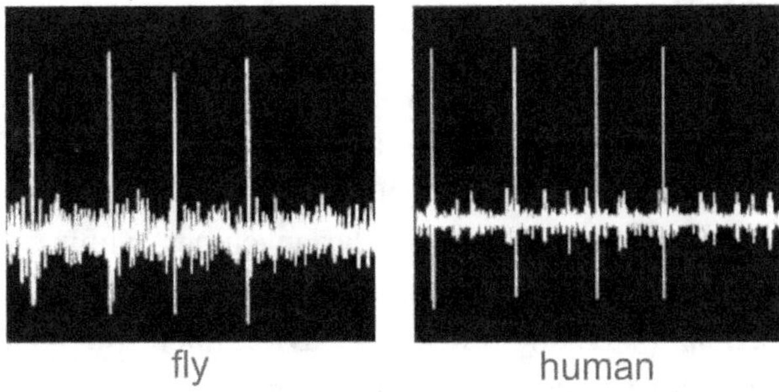

Figure 2.   Example recordings of the brief trains of action potentials recorded from a neuron in the fly visual system (adapted from Rieke *et al.* [1999]) and from an axon supplying a tactile receptor in the skin of the human hand (from the author's laboratory).

that make it possible to begin to understand some aspects of how it works. First, the individual neurons (the building blocks of the nervous system) are roughly similar in terms of their structural and functional organizations. Second, communication among neurons, which is typically in the form of electrical impulses, is similar not only among various neurons within an organism but also across widely different species. For example, as shown in Figure 2, the electrical impulses recorded from a neuron in the visual system of a fly is, for all practical purposes, indistinguishable from that recorded from a tactile neuron arising from the fingertip of a human subject. This means that we can understand a great deal about the workings of the nervous system by studying neural function in simpler organisms.

The **electrical impulses** are referred to by a number of names (*spikes, action potentials, discharges, impulses*) and are used interchangeably. The patterns of these impulses generated by neurons can be thought to represent the vocabulary of the nervous system by which neurons communicate. In some respects, *neurophysiology* can be considered as the study of this communication and the associated processing of information in the nervous system by analyzing electrical signaling within and among neurons. As such, it is crucial for anyone attempting to understand neurophysiology to have a reasonable conceptual grasp of electricity and simple electronics. Accordingly, Appendix A provides a general overview of these topics. Anyone without a solid background in these topics (or who has forgotten their physics!) is urged to review Appendix A.

Dawn of Modern Neuroscience

The broad topic of neurophysiology is centrally situated among an array of overlapping subdisciplines within the field of neuroscience. These subdisciplines range from molecular neurobiology—used to understand the structure and function of the molecular machines within neurons—to psychology—used to make important inferences about the organization of the brain based on systematic study of behavior. Interestingly, the study of the nervous system lagged behind that of other physiological systems. Indeed, it wasn't until well into the 20th century that it was even accepted that the nervous system was composed of distinct cells. Instead, the largely accepted view was that which was embodied in the **Reticular Theory**, which states that the *nervous system is a continuous meshwork (i.e., a "reticulum") with one element in direct continuity with the next.* As shown in Figure 3, taken from a famous textbook published in 1867, the nervous system was represented as a continuous system not unlike that of a vascular network. Furthermore, nervous signals were thought to be able to flow in any direction within the network.

One major reason why the study of the nervous system was impeded is that nervous tissue is inherently difficult to study under the microscope. On its own, a section of the nervous system is translucent, and it is challenging to identify individual cells. When various substances were applied to nervous-system sections to stain cells, typically only parts of neurons (such as the nucleus) would be stained. As a consequence, little was known throughout most of the 19th century about the structure of neurons or their physical interrelationships with one another. Therefore, it was one of the major breakthroughs in neuroscience when, in 1873, Camillo Golgi of Italy discovered that the application of a silver nitrate solution to sections of neural tissue yielded highly detailed labeling of individual neurons (Figure 4). There were a number of remarkable features of Golgi's stain. First, the cells turned a deep black with the entire cell down to its finest processes sharply stained. Second, only a fraction of the cells in a section took up the stain. This enabled a clear and unobstructed view of entire neurons. Had all the cells taken up the stain, it would be nearly impossible to distinguish one cell from another given the density of cells and the extensive spatial overlap of their processes. Furthermore, there did

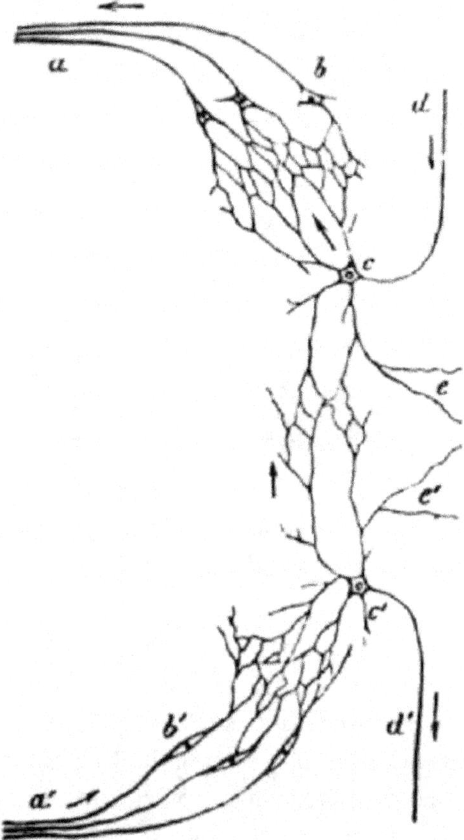

Figure 3.   Illustration taken from Kölliker A, Handbuch der Gewebelehre des Menchen (1867), showing continuous network (reticulum) of connections among neural elements. Signals are shown to flow in many directions within the network. For example, the arrow at a′ is directed toward the neuron c′, whereas the arrows at d′ and across from e′ are directed in opposite directions away from neuron c′. (Adapted from Shepherd [1991].)

not appear to be any particular bias as to what types of neurons took up the stain. As such, the neurons that were stained provided a more or less representative sample of the neural population within the section. Upon viewing a section labeled with his stain, it was immediately obvious to Golgi that there were distinctly different types of neurons with particular spatial relationships to one another and that fine processes seemed to link some neurons to others.

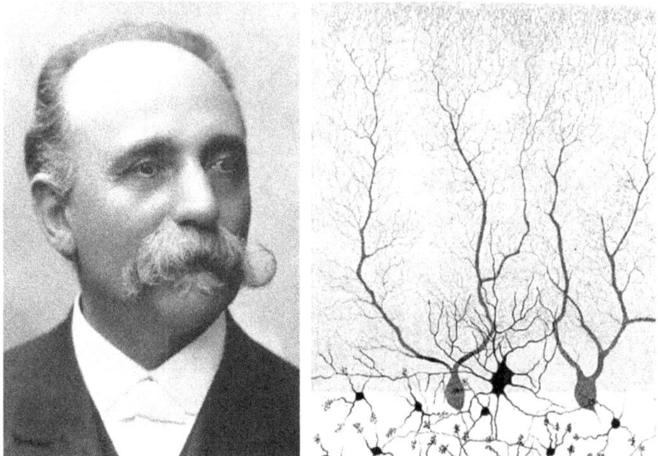

Figure 4.   Camillo Golgi, discoverer of silver nitrate stain that enabled a detailed view of individual neurons. Drawing made by Golgi of a section stained with his method showing distinct types of neurons within the cerebellum.

The discovery by Golgi threw open the doors to systematic investigation of the nervous system and ushered in the modern era of neuroscience. And it was the great Spanish anatomist, Santiago Ramon y Cajal (Figure 5) whose extensive use of the Golgi stain in the late 19th century advanced the field of neuroscience more than any other investigator past or present. His observations of neurons in multiple regions of the nervous system across many species and at various stages of development led Cajal to reject the Reticular Theory. Instead, Cajal proposed the **Neuron Doctrine**, which simply states that *the basic signaling units of the nervous system are the neurons and each neuron is a distinct entity*. Furthermore, Cajal added a corollary to the Neuron Doctrine referred to as the **Principle of Dynamic Polarity**, which states that *information flows in one direction only within a neuron*. Figure 5 shows one of the many extraordinary schematic diagrams made by Cajal (who was also an artist), vividly depicting the interrelationships among neurons, illustrating each neuron as a discrete entity, and designating the flow of information to be in one direction only. These principles are the foundations of neuroscience and both Cajal and Golgi were awarded the Nobel Prize in 1906 for their contributions toward laying these foundations. Surprisingly, Golgi remained a steadfast

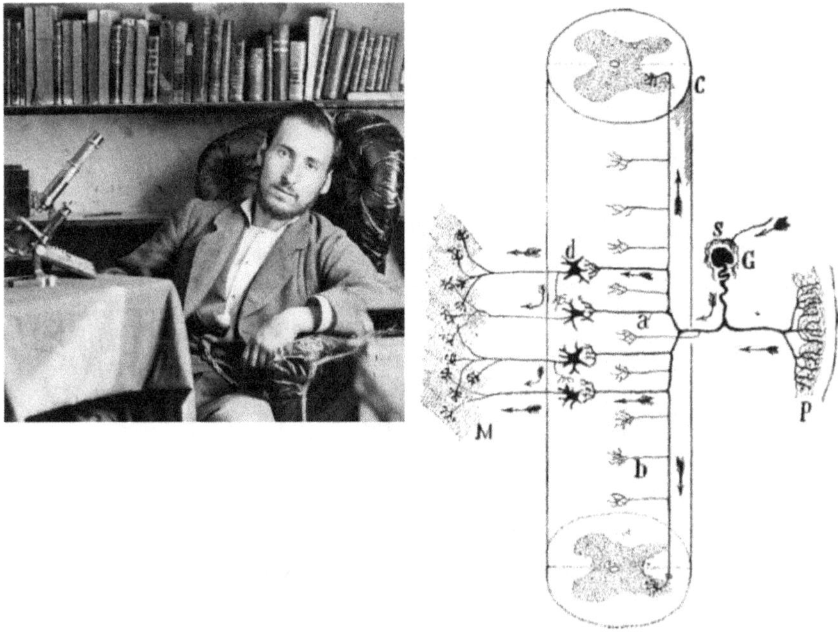

Figure 5.   The father of modern neuroscience, Santiago Ramon y Cajal. Drawing of the spinal cord made by Cajal showing each neuron as a distinct entity (according to his Neuron Doctrine) and information flowing in one direction only within neurons (according to his Principle of Dynamic Polarity).

proponent of the Reticular Theory and challenged the Neuron Doctrine in his Nobel lecture (Seal 2023).

Modern View of the Anatomy of a Neuron

Extensive investigation throughout the first half of the 20th century, including the emergence of new methods (e.g., intracellular recording of electrical signals in living neurons, electron microscopy), led to a consolidated view of the key anatomical components (and their functions) associated with most neurons. Figure 6 shows those components for a typical neuron. The **soma**, or *cell body, houses the nucleus with the genetic material and organelles* needed to keep the neuron alive. *Emerging from the soma are many thin processes* called **dendrites**. The form of the dendritic branches

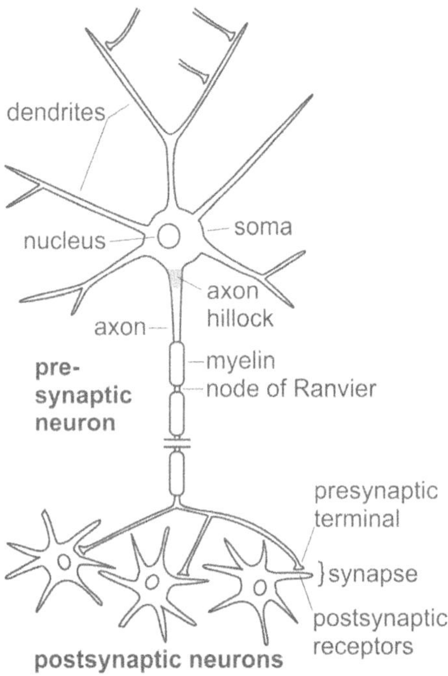

Figure 6.   Anatomical components of a typical neuron. (Adapted from Kandel *et al.* [2012].)

can vary markedly across different types of neurons—some have elaborate branching patterns whereas others have meager arbors. Indeed, the distinctive profiles of dendritic arbors are often used to identify different types of neurons. The dendrites function as the input apparatus for a neuron by gathering synaptic information from many other neurons, not unlike wide astronomical antennae sampling signals from a large array of stars.

One additional process that issues from the soma is the axon. *The region from which the axon emerges from the soma* is sometimes called the **axon hillock** out of which extends the **initial segment of the axon**. This rather humble anatomical region is actually the site of decision-making by most neurons. As we shall see, it dictates whether, and to what degree, a neuron sends signals to other neurons. As such, *it is also referred to by the function it performs* (rather than by its anatomical features) as the **spike-initiating zone**.

The **axon** itself *serves as the communication link between the spike-initiating zone and the output apparatus of a neuron.* Depending on the type of neuron, single axons can have an enormous range of lengths, from less than a millimeter to the total distance from toe to head. Some axons possess a kind of *insulating material that encircles the exterior of the axon called* **myelin** whereas others do not. In myelinated axons, there are *small breaks in the myelin at regular intervals,* called the **nodes of Ranvier** that serve to boost the signals propagated along axons.

Near the end of the axon, many branches are given off that *terminate with specialized swellings* called **presynaptic terminals**. The presynaptic terminals house the output equipment of a neuron that governs the release of chemical signals transmitted to and sensed by other neurons and cells. This *site of exchange of information between neurons* is called the **synapse**, which has two parts: (1) the presynaptic terminal and (2) the **receptors** for the chemical message on the **postsynaptic membrane**. It should be noted that the terms **presynaptic** and **postsynaptic** are relative terms; the neuron depicted in Figure 6 is the presynaptic neuron relative to the synapses indicated at the bottom of the diagram but is the postsynaptic neuron relative to the synapses shown at the top.

General Types of Neurons

In the broadest terms, neurons can be categorized into three general types (Figure 7). **Primary sensory neurons** *gather information from the environment and deliver it to the spinal cord or brainstem* and, as such, can be considered as *input* neurons. **Motor neurons** *carry commands away from the nervous system to activate muscles and therefore are output neurons. All neurons that are not primary sensory neurons or motor neurons are lumped into a huge category* called **interneurons** that carry out the manifold operations within the nervous system. Those *interneurons involved in processing information within a small region of the nervous system* and that have relatively short axons are called **local interneurons** while those that are involved in *communication across regions of the nervous system* and that have longer axons are called **projection interneurons**.

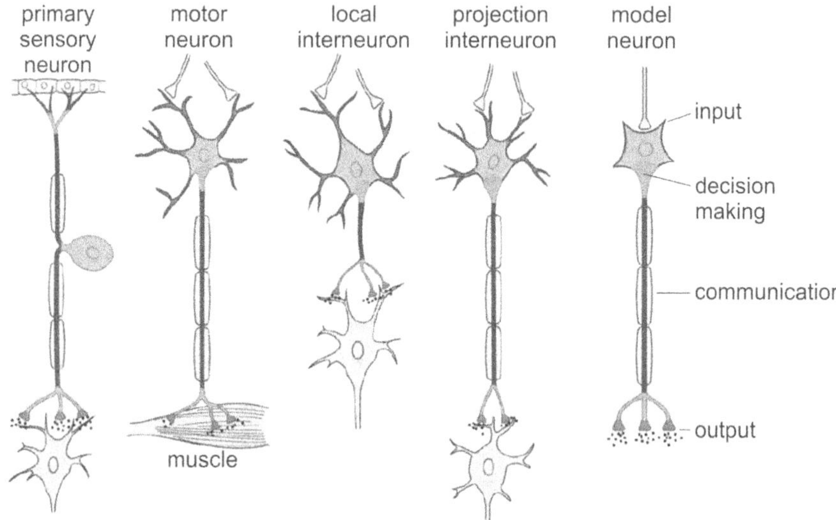

Figure 7.   General types of neurons and a model neuron showing functional components. (Adapted from Kandel *et al.* [2012].)

Regardless of the neuron type, most neurons possess four **functional components** (model neuron, right side of Figure 7). One is an **input** apparatus, which typically is the dendrites but this is not always the case. For example, primary sensory neurons do not have dendrites. Instead, they possess specialized structures for taking in information from the environment. Two is a **decision-making** site (equivalent to the spike-initiating zone) that is usually housed near the emergence of the axon from the soma but not always. For example, the decision-making site is not found near the soma in primary sensory neurons. The third component is a **communication** path (the axon) by which signals set up at the decision-making site are delivered to the fourth component, the **output** element (the pre-synaptic terminal) of the neuron.

Glia

There is another class of cells in the nervous system that outnumbers the neurons—the **glia** (Figure 8). *While glia means "glue," the function of the glia is not simply to provide structural support to the nervous system.*

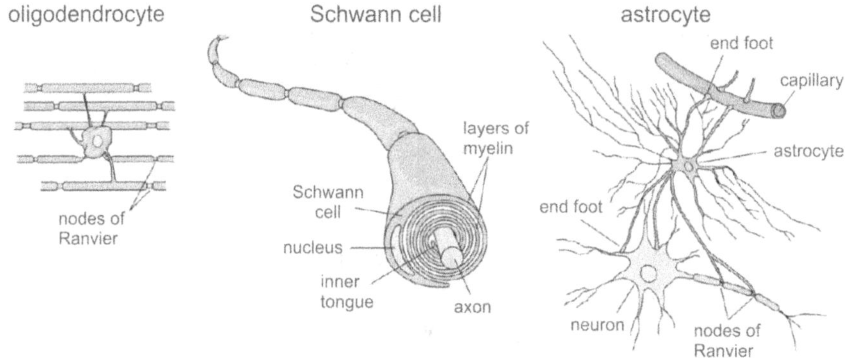

Figure 8.   Examples of glial cells that carry out numerous supportive functions in the nervous system. (Adapted from Kandel *et al.* [2012].)

Indeed, there are several subtypes of glia each of which play an important role in maintaining the operations of the nervous system. For example, **oligodendrocytes** *provide myelin insulation to axons within the central nervous system* whereas **Schwann cells** *perform the same function for axons of the peripheral nervous system.* It should be noted that the term **central nervous system** (CNS) *refers specifically to the brain and spinal cord* whereas the **peripheral nervous system** (PNS) refers to the nerves and *neurons outside of the brain and spinal cord.*

One of the *most numerous of the glial cells* is the **astrocytes**, so named because of their *star-shaped radial extensions* (Figure 8). Many supportive functions have been ascribed to astrocytes. For example, astrocytes are thought to take up potassium ions that are released during neural activity. This buffering action is important because the build-up of potassium in the extracellular space can severely impair the ability of neurons to generate action potentials. The potassium taken up by the astrocytes is then conveyed to nearby blood vessels where it can be removed. Interestingly, potassium is also a vasoactive substance and can cause arterioles to dilate (Longden *et al.* 2017). Such dilation causes localized increases in blood flow and thereby increases oxygen and nutrient delivery to active regions of the brain. As such, astrocytes play an important link in directing blood flow to the areas of the brain that need it at any moment. This tight coupling between brain activity and blood flow is the basis of functional magnetic resonance imaging, which detects changes in oxygenated blood delivered to different regions of the brain, thereby indirectly indicating which regions of the brain are active at a given moment.

Summary

Neurons are diminutive information-processing machines that communicate with other neurons through electrical and chemical signaling. As originally articulated by Cajal, neurons are the basic operational elements of the nervous system. Each neuron possesses a few key functional components: an input apparatus, a decision-making region, a communication line, and an output device. In the following few chapters, the mechanisms underlying electrical signaling and communication among neurons are laid out. These functions are the foundations of neurophysiology and need to be understood in order to comprehend how the nervous system processes sensory information, makes decisions, and generates movements.

References

Kandel ER, Schwartz JH, Jessell TM, Siegelbaum SA & Hudspeth AJ (2012). Principles of Neural Science (5th Edition). McGraw-Hill.

Longden TA, Dabertrand F, Koide M, Gonzales AL, Tykocki NR, Brayden JE, Hill-Eubanks D & Nelson MT (2017). Capillary K+-sensing initiates retrograde hyperpolarization to increase local cerebral blood flow. *Nature Neuroscience* **20**, 717–726.

Rieke F, Warland D, Van Steveninck RD & Bialek W (1999). Spikes: Exploring the Neural Code. MIT Press.

Seal B (2023). *A cold day in Stockholm.* Distillations Magazine: Science History Institute. https://www.sciencehistory.org/stories/magazine/a-cold-day-in-stockholm/.

Shepherd GM (1991). Foundations of the Neuron Doctrine. Oxford Press.

Chapter 2

Ion Channels

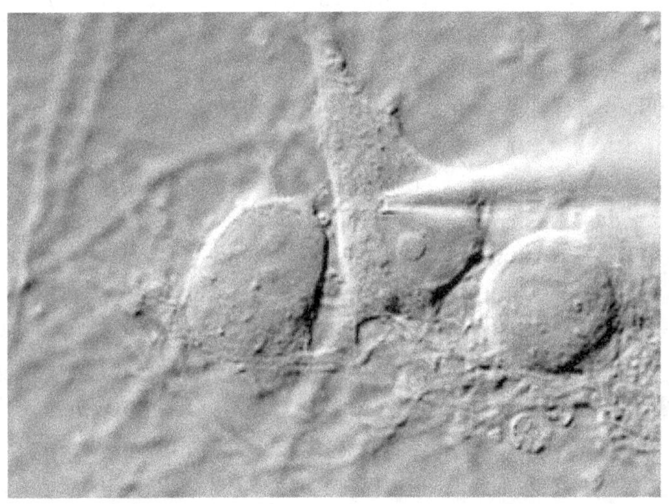

Micropipette electrode patched onto the membrane of a neuron through which activities of single ion channels can be recorded.

Source: http://www.physiologie.uni-freiburg.de/research-techniques/electrophysiology

Electrical activity in neurons and muscle fibers depends on the movement of charge across the cell membrane. Charge is carried by the inorganic ions sodium (Na^+), potassium (K^+), chloride (Cl^-), and calcium (Ca^{2+}). The ions can only readily cross the membrane (a lipid bilayer that is also a good electrical insulator) at specialized proteins embedded in the membrane called ion channels (Figure 1). An ion channel forms a water-filled

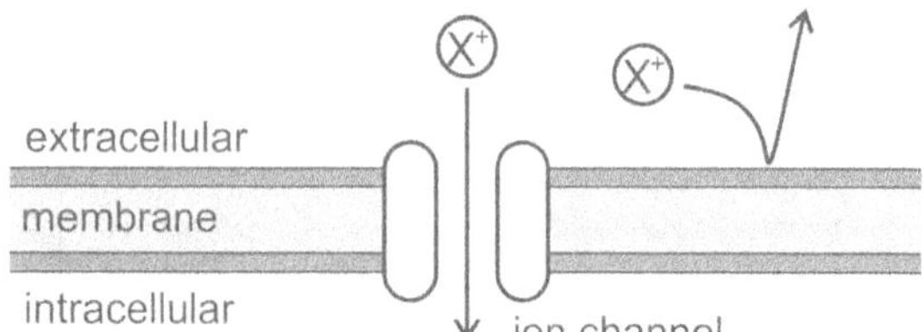

Figure 1.   Ions carry electrical charge across nerve cell membranes at specialized proteins called ion channels. Such movement of charge is the basis of electrical signaling by neurons. (Adapted from Levitan and Kaczmarek [2001].)

conduit across the membrane through which ions can pass. For consistency throughout this book, the extracellular space will typically be represented above the membrane and the intracellular space below.

Ion channels have two key properties. First, they tend to be selective for specific ions. For example, certain types of ion channels primarily allow Na^+ ions to pass but not other ions. Second, they can be "gated" (opened and closed) by specific types of signals. In general, there are three main types of ion channels based on the signals that gate the channel: **voltage-gated** channels, opened by electrical signals, **ligand-gated** channels, opened by chemical signals, and **mechanically-gated** channels, opened by stretch or pressure. In addition, there are **non-gated** (also called "**leak**") channels that tend to be always open. Typically, a given channel is gated by only one type of signal. Given their specificity for the type of gating signal and for the ions they let pass, ion channels are usually named based on these two attributes; for example, "voltage-gated Na^+ channel" or "ligand-gated Cl^- channel."

Gating

The process by which ion channels are gated is highly complex and is not yet completely understood. In general, the activating signal induces a conformational change in the atoms making up the ion channel molecule that, in turn, leads to the opening of a pore through the molecule. Such gating is shown schematically for ligand-gated, voltage-gated, and mechanically gated channels in Figure 2. In ligand-gated channels, the

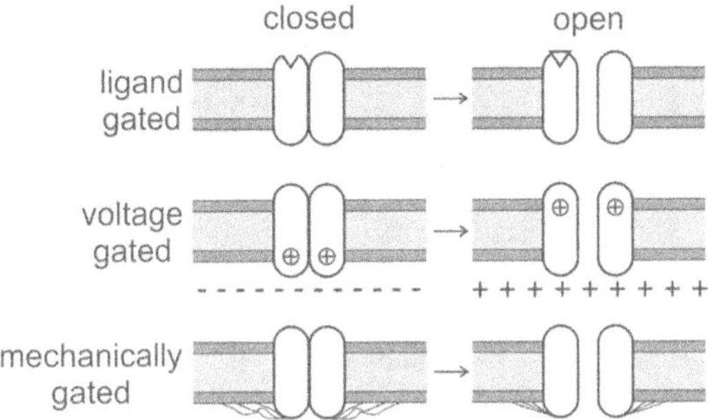

Figure 2.   Schematic diagram showing channel gating in response to chemical (top), electrical (middle), and mechanical (bottom) signals. (Adapted from Kandel *et al.* [2012].)

energy liberated by the binding of the chemical substance to the receptor site triggers the conformational change. For voltage-gated channels, charged components of the ion channel may be repulsed by an increase in similar charge along the interior of the membrane to actuate the conformational change. And for mechanically-gated channels, the channel may be tethered to the membrane through cytoskeletal filaments that are pulled taut when the membrane is stretched or deformed. Also, stretch on the lipid membrane by itself may also cause these channels to open.

Figure 3A shows a generic ion channel undergoing simple gating. When the closed channel receives its appropriate signal (chemical, electrical, or mechanical), it experiences a conformational change and opens a pathway that enables ionic current to flow across the membrane in a process referred to as **activation**. In these depictions, the channel is schematically portrayed as a passageway having a gate that is opened by activation. When the signal is removed, the gate shuts and restores the channel to the original closed configuration. This process of closing a channel by removing (detaching) the activating signal is called **deactivation**.

Many ion channels, however, go through a more complex gating process. Figure 3B schematically depicts such gating for a channel having two gates: an outer and an inner gate. If either is shut, then no ions can move through the channel. In the resting state, the outer gate is closed, and the inner gate is open. Upon receipt of the appropriate signal, a conformational change is induced causing the outer gate to open allowing ionic current to flow through the channel. As with simple gating, this process is

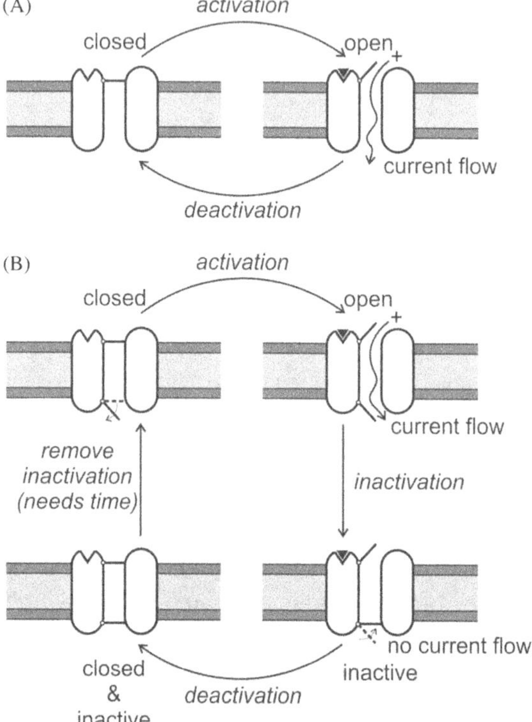

Figure 3.   (A) Simple and (B) complex gating of ion channels. Extracellular space is above the membranes and intracellular below.

called **activation**. However, in this case, the very signal that caused the outer gate to open causes the inner gate to close (bottom right, Figure 3B). As such, there is only a brief moment when both gates are open and ionic current can flow. The closure of the channel in the *presence* of the activating signal (i.e., the signal is still <u>in</u> place) is referred to as **inactivation**.

To restore the channel to its original configuration and to enable it to respond to another incoming signal, two things must occur. First, the original activating signal must be removed (i.e., <u>de</u>tached).Such **deactivation** causes the outer gate to close (bottom left, Figure 3B). Second, a certain amount of time must elapse before the inner gate returns to its original open configuration. At all times when the inner gate is closed, the channel is unresponsive (**refractory**) to any additional activating signal.

Many types of ion channels go through such complex gating including a key channel that underlies the action potential (as will be discussed).

Agonists and Antagonists

It is interesting that many of the poisons developed by organisms to disable prey or to ward off intruders do so by interfering with the normal operation of ion channels in the nervous system. Some of these substances work by preventing the opening of specific ion channels in the targeted creature. These substances are broadly referred to as **<u>exogenous</u>** (i.e., from outside the organism) **antagonists.** For example, **curare** is a substance derived from one of several tropical plants used by indigenous South Americans as a poison placed on the tip of arrows to immobilize prey. Curare binds to the receptor site of ligand-gated channels at the neuromuscular junction of skeletal muscles. The binding of curare, however, does not provoke a conformational change and the associated opening of a channel. Instead, it prevents the naturally occurring chemical signal within the organism (i.e., the **<u>endogenous agonist</u>** — in this case, acetylcholine) from activating the channel and thereby causes paralysis.

Likewise, there are many substances that mimic, rather than obstruct, the action of naturally occurring gating signals. Such substances are called **exogenous agonists**. For example, **muscimol** is a chemical found in certain types of mushrooms that activates ligand-gated channels at *inhibitory* synapses. Therefore, ingestion of muscimol leads to the widespread inhibition of neural activity throughout the central nervous system and can severely disrupt normal brain function. It should also be pointed out that many of the medicines used to treat disorders of the nervous system operate as exogenous agonists or antagonists.

Ionic Current Through Channels

In the 1970s, Erwin Neher and Bert Sakmann of Germany developed a method that made it possible to measure the ionic current passing through single ion channels. This method, called **patch-clamp** recording, involves placing the tip of a glass micropipette that has been pulled out to a very

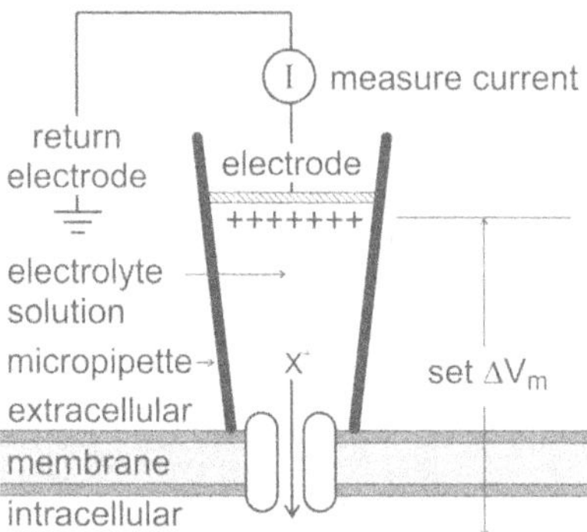

Figure 4.   Patch clamp recording that can be used to monitor the ionic currents passing through a single ion channel.

small diameter (as small as 1 µm) against a *patch* of cell membrane to enclose one or a few ion channels (Figure 4; also see image at beginning of this chapter). Under gentle suction, the patch of membrane is partially pulled into the pipette to make a tight seal between the pipette and the membrane in order to prevent ions from entering or escaping at the pipette–membrane interface. The pipette is filled with an electrolyte solution (a good conductor) and contains an electrode that enables the experimenter to set and hold (i.e., to "*clamp*") the difference in potential across the membrane (ΔV_m) at a desired level. If the channel is ligand-gated, some of the ligand (or an exogenous agonist) can be added to the pipette to induce activation of the channel. Upon opening of the channel, the ionic current passing through the channel can be measured with a highly sensitive ammeter connected to the electrode. As such, the actual operation of single ion channels can be monitored in living cells and in real time. Patch-clamp recording is an indispensable tool used by electrophysiologists and has provided key insights into the mechanisms of electrical signaling in excitable cells. For this advancement, Neher and Sakmann were awarded the Nobel Prize in 1991.

Before considering the type of results obtained with patch-clamp recording, it is instructive to first think about the measurement of current in a simple electrical circuit (see Appendix A for a refresher on electrical

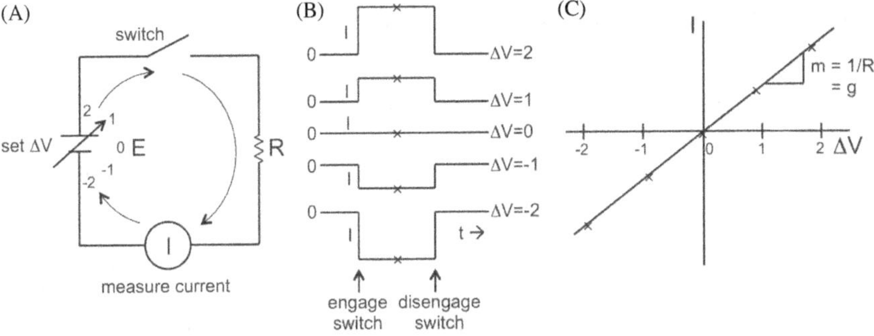

Figure 5.   (A) Circuit with a single resistor in which the experimenter sets the voltage to various values and measures the associated current when the switch is engaged. (B) Time courses of the measured current when the difference in potential (ΔV) is set to specific values. The "x"s indicate measured current during steady-state periods. (C) Current–voltage plot indicates measured current for different set values of voltage. Slope (m) is equivalent to $1/R$ and to the conductance, g.

circuits, if needed). This circuit has a single resistor connected to a voltage generator (Figure 5A). A switch is included that allows current to flow when engaged. Upon setting the difference in potential at a desired level, the switch is engaged and the resulting current flowing through the circuit can be measured before the switch is disengaged. Because there is no capacitance in the circuit, upon engaging the switch, a current is instantaneously established at a constant level until the switch is disengaged, when it immediately falls back to zero. This gives rise to rectangular-shaped current pulses (Figure 5B). On repeated trials, the experimenter can set the voltage generator to several different levels of potential difference and measure the associated current for each level. For example, when the potential difference is set to 0 V, no current flows when the switch is engaged. When the potential difference is set to 1 V, a certain level of current is measured. When the potential difference is doubled to 2 V, then the measured current is doubled. The experimenter can even invert the potential difference such that the high potential side is switched from the "top" of the voltage generator to the "bottom." Such a change is registered as a negative potential difference when measured by a voltmeter. In this negative voltage configuration, the charge will now move in the opposite direction through the circuit compared to that when the potential difference was positive. This reversal in the direction of charge movement (i.e., current) is denoted as a change in the polarity of current from positive to negative.

The experimenter can then plot the measured current for each level of potential difference set across all of the trials (Figure 5C). In this case, the resulting current-voltage plot (one of the most prevalent and important types of plots used in cellular electrophysiology) is a straight line (i.e., $Y = mX + b$). I is the Y variable, ΔV is the X variable, and b is zero, yielding the equation $I = m\Delta V$. Because the relationship between current and potential difference is dictated by Ohm's law in this situation, the slope, m, must be equal to $1/R$, giving $I = (1/R)\Delta V$. Because electrophysiologists prefer to consider how readily an ion channel conducts ionic current rather than how much it resists it, they refer to the **conductance** of ion channels. *Conductance is simply the inverse of resistance* and is represented by the symbol g. As such, the slope of the current–voltage relationship is given by $m = 1/R = g$ (Figure 5C). The steeper the slope, the more current will flow for a given change in membrane potential. The *unit* of conductance is equivalent to 1/ohm, and for a long time was referred to as a mho ("ohm" written backward!). Eventually, mho was renamed **siemens** (S), after the 19th-century electrical inventor Werner von Siemens.

Now, let's examine the outcome of a patch-clamp recording experiment. Figure 6A shows recordings of the current passing through an ion channel when the difference in potential across the membrane was held (clamped) at nine different levels from +100 mV to −80 mV. For positive membrane potentials, the magnitude of the current increased in proportion to the difference in potential. Likewise, the magnitude of the current increased with increasingly negative membrane potentials except that the ionic current across the membrane flowed in the opposite direction. As such, the current is indicated as negative. Note that when the channel opened, the measured current immediately reached a new steady level and when the channel closed, the current abruptly dropped to zero. The duration that a channel stays open varies randomly from opening to opening.

A plot of the channel current measured as a function of the difference in potential across the membrane yields a linear relationship (Figure 6B). The *slope* (m) of the line indicates the single channel conductance, g, and

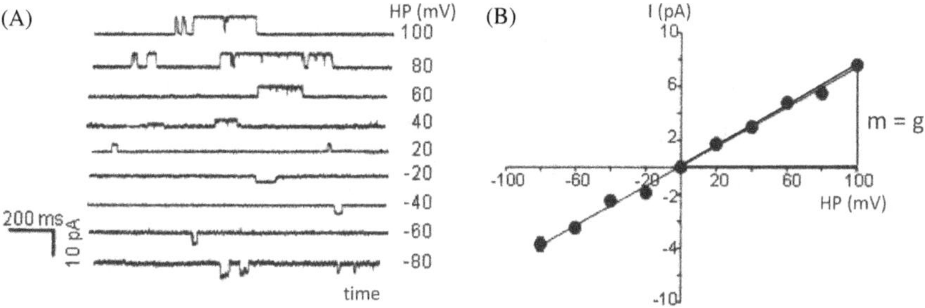

Figure 6.   Ionic current measured through a single ion channel using patch-clamp record-ing. (A) Nine trials (each trace) during which current was measured while membrane potential was held (holding potential, HP) at different values. (B) Plot of steady-state current versus holding potential for ion channel shown in panel A. Slope of the line (m) is equivalent to the conductance (g) of the channel.

is given as $g = \Delta I/\Delta V$ (i.e., rise over run) $\approx$ 7.5 pA/100 mV = 7.5×10^{-12} A/100 $\times 10^{-3}$ V = 75×10^{-12} A/V = 75×10^{-12} S = 75 pS—an extremely small value of conductance. On the other hand, the resistance (the inverse of conductance) of the single channel is enormous, namely $R = 1/g = 1/(75 \times 10^{-12}$ S$) \approx 13 \times 10^{9}$ ohms! This very high resistance is due to the minuscule cross-sectional area of the channel (remember from Appendix A that the resistance is inversely related to the cross-sectional area). Most importantly, such patch-clamp experiments on single channels indicated that when open, most ion channels operate more or less like simple resistors (note the similarity of the responses in Figure 5C to that of Figure 6B). As such, we can model electrical signaling in neurons by assuming that ion channels function like resistors. Furthermore, to obtain a reasonable level of ionic current in a neuron, thousands of ion channels must be opened together (keeping in mind that as more resistors are "added" in parallel, the lower the effective resistance; alternatively, conductances in parallel add up algebraically).

Summary

Ion channels are the molecular machines that enable signaling in neurons. Different types of channels open in response to chemical, electrical, or mechanical signals and typically allow only specific ions to flow across the membrane. The process of opening (gating) ion channels can be simple or complex. The electrical properties of single ion channels, studied using patch-clamp recording, indicate that they behave like that of a simple electrical resistor. In Chapter 3, we discuss how the leak (non-gated) ion channels play a crucial role in setting the resting potential of neurons.

References

Kandel ER, Schwartz JH, Jessell TM, Siegelbaum SA & Hudspeth AJ (2012). Principles of Neural Science (5th Edition). McGraw-Hill.

Levitan IB & Kaczmarek LK (2001). The Neuron: Cell and Molecular Biology (3rd Edition). Oxford University Press.

Chapter 3

Resting Membrane Potential

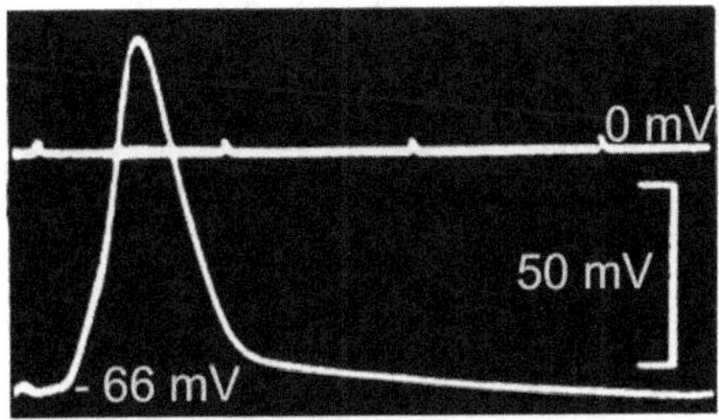

One of the first intracellular recordings showing the resting membrane potential (–66 mV) and action potential in a mammalian neuron of the central nervous system. Time between ticks on horizontal line is 1 ms. (Adapted from Brock LG, Coombs JS & Eccles JC [1952]).

As mentioned in Chapter 2, all electrical signaling in neurons and muscle fibers comes about by the movement of charged ions across the cell membrane through open ion channels. To understand what compels ions to move through channels, we need to understand how neurons (and other cells) come to possess a difference in electrical potential across the membrane even when the neuron is not signaling (i.e., at "rest"). This so-called **resting membrane potential** provides one of the main forces driving ions to move across the membrane.

In all neurons and muscle fibers (and other cells as well) at rest, there is a thin layer of positive charge on the outside of the membrane and a thin layer of negative charge on the inside (Figure 1). The lipid bilayer keeps the charges separated. As a consequence, the membrane is polarized — just like a magnet or a battery; it has a positive pole and a negative pole.

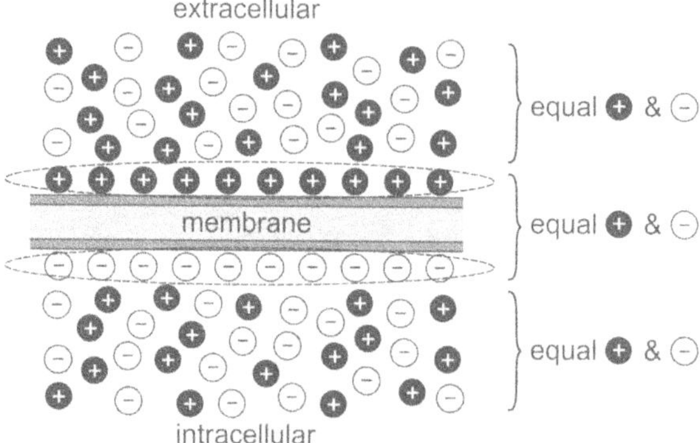

Figure 1.   Distribution of positive and negative charges across the nerve (or muscle) membrane. In the resting state, there is a thin layer of positive charges along the outside of the membrane and a thin layer of negative charges along the inside, making the membrane "polarized." Otherwise, there are equal numbers of positive and negative charges inside and outside the cell (adapted from Kandel *et al.* [2012]).

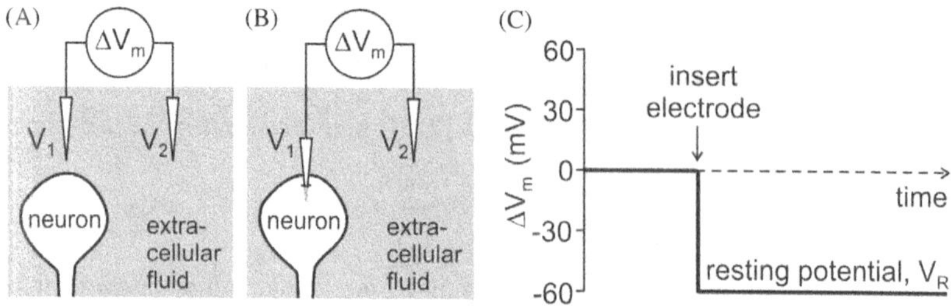

Figure 2.   Recording resting membrane potential. (A) Initially, two probes of a voltmeter (V_1 and V_2) are both in the extracellular fluid. Then (B) the V_1 probe is inserted through the membrane of the neuron. (C) When both probes are outside the neuron, the detected membrane potential ($\Delta V_m = V_1 - V_2$) is 0 mV. When the V_1 probe is inserted into the neuron, the membrane potential now registers as ~−60 mV, referred to as the resting membrane potential, V_R (adapted from Kandel *et al.* [2012]).

It is important to keep in mind (and something we shall return to) that the number of ions associated with this charge separation at the membrane is very small in comparison to the relatively huge volumes of ions filling the extracellular and intracellular spaces.

We can measure this difference in electrical potential across the membrane of a neuron with an amplified voltmeter (Figure 2A). If the two probes of the voltmeter are initially situated in the extracellular fluid, then no difference in potential is detected. Because the extracellular fluid is an excellent conductor, this situation is analogous to placing both probes of a voltmeter on a large copper wire extending off the top of a battery. Each probe detects the potential stored on the top pole of the battery and therefore no *difference* in potential is registered.

If one of the probes (V_1) is inserted through the membrane (Figure 2B), it now tastes the potential on the inside of the neuron. As a consequence, a difference in potential ($V_1 - V_2$) is now indicated by the voltmeter. The convention in electrophysiology is to measure the potential on the inside of the membrane relative to that on the outside. For a typical neuron at rest with an interior potential of ~−30 mV and an exterior potential of ~+30 mV, the difference in potential across the membrane is: $\Delta V_m = V_1 - V_2 = $ (−30 mV) − (+30 mV) ≈ −60 mV (Figure 2C). This steady difference in potential is referred to as the resting membrane potential, V_R.

It is *very advantageous*, however, to consider all of the potential underlying the difference in potential to be concentrated on the *inside* of the neuron. Keep in mind that a typical 12 V battery is one that has +6 V of potential on one pole and −6 V on the other. The operation of this battery in a circuit will be *identical* to one that has +12 V of potential on one pole and 0 V of potential on the other. Likewise, a membrane with −60 mV of potential on the inside and zero on the outside will function identically to one with −30 mV inside and +30 mV outside because it is the *difference* in potential that dictates movement of charge (see Appendix A). This greatly simplifies our thinking about membrane potential since one only needs to keep track of what takes place on the inside of the membrane.

If one now uses a current generator to inject negative current inside the neuron (think of it as a little hose spraying negative charges inside the cell; Figure 3A), then the interior of the membrane will become more negative than that associated with the resting membrane potential. This means the *membrane is now even more polarized than at rest*, and as such, is referred to as being **hyperpolarized**. If the magnitude of this negative current is increased, then there is a proportional increase in the degree of hyperpolarization (Figure 3B). Note that when the current generator is turned off (injected current goes to zero) the membrane potential returns

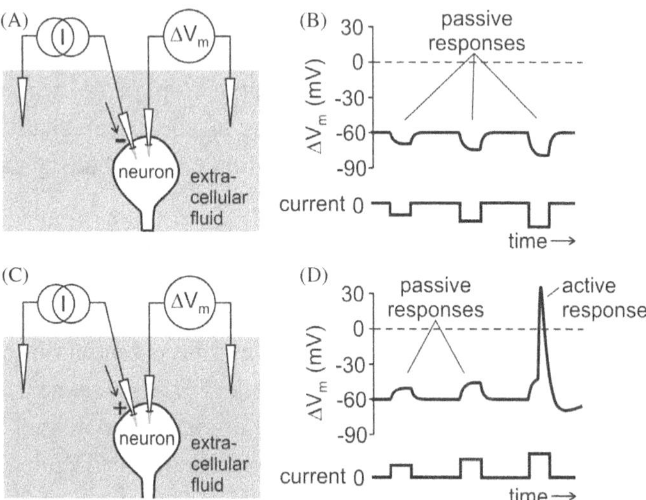

Figure 3.   (A) Injection of negative current into a neuron using a current generator causes (B) the measured membrane potential to become more negative (hyperpolarized) than the resting potential. The magnitude of the hyperpolarized responses is proportional to the amplitude of the negative current injected. These responses are dictated by passive neuron properties (static features such as neuron geometry and leak channels) and are referred to as passive responses. (C) Injection of positive current causes (D) the membrane potential to become less negative (depolarized). The depolarized responses are proportional to the amplitude of the injected current and are determined by passive properties only up to a certain level, beyond which the response is no longer proportional to the input current. Such an active response is due to the activation of ion channels that otherwise are quiescent, for example, as occurs during an action potential (adapted from Kandel *et al.* [2012]).

to the resting membrane potential. Why is that? We will address that question later in this chapter.

Likewise, when the current generator is used to *deliver positive charge inside the cell* (Figure 3C), *it reduces the difference in potential between the inside and outside (i.e., it reduces the degree of membrane polarization)* and is referred to as being **depolarized**. However, in the case of depolarization, the magnitude of the detected change in potential is proportional to the intensity of current injected only up to a certain level. Beyond that level, there is a dramatic change in potential that is no longer proportional to the injected current (Figure 3D). Indeed, the magnitude of this new response does not change appreciably even with increasing intensities of current injection. This large and transient change in membrane potential is that associated with the production of an **action potential** (the mechanisms of which are discussed in Chapter 4). The hyperpolarizing and depolarizing responses that are *proportional* to the current injected are mediated by so-called **passive processes** (Figures 3B and 3D). These processes are related to *properties of the cell that do not change moment-by-moment, such as the geometry of the cell, the cell membrane, and the non-gated (leak) channels in the membrane.* The non-proportional responses, such as the action potential, involve **active processes**, which primarily *arise from the opening of ion channels that are otherwise closed.*

Genesis of the Resting Membrane Potential

A fundamental question in electrophysiology relates to how the resting membrane potential gets established in the first place. As we shall see, the resting membrane potential largely depends only on passive processes. Therefore, we can ignore the active process for the time being. One critical factor underlying the genesis of the resting membrane potential is the unequal distribution of ions on either side of the cell membrane (Figure 4). The extracellular fluid has relatively high concentrations of Na^+ and

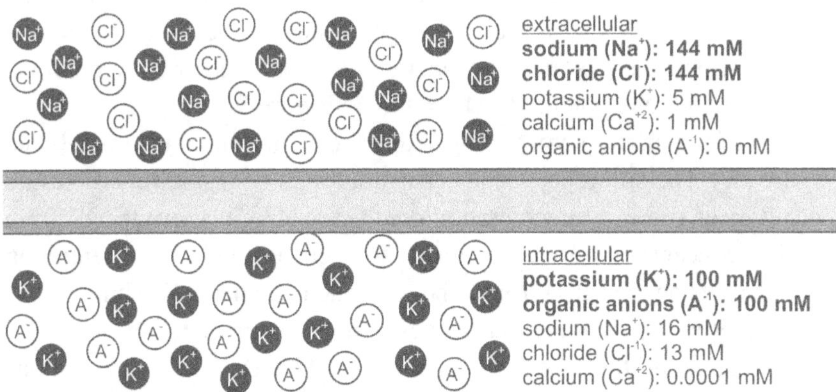

Figure 4.   Concentrations of key ions inside (below membrane) and outside (above membrane) a typical neuron.

Cl$^-$ ions whereas the intracellular fluid has high concentrations of K$^+$ ions and negatively charged organic anions, A$^-$ (such as proteins and amino acids). Ca^{2+} is also in relatively high concentration in the extracellular fluid.

Perhaps one way to remember these concentration differences is to consider that the evolution of the first single-cell organisms likely occurred within the waters of primordial seas. Seawater is salty (i.e., high concentrations of Na$^+$ and Cl$^-$). As these organisms evolved into multicellular creatures, seawater was probably hemmed in between the cells and as such constituted the extracellular fluid. It seems likely that our own extracellular fluid, also with high concentrations of Na$^+$ and Cl$^-$ (albeit more diluted than seawater), is a remnant of that early evolution.

Resting Membrane Potential of a Cell Permeable to Just One Ion

How does the unequal distribution of ions across the membrane lead to the resting membrane potential? To understand this, let's build a simple cell from the ground up. (We will address the slightly more complicated case of a real neuron later.) To begin, assume the cell membrane has no ion channels (Figure 5A). The intracellular fluid has a high concentration of K$^+$ ions and inorganic anions A$^-$, whereas the extracellular fluid, like seawater, has high Na$^+$ and Cl$^-$ concentrations. At this stage, there are equal numbers of positive and negative charges inside the cell and outside the cell. Therefore, there is no excess charge on either side of the membrane and zero membrane potential ($\Delta V_m = 0$ mV; Figure 5A).

Now, let's insert some non-gated K$^+$ channels into the membrane (Figure 5B). The difference in the concentration of K$^+$ inside versus outside the cell gives rise to a concentration gradient tending to drive the K$^+$ from the high concentration location (inside the cell) to the low concentration location (outside the cell) through the non-gated K$^+$ channels. Think of this diffusion process as a force that propels ions from one location to another with a magnitude that is proportional to the difference in concentrations between the two locations. We will refer to this as the **chemical force**, F_C, and represent it as a vector with a length indicating its magnitude, and the arrowhead pointing in the direction from high to low concentration.

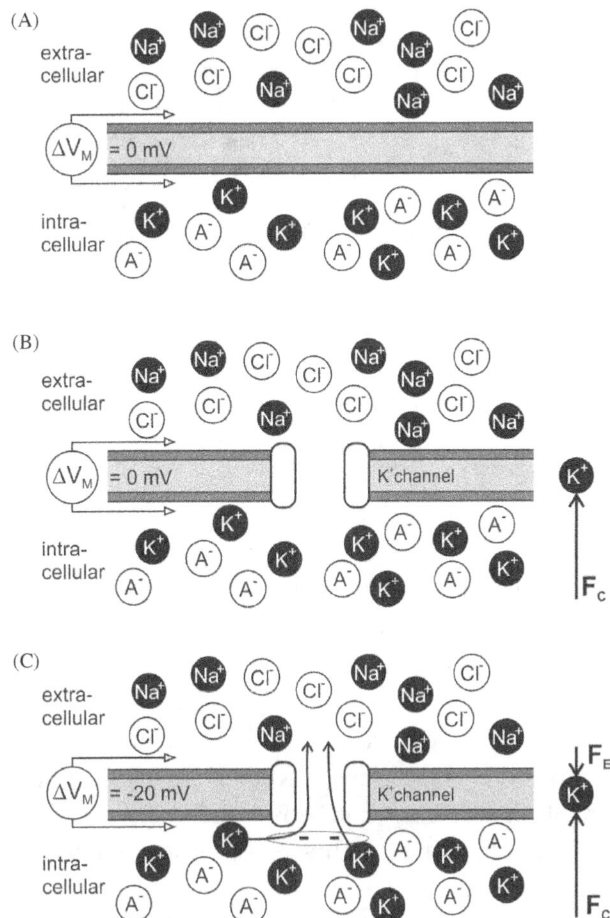

Figure 5. Development of the resting membrane potential in a cell permeable to K^+ ions only. (A) Initially, there are no channels in the membrane and the resting potential is 0 mV. (B) The moment K^+ leak channels are inserted into the membrane. The difference in concentrations of K^+ inside and outside the cell causes a chemical force, F_C, that acts to drive K^+ out of the cell. For clarity, F_c is shown to the right of the membrane. (C) As K^+ ions leave the cell, companion organic anions are left behind depositing negative charge along the interior of the membrane. This initial small buildup of negative charge causes a weak electrical force, F_E, to partially oppose the exit of K^+ ions driven by F_C. The small negative charge inside the membrane is detected as a modest membrane potential of −20 mV. (D) As more K^+ ions exit, the buildup of negative charge along the interior of the membrane increases, which increases F_E. Eventually, F_E will be equal but opposite to F_C, causing all movement of K^+ ions to halt. The membrane will persist indefinitely in this state with a resting membrane potential of about −75 mV.

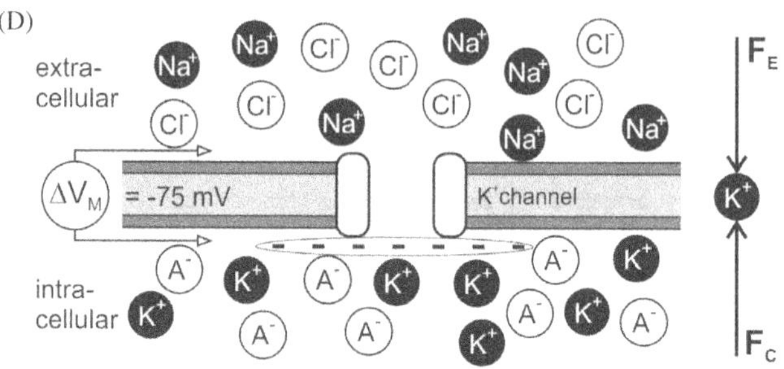

Figure 5.   (*Continued*)

In Figure 5B, this force is shown operating on a K^+ ion off to the right side (so as to not overly clutter the diagram), but think of the ion situated near or in the pore of the open channel.

As the K^+ ions are driven out of the neuron by the chemical force, F_C, their companion A^- anions are carried along for the ride but are not allowed to pass through the K^+ selective channel (Figure 5C). As such, they accumulate near the membrane and excess negative charges begin to build up on the inside of the membrane (shown as a thin cloud of negative charges). In reality, there is also an equivalent thin cloud of positive charges building up on the outside of the membrane associated with the efflux of K^+. However, as mentioned earlier, if we consider that the difference in potential across the membrane is entirely due to the accumulation of charge on the inside of the membrane, we greatly simplify our thinking about membrane potential and associated ionic currents.

Now, this excess of negative charge along the interior of the membrane will begin to impede the exit of positively charged K^+ ions. This is due to another force operating on the ions, the **electric force, F_E** (the nature of which is described in Appendix A). Keep in mind that the magnitude of the electric force set up between two objects is directly proportional to the product of the charge on one object (q_1) and that on the other (q_2): $F_E \propto q_1 \bullet q_2$. In our case, the two objects are (1) the *inside of the membrane*, with a charge equivalent to the excess negative charge along the interior of the membrane (let's call it q_1), and (2) the K^+ *ion itself*, with a charge equivalent to +1 proton (let's call it q_2). The direction of F_E is to pull the two objects toward one another if they have opposite signs and to repel if they have the same sign.

At the moment depicted in Figure 5C, only a few K^+ ions have exited the cell and thereby have left behind relatively few negative charges along the inside of the membrane. Therefore, the magnitude of the electric force, F_E, (shown operating on the K^+ ion at the right side of Figure 5C) is relatively small because q_1 is small. The direction of F_E acting on the K^+ ion is to pull it toward the negatively charged interior of the membrane. The net force (sometimes referred to as the *electrochemical* driving force) is the vector sum of F_E and F_C. In this case, $F_C > F_E$ and therefore the movement of K^+ ions is in the direction of F_C, namely, out of the cell. Keep in mind that the *net* force associated with the situation in Figure 5C is smaller than that in Figure 5B (where no electric force opposes F_C), and therefore, the movement of K^+ ions out of the cell is slower in Figure 5C than in Figure 5B. It is also important to note that because of the small excess negative charge on the inside of the membrane, we now detect a small difference in potential across the membrane, ΔV_m, let's say of -20 mV (Figure 5C).

As this process continues, more K^+ ions move out of the cell and the interior of the membrane becomes more negative. This leads to a progressive increase in the magnitude of F_E slowing the exit of K^+ ions. Eventually, F_E attains a magnitude that is equal to that of F_C but is in the opposite direction (Figure 5D). When this occurs, all movement of K^+ ions halts and the membrane can remain indefinitely in this state of affairs without expenditure of energy. We've just created a cell with a resting membrane potential. In this case (namely a cell with a membrane that is exclusively permeable to K^+ ions), the difference in potential across the membrane, ΔV_m, will have a value of about -75 mV. This is not unlike certain glial cells whose cell membrane is selectively permeable to K^+ ions and has a membrane potential of ~-75 mV.

The most common questions raised at this point are: *why did the chemical force acting on K^+ ions not diminish as K^+ left the cell? Wouldn't this reduce the concentration gradient acting on K^+ ions, and thereby reduce F_C?* There are two reasons why the concentration gradient, and therefore F_C, remains effectively constant. First (as discussed in Appendix A), electrical forces are incredibly strong. As such, only a minuscule number of charged ions need to be moved from the inside to the outside of the cell (or vice versa) in order to develop significant electrical forces.

This number of ions is a drop in the bucket compared to the vast quantities of ions in the extracellular and intracellular spaces. Therefore, the tiny change in concentrations associated with such movement is virtually undetectable. Second, there are processes (that we will mention later) that operate in the background to ensure that concentration gradients are maintained, thereby keeping F_C practically constant.

Equilibrium Potential

In the situation depicted in Figure 5D, the chemical force is perfectly counteracted by an opposing electrical force leading to no movement of K^+ ions. We refer to this situation as the ion being in **equilibrium**. The *membrane potential at which the associated electrical force perfectly opposes the chemical force* acting on some ion X is called the **equilibrium potential, E_X**. It is very important to remember that membrane potential is directly proportional to the charge on the membrane, that is, $\Delta V_m \propto q_1$. Furthermore, as we discussed earlier, the electric force, F_E, is directly proportional to $q_1 \cdot q_2$. Because the charge on an ion (q_2) doesn't change, we can also say that, in this case, $F_E \propto q_1$. Therefore, because both F_E and ΔV_m are proportional to q_1, we can conclude that the *electrical force, F_E is directly proportional to the membrane potential, ΔV_m.* As a consequence, the electrical force acting on an ion walks hand-in-hand with the membrane potential: if the membrane potential doubles, then the electrical force will also precisely double. If the membrane potential is zero, then the electrical force is also zero. On the other hand, as mentioned above, the *chemical force, F_C, normally does not change.* These two principles (as we shall see) are essential to keep in mind when attempting to understand ionic current flow across the cell membrane.

The **equilibrium potential** (i.e., the membrane potential at which the electrical force perfectly opposes the chemical force) for any ion can be estimated from an equation developed by the Nobel laureate Walther Nernst in the latter part of the 19th century. This equation, the so-called **Nernst equation**, is:

$$E_X = \frac{R \cdot T}{Z \cdot F} \ln \frac{[X]_{out}}{[X]_{in}}$$

where R is the gas constant, T is the temperature in degrees Kelvin, Z is the valence of the ion (e.g., +1, +2, −1), F is Faraday's constant, ln is the natural logarithm, $[X]_{out}$ is the concentration of ion X outside the cell, and $[X]_{in}$ is the concentration of ion X inside the cell. The Nernst equation can be simplified to the following (see Appendix B for derivation of the simpler form, a description of the constants, their units, and other considerations):

$$E_X = \frac{57.5\ mV}{Z} \log_{10} \frac{[X]_{out}}{[X]_{in}}$$

Now, let's use the Nernst equation to find the equilibrium potential for each of our key ions, K^+, Na^+, Cl^-, and Ca^{2+} using the concentrations for each ion for a typical neuron shown in Figure 4 and their valences, Z:

$$E_{K^+} = \frac{57.5\ mV}{+1} \log_{10} \frac{[5\ mM]_{out}}{[100\ mM]_{in}} = -75\ mV$$

$$E_{Na^+} = \frac{57.5\ mV}{+1} \log_{10} \frac{[144\ mM]_{out}}{[16\ mM]_{in}} = +55\ mV$$

$$E_{Cl^-} = \frac{57.5\ mV}{-1} \log_{10} \frac{[144\ mM]_{out}}{[13\ mM]_{in}} = -60\ mV$$

$$E_{Ca^{2+}} = \frac{57.5\ mV}{+2} \log_{10} \frac{[1\ mM]_{out}}{[0.0001\ mM]_{in}} = +115\ mV$$

It will be important to have these values of the equilibrium potentials for each ion in mind as we go forward.

Ion Flux

The rate at which an ion flows across a membrane is referred to as the **ion flux**. Ion flux depends on *three factors*. One is the *concentration gradient*, which is due to the difference in concentrations of the ion outside and inside of the cell, giving rise to the chemical force, F_C. Remember that under normal circumstances F_C does not change. Two is the *membrane* *potential*, which gives rise to and is directly proportional to the electrical force, F_E. And three is the *permeability*, P, of the membrane to the ion, which is directly related to the number of channels specific to the ion that are open.

As such, the flux of some ion A can be considered proportional to:

$$\text{Flux}_A = (F_C + F_E) \times P_A$$

This relationship should be considered conceptual rather than strictly quantitative but turns out to be very useful in understanding electrical signaling in excitable cells. From this relationship, it should be clear that there are two ways to bring the flux of an ion to zero. One is if P_A is zero; meaning simply that there are no channels open through which ion A can pass. And two is if the sum $F_C + F_E = 0$. This is possible because these forces can be of different directions and therefore possess opposite signs. This occurs when the electrical force, F_E, is of the same magnitude but in the opposite direction of F_C, namely, when the membrane potential is at the equilibrium potential for the ion.

Resting Membrane Potential for a Cell Permeable to More than One Ion

Now let's tackle the resting membrane potential for a real neuron that is permeable, in the resting state, to Na^+ and Cl^- in addition to K^+ ions. To simplify this somewhat, we will first consider the case for a neuron permeable to just Na^+ and K^+. To begin, let's pick up where we left off in Figure 5 with a membrane that is only permeable to K^+ ions. In this case, the resting membrane potential is equivalent to the equilibrium potential of K^+ (i.e., -75 mV; Figure 6A). From the above equation, the flux in this situation is given by $\text{Flux}_{K^+} = (F_C + F_E) \times P_{K^+} = 0 \times P_{K^+} = 0$. Now, let's make the membrane slightly permeable to Na^+ by inserting a few non-gated Na^+ channels. Typically, there are about 30 times more non-gated K^+ than Na^+ channels, and as such, the membrane permeability for K^+ is much greater than for Na^+. This is symbolically represented in Figure 6B by depicting the K^+ channel as wider than the Na^+ channel.

Now that there is a pathway for Na^+ ions to move, Na^+ ions will flow into the cell driven by a chemical force (due to the high concentration of

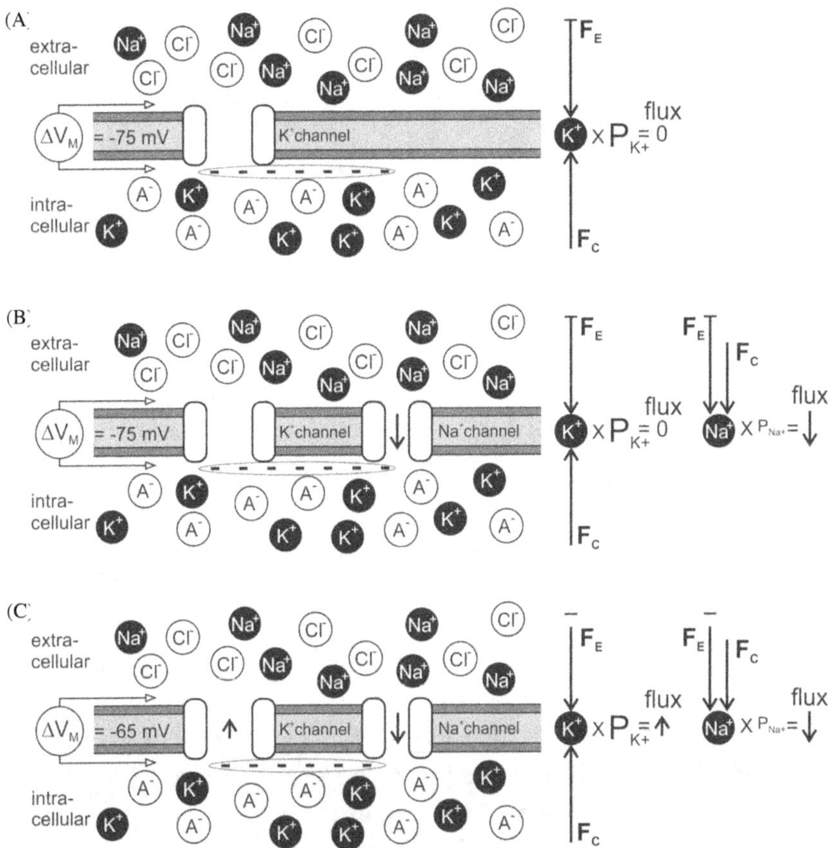

Figure 6.   Genesis of resting membrane potential. (A) Equilibrium of chemical, F_C, and electrical, F_E, forces in a cell permeable only to K⁺ ions with a resting potential of −75 mV. (B) Moment at which Na⁺ leak channels are inserted into the membrane. The small permeability of Na⁺ relative to K⁺ is due to fewer leak channels for Na⁺. Large F_C and F_E drive Na⁺ into the neuron but when multiplied by the small permeability, $P_{Na}{}^+$, leads to the modest influx of Na⁺ (arrow in channel). The entry of positively charged Na⁺ (C) reduces the net negative charge on the membrane and decreases the membrane potential to −65 mV. This slightly reduces F_E acting on both Na⁺ and K⁺ ions and slightly decreases the net electrochemical force acting on Na⁺ to slightly reduce Na⁺ influx. The equilibrium for K⁺, however, is now disrupted with F_C slightly larger than F_E, leading to a very small efflux of K⁺. This efflux is smaller than the influx of Na⁺ (see arrows in channels). Therefore, there will be a small net influx of positive charge to further reduce membrane potential to (D) −60 mV. F_E is again reduced for both K⁺ and Na⁺. This causes the electrochemical force (and associated flux) to slightly increase for K⁺ and decrease for Na⁺, such that now their fluxes are equal but in opposite directions. In this steady state, there is no net ion flux and the membrane potential stabilizes at this level—the resting membrane potential.

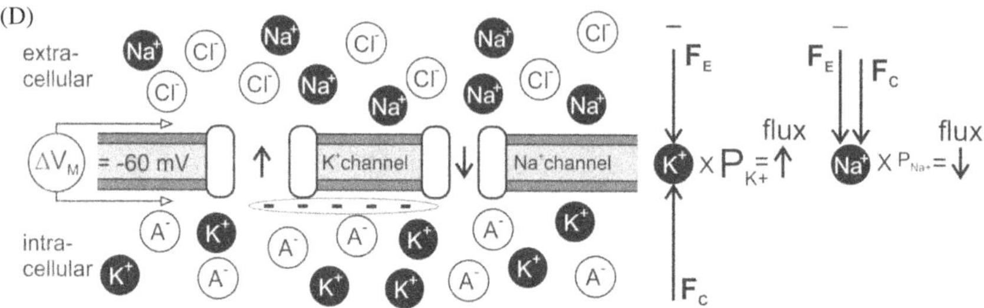

Figure 6.   (*Continued*)

Na$^+$ outside the cell) and an electrical force set up by the negatively charged interior of the membrane pulling positively charged Na$^+$ ions into the cell (Figure 6B). These two forces (shown acting on a Na$^+$ ion off to the right of the diagram) operate in the same direction to provide a strong net force to drive Na$^+$ ions into the cell. It should be noted that the *electric force* applied to the Na$^+$ ion is *identical* to that acting on the K$^+$ ion. Recall that the electrical force $F_E \propto q_1 \bullet q_2$. We consider q_1 to be the charge on the membrane (that associated with a membrane potential of -75 mV at this moment) whereas q_2 is the charge on the ion, which is $+1$ proton for both Na$^+$ and K$^+$. Because the same membrane charge acts on both ions and both ions have the same charge, the electric force must be the same acting on both ions. It should also be noted that the magnitude of the chemical force acting on Na$^+$ is smaller than that acting on K$^+$ ions. This is because the difference in concentration across the membrane is greater for K$^+$ than for Na$^+$ ions.

Now, despite the large electrochemical force acting on Na$^+$ ions when the membrane potential is -75 mV (Figure 6B), the actual inward flux of Na$^+$ is relatively small because the permeability (P) of the membrane to Na$^+$ is small (remember, Flux $= (F_C + F_E) \times P$). This small influx is depicted as a short arrow inside the Na$^+$ channel. Also, at the moment when we first insert Na$^+$ channels into the membrane, the membrane potential is still at -75 mV and, as such, the electrical and chemical forces acting on K$^+$ ions are equal and opposite, and therefore, the K$^+$ flux is zero.

In the next moment, the small influx of Na$^+$ ions will cancel out some of the excess negative charge on the inside of the membrane. This will slightly depolarize the membrane. Let's freeze this process at this stage and examine what is taking place (see Figure 6C). Let's say the membrane potential is now −65 mV rather than −75 mV. The amount of negative charge on the inside of the membrane is slightly less than it was at the outset. Therefore, the electric force, F_E, acting on Na^+ is also slightly less than it was at the start (indicated by the small horizontal tick mark). The chemical force has not changed, nor the permeability, and therefore the inward flux of Na^+ is slightly less than it was before (shown as a slightly smaller arrow inside the Na^+ channel).

Most interesting is that the balance between electrical and chemical forces acting on K^+ has now been disrupted. The chemical force acting on K^+ has not changed but the electrical force has been slightly reduced indeed, to exactly the same degree as that for the Na^+ ion. At this moment, the chemical force driving K^+ out of the cell is slightly larger than the electrical force pulling K^+ into the cell. This leads to a small efflux of K^+ but the magnitude of that efflux is slightly smaller than the influx of Na^+ (compare flux arrow lengths inside the K^+ and Na^+ channels in Figure 6C).

Now there will be very slightly more positively charged Na^+ ions entering the cell than positively charged K^+ ions exiting. The net effect will be to slightly depolarize the membrane further (Figure 6D). Such a depolarization will slightly reduce the electric forces acting on Na^+ and K^+ ions (remember that the electrical forces are tied to the membrane potential). As a consequence, the net force acting to drive Na^+ ions into the cell will be slightly reduced and the net force driving K^+ ions out of the cell will slightly increase. Indeed, at this stage, the magnitude of the influx of Na^+ ions will be exactly equal to the efflux of K^+ ions. Note that the equivalence in flux magnitudes comes about for quite different reasons for the two ions. For Na^+, the net electrochemical force is large but when multiplied by a small permeability yields a modest flux. For K^+, the net electrochemical force is small but the permeability is high, also yielding a modest flux.

Most crucially, in this state of affairs, for every K^+ ion that walks out its door to leave the cell, a Na^+ ion walks in its door to enter the cell. As a consequence, the membrane potential now does not change. The membrane potential "locks in" at this new value and remains at this value indefinitely. The value of the membrane potential when this occurs is around −60 mV (Figure 6D), which is approximately the value of the resting membrane potential for most neurons. It is important to note that at the resting membrane potential, Na^+ and K^+ ions are not in equilibrium (i.e., the chemical and electrical forces do not balance one another). Instead, there is a *steady* (but small) influx of Na^+ ions and a *steady* (and equally small) efflux of K^+ ions leading to no net change in the membrane potential. This situation is referred to as the membrane being in a **steady state**.

Ion Flux — Membrane Potential Relation

A good way to visualize how concurrent Na^+ and K^+ fluxes shape the resting membrane potential is to draw a plot of ion flux versus membrane potential (Figure 7). To do this, let's consider the electrical and chemical forces acting on K^+ and Na^+ ions at different values of membrane potential. From these forces, and the knowledge of the permeabilities of the membrane to the two ions, we can calculate the fluxes for each ion. To do this, imagine that we "clamp" the membrane potential of the neuron at different values (indicated along the horizontal axis in Figure 7) and then work out, for each ion, the forces and the associated fluxes (represented on the vertical axis). We denote the **influx** of an ion in the "negative" direction, that is, pointed downward and into the cell (keeping in mind that we typically draw intracellular space below the membrane), whereas the **efflux** is indicated as "positive," simply meaning the ions move "upward" and out of the cell. It is also important to remember that we are still dealing only with the passive operations of the membrane, namely, those involving leak channels (in Chapter 4, we address active processes associated with the action potential).

Let's begin by first just considering the K^+ flux (Figure 7A); a good place to start is at the equilibrium potential (i.e., −75 mV). We know that when the membrane is held at the equilibrium potential, the electrical and chemical forces acting on the ion must be equal and opposite. Because K^+ is a positively charged ion, it will be attracted toward the negative charge

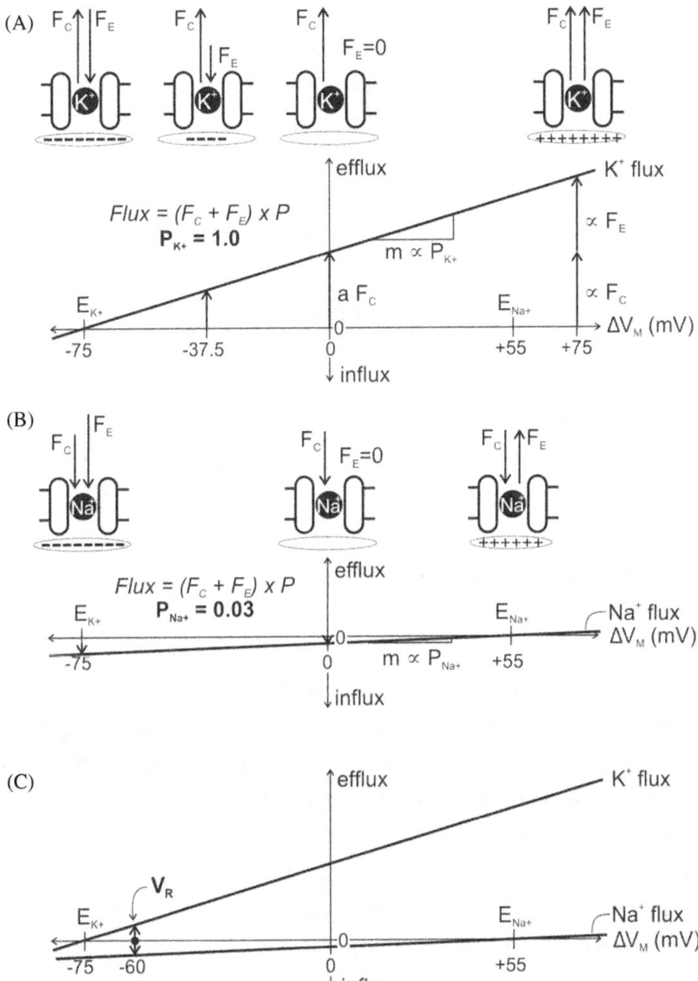

Figure 7.   (A) Top: Depiction of chemical, F_C, and electrical, F_E, forces acting on K^+ ion at different membrane potentials. Bottom: Plot of ion flux versus membrane potential for K^+. Slope of line, m, is proportional to the permeability of the membrane to K^+, P_K^+. (B) Same as in panel A but for Na^+. (C) Plot of ion flux versus membrane potential for both K^+ and Na^+. At only one level of the membrane potential, -60 mV, will magnitude of K^+ efflux equal that of Na^+ influx. Because there is no net flux of ions at this level, the membrane will stabilize at this potential—the resting membrane potential, V_R.

on the inside of the membrane (depicted at the top left of Figure 7A representing the membrane at −75 mV). Therefore, the direction of the electric force vector, F_E is toward the inside of the cell (downward). Because we are at equilibrium, the chemical force vector, F_C must be the same magnitude but in the opposite direction (outward). We can confirm that this direction is correct by recalling that K^+ ions are in high concentration inside the cell, and therefore, the chemical force is to drive K^+ out of the cell. Now, remembering that Flux $= (F_C + F_E) \times P$, and that $F_C + F_E = 0$ at −75 mV for K^+ ions, then the flux must equal zero. This is indicated in Figure 7A with the K^+ flux line passing through zero flux at −75 mV.

Now, let's consider the forces and flux at a more depolarized membrane potential, say at −37.5 mV (half that at −75 mV). Identifying the chemical force is easy, because it does not change, and therefore it is exactly the same as it was at −75 mV (see second image from the left at the top of Figure 7A). For the electrical force, recall that it is tied to and directly proportional to the membrane potential. As such, when the membrane potential is cut by half going from −75 to −37.5 mV, the electric force is also reduced precisely by half. The electrical and chemical forces are now no longer in balance. Indeed, the resultant vector associated with the sum of the electrical and chemical forces in this situation will point in the outward (efflux or up) direction with a magnitude half that of the chemical force. According to the flux equation (Flux $= (F_C + F_E) \times P$), we must multiply that sum by the permeability of the membrane to K^+, that is, P_K^+. Remember that permeability relates to the number of ion channels that are open in the membrane for a particular ion. In this case, we are considering only the K^+ leak channels. For ease of calculations, let's assign a *relative* permeability value for K^+ as $P_K^+ = 1.0$. Consequently, the amount of flux of K^+ at −37.5 mV is simply equivalent to the vector sum of $F_C + F_E$ (shown as an arrow pointing upward at −37.5 mV) indicating that K^+ flows out of the neuron when the membrane is held at this membrane potential.

Similarly, if we now hold the membrane potential at 0 mV, the chemical force again remains the same and the electric force is now zero. Recall that the electric force is proportional to $q_1 \times q_2$ where q_1 can be considered the excess charge on the membrane. At 0 mV, the excess charge on the membrane q_1 is precisely zero, and therefore the electric force is also precisely zero. As such, the flux is directly proportional to the chemical force by itself, shown as an upward arrow at 0 mV in Figure 7A. Indeed, when examining *any* flux—membrane potential (or current–membrane potential) plot—the flux at 0 mV provides a unique indicator of how chemical forces alone drive ions across the membrane.

To continue in this vein, let's now consider K^+ flux at a positive membrane potential, say +75 mV. Again, the chemical force is the same as in previous situations. The electric force will now have a magnitude exactly equal to that at −75 mV but will now drive K^+ out of the cell (see the rightmost image at the top of Figure 7A) because the positively charged membrane potential will repel the positively charged K^+ ions. In this case, the chemical and electrical forces have the same magnitude, and both point in the same direction to potently drive K^+ ions out of the cell. If we connect the values of flux across these different values of membrane potential, we get a straight line with a slope (m) that is proportional to the permeability of the membrane to K^+, P_{K^+}.

Now, let's apply this same approach for Na^+ ions. The best place to begin is at the equilibrium potential, $E_{Na^+} = +55$ mV (right side of Figure 7B). We know that the chemical and electrical forces acting on Na^+ ions must be equal and opposite at this membrane potential. When the membrane potential is positive, the direction of the electrical force acting on positively charged Na^+ ions is to drive them out of the cell. We also know that the chemical force is to drive Na^+ into the cell because of the relatively higher concentration of Na^+ outside compared to inside. The vector sum of these two forces is zero, and therefore the flux is zero at +55 mV for Na^+.

If we now consider Na^+ flux at 0 mV, we know that the electric force is also zero. The chemical force is exactly the same as it was at +55 mV and tends to drive Na^+ into the cell. Therefore, in this case, Flux = $(F_C) \times P_{Na^+}$. The leak permeability of the membrane to Na^+, however, is only about 3% (i.e., 0.03) that for K^+. Therefore, the flux of Na^+ ions at 0 mV is proportional to just a small fraction of F_C, shown as a barely visible small arrow pointed downward (inwardly) at 0 mV (Figure 7B).

When the membrane potential is at −75 mV, the chemical force is the same as it was at +55 mV, but now the electric force is large and acts to pull Na^+ ions inwardly (leftmost image in Figure 7B). Note that the electric force operating on Na^+ ions is identical to that shown acting on K^+ ions at -75 mV in Figure 7A. In this situation, the chemical and electrical forces are collaborating to strongly drive Na^+ into the cell. However, this relatively large electrochemical driving force when multiplied by the small permeability yields a relatively modest influx. The line connecting the flux values of Na^+ (Figure 7B) has a shallow slope (proportional to the small P_{Na}^+) and passes through zero flux at the equilibrium potential for Na^+ ($+55$ mV).

Keep in mind that the membrane is simultaneously permeable to both Na^+ and K^+. Therefore, let's put the flux versus membrane potential relations for both these ions on the same plot (Figure 7C). It turns out that there is only one value of membrane potential (i.e., position along the horizontal axis) where the flux of Na^+ ions is equal but opposite to that of K^+ ions—and that is at the resting membrane potential, V_R (~-60 mV). As a consequence, when the membrane is at V_R, there will be no change in membrane potential because there is no *net* flux of ions (even though there is a steady but small efflux of K^+ ions matched by a small steady influx of Na^+ ions).

The Role of Chloride Permeability

Until now, we have conveniently neglected that the membrane of neurons is also permeable to Cl^- ions in the resting state. The permeability of the membrane associated with Cl^- leak channels is about half that of K^+ leak channels. Therefore, it is not negligible. Interestingly, the equilibrium potential for Cl^- in neurons (see calculations performed earlier in this Chapter using the Nernst equation) is close to the resting potential, namely, around -60 mV. At -60 mV, the chemical force driving Cl^- ions into the cell is opposed by an equal magnitude electrical force repelling negatively charged Cl^- ions from entering the cell (leftmost image, Figure 8). Consequently, at the resting potential (-60 mV), there is little or no flux of Cl^- ions. If the membrane was held at 0 mV (middle image, Figure 8), then only the chemical force operates. When this force is multiplied by an intermediate permeability of the membrane to Cl^-, then there is a moderate influx of Cl^- ions. If instead, the membrane was held at the

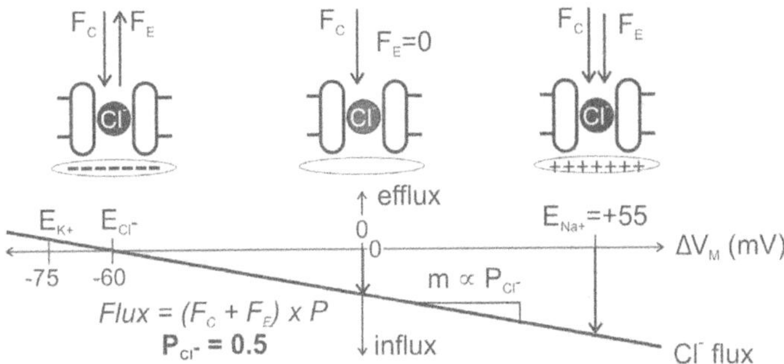

Figure 8.   Top: Depictions of chemical, F_C, and electrical, F_E, forces acting on Cl$^-$ ion at different membrane potentials. Bottom: Plot of ion flux versus membrane potential for Cl$^-$. Magnitude of slope m, is proportional to the permeability of the membrane to Cl$^-$, P_{Cl^-}.

equilibrium potential for Na$^+$ (+55 mV, right image, Figure 8), then the electrical force operating on Cl$^-$ ions would be in the same direction as the chemical force and almost as big. Therefore, there would be a large electrochemical driving force at this membrane potential. When this large net force is multiplied by an intermediate permeability, then there would be a large influx of Cl$^-$ ions. It is important to recognize that an influx of Cl$^-$ ions will tend to cause the membrane to *hyperpolarize* whereas an efflux of negatively charged Cl$^-$ ions (at membrane potentials to the left of E_{Cl}^-) will act to *depolarize* the membrane.

Summary of Forces and Fluxes at the Resting Membrane Potential

Figure 9 provides a summary of the forces and fluxes associated with the resting membrane potential. The large chemical force tending to drive K$^+$ out of the cell is nearly balanced by the large electrical force acting to drive the positively charged K$^+$ ions toward the negative charges on the inside of the membrane. The small net electrochemical force is multiplied by a large permeability to yield a modest net efflux of K$^+$ (small arrow). For Na$^+$, the chemical and electrical forces both act to drive Na$^+$ into the cell. The large net electrochemical force is multiplied by a small permeability to produce a small influx of Na$^+$ (small arrow). This influx of Na$^+$

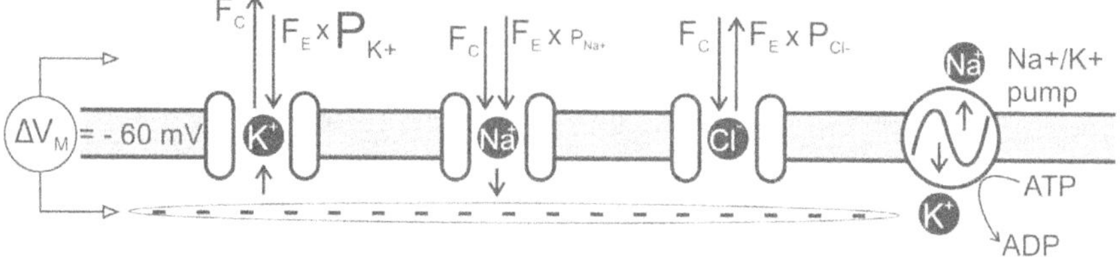

Figure 9.   Chemical (F_C) and electrical (F_E) forces, permeabilities (P), and fluxes (small arrows) for K⁺, Na⁺, and Cl⁻ ions at the resting membrane potential (~−60 mV). The small efflux of K⁺ is matched by the small influx of Na⁺ such that there is no net flux. Because −60 mV is approximately equal to the equilibrium potential for Cl⁻, there is no Cl⁻ flux. The Na⁺/K⁺ pump, fueled by the breakdown of adenosine triphosphate (ATP), operates slowly in the background to return Na⁺ to the extracellular space and K⁺ to the intracellular space, and thereby maintain the concentration gradients.

is equal to the efflux of K⁺. Chloride is approximately in equilibrium at the resting potential, such that the chemical force tending to propel Cl⁻ ions into the cell is counterbalanced by the electrical force driving the negatively charged Cl⁻ ions out of the cell. Consequently, there is no flux of Cl⁻ at the resting potential.

When we initially discussed the genesis of the resting membrane potential in the context of a simple cell permeable to one ion (Figure 5), we argued that the number of ions that would need to cross the membrane in order to develop a significant electrical force would be very small. As a consequence, there would be no detectable change in concentration gradient. While true for that transient situation, in the case of a neuron (Figure 6D), the persistent (albeit small) efflux of K⁺ and influx of Na⁺, if left unchecked, would eventually erode the concentration gradients. This in turn would dwindle the equilibrium potentials and completely disable electrical signaling in neurons. To counteract this, neuron and muscle membranes possess molecular pumps (Na⁺/K⁺ pump; Figure 9) that slowly operate in the background to move Na⁺ ions out of the cell and to bring K⁺ ions into the cell. This process requires energy (provided by the breakdown of adenosine triphosphate [ATP] to adenosine diphosphate [ADP]) to drive those ions against their concentration gradients. Indeed, one of the major sources of energy consumption by neurons is that needed to fuel the Na⁺/K⁺ pump.

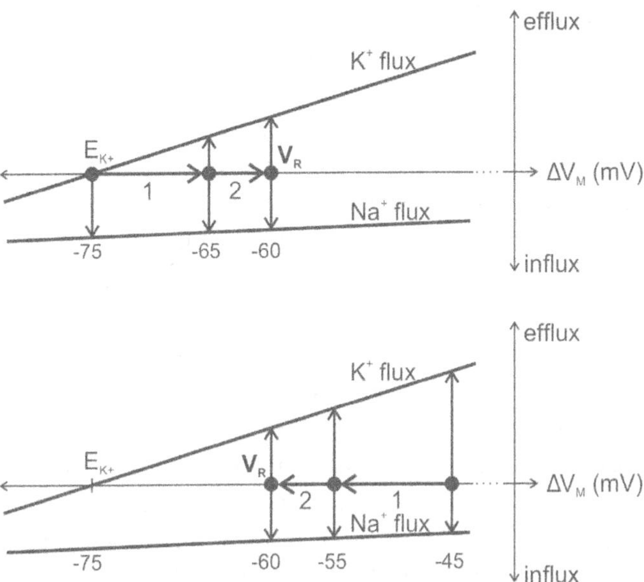

Figure 10.   (A) Return of membrane potential to resting potential, V_R, after the membrane potential had been displaced in hyperpolarizing direction to –75 mV. At –75 mV, Na⁺ influx drives the membrane in the depolarizing direction (arrow 1). At –65 mV, a small K⁺ efflux and reduced Na⁺ influx diminishes the magnitude of the net influx of positive charge to drive the membrane in the depolarizing direction. When at –60 mV, that is, the resting potential, the influx of Na⁺ equals the efflux of K⁺ and therefore, there is no further change in membrane potential. (B) Return of membrane potential to resting potential, V_R, after membrane potential had been displaced in depolarizing direction to –45 mV. At –45 mV, K⁺ efflux is larger than Na⁺ influx, and therefore the membrane potential is driven in the hyperpolarizing direction (arrow 1). At –55 mV, while the efflux of K⁺ is reduced and the influx of Na⁺ increased, K⁺ efflux remains slightly larger than Na⁺, leading to a net efflux of positive charge to drive the membrane in the hyperpolarizing direction (arrow 2). When at –60 mV, that is, the resting potential, the influx of Na⁺ equals the efflux of K⁺ and no further change in membrane potential occurs.

Why the Membrane Potential Returns to the Resting Membrane Potential

When the membrane is at the resting potential, there is no *net* flux of ions, and therefore, no change in membrane potential. At any other membrane potential, however, the imbalance of fluxes will lead to a change in membrane potential if the membrane is not artificially "clamped" by external sources. Indeed, let's take a look at what happens when we displace the membrane potential away from the resting potential by injecting current into the cell with an electrode and then turn off the current injection (like that depicted in Figures 3A and 3B). Let's again begin by just considering the roles played by K^+ and Na^+. Furthermore, to better visualize the process, let's zoom in on the region of the ion flux—membrane potential relations close to the resting membrane potential (i.e., in the neighborhood of −60 mV; Figure 10). First, let's displace the membrane potential away from the resting potential to a more hyperpolarized value, say −75 mV (Figure 10A) and then switch off the current injection. What will happen? We know that −75 mV is equivalent to the equilibrium potential for K^+ and therefore, there will be no flux of K^+ ions at this membrane potential. However, there is a small influx of Na^+ ions at this membrane potential (as shown by the downward arrow in Figure 10A). This influx of positively charged ions into the cell will modestly depolarize the membrane (i.e., shift it in the rightward direction, as indicated by the horizontal arrow 1), say to a value of −65 mV. When the membrane potential is now at −65 mV, there will be a small efflux of K^+ (indicated by the upward arrow) but a slightly larger influx of Na^+. Consequently, the *net* flux at this membrane potential will be a slight inward movement of positive charge. This in turn will again slightly depolarize the membrane potential (arrow 2), say to −60 mV. At −60 mV, the influx of Na^+ is perfectly balanced by the efflux of K^+. As such, there is no net charge passing across the membrane and, no further change in membrane potential.

Let's now repeat this process but begin by displacing the membrane potential in the opposite direction to a more depolarized state (say to −45 mV; see Figure 10B). At the moment we switch off the current injection and the membrane is sitting at −45 mV, there will be a fairly large efflux of K^+ (upward arrow at the right of Figure 10B), and a small influx of Na^+. Therefore, the *net* flux is an outward movement of positive charge. Tossing positive charges out of the cell will cause the interior of the membrane to become more negative. This will shift the membrane potential to the left to become more hyperpolarized, say to a value of −55 mV (arrow 1, Figure 10B). At this new membrane potential, the efflux of K^+ is smaller than it was at −45 mV, and the influx of Na^+ is slightly larger, but the *net* flux is still in the outward direction. Consequently, the membrane will be further hyperpolarized (arrow 2, Figure 10B), say to −60 mV. Now we are back at the resting membrane potential where no further change in membrane potential will occur. It is as though when we displace the membrane potential in either direction and then "let it go," the membrane potential "springs" back to the resting potential. The membrane potential will then remain indefinitely at the resting potential until some external agent (electrode or other neurons) delivers charge (positive or negative) to the interior of the membrane to displace the membrane potential away from the resting potential.

While not illustrated in Figure 10, chloride flux will also help restore the membrane potential to the resting potential from hyperpolarized or depolarized positions. As shown in Figure 8, if the membrane is hyperpolarized from the resting potential (equivalent to the equilibrium potential for Cl^-), then Cl^- ions will exit the cell. Such removal of negative charge will depolarize the membrane, returning it back toward the resting potential. Likewise, depolarizing the membrane away from the resting potential, will lead to an influx of Cl^- ions and thereby drive the membrane in the hyperpolarizing direction back toward the resting potential.

Summary

In this chapter, we have described the mechanisms that underlie the resting membrane potential. The resting membrane potential endows excitable cells like neurons and muscle fibers with the electromotive force needed to drive ions across the membrane that is the basis of electrical signaling. As such, the resting membrane potential is one of the most important functional properties of neurons and muscle fibers.

There are a few key ingredients that give rise to the resting membrane potential. First, is the unequal distribution of ions on either side of the membrane. This gives rise to chemical forces that drive ions from the high concentration side to the low concentration side of the membrane. Second is the relatively higher resting permeability (due to leak channels) of the membrane to K^+ than to other ions. Indeed, we showed that a cell that is only permeable to K^+ readily establishes a resting membrane potential at the equilibrium potential for K^+ (−75 mV). The equilibrium potential itself can be calculated using the Nernst equation and represents the membrane potential at which the associated electrical force precisely counteracts the chemical force for a particular ion, thereby halting flux (movement) of the ion across the membrane. In general, the flux of an ion is proportional to the sum of the chemical and electrical forces acting on the ion (i.e., the electrochemical force) multiplied by the permeability of the membrane to the ion (related to the number of ion-specific channels open). A third ingredient is that the resting permeability of Na^+, while small, is not negligible. As such, there exists only one level of membrane potential at which the small efflux of K^+ is perfectly balanced by a small influx of Na^+ such that there is no *net* movement of charge across the membrane. When there is no net movement of charge, the membrane potential remains fixed. This stable value of membrane potential, referred to as the resting membrane potential, occurs at about −60 mV in neurons.

In Chapter 4, we will see how abrupt changes in the permeability of the membrane launch large swings in membrane potential away from the resting potential associated with the generation of an action potential.

References

Brock LG, Coombs JS & Eccles JC (1952). The recording of potentials from motoneurones with an intracellular electrode. *Journal of Physiology* **117**, 431–460.

Kandel ER, Schwartz JH, Jessell TM, Siegelbaum SA & Hudspeth AJ (2012). Principles of Neural Science (5th edition). McGraw-Hill.

Chapter 4

Action Potential

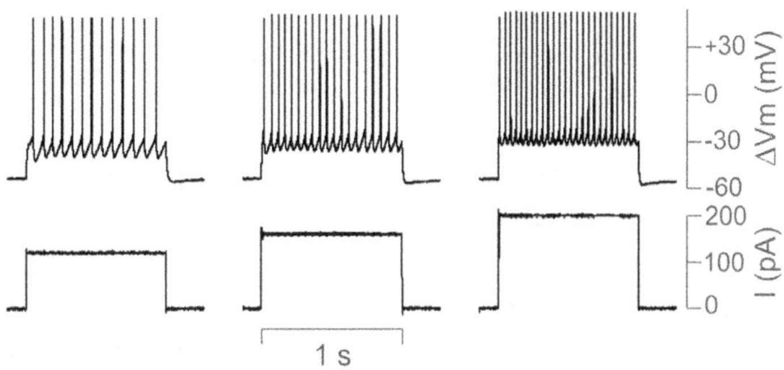

Action potential trains evoked in a motor neuron of a neonatal rat in response to three different levels of injected current. From the author's laboratory in collaboration with Dr. Ralph Fregosi.

What was discussed in Chapter 3 related to the effects of the *leak* channels for K^+, Na^+, and Cl^- on membrane potential. The *number* of these open channels remains relatively constant and determines the resting *permeability* of the membrane for these ions. Furthermore, the *permeabilities* of the membrane to these ions dictate the *slopes* of the membrane potential–ion flux relations shown in Figure 7C (for K^+, Na^+) and Figure 8 (for Cl^-) of Chapter 3. Remember, however, that neurons possess many types of *gated* ion channels that can be opened with an appropriate stimulus. If these channels are opened and are also permeable to Na^+, K^+, or Cl^-, then the slopes of the membrane potential–ion flux relations will increase. How can we now start to account for the effect of these changing permeabilities on the membrane potential?

Effects of Changes in Permeability on Membrane Potential

One way to visualize the effects of changing permeability on membrane potential is to consider the membrane potential–ion flux line as a stick that is nailed to the membrane potential axis at the equilibrium potential for each ion. As such the stick can rotate about the hinge point provided by the nail. Rotating the stick is associated with a change in slope and represents a change in the permeability of the membrane to a particular ion. For example, let's consider what would happen to the membrane potential if we increased the permeability of the membrane to Na^+ such that it now has a permeability equal to that of K^+ (Figure 1A). This would be associated with a rotation of the Na^+ flux line about the equilibrium potential for Na^+ (the hinge point) from its low slope resting position (dashed line) to a steeper inclination. If the membrane potential were initially sitting at the resting potential (−60 mV) when this happens, then there would be a significant influx of Na^+ that would depolarize the membrane, driving it to the right along the membrane potential axis. Indeed, it would move rapidly to a new steady-state position where Na^+ influx is balanced by an equivalent magnitude K^+ efflux (for simplicity, we again neglect the influence of Cl^-). In this case, the new membrane potential, V_M, will be at *half* the distance along the membrane potential axis between the equilibrium potentials for K^+ and Na^+ (E_K^+ and E_{Na}^+).

If the membrane now becomes very permeable to Na^+ such that P_{Na}^+ is much greater than P_K^+, then the slope of the Na^+ flux line (hinged at E_{Na}^+) will become very steep (Figure 1B). The new balance point where Na^+ influx is equal but opposite to K^+ efflux and sits very close to the equilibrium potential for Na^+. It is as if there is a tug-of-war between a potassium team and a sodium team (Figure 1C). Each team pulls the membrane potential toward their equilibrium potential. The *number* of players on each team, and the associated strength with which the team pulls on the membrane potential is equivalent to the *number* of channels that are open for their ion (i.e., the permeability of the membrane to the ion). In the case of the resting membrane potential, V_R, as depicted in Figure 1C, the number of open K^+ channels far outweighs the number of

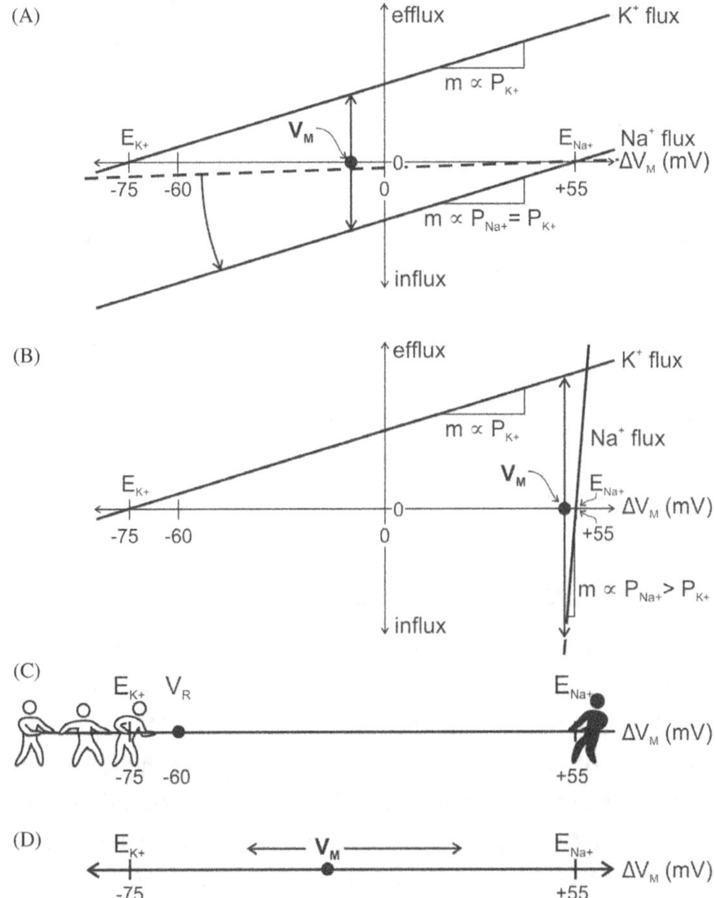

Figure 1.   Effect of change in permeability on membrane potential. (A) Flux–membrane potential relations for K^+ and Na^+ for cases in which Na^+ permeability equals that of K^+. The steady-state membrane potential (V_m, black dot) would reside halfway between the equilibrium potentials for K^+ (E_{K+}) and Na^+ (E_{Na+}). (B) Flux–membrane potential relations for cases in which the permeability to Na^+ is much greater than that of K^+. In this situation, V_m would sit close to E_{Na}^+. (C) At rest, V_M (black dot) sits close to the E_K^+ because of the higher permeability of the membrane to K^+. It is as though there is a tug-of-war between K^+ and Na^+ on V_M, where the strength of the pull is directly related to the number of channels open (i.e., the permeability) for each ion. (D) From moment to moment, V_M can shift anywhere between E_K^+ and E_{Na}^+ depending on changing permeabilities to K^+ and Na^+ (and Cl^-, not shown).

open Na^+ channels, and therefore the membrane potential is pulled quite close to the equilibrium potential for K^+. If there were equal numbers of players on each team, then the membrane potential would be pulled to a position halfway between E_K^+ and E_{Na}^+.

Therefore, one way to understand changes in membrane potential, V_M, that occur over time is to imagine the ball on the tug-of-war rope moving along the membrane potential axis driven by the relative permeabilities (i.e., the strength of the pulls toward the respective equilibrium potentials) at any moment (Figure 1D). Although not shown in Figure 1, chloride also has a team in this game and will pull the membrane potential toward its equilibrium potential at −60 mV. As such, we have a three-way tug-of-war, with each ion pulling the membrane potential toward its equilibrium potential with strengths equivalent to the number of ion channels open for each ion at any moment.

Goldman-Hodgkin-Katz Equation

The concepts just discussed were formalized into an equation derived by David Goldman and Nobel laureates Alan Hodgkin and Bernard Katz. The so-called Goldman-Hodgkin-Katz equation (**GHK equation**) estimates the value of the membrane potential, V_M, given the relative permeabilities, P, of the membrane to K^+, Na^+, and Cl^-. The equation looks very similar to the Nernst equation except that it simultaneously takes into account the permeabilities and concentrations of all three ions:

$$V_M = 57.5\,mV \cdot \log_{10}\left(\frac{P_K\left[K^+\right]_{out} + P_{Na}\left[Na^+\right]_{out} + P_{Cl}\left[Cl^-\right]_{in}}{P_K\left[K^+\right]_{in} + P_{Na}\left[Na^+\right]_{in} + P_{Cl}\left[Cl^-\right]_{out}}\right).$$

Note, however, that the valence, Z, is not shown explicitly as a denominator in the GHK equation as it is in the Nernst equation. This is because the valence for K^+ and Na^+ is +1 and, therefore, will not affect the calculated value of V_m if left out. The −1 valence for chloride, however, is accounted for in the GHK equation by cleverly inverting the ratio of the concentrations for Cl^- such that the numerator represents the concentration **in**side and the denominator the concentration **out**side the cell.

One should also notice that if the permeabilities are set to zero for two of the three ions, then the GHK equation is equivalent to the Nernst equation for the other ion. For example, if $P_{Na} = P_{Cl} = 0$, then the resulting equation is indeed the Nernst equation for K^+ with a calculated value of $V_M = -75$ mV. If one inserts the values of the concentrations outside and inside the cell for each ion, and the relative permeabilities of the membrane associated with the resting state (namely, $P_K = 1.0$, $P_{Na} = 0.03$, $P_{Cl} = 0.5$) then the calculated value of the membrane potential will be:

$$V_M = 57.5\,mV \cdot log_{10}\left(\frac{1.0[5mM]_{out} + 0.03[144mM]_{out} + 0.5[13mM]_{in}}{1.0[100mM]_{in} + 0.03[16mM]_{in} + 0.5[144mM]_{out}} \right)$$

$$V_M = 57.5\,mV \cdot log_{10}\left(\frac{15.2}{165.3} \right) = -59.6\,mV \cong -60\,mV$$

Action Potential

When the spike-initiating zone (initial segment of the axon) is depolarized beyond a certain level called **threshold** (V_{Th}, usually 15 to 20 mV above the resting potential), dramatic changes occur in the membrane potential. These changes in membrane potential, called the **action potential**, come about due to rapid and large changes in the permeability of the membrane to Na^+ and K^+. It is as though the ball on the membrane potential axis (Figure 1D) gets rapidly propelled toward the equilibrium potential for Na^+ and then gets pulled back just as quickly toward the equilibrium potential for K^+. It is the action potential that enables long-distance signaling along the axon between the soma or spike-initiating zone and the presynaptic terminals at the synapses with other neurons or muscle fibers.

To understand how the action potential evolves over time, let's flip the membrane potential axis vertically and have time represented along the horizontal axis (Figure 2A). The membrane potential axis is labeled with those critical levels (i.e., E_K^+, V_R, V_{Th}, E_{Na}^+) that dictate the progression of the action potential. Initially, the membrane potential sits at a value close to -60 mV (V_R), which is close to E_{K+} because of the much higher permeability of the membrane to K^+ than to Na^+. Then, in order to trigger an

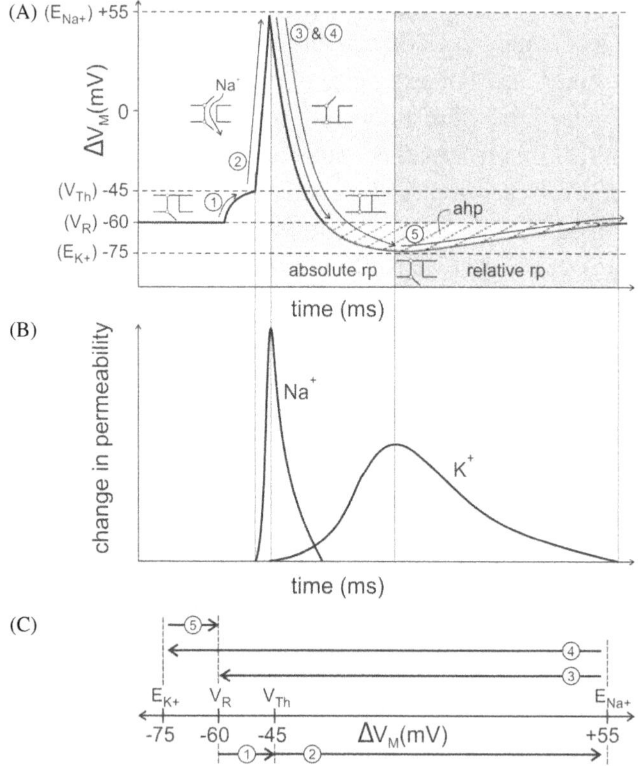

Figure 2.   Channel events underlying the action potential. Changes in membrane potential (A) and permeability (B) as a function of time. **1**. External source depolarizes membrane from resting potential (V_R) to threshold voltage (V_{TH}). **2**. Large number of voltage-gated Na^+ channels open, Na^+ permeability greatly increases (B), which leads to a large influx of Na^+, driving the membrane potential toward equilibrium potential for Na^+ (E_{Na}^+). **3**. Voltage-gated Na^+ channels inactivate, rapidly reducing permeability to Na^+ (B), driving the membrane potential back toward V_R. **4**. Activation of delayed voltage-gated K^+ channels, gradually increases permeability to K^+ (B), leading to efflux of K^+ ions, driving the membrane toward equilibrium potential for K^+ (E_K^+). **5**. Voltage-gated K^+ channels deactivate, gradually reducing permeability to K^+, and restoring the membrane potential back to V_R. Diagrams represent the state of voltage-gated Na^+ channels at different stages. AHP — afterhyperpolarization, rp — refractory period. (C) Schematic showing the same five events as in (A) but on a horizontal membrane-potential (ΔV_M) axis.

action potential, the membrane must be depolarized up to the critical level, V_{Th} (arrow 1 in Figure 2A). But how does this happen? Typically, this occurs through the opening of ligand-gated channels at the synapses on the dendrites and soma that deliver positively charged ions into the neuron. Experimentally, this can also occur by injecting a positive current through an electrode that has been inserted into a neuron (like in Figure 3C of Chapter 3). In a nutshell, the first process (**arrow 1**) requires an external source (other neurons or an electrode injecting positive current) to depolarize the membrane by about 15 mV (up to V_{Th}).

If the membrane potential reaches V_{Th}, then a set of processes (arrows 2 to 5, Figure 2A) play out in rapid succession. First, an enormous number of *voltage-gated Na$^+$ channels* located at the spike-initiating zone (or elsewhere on the axon) spring open (i.e., voltage-gated Na$^+$ channels become activated, **arrow 2**). This causes the membrane to become highly permeable to Na$^+$ (Figure 2B). Because of the large electrical and chemical forces acting to drive Na$^+$ into the cell and now the immense permeability, there will be a massive influx of positively charged Na$^+$ ions to depolarize the membrane toward the equilibrium potential for Na$^+$ (top of arrow 2, Figure 2A).

Keep in mind the channels that instigated the large influx of Na$^+$ (voltage-gated Na$^+$ channels) are opened by the membrane becoming depolarized by about 15 mV above rest. But now the membrane potential is about 100 mV above that level. As such, the activating signal is extremely potent and, if nothing else were to occur, these channels would remain open, and the membrane would "lock in" at a new membrane potential close to +55 mV. In essence, we would get one action potential and then no more. To prevent this from happening and to enable repetitive generation of action potentials, two processes occur more or less in parallel. One is that the *voltage-gated Na$^+$ channels undergo the process of inactivation* (**arrow 3**, Figure 2A). Recall from Figure 3B of Chapter 2 that for some channels, the same signal that opens the channels also causes them to close rapidly. As such, the membrane permeability to Na$^+$

falls steeply (Figure 2B). This in turn drives the membrane potential back toward the original *resting level*.

Interestingly, at about the same time, there is a marked but slower increase in the permeability of the membrane to K^+ (Figure 2B). How does this come about? It turns out that membrane depolarization from rest by about 15 mV also activates another class of ion channels. However, these channels are permeable to K^+ but they are relatively slow to open. Therefore, *activation of these delayed, voltage-gated K^+ channels* greatly increases the permeability of the membrane to K^+ beyond that found in the resting state. This pulls the membrane potential below the resting potential to approach the equilibrium potential for K^+ (**arrow 4**, Figure 2A). When the membrane potential drops below the threshold, these *simple-gated* channels no longer have their activating signal. As such, with a delay, these *voltage-gated K^+ channels slowly deactivate* causing the excess permeability of the membrane to K^+ to fall (Figure 2B), returning the membrane potential back to its original resting level (**arrow 5**, Figure 2A).

The entire period of time during which the membrane potential sits lower than the resting potential due to the excess permeability of the membrane to K^+ is referred to as the **afterhyperpolarization** (AHP) period. The duration of the action potential up to the onset of the AHP may be only a few milliseconds. The AHP itself, however, may last tens of milliseconds. If drawn to scale, the AHP period would be about 10 times longer than that shown in Figure 2A.

The British scientists Alan Hodgkin and Andrew Huxley first described the sequence of events that underlie the action potential in the 1950s for which they were awarded the Nobel Prize. We can summarize these events by simply considering how each process shifts the membrane potential. To do this, let's return to a horizontal membrane potential axis and visualize how the membrane potential is displaced (shown with arrows in Figure 2C) in response to each of the following processes: (1) an external source depolarizes the membrane from rest to threshold, (2) voltage-gated Na^+ channels *activate*, pushing the membrane toward E_{Na}^+, (3) voltage-gated Na^+ channels *inactivate*, driving the membrane potential back toward the resting potential, (4) delayed voltage-gated K^+ channels *activate*, driving the membrane potential toward E_K^+, and (5) delayed voltage-gated K^+ channels *deactivate*, returning the membrane back to the resting potential.

The voltage-gated Na^+ channels are the linchpins of the action potential. Without high densities of these channels concentrated in certain locations, action potentials will not be produced in neurons (or muscle fibers). It is instructive, therefore, to inspect the different states that these channels undergo throughout the sweep of an action potential. At rest, and up until the membrane exceeds the threshold, these channels are in a closed state. We can think of these channels as having two gates (image to the left of arrow 1, Figure 2A), with the inner gate open and the outer gate closed at rest. When the membrane potential exceeds the threshold level, the channel molecule undergoes a conformational change to open a pathway through the membrane. We can think of this as the opening of the outer gate (image to the left of the arrow 2, Figure 2A). Sodium ions dash through the briefly opened pathway. Now, the same voltage signal that caused the outer gate to open, rapidly closes the inner gate, shutting off the flux of Na^+. These channels are now in an *inactive* state (image to the right of arrow 4, Figure 2A). These channels will remain in this state as long as the depolarizing signal remains in place. Therefore, to reset these channels (i.e., remove the inactivation), the membrane potential first needs to drop below the threshold potential (image to the right of the action potential and below threshold). This eliminates the original activating signal and the outer gate closes. However, to completely restore the voltage-gated Na^+ channels to their original state, a certain amount of time must elapse following the removal of the activating signal in order for the inner gate to open (image below the action potential during the AHP period).

During the time that the voltage-gated Na^+ channels are in the inactive state, *it is impossible to ignite another action potential.* This period of time, starting roughly at the peak of the action potential and ending sometime during the AHP period, is referred to as the **absolute refractory period** (light gray region, Figure 2A). This period sets a limit on how close in time a subsequent action potential can occur following an action potential and is typically on the order of 2 to 5 ms. Immediately following the absolute refractory period, the neuron enters another phase referred to as the **relative refractory period** (dark gray region, Figure 2A). During this phase, the membrane is hyperpolarized. As a consequence, *the magnitude of a signal arising from an external source must be larger than that in the resting state in order to trigger an action potential.* For example, the original signal that brought the neuron to the threshold in the first place (arrow 1, Figure 2A) caused a depolarization of about 15 mV. However, at the outset of the relative refractory period, that same signal would only bring the membrane potential back to near the resting potential. Indeed, at that time early on in the relative refractory period, a signal nearly double in strength to that which originally triggered the action potential would be needed to evoke a second action potential. The duration of the relative refractory period can last as long as 100 ms in some neurons.

Mechanisms of Repetitive Firing

Neurons rarely fire just a single action potential. Instead, sequences (or trains) of action potentials are produced by neurons in response to depolarizing synaptic input from other neurons or injected current through a microelectrode (see frontispiece at beginning of this chapter). Indeed, it is through such repetitive firing of action potentials that information is encoded and transferred from one neuron to another.

To understand how information is represented in sequences of action potentials, let's first address the mechanisms underlying the repetitive firing of action potentials. A single action potential (top trace) is shown on the left side of Figure 3A in response to a rather un-physiological brief pulse of depolarizing current (lower trace). As we have discussed previously, the membrane potential returns to the resting potential (i.e., the steady-state condition) following the AHP period. Also shown (the thick line) is the change in membrane potential that would occur in response to the current injection if no voltage-gated channels were opened. Indeed, it is possible to disable the operation of the voltage-gated channels involved in the action potential experimentally by adding the antagonist tetrodotoxin (**TTX**) to *block voltage-gated Na^+ channels* and tetra-ethyl-ammonium (**TEA**) to *block voltage-gated K^+ channels*. Therefore, the thick trace at the left of Figure 3A shows the membrane depolarization that would occur in the presence of TTX and TEA. When the current is turned off, the

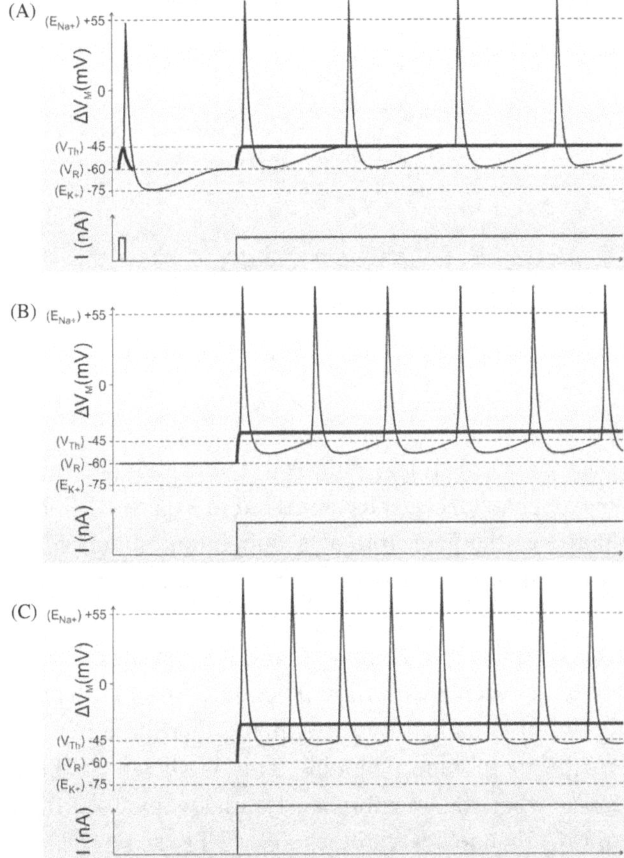

Figure 3.   Repetitive firing. (A) Left — brief pulse of injected current just sufficient to elicit an action potential (thin line). The thick line indicates membrane potential if no voltage-gated channels are activated. Right — membrane potential response to sustained current injection just sufficient to bring the membrane to the threshold (V_{Th}). The thick line indicates the new steady state, namely, the potential at which the membrane would remain if only leak channels were available. Action potentials "ride" upon this new steady state. Note that at the end of the AHP period, the membrane potential is at V_{Th} and another action potential is ignited. (B) Response to stronger current injection. The new steady state (thick line) is more depolarized than in (A). The vertical "distance" that the membrane potential needs to traverse from the depth of the AHP to V_{Th} is less than that in (A). Therefore, less time elapses between action potentials, leading to increased firing rate. (C) Response to even stronger current injection, with very little vertical distance from the bottom of AHP to V_{Th}. As such the time between action potentials is short and the firing rate is high. (D) If the current injection is too high, then following the first action potential, the membrane potential does not go below V_{Th} during the AHP. This keeps the voltage-gated Na^+ channels in an inactive state, preventing the generation of further action potentials.

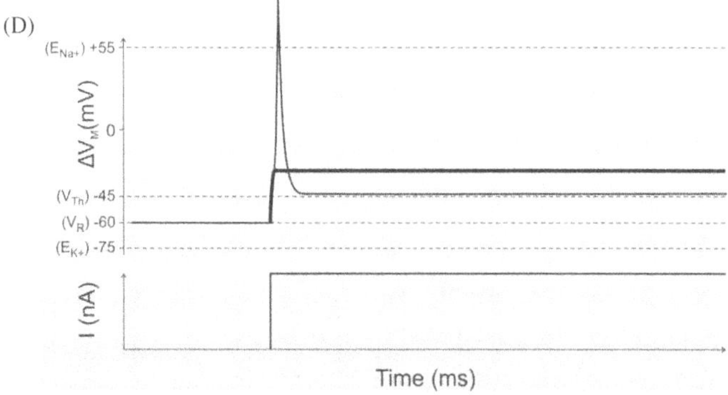

Figure 3.   (*Continued*)

membrane potential then simply returns to the resting potential under the action of the leak channels (just as described in Figure 10B of Chapter 3).

The response of the neuron to a sustained (and more physiologically realistic) current injection is shown on the right side of Figure 3A. The level of current injected is just sufficient to bring the neuron to threshold. Now a repeated sequence of action potentials is produced. What dictates the time elapsed between each action potential? An important insight into the timing question is gained by recognizing that there is a new steady-state level of the membrane potential. This is shown as the thick line, which represents where the membrane potential would "sit" if the voltage-gated Na^+ and K^+ channels were blocked by TTX and TEA, respectively. It is steady state because the action of the leak channels tending to drive the membrane potential back toward the resting potential is counterbalanced by the steady depolarizing current injected through the microelectrode. In some respects, it is as if we have a new resting potential or baseline upon which all changes in potential are superimposed. Indeed, the voltage changes that occur during the action potential are partially shifted to a more depolarized level associated with the new baseline. Note, for example, that at the depth of the AHP, the membrane potential is about 15 mV below the new baseline, just as it was for the single action potential. But now this level is roughly at the resting potential rather than at E_{K+} (Figure 3A). As the AHP dissipates, the membrane returns to the new baseline. But just when the AHP period ends, the membrane potential (as it approaches the new baseline) is at the threshold and a new action potential is ignited. This process will repeat itself indefinitely as long as the current injection is maintained. In this case, and as demonstrated by Daniel (Kernell 1965), the time *interval between each successive action potentials is determined by the duration of the AHP*. Furthermore, these intervals are the longest, and the associated firing rate is the lowest that the neuron can produce under steady-state conditions. If we drop the level of the current injection slightly, then the neuron does not reach the threshold and no action potentials are produced.

What happens if we increase the magnitude of the injected depolarizing current? Figure 3B shows such a case where the level of injected current is moderately increased above that shown in Figure 3A. This leads to a more depolarized steady state (baseline) level (thick line, Figure 3B) upon which changes in the membrane potential are superimposed. It is as if the action potential is shifted "northward." Following the spike of the first action potential in the sequence, the AHP begins to die out bringing the membrane potential back toward the new baseline. However, before the baseline level (thick line) is reached, the membrane potential passes through the threshold, triggering another action potential. The extent of membrane potential that needs to be traversed from the depths of the AHP to the threshold is less for the situation in Figure 3B compared to that in Figure 3A. Therefore, the time to reach the threshold is less and the associated *firing rate is higher*.

Figure 3C shows the case for an even stronger level of current injection. Once again, under the higher level of injected current the baseline level (thick line) is shifted to a more depolarized level. Keep in mind that this is where the membrane potential would reside if there were no voltage-gated channels activated. After the first spike, the membrane potential barely starts to recover from the deepest part of the AHP and is headed toward the baseline level when the threshold is crossed, and another action potential is triggered. Therefore, the time interval between action potentials is brief and the associated firing rate is high.

If we inject even higher levels of depolarizing current, then something unexpected occurs. Such a case is illustrated in Figure 3D. An action potential is evoked at the onset of current injection. But because the baseline is shifted so high, the membrane potential associated with the AHP now does not cross below the threshold voltage, V_{Th}. Consequently, the voltage-gated Na^+ channels remain in an inactive state. Remember from Figure 2A that once these channels inactivate, they can only be reset and ready to produce another action potential if the original activating signal (namely, the membrane depolarized ~15 mV above the resting potential) is removed. Under such strong depolarizing current, the membrane potential cannot be pulled below this level even under the action of the voltage-gated K^+ channels. Interestingly, the voltage-gated K^+ channels are the type of channel that undergoes simple gating: they activate (albeit slowly) when they are depolarized (by ~15 mV) and deactivate when that depolarization is removed. In this case, however, the depolarization cannot be removed and therefore they remain in a relatively persistent active state. It is as if they are continuously struggling to pull the membrane potential below the threshold level but can't quite make it because of the overpowering influence of the injected depolarizing current. Therefore, the firing of action potentials is arrested and the membrane potential sits below the baseline level (remember, this level is where the membrane potential would dwell if no voltage-gated channels were activated) because of the persistent activation of the voltage-gated K^+ channels.

There is some question as to whether under natural circumstances such high levels of depolarizing current from synaptic sources could occur to push the membrane potential into the arrested state shown in Figure 3D. Nevertheless, it provides a good illustration of the importance and function of the voltage-gated K^+ channels. Their job is to pull the membrane potential below the threshold level after each action potential in order to remove inactivation on voltage-gated Na^+ channels. Without these K^+ channels, the membrane would readily succumb to an arrested state even for modest levels of membrane depolarization.

Rate Coding

Once above the threshold, the firing rate increases more or less in direct proportion to the amplitude of the depolarizing current delivered (see frontispiece at beginning of this chapter). As such, neurons transform ("encode") the input received from upstream sources into a reliable output message (frequency of action potentials) that it sends to its downstream targets. The code is a relatively simple one: namely, the *frequency of action potentials delivered to other neurons (or muscle fibers) is proportional to the intensity of excitation received*. This method of conveying information is referred to as **rate coding**. In later chapters, we will see a number of cases of rate coding in both sensory and motor systems.

It is also important to recognize that the existence of a *threshold* is important to ensure that only information of sufficient importance is communicated. For depolarization levels lower than ~15 mV, no action potentials are generated. Without such a threshold, neurons would be chattering all of the time and our nervous system would become swamped with activity. This is not so different from our use of cell phones. We don't call up our friends and inform them of each insignificant detail that we encounter (or at least most of us don't), such as "Hey, I just saw a tree!" or "I just went outside, and the sky is blue!" Thankfully, we have a threshold for the importance of information to convey, below which we don't go through the effort to phone. Otherwise, everyone would be calling everyone else all the time and the phone networks would become completely overloaded and stop operating.

Summary

Action potentials are the brief, large changes in membrane potential that serve as the main vehicle for delivering signals along the axon from the soma or spike-initiating zone to the presynaptic terminals. These electrical impulses occur due to rapid, massive, and sequential changes in the permeability of the membrane to Na^+ and K^+ ions—driving the membrane potential first toward the equilibrium potential of Na^+ and then back toward the equilibrium potential of K^+. Action potentials rarely occur as singular events. Instead, they arise as a procession of impulses, the frequency of which provides one of the main codes by which the brain processes information.

References

Kandel ER, Schwartz JH, Jessell TM, Siegelbaum SA & Hudspeth AJ (2012) Principles of Neural Science (5th Edition). McGraw-Hill.

Kernell D (1965). The limits of firing frequency in cat lumbosacral motoneurones possessing different time course of afterhyperpolarization. *Acta Physiologica* **65**, 87–100.

Chapter 5

Conduction of Electrical Signals

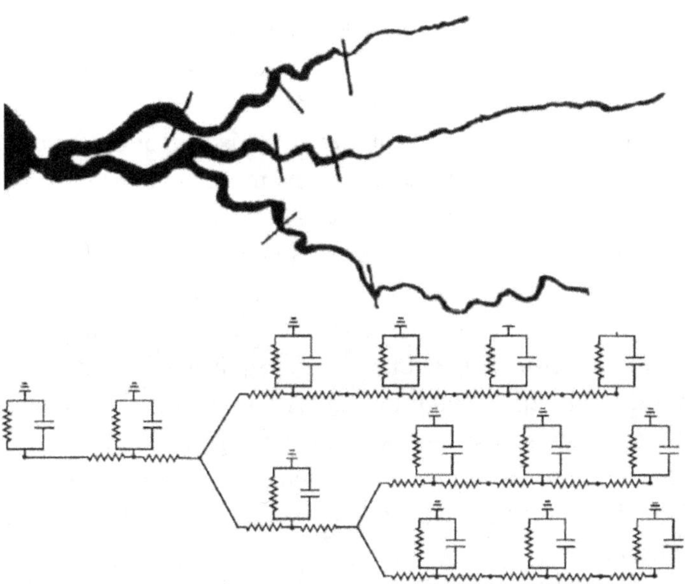

Part of soma and dendrites of a motor neuron and the circuit representing the electrical properties of this system. (Adapted from Segev et al. [1992].)

In Chapters 3 and 4, we discussed how the membrane potential can change at a particular *location* in a neuron. But how do membrane potential signals travel from one location to another within a neuron? Perhaps surprisingly, the passive electrical properties of neurons play a dominant role in shaping how electrical signals get delivered to different locations. As we discussed earlier, these **passive properties** are associated with the features of neurons that do not change from moment to moment, namely, the *physical geometry* of the cell, the *lipid bilayer membrane*, and *non-gated leak channels* in the membrane.

Electrical Model of Neuron Segment

To understand how these passive properties affect electrical signaling, let's begin by constructing an electrical circuit that represents a small segment of a neuron, for example, a small segment of dendrite (Figure 1). The dendritic segment possesses mainly leak channels with relatively few voltage-gated channels. If we slice the membrane along one side (dashed line, Figure 1A) and unfurl the membrane, we end up with a slab of membrane like that shown in Figure 1B. As we discussed in Chapter 2 (Figure 6), ion channels can be represented electrically as resistors. Therefore, our slab of membrane has many resistors passing through, connecting the inside of the cell (below the membrane) to the outside (above the membrane). Both the extracellular and intracellular fluids are good conductors (Figure 1C), so they connect together the tops and bottoms of the many resistors. In this way, leak channels are like many resistors configured in parallel. We can use our rule for resistors in parallel (see Appendix A) to come up with a single equivalent resistance passing through the membrane (Figure 1D). As you might remember from Appendix A, the more resistors "added" in parallel, the lower the effective resistance. As such, the equivalent resistance representing all of the leak channels in the membrane segment will be much lower than the resistance of a single channel.

Now, we can't forget that sitting above and below the membrane are the extracellular and intracellular electrolyte solutions. The faces of these conductive solutions on either side of the lipid membrane function just like two large plate conductors separated by an insulator (Figure 1E). Such an arrangement behaves like an electrical capacitor (Appendix A). As such, our dendritic segment can be represented as a capacitor with a resistor passing through a hole drilled in the capacitor plates (Figure 1F). Now, extending outward from the faces of the electrolyte solutions at the membrane is more electrolyte solution (Figure 1G). These big volumes of

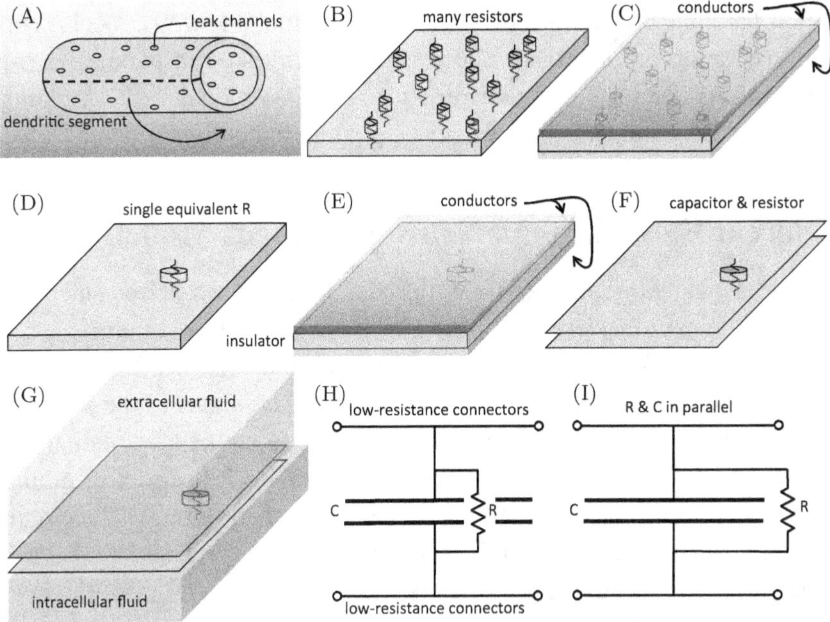

Figure 1.   Electrical circuit representing a segment of a dendrite. (A) Dendritic segment is unfurled. (B) Leak channels in membrane represented as an array of resistors. (C) Intracellular and extracellular solutions are good conductors linking together the transmembrane resistors into a parallel array. (D) Parallel transmembrane resistors denoted as a single equivalent resistance. (E) Lipid bilayer membrane is a good insulator sandwiched between conductive sheets of electrolyte solution. (F) Such an arrangement shown in (E) can be represented as a capacitor with a resistor passing through a hole in the capacitor. (G) Above and below the electrolyte sheets that serve as part of the capacitor are volumes of electrolyte solution (extracellular and intracellular fluid). (H) The electrolyte volumes shown in (G) serve as low-resistance connectors linking the resistor and capacitor circuit to neighboring regions. (I) The equivalent resistance is "moved" outside the hole in the capacitor plate to yield a parallel resistor-capacitor (RC) circuit representing the electrical properties of the dendritic segment.

electrolyte function like big copper bars soldered to the plates of the capacitor and to the resistor. Such large conductors can be represented as low-resistance wires (connectors) to which other electrical components can be attached (Figure 1H). Lastly, we can simply reposition the resistor from the little hole through the capacitor plates to "outside" the plates, which has no effect on the function of the circuit (Figure I). We end up with a circuit with a resistor and capacitor configured in parallel as the electrical model for a segment of a neuron. This model is the building block needed to understand electrical signaling in neurons.

Current Flow through Neuron Segment Model

To understand how the passive properties of a neuron affect electrical signaling in neurons, let's begin by injecting a steady level of current, I_{CC}, into a neuron segment through a microelectrode using a constant current device (Figure 2A). To start, we assume that the two ends of the segment are sealed. A "return" electrode is placed outside the neuron segment to connect the constant current device to the low-resistance extracellular fluid surrounding the segment in order to complete the circuit. The circuit representation of our situation is shown in Figure 2B. When the switch is engaged, then a steady current (I_{CC}) is delivered to the interior of the neuron segment (Figure 2C). The injected current splits into two parts: one to charge the membrane capacitance (I_C) and the other passing through the leak channels in the membrane (I_R). It is important to recognize that the sum of I_C and I_R will equal I_{CC} at all times (in accordance with Kirchhoff's Second Law). As discussed in Appendix A, at the moment the current begins to be injected (Figure 2D), all the current will be directed toward the capacitor (toward the "ice-skating pond with no skaters on it"). This means that initially, no current passes through the ion channels. In other words, at time $t = 0$, $I_C = I_{CC}$ and $I_R = 0$.

As charge starts to build up on the capacitor, those charges tend to repel the addition of further charge. As such, the current directed toward the capacitor begins to modestly decrease (Figure 2E), which means a small current will now start to pass through the ion channels (keep in mind that if I_C drops by a certain amount, I_R must increase by exactly that same amount such that $I_C + I_R$ = a constant = I_{CC}). Eventually, so much charge is built up on the capacitor that the "push back" of those charges equals the push forward generated by the constant current device. When this occurs, no further current goes toward the capacitor and all of the injected current (I_{CC}) passes through the ion channels (I_R) in the membrane (Figure 2F). If the current injection is maintained, then this state of affairs will persist indefinitely. Furthermore, in this state, no action takes place in

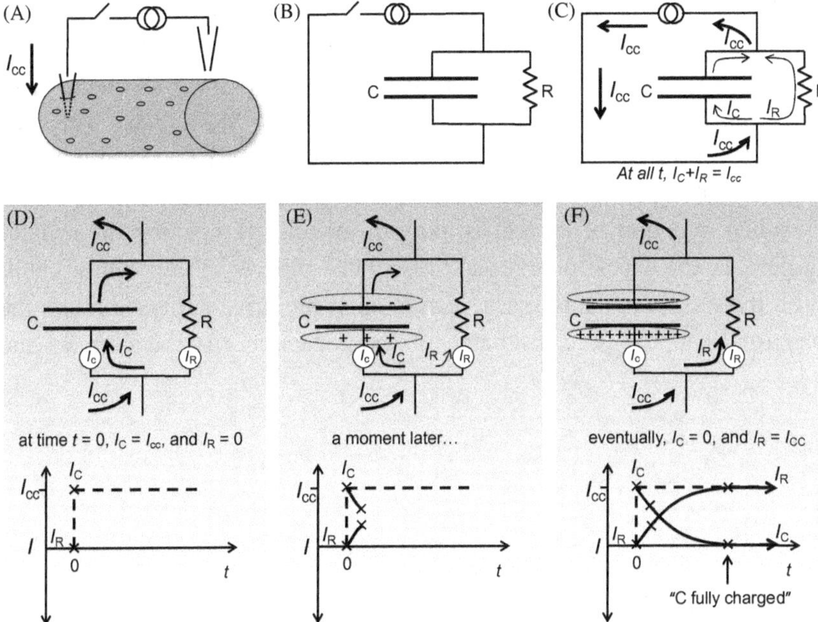

Figure 2.   Current flow in a dendritic segment during current injection. (A) A current generator is used to deliver current into a "sealed" segment of a dendrite. (B) The circuit representation of panel A. (C) When a switch is engaged, a steady level of current, I_{CC}, is delivered to the circuit, some of which goes to charge the membrane capacitance, I_C, and the remainder passes through the membrane resistance, I_R. The total current I_{CC} is always equal to $I_C + I_R$. (D) At the outset, all of the injected current (dashed line) is directed to the membrane capacitance. (E) As charge builds up on the capacitor (which partially repels the addition of further charge), some of the current gets directed through the membrane resistance. (F) At some time point, the strength of the repulsive forces built up on the capacitor prevents further addition of charge, thereby directing all of the injected current through membrane resistance. The capacitor is referred to as being fully charged in this situation. Note that the capacitor current, I_C, falls off exponentially whereas the current through the resistor increases exponentially to reach a new steady state.

the capacitor segment of the circuit. As such, this circuit now behaves like a simple one with just a resistor connected to the constant current device, where the capacitor plays no role.

As discussed in Appendix A, the capacitive and resistive currents follow profiles of falling and rising exponentials, respectively, with a time constant equivalent to the product of the membrane capacitance and membrane resistance, that is, $\tau = C_m \times R_m$. It takes about four time constants for the membrane to reach the fully charged state. In such a small neuron segment, the capacitance is small (the area of the capacitor "plates" is tiny) whereas the resistance is very high (relatively few leak channels in such a small membrane segment). A typical time constant for a neuron might be approximately 10 ms but this can vary widely depending on the properties of the neuron.

When injection of current is abruptly halted (by opening the switch; Figure 3A), the excess charge (and associated difference in potential) built up on the membrane capacitance can temporarily drive current through the open ion channels (i.e., discharge of the capacitor). At the moment the

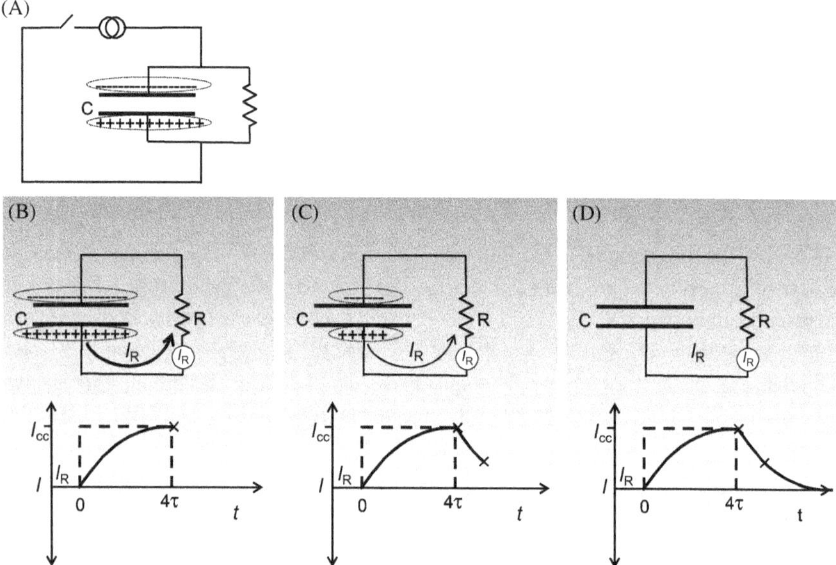

Figure 3.   Current flow in the dendritic segment when current injection ceases. (A) Circuit representation of dendritic segment at the moment when current injection is halted by disengaging the switch. (B) At the instant when current injection is halted, a large current, I_R, flows from the positively charged plate of the capacitor (representing the interior of the membrane) toward the negative plate (representing the exterior of the membrane) through the membrane resistance (R, leak channels). (C) The magnitude of the current diminishes as charge is lost from the interior plate of the capacitor and the negative charge on the exterior is canceled leading to a reduction in the difference in potential across the membrane. (D) Eventually (four time constants after the switch was disengaged), all the excess charge is lost from both plates of the capacitor leading to the cessation of current flow.

current injection is switched off (say four time constants after the current was switched on), the magnitude of that capacitive current is high (Figure 3B). As the excess charge on the membrane capacitance exits through the membrane resistance, the current progressively weakens (Figure 3C). Eventually (approximately four time constants later), no excess charge will remain on the capacitor and current flow will halt (Figure 3D).

Membrane Potential Change in Neuron Segment

How do such time-dependent changes in current alter the membrane potential? As discussed in Chapter 2, the convention in electrophysiology is to measure the membrane potential, ΔV_{m}, as the difference between the potential on the inside of the membrane (V_i) and that on the outside (V_O), that is, $\Delta V_m = V_i - V_O$ (Figure 4A). In addition, for simplicity, we consider here only the *changes* in membrane potential away from the resting potential. From Kirchhoff's Second Law (see Appendix A), we know that the difference in potential across the membrane capacitance (ΔV_C) must be equal to the change in membrane potential across the membrane resistance (ΔV_R), and that both of these are equivalent to ΔV_m. From Ohm's law, we know that the change in potential across a resistor is simply the product of the current flowing through the resistor and the resistance, namely, $\Delta V_R = I_R \times R_m = \Delta V_m$. Therefore, how the membrane potential varies as a function of time looks exactly like that of the resistive current, I_R. As redrawn from Figure 3D, the resistive current first increases and then decreases exponentially in response to a rectangular pulse of current (Figure 4B, top). Consequently, the membrane potential must follow this identical profile (Figure 4B, bottom). One important outcome of these electrical properties (as we shall discuss momentarily) is that for a relatively brief pulse of current injected into a neuron (the "input"; Figure 4B), the voltage response of the neuron ("output"; Figure 4B) is extended in time.

Ion Channel Currents Are Pulse-Like

As discussed in Chapter 2, the current that passes through an ion channel has the form of a brief, small, rectangular pulse (Figure 5A), not unlike that injected by a constant current device. If the movement of positive

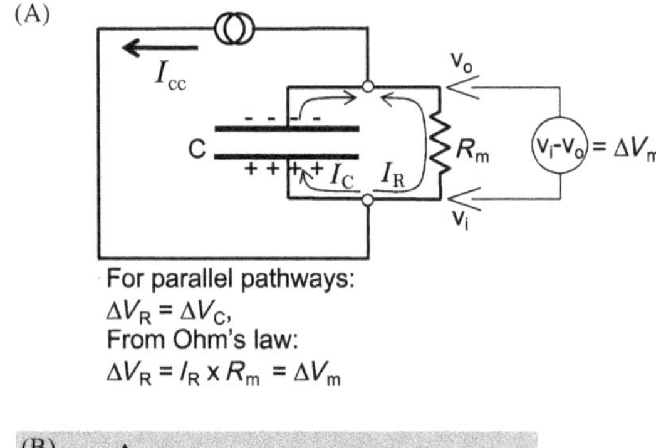

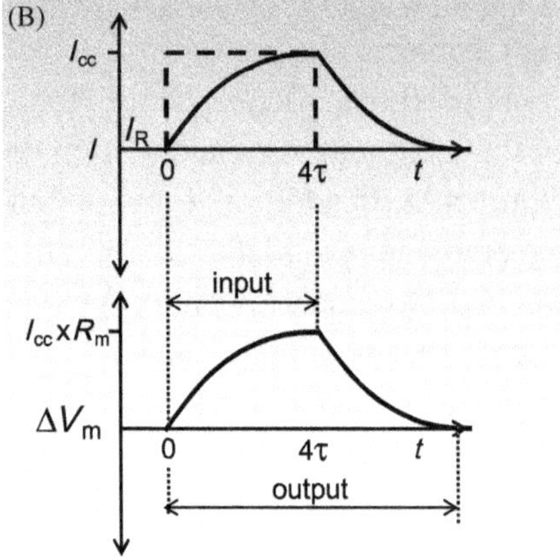

Figure 4. Membrane potential response to injection of a depolarizing current pulse. (A) Circuit representation of a dendrite segment receiving a pulse of depolarizing current, I_{CC}, delivered by a constant current device. A voltmeter measures the difference in potential across the membrane, ΔV_m. From Ohm's law, $\Delta V_m = I_R \times R_m$, and therefore, ΔV_m will be directly proportional to I_R. (B) Current flow (top) through membrane resistance, I_R, in response to a pulse of current with a magnitude of I_{CC} (from Figure 3D). The current pulse is halted after a period of four time constants (τ) when I_R has just reached a new steady state. Membrane potential (bottom) is directly proportional to I_R and reaches a maximum value of $I_{CC} \times R_m$. Note that the duration of the membrane potential response (output) is extended in time compared to the duration of the current pulse (input).

charge is in the "upward" direction (i.e., from inside to outside the cell), then such a current is conventionally (although not always) designated as a "positive" current (left side of Figure 5B). Such a current will act to hyperpolarize the membrane (removing the positive charge from inside the cell will increase the net negative charge inside the membrane). Recall

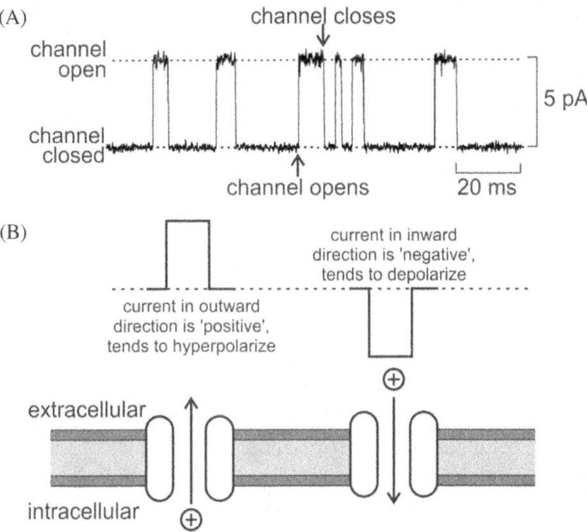

Figure 5.   (A) single ion channel current (recorded with a patch-clamp apparatus). When the channel opens, the current immediately reaches a new steady level; when the channel closes, the current instantaneously drops to zero. Small fluctuations in the signal represent electronic noise picked up by the recording system. (B) Current responses as depicted in panel A can be represented as rectangular pulses of current. Positive current indicates positive charges are exiting the cell, whereas negative current indicates positive charges enter the cell.

from Appendix A that the polarity of current (i.e., positive or negative) simply indicates the *direction* that positive charge flows. Consequently, when charges move in the opposite "downward" direction (from outside to inside the cell), then the polarity flips, and the current is indicated as negative (right side of Figure 5B). Somewhat confusingly, such a negative current will tend to depolarize the membrane (injecting more positive charge to the interior of the membrane).

Temporal Summation

One consequence of the passive electrical properties (like that shown in Figure 4) is that it affects the *efficacy by which synaptic inputs arriving at different times sum to produce an overall change in membrane potential*. This so-called **temporal summation** is highly dependent on the

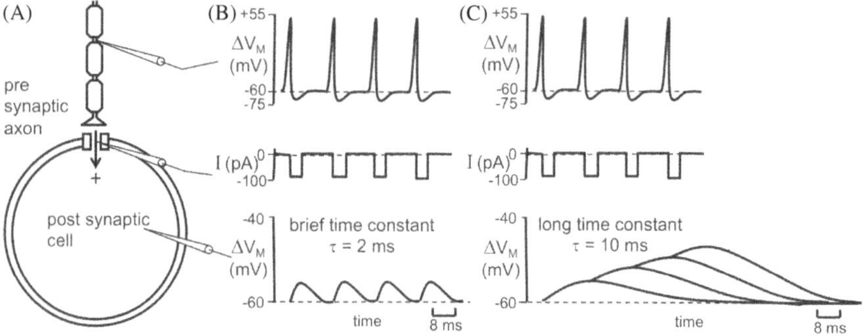

Figure 6.   Temporal summation of synaptic potentials. (A) Electrodes placed to record action potentials in presynaptic axon, ionic current through ligand-gated ion channels, and associated change in potential in postsynaptic cell. (B) Sequence of four action potentials in the presynaptic axon, leads to four inward (depolarizing) pulses of ionic current into the postsynaptic cell, which causes four brief changes in membrane potential in the cell with a brief time constant. (C) In a cell with a long time constant, the same inputs cause long-lasting changes in membrane potential, enabling individual responses to summate with preceding responses. This temporal summation helps drive the overall membrane potential in the depolarizing direction.

membrane time constant, τ, which by itself is determined by membrane capacitance and resistance. Because different types of neurons can possess substantial differences in membrane capacitance and resistance, the temporal summation capabilities can also vary widely across neurons. For example, the presynaptic neuron shown in Figure 6A delivers four action potentials in succession to its presynaptic terminal (Figure 6B, top trace). Each action potential causes the release of a small puff of neurotransmitter that then causes ligand-gated channels in the postsynaptic membrane to open briefly. In this case, these channels enable the flow of positive charge into the cell. As shown in Figure 6B (middle trace), a recording of the associated ionic current shows four brief negative (inward-going) pulses. In a cell with a very brief time constant (due to small capacitance, low resistance, or both), the change in membrane potential associated with each current pulse will also be brief (Figure 6B). As a consequence, the membrane potential returns to the resting potential before the next action potential arrives, and no temporal summation occurs.

On the other hand, if the same four pulses of ionic current are delivered to a cell with a long time constant (Figure 6C), then the change in membrane potential associated with each pulse will be prolonged. In this case, the change in membrane potential caused by one pulse will "stack" upon that of the preceding pulses. Such temporal summation effectively drives the membrane to a more depolarized level than could be accomplished by any pulse by itself. As we shall discuss in a later chapter, temporal summation is one of the key mechanisms by which the spike-initiating zone can be brought to threshold for generating an action potential.

Cable Model

As mentioned at the outset of this chapter, passive properties dictate how electrical signals are conveyed from one location to another in neurons. To understand how this occurs, let's begin by constructing an electrical model for a dendrite. Because dendrites do not have the high densities of voltage-gated channels found in axons, as a first approximation, they can be considered to operate largely as passive structures.

To build our model, we first must add a component to our model of a neuron segment. This is necessary because now we are interested in how electrical signals travel from one segment to the next. As shown in Figure 7A, this additional passive feature is *the resistance to current flow along the long axis of the interior of the segment*, the **axial resistance**. The interior of the segment is an electrolyte-filled cylinder and as such, operates much like a very thin wire. As described in Appendix A, the

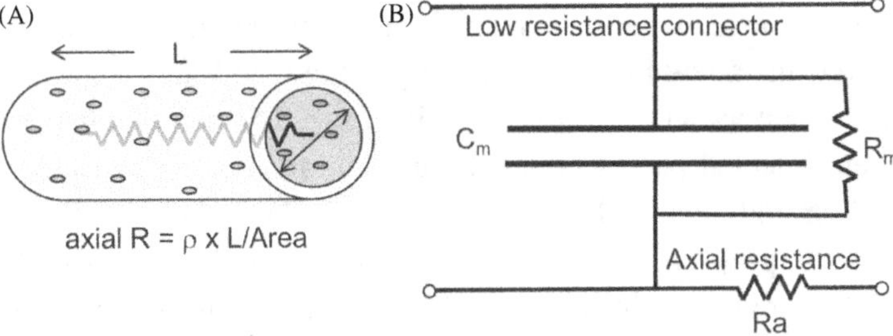

Figure 7.   (A) Small segment of neuron depicting resistor to represent resistance to current flow along the axis of the segment. (B) Incorporation of axial resistance into circuit representation of neuron segment. Cm — membrane capacitance, Rm — membrane resistance.

resistance of a cylinder, in this case, the axial resistance, R_a, is given by $R_a = \rho \times L/A$, where ρ is the resistivity (related to how well the material conducts electricity), L is the length of the segment, and A is the cross-sectional area. Because the diameter of a dendrite is tiny (a few micrometers), the cross-sectional area is very small. This means that the axial resistance is significant and cannot be neglected. Therefore, the neuron segment model now includes an additional resistor to represent the axial resistance (Figure 7B).

To create our electrical model of a dendrite, we simply link together several of the segment models together into a long chain called the cable model (Figure 8A; also see the frontispiece of this chapter for a more complex cable model for branching dendrites). A microelectrode, connected to a constant current device, is inserted into the leftmost dendritic segment. A second electrode also connected to the constant current device is placed in the extracellular fluid, thereby connecting it to the low-resistance wire of the segment models to complete the circuit. A key feature of the cable model is that it helps us to understand how current delivered at one site gets distributed to downstream locations.

When the switch is engaged, a steady level of current is injected into the first (leftmost) dendritic segment (Figure 8A). At the outset, that current has three different paths it can take: it can charge the membrane capacitance, it can pass through the leak channels (i.e., the membrane resistance) in that segment, or it can pass through the axial resistance into the next segment. The current that passes into the next segment can then follow the same three paths in its segment — charge capacitance, pass through the membrane resistance, or move along the axial resistance, and so on — down the line.

If one waits a few moments (namely, more than four time constants), then the capacitors will be close to fully charged. When that happens, all the current injected passes either through the membrane resistance or is delivered through the axial resistance (Figure 8B). In essence, the capacitors no longer play a role in dictating current flow and we can simplify the circuit by removing them (Figure 8C). We can now use the resulting circuit (Figure 8D) to estimate how much current there is in each branch of the circuit.

For example, let's assume that the constant current device in Figure 8D delivers 16 nA of current into the first segment (the length of

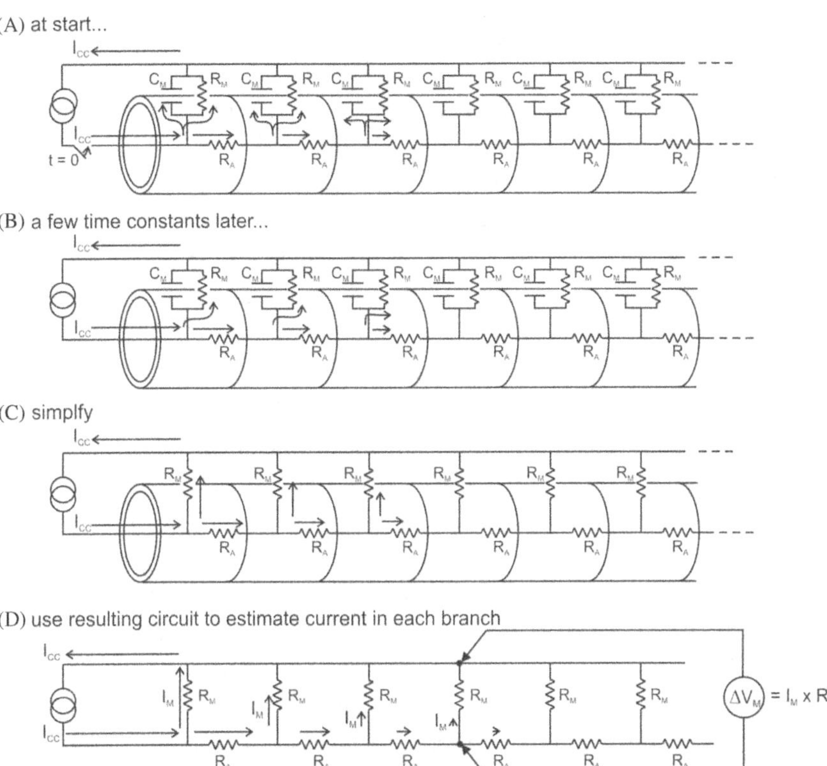

Figure 8.   Cable model. (A) Many segment-circuit models are linked together into a chain to represent the length of the dendrite. Injection of current, I_{CC}, via a constant current device at one location in the circuit. At the outset, that current gets distributed to the membrane capacitance, C_M, through the membrane resistance, R_M, and advanced along the axial resistance, R_A, into the next segment, and so on down the length of the circuit. (B) After approximately four time constants, the capacitances are fully charged. As such, no additional current flows toward them and all the current is directed to membrane and axial resistances. (C) As a consequence, we can then simplify the circuit to one that only possesses membrane and axial resistances. (D) If a steady level of current, I_{CC}, is injected into the circuit and if the $R_M \cong R_A$, then at the first node, approximately half of the current will leak out across the membrane through R_M, and the other half will be advanced to the next segment. That advanced current will then divide at the next node, where again half will exit through R_M and the other half will be advanced into the next segment. This process continues down the length of the dendrite until there is virtually no current left to advance. The membrane potential, ΔV_M, measured at any site along the length of the dendrite will be equivalent to the magnitude of the current exiting across the membrane, I_M, at that location times the membrane resistance, R_M.

the arrow is proportional to the amount of current). For simplicity, let's also assume that the membrane resistance is equal to the axial resistance. We know from one of our rules of thumb about current flow (Appendix A) that current tends to take the path of least resistance. If the two paths have equal resistance, then half of the current goes down one path and the other half goes down the second path. As such, the current would divide such that 8 nA goes out through the leak channels (R_m) in the first segment, and 8 nA gets carried along the axial resistance into the second segment.

The 8 nA that passes through the leak channels ends up in the extracellular fluid and is delivered back to the constant current device. The 8 nA that is delivered via the axial resistance into the next segment then splits into two equal halves: 4 nA exits through the leak channels and 4 nA passes down into the third segment. This process continues with the 4 nA splitting into two 2 nA components with the component that is advanced into the next segment splitting into two 1 nA components, and so on, until at some location, virtually no current remains to be advanced.

Recall from Figure 4A that the change in potential across the membrane at any location along the dendrite is equal to the product of the current passing through the membrane at that site (I_m) and the membrane resistance (R_m), namely, $\Delta V_m = I_m \times R_m$. Note that in Figure 8D, the membrane current, I_m, is cut in half for each segment advanced along the dendrite. Because the membrane resistance remains relatively constant from segment to segment, this means that the change in membrane potential also gets reduced by half from segment to segment. For example, Figure 8D shows the membrane potential being measured in the fourth segment with an I_m value of 1 nA. The membrane potential at this location would be only one-eighth that measured at the first segment with an I_m value of 8 nA.

Electrotonic Conduction

The fall in membrane potential with distance from the site of current injection is illustrated in Figure 9. In this figure, the membrane potential is measured simultaneously at different locations along the length of the

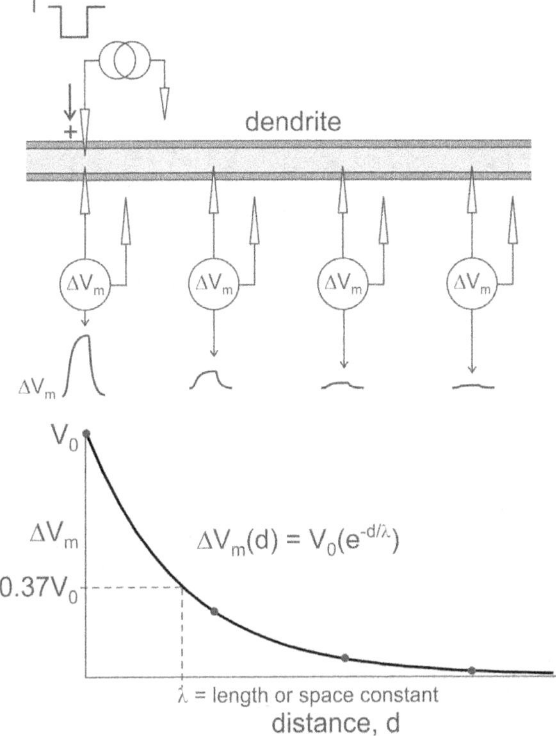

Figure 9.   Electrotonic conduction. (Top) Change in membrane potential, ΔV_m, measured at different locations along the length of dendrite in response to depolarizing current injected at one location. (Bottom) Peak membrane potential plotted as a function of distance, d, from the site of current injection. Decaying voltage response with distance characterized with an equation for a falling exponential. The length constant, τ, represents the distance from the site of injection where membrane potential drops to a value 37% of that detected at the site of injection, V_0.

dendrite in response to a pulse of depolarizing current delivered at one end. If we plot the peak voltage detected at each location as a function of the distance from the site of current injection, we obtain a falling exponential function. This exponential decay is just like that described in the Appendix and in Figures 2F and 3D of this chapter except that it is a function of *distance* rather than *time*. As such, the distance away from the site of current injection at which the membrane potential drops to 37% of the initial value (i.e., $0.37V_0$) is referred to as the *length* or *space* constant, λ. The function describing this decay is given by:

$$\Delta V_M(d) = V_0 \cdot e^{-d/\lambda}$$

where V_0 is the value of the membrane potential detected at the site of current injection and d is the distance from the site of current injection.

What is important to recognize is that this rather inefficient means of delivering electrical signals from one location to another is the main mechanism by which information gets transferred within neurons. This *passive means of conveying electrical signals is referred to as* **electrotonic conduction**. For example, an action potential arriving at a presynaptic terminal will lead to an ionic current pulse delivered into the postsynaptic dendrite (Figure 10). This current pulse will cause a localized change in the membrane potential detected with an intracellular electrode (trace on left side of Figure 10). Some of that injected current

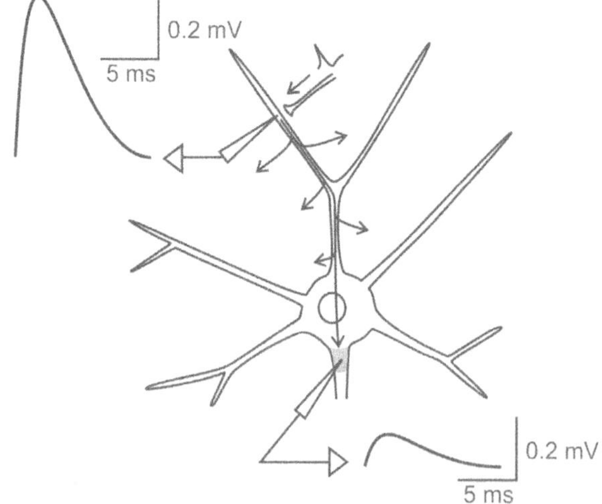

Figure 10.   Electrotonic conduction from synapse on dendrite to spike-initiating zone. Microelectrode inserted into a dendrite will detect a change in the membrane potential associated with the ionic current delivered by a nearby active synapse. That ionic current advances electrotonically, with some of the current exiting through leak channels, leaving a fraction remaining at the spike-initiating zone, where it is detected as a small change in membrane potential.

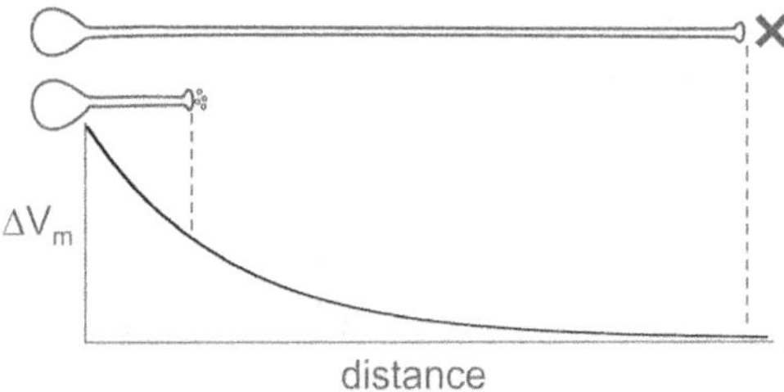

Figure 11.   Electrotonic conduction is sufficient to trigger neurotransmitter release from a short axon but not from a long axon.

leaks out across the membrane and some gets advanced along the dendrite. At the spike-initiating zone, the amount of current crossing the membrane and the associated change in potential will be substantially smaller than that at the synaptic input site.

Not only do dendrites rely on electrotonic conduction for signaling to the spike-initiating zone but some neurons only use electrotonic conduction to send signals along the axon (Figure 11). Such neurons (lower neuron, Figure 11) have short axons. Therefore, there is sufficient depolarization at the presynaptic terminal to provoke the release of neurotransmitters. However, for most neurons with longer axons, the electrotonic signal would largely dissipate before arriving at the presynaptic terminal and therefore, would not be capable of triggering neurotransmitter release. Because of this, neurons evolved the ability to produce action potentials in order to send robust electrical signals over large distances. Nevertheless, as we shall see, even the delivery of action potentials relies heavily on electrotonic conduction.

Factors Affecting the Length Constant

The efficacy by which dendrites and axons deliver electrical signals is highly dependent on the electrotonic length constant. The larger the length constant, the farther the signal will travel before dropping to 37% of the initial value. But what factors determine the value of the length constant? To understand this, let's go back to the cable model (Figure 8D). In general, a longer length constant will occur when little of the current leaks out across the membrane resistance and more gets delivered downstream along the axial resistance. As such, and keeping in mind the rule of thumb that current tends to follow the path of least resistance, there are two main ways to increase the length constant: *increase* the membrane resistance R_m or *decrease* the axial resistance R_a.

Biologically, this can be accomplished in different ways. For example, one way to significantly increase the effective membrane resistance in axons is to add myelin. Myelin contains a great deal of lipid, which is a good insulator. Therefore, when an axon possesses myelin, it is as though the leak channels are covered by an insulator, which greatly increases the membrane resistance. As such, most of the current delivered into a myelin-coated segment is advanced forward (along the intracellular electrolyte "wire" — the axial resistance) with only a modest amount of current leaking out of the membrane.

Another biological strategy to increase the length constant is to decrease the axial resistance by increasing the diameter of the axon or dendrite. Indeed, as we shall see later, neurons possess a wide range of axon diameters. Neurons with large-diameter axons conduct signals more effectively than those with small-diameter axons. Figure 12 shows the electrotonic conduction profiles for a thin axon without myelin, a thick axon without myelin, and a thick axon with myelin. Quantitatively, the length constant λ can be estimated as:

$$\lambda = \sqrt{\frac{\rho_m}{R_a}}$$

where ρ_m is the resistivity of the membrane (units $\Omega \cdot m$) and R_a is the axial resistance normalized to the length of the resistor (units Ω/m). From this

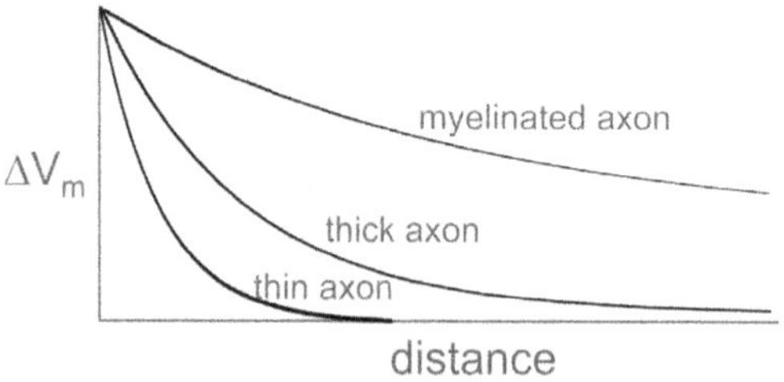

Figure 12.   Electrotonic conduction profiles for a thin, unmyelinated axon, for a thicker, unmyelinated axon, and a thick myelinated axon.

equation, we can see that axons (or dendrites) with higher membrane resistances have longer length constants whereas neurons that have higher axial resistances (narrower diameters) have shorter length constants. Also, note that the units for λ reduce to meters (m) as it should for a length measurement.

Conduction of Action Potentials in Myelinated Axons

To understand how action potentials travel along axons, we need to combine the concepts of electrotonic conduction and threshold for opening voltage-gated Na^+ channels. To do this, let's track the change in membrane potential detected with an array of voltmeters inserted at multiple locations along the length of a myelinated axon (Figure 13). Think of these voltmeters as little thermometers that detect the maximum "temperature" (i.e., the maximum membrane potential) at each location. In a myelinated axon, the only locations where there is a high enough density of voltage-gated Na^+ channels (shown as little black dots in the image of the neuron in Figure 13) to produce an action potential are at the nodes of Ranvier.

If the collective action of the synaptic inputs on the dendrites (left side of membrane potential–distance plot, Figure 13), conveyed by electrotonic conduction is large enough to just exceed the threshold at the spike-initiating zone, then an action potential is ignited and a large number of voltage-gated Na^+ channels open in the initial segment. This will cause a massive influx of Na^+ ions, driving the membrane toward the equilibrium potential of Na^+ (+55 mV). This rapid influx of Na^+ ions acts like an injection of depolarizing current into the axon at the initial segment. That current then *passively* (electrotonically) spreads down the length of the axon. Because of the myelin coating (providing a high membrane resistance), most of the current advances forward but some nevertheless leak out across the membrane. This causes the detected membrane potential to fall exponentially with distance but with a relatively long length constant.

Before the membrane potential associated with this electrotonically advanced signal falls below the threshold level, there is a break in the myelin where a high density of voltage-gated Na^+ channels are embedded in the membrane at the node of Ranvier. This means that an action potential now gets instigated at this node of Ranvier, actively boosting the membrane potential back up to around +55 mV. The influx of ionic

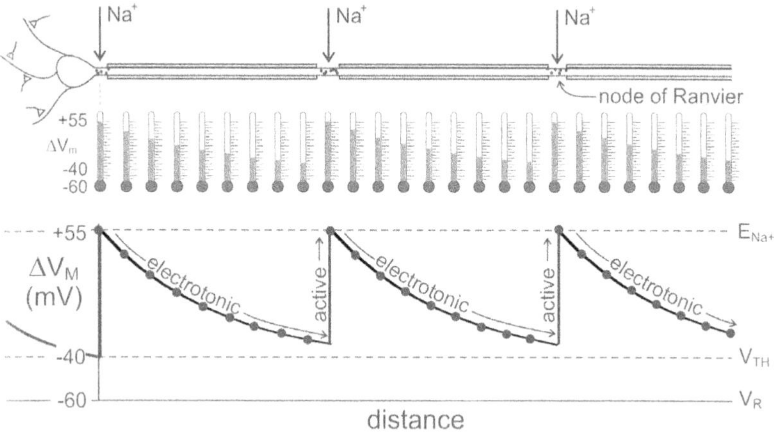

Figure 13.   Conduction of electrical signals in a myelinated axon. Synaptic inputs on dendrites conducted electrotonically toward the spike-initiating zone (left side of membrane potential vs. distance graph at bottom). If that signal is large enough to exceed the threshold (V_{TH}), then activation of voltage-gated Na⁺ channels (small black dots in the axon) associated with an action potential at the first segment of the axon will drive the membrane potential toward the equilibrium potential for Na (E_{Na}^+). The image of thermometers represents the maximum membrane potential measured at each location (shown as large dots on the membrane potential–distance graph). The influx of Na⁺ current at the initial segment is advanced electrotonically. Despite the decay in voltage with distance, there is sufficient membrane potential at the next node of Ranvier to exceed the threshold and to ignite an action potential at that location. This process continues unabated down the entire length of the axon. The spatial profile of conduction can be thought of as an active boost of membrane potential at each node of Ranvier followed by a diminishing electrotonic glide toward the next node of Ranvier.

current then again gets electrotonically conveyed forward to the next node of Ranvier where the next action potential gets activated. This process then continues down the entire length of the axon to the presynaptic terminals.

It is important to note that action potentials only occur at the nodes of Ranvier. Most of the distance that the signal travels along the axon is mediated entirely by passive (electrotonic) conduction. As such, in myelinated axons, the profile of the membrane potential as a function of distance (Figure 13) has a repeating sawtooth form. This type of conduction is sometimes referred to as **saltatory** ("jumping") conduction. While such a term has historical precedent, it may be conceptually more useful to think of this conduction as *"boost and glide,"* namely, an active boost of the membrane potential at the nodes of Ranvier followed by a passive glide of the signal forward to the next node of Ranvier.

Conduction of Action Potentials in Unmyelinated Axons

There are many important types of neurons with thin axons that possess no myelin. As shown in Figure 12, these axons have relatively small length constants and conduct signals somewhat inefficiently. As we shall see directly, the profile of membrane potential as a function of distance in unmyelinated axons is markedly different than that of myelinated axons.

The top part of Figure 14A shows an image of an unmyelinated axon. Voltage-gated Na^+ channels are distributed along the entire length of the axon. Now, if the collective action of synaptic inputs, electrotonically conducted to the spike-initiating zone, is sufficient to exceed the threshold (left side of Figure 14A), an action potential will be instigated at this location. The associated influx of Na^+ ions is then electrotonically conveyed forward along the axon (lower part, Figure 14A). Because of the short length constant associated with a leaky membrane (i.e., one with a low membrane resistance), the membrane potential decays steeply with distance. Indeed, only up through a relatively short distance d will the membrane potential exceed the threshold. This distance d is directly related to the length constant.

In the next time step, voltage-gated Na^+ channels will open up only through this distance d (Figure 14B). The associated influx of Na^+ ions will boost the membrane potential up toward E_{Na}^+ along this stretch of axon from the otherwise decaying membrane potential signal (dashed curve, Figure 14B). The most forward location that generated an action potential along this stretch of axon and within this time segment will advance its ionic current electrotonically. This will be associated with a decaying membrane potential forward of this location. In the next time step, the process repeats (Figure 14C) with action potentials now produced along the next d — length of axon segment. This continues along the entire length of the axon. When complete, the maximum membrane potential ("temperature") detected will have reached ~+55 mV at every

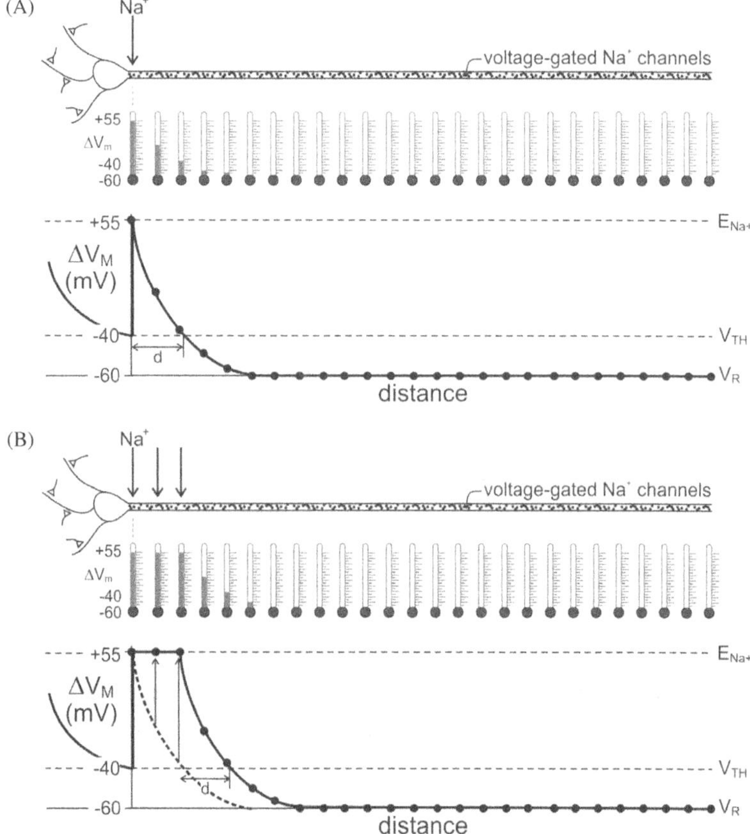

Figure 14.   Conduction of electrical signals in an unmyelinated axon. The layout is the same as in Figure 13. (A) Synaptic inputs are just sufficient to bring the initial segment to the threshold. The Na$^+$ influx associated with an action potential at that location drives the membrane potential to near $E_{Na}{}^+$. That ionic current is advanced electrotonically down the axon. Because of the low membrane resistance in the absence of myelin, the length constant is short. As such, only a short span of the axon, d, will be brought above the threshold in the next time instant. (B) Influx of Na$^+$ associated with action potentials instigated along the region of the axon brought above threshold in panel A. This boosts the membrane potential toward $E_{Na}{}^+$. The ionic current is advanced electrotonically forward such that up through another distance d, the membrane will be brought above the threshold in the next time instant. (C) The process shown in (B) is repeated for the next region of the axon. This continues down the entire length of the axon such that the membrane potential at every site along the axon attains a value near E_{Na}.

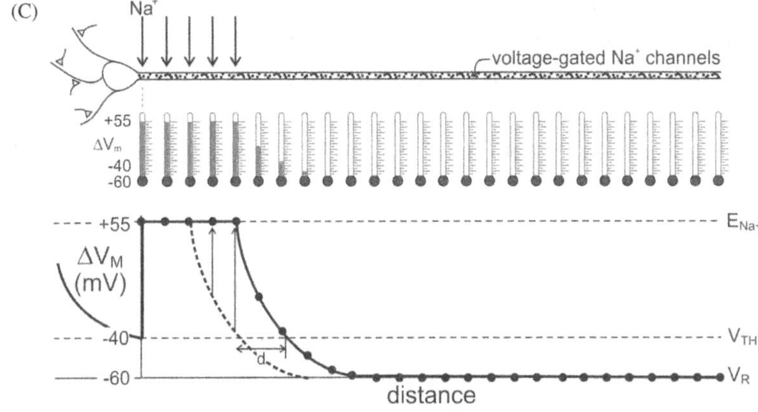

Figure 14.   (*Continued*)

location. As such, the profile of membrane potential versus distance will be a flat line at +55 mV over the entire length of the axon — markedly different than the sawtooth form for a myelinated axon (Figure 13).

Conduction Velocity

The conduction of an action potential along an unmyelinated axon is analogous to a flame traveling along a long fuse of a firecracker. If the heat applied at one end is above the threshold for igniting the combustible material of the fuse, then the fuse flames at that location, driving the temperature to a high value. That high temperature associated with the flame will radiate away from the flame in a decaying fashion. Nevertheless, the temperature in a small region just forward of the flame will be hot enough to exceed the ignition threshold and it will then combust. This process will continue along the entire length of the fuse moving at a more or less constant speed, with every region successively reaching the high temperature associated with the flame. In a myelinated axon, the "flame" only occurs at the nodes of Ranvier.

The speed at which an action potentials travels along an axon depends on two key factors. One has to do with *how far forward* an action potential at a given instant can drive the membrane potential above the threshold (e.g., the distance d in Figure 14A). And two, the *time delay*, t_d, associated with raising the membrane to threshold in response to the injection of ionic current associated with the action potential (like the delay in the rise of membrane potential shown in Figure 4B). As such, one can write an expression for the conduction velocity (CV) of an action potential along an axon simply as:

$$CV = d/t_d.$$

The distance d is directly related to the *length constant*, λ. As discussed earlier, unmyelinated axons have small length constants whereas large-diameter myelinated axons have long length constants. Therefore, the conduction velocity of myelinated axons will be higher than in unmyelinated axons.

The time delay, t_d, is related to the *time constant* of the membrane, τ. As shown in Figure 4B, the increase in membrane potential in response to a pulse of depolarizing current rises gradually, dictated by the time constant. We know that the time constant is given by $\tau = R_m \times C_m$ where R_m is the membrane resistance and C_m is the membrane capacitance. If the value of τ gets larger, then t_d would also get larger, which in turn would be associated with a *slowing* of conduction velocity. At first glance then, it may seem as though we have a paradox: myelin *increases* R_m, which should increase τ, thereby increasing t_d, and leads to a slowing in conduction velocity. However, myelin even more greatly *reduces* the membrane capacitance. From Appendix A (see Figure 25 in Appendix A), we know that capacitance is *inversely* proportional to the thickness of the insulator separating the two conductive sheets. In the case of a myelinated axon, the insulator thickness includes both the axon membrane and the wide myelin sheath, whereas in unmyelinated axons, the insulator thickness is just that provided by the thin lipid bilayer of the axon membrane. Indeed, the insulator thickness provided by myelin can be 100 times greater than that of just the axon membrane alone. This gives rise to a very small value of C_m in myelinated axons, which in turn yields a briefer time constant in myelinated axons as compared to unmyelinated axons. Collectively, the larger length constant (yielding a larger value of d) and the smaller time constant (yielding a smaller value of t_d) in myelinated axons means that they conduct action potentials much faster than unmyelinated axons, indeed in some cases, more than 100 times faster.

Failure of Conduction In Demyelinating Diseases

There are a variety of neurological disorders in which the myelin surrounding axons degenerates. The most common of these diseases is **multiple sclerosis (MS)**. In MS, *myelin degenerates in localized patches of white matter (axon tracts) within the* **central nervous system (CNS)**. These regions of demyelination (also called lesions) can occur in a variety of regions of the brain and spinal cord and can be visualized using magnetic resonance imaging (Figure 15). While the specific cause of MS is unknown, it appears to be an autoimmune disease in which the immune system attacks and destroys myelin produced by oligodendrocytes. Depending on the sites of the lesions, MS can lead to a host of impairments, including visual problems, numbness, weakness and fatigue, bladder and bowel dysfunction, and cognitive deficits. Unfortunately, there is no cure for MS.

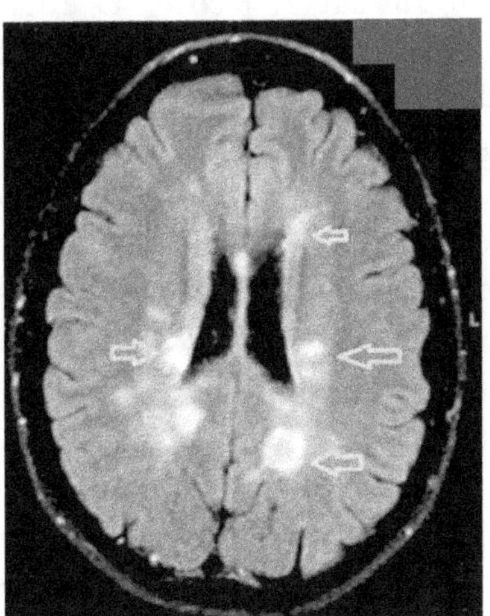

Figure 15.   Magnetic resonance image of the brain showing numerous lesions (white areas, arrows) in a patient with MS.

Source: www.mslivingwell.org

But why does removal of myelin from small stretches of axons lead to such devastating consequences? To understand why, let's reexamine conduction of an action potential along a myelinated axon with myelin removed from a segment of the axon (Figure 16A). An action potential instigated at the spike-initiating zone will propagate along the axon, with a boost and electrotonic glide profile. When the signal arrives at the node of Ranvier on the segment that has lost its myelin, voltage-gated Na^+ channels will still open to boost the membrane potential to a value close to the equilibrium potential for Na^+(Figure 16A). However, the Na^+ current that enters at that location will be advanced electrotonically with a relatively short length constant. This is because the denuded section of the axon still possesses ample leak channels but few voltage-gated Na^+ channels. As a consequence, the membrane resistance is low and much of the current exits through the leak channels. This means that the membrane potential at the next node of Ranvier will be below the threshold for activating voltage-gated Na^+channels. Consequently, signaling will halt at that point. As such, demyelination can completely disable action potential propagation in the affected neurons.

Interestingly, many patients with MS undergo periods of remission during which function can largely recover. One mechanism thought to underlie remission is the upregulation and expression of voltage-gated Na^+ channels along the demyelinated regions of the axon (Waxman 2006) (Figure 16B). The axon then becomes like a hybrid of myelinated and unmyelinated axons. In the unmyelinated sections, action potential conduction is slower and has the flat spatial profile like discussed for unmyelinated axons in Figure 14. This enables conducted signals to bridge the unmyelinated sections and restore conduction of action potentials along the entire length of the axon.

Summary

To understand how electrical signals are conveyed in dendrites and axons, we constructed a simple circuit that represents the electrical properties of a small segment of a neuron. The circuit consisted of membrane resistance (representing leak channels in the membrane), membrane capacitance

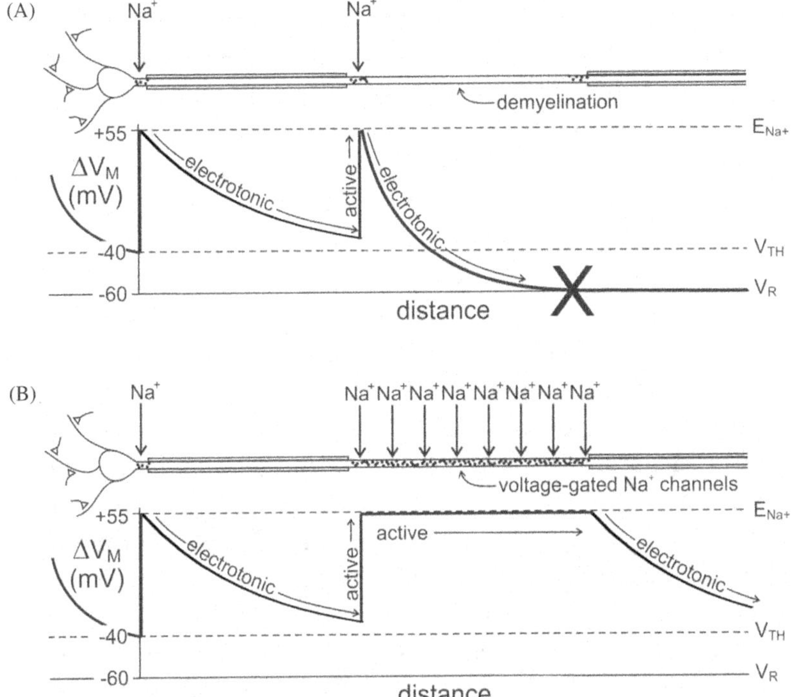

Figure 16.   (A) Arrest of signal conduction in demyelinating disease such as MS. Layout as in Figures 12 and 13. When an action potential is initiated at a node of Ranvier immediately adjacent to the axon segment that has lost its myelin, the subsequent electrotonic conduction diminishes sharply with distance due to the relatively low membrane resistance. As such, the magnitude of depolarization at the next node of Ranvier (the only site with significant density of voltage-gated Na$^+$ channels) is below the threshold. This prevents the signal from being advanced farther down the axon. (B) Potential mechanism underlying remission of symptoms in MS. Voltage-gated Na$^+$ channels eventually populate denuded stretches of the axon. These regions now function like unmyelinated axons to bridge signal conduction across demyelinated segments of the axon, and thereby restore signaling.

(representing the lipid bilayer sandwiched between conductive, electrolyte layers), axial resistance (representing the resistance along the length of the electrolyte interior of dendrites or axons), and a low-resistance connector (representing the extracellular fluid). We used this circuit to show that a brief pulse of current into a neuron is transformed into a change in membrane potential that is extended in time compared to the duration of the current pulse. Such elongation of the voltage response helps facilitate temporal summation of synaptic inputs at the spike-initiating zone.

When many segment circuits were linked together in a chain, we obtained a model (the cable model) that revealed how electrical signals are conveyed passively from one location to another. The main feature of such electrotonic signaling is that the strength of the signal diminishes exponentially with distance. The extent of signal decay can be lessened by increasing membrane resistance (e.g., with myelin) or decreasing axial resistance (e.g., by having larger axon or dendrite diameters). And while electrotonic signaling may be sufficient over short distances (e.g., in dendrites or very short axons), it is ineffective, by itself, for signaling in most axons. As such, typical axons have high densities of voltage-gated Na^+ channels embedded in the axon membrane to produce action potentials to boost otherwise decaying electrotonic signals. In unmyelinated axons, these channels are distributed along the entire length of the axon. In myelinated axons, these channels are clustered at the nodes of Ranvier between regions of the axon enveloped in myelin. Despite the importance of the action potential, electrotonic conduction is still largely responsible for advancing electrical signals down the axon. In demyelinating diseases, loss of myelin shortens the effective distance signals that can be conveyed electrotonically. Therefore, the depolarizing signal may be too weak to activate voltage-gated Na^+ channels at downstream nodes of Ranvier, which halts signal conduction and interrupts signal processing in the CNS.

References

Kandel ER, Schwartz JH, Jessell TM, Siegelbaum SA & Hudspeth AJ (2012). Principles of Neural Science (5th Edition), McGraw-Hill.

Segev I, Fleshman JW & Burke RE (1992). Compartment models of complex neurons. In: Koch C & Segev I (eds.), Methods in Neuronal Modeling, MIT Press.

Waxman SG (2006). Axonal conduction and injury in multiple sclerosis: the role of sodium channels. *Nature Reviews Neuroscience* 7, 932–941.

Chapter 6

Synaptic Transmission

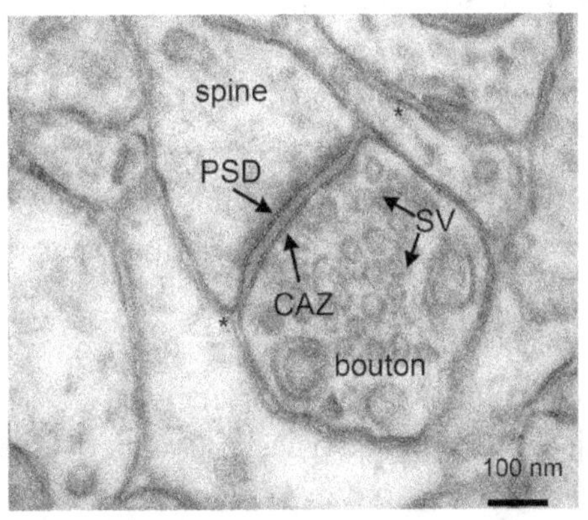

Electron micrograph in rat cerebral cortex showing the presynaptic terminal (bouton) possessing numerous synaptic vesicles (SV) and cytomatrix of the active zone (CAZ). The membrane of the dendritic spine on the postsynaptic neuron shows a darkened region (the postsynaptic density [PSD]) containing postsynaptic receptors. (With permission, from Dieterich & Kreutz [2016].)

As discussed in Chapter 1, it was not until well into the 20th century that Cajal's idea that neurons are distinct entities was fully accepted. Part of the reason for this was that until the advent of the electron microscope in the 1950s, microscopes did not have the resolution to discern the physical separation between neurons at synapses. Charles Sherrington, a British scientist (and Nobel Prize winner) working during the early part of the 20th century, used neurophysiological methods, such as electrically stimulating nerves and measuring the evoked responses in muscles, to understand the basic operations of the nervous system. Based on his observations and appreciation of Cajal's ideas, Sherrington proposed that at the site of contact between neurons (or between neurons and muscle fibers), there must exist a *specialized structure that he likened to a one-way valve that allows unidirectional conduction from one neuron to another.* Sherrington called this entity a "**synapse**" from the Greek word for clasp.

Just as two hands are needed to form a clasp or handshake, two components are needed to form a synapse (Figure 1). The "sender" of the information is the presynaptic terminal and the "receiver" is the postsynaptic receptors embedded in the membrane of the target cell. Sherrington also proposed that synapses come in two main types: **excitatory**—*that tend to activate the postsynaptic cell*—and **inhibitory**—*that tend to suppress activity in the postsynaptic cell.*

Throughout the first half of the 20th century, there was substantial debate over the mechanisms by which the presynaptic neuron delivers signals to postsynaptic cells. One idea was that electrical signals in the presynaptic neuron directly induce electrical signals in the postsynaptic cell. The other idea was that the presynaptic neuron releases a chemical that influences the activity of the postsynaptic cell. The first definitive evidence of chemical signaling at synapses was provided by the Viennese scientist Otto Loewi, for which he won the Nobel Prize. He excised two hearts from frogs and kept them alive by placing them in two separate chambers of physiological solution. Because of intrinsic pacemaker cells, the hearts continued to beat while maintained in the solution. He then electrically stimulated the vagus nerve supplying one of the hearts. This stimulation caused the strength of cardiac contractions to diminish and the

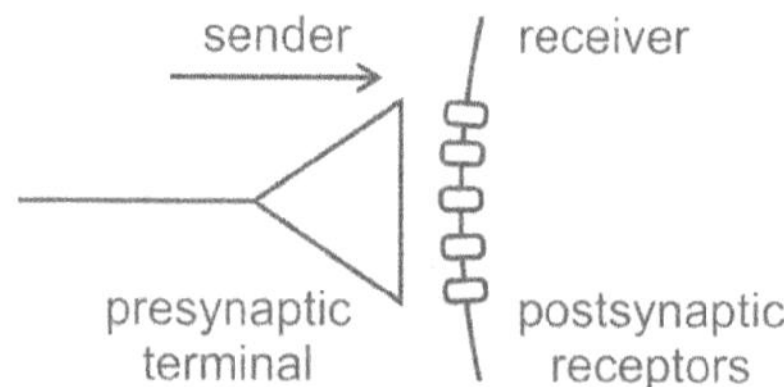

Figure 1.   A synapse has two parts: a presynaptic terminal that sends information and receptors that receive the information on the postsynaptic cell.

beating to slow. He then transferred some of the solution surrounding the heart whose nerve he had just stimulated into the chamber containing the other heart. That heart then also slowed its beating. The only logical interpretation of this elegant experiment was that stimulating the nerve had caused the release of a substance, some of which spilled out into the bathing solution, and when transferred to the other chamber, led to the inhibition of the heart activity. Loewi simply called the unknown substance "Vagusstoff." Later, it was determined to be acetylcholine (Ach), the first identified neurotransmitter. Eventually, it was established that most synapses use chemical transmission.

Beyond the fundamental importance of Loewi's discovery, his finding also highlights another important principle. In Loewi's experiment involving the vagus nerve, the release of Ach was associated with the *inhibition* of the heart. However, the release of Ach at the neuromuscular junction (NMJ) is known to cause *excitation* of skeletal muscle. Therefore, it is not the neurotransmitter itself that determines whether a synapse is excitatory or inhibitory but the characteristics of the receptors on the postsynaptic cell. In the heart, Ach binds to muscarinic receptors, which leads to the gating of K^+ channels, whereas in the skeletal muscle, Ach binds to nicotinic receptors on ligand-gated channels that increase the permeability to Na^+. The terms muscarinic and nicotinic are derived from the specific exogenous agonists (muscarine and nicotine) whose actions mimic those of Ach at those two sites.

Neurotransmitter Release

Once it was accepted that most synapses use chemical neurotransmission, attention turned to the question as to how the entry of an action potential (AP) into the presynaptic terminal provokes the release of a neurotransmitter. The basic mechanisms by which this occurs were largely revealed through investigations led by Bernard Katz (Figure 2), who won the Nobel Prize in 1970. Katz and his colleagues studied synaptic transmission at the NMJ—the synapse between a motor neuron and a muscle fiber. They selected this synapse because it was relatively easy to study: muscle fibers are reasonably large and a microelectrode can be readily inserted into them to record changes in membrane potential associated with synaptic

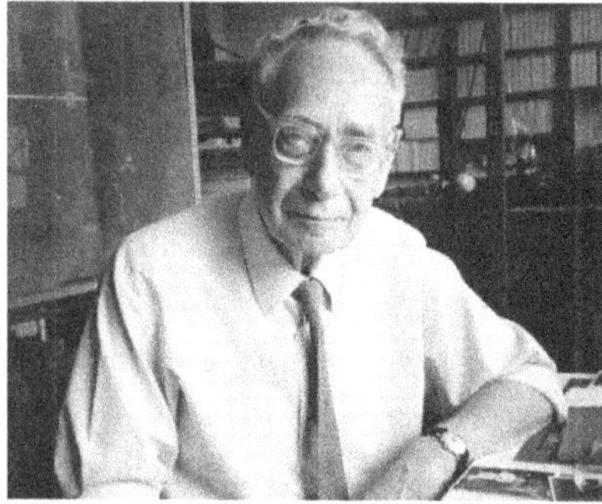

Figure 2.   Sir Bernard Katz, the 1970 Nobel Prize winner for discoveries related to synaptic transmission.

transmission. In addition, the synapse can be visualized with a regular light microscope, and importantly, muscle fibers only receive a single synaptic contact (compared to thousands on typical neurons).

Previous work had led Katz to believe that Ca^{2+} ions might be important in this process. To test this idea, Katz dissected a muscle and its motor nerve and placed them into a bathing solution containing no Ca^{2+}. Katz then stimulated the motor nerve to initiate an AP and recorded the associated change in membrane potential inside a muscle fiber (Figure 3). This was done with a microelectrode inserted into the muscle fiber near the end-plate zone, a small depression in the muscle fiber immediately opposite the presynaptic terminals. Changes in membrane potential at this location were referred to as end-plate potentials (EPPs). As shown in Figure 3A, no EPP was detected in response to the AP entering the presynaptic terminal in the zero $[Ca^{2+}]$ solution. This meant that the large depolarization associated with an AP entering the presynaptic terminal was not sufficient, by itself, to trigger a synaptic transmission. Katz next simply spritzed a high $[Ca^{2+}]$ solution from a micropipette positioned near the NMJ (Figure 3B). Again, no change in membrane potential was detected in the muscle fiber. That meant that Ca^{2+} ions alone were not sufficient to trigger the release of neurotransmitters needed for synaptic transmission. Lastly, Katz spritzed the Ca^{2+} solution near the NMJ immediately prior to stimulating the nerve (Figure 3C). In this case, a robust EPP was measured. The most logical interpretation of these results was that the large depolarization provided by the AP entering the presynaptic

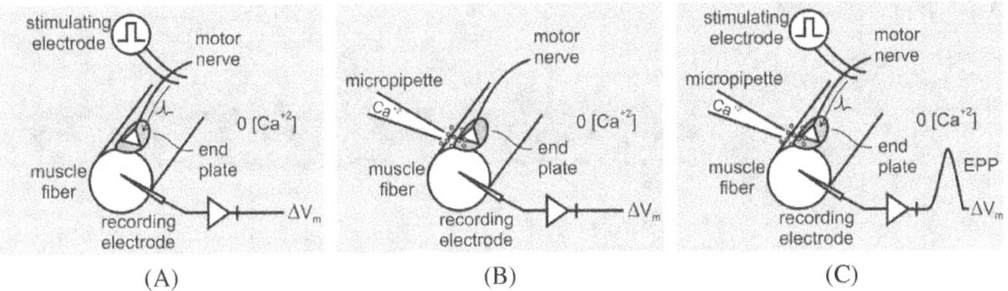

Figure 3.   Katz's demonstration of the importance of Ca^{2+} in mediating the release of neurotransmitters at the NMJ. Muscle fiber and motor nerve were dissected and placed in a bathing solution with no Ca^{2+}. (A) Stimulating the nerve to initiate an AP caused no detectable change in membrane potential (ΔV_m) in the muscle fiber. The vertical tick mark in the ΔV_m record indicates the time at which the nerve was stimulated. (B) Puffing a high $[Ca^{2+}]$ solution onto the NMJ with a micropipette also caused no measurable change in the membrane potential. (C) Stimulating the nerve immediately after a high $[Ca^{2+}]$ solution had been puffed near the NMJ caused a large change in membrane potential in the muscle fiber. This change in membrane potential is referred to as an EPP.

terminal activated voltage-gated Ca^{2+} channels in the terminal. Because of the extremely high concentration gradient for Ca^{2+}, opening these channels caused a brief strong influx of Ca^{2+} into the presynaptic terminal, which in turn, triggered the release of neurotransmitters. Eventually, it was later discovered that Ca^{2+} entry into the presynaptic terminal is indeed the trigger for neurotransmitter release at virtually all chemical synapses.

Quantal Release

Another question tackled by Katz relates to the nature by which a neurotransmitter is expelled from the presynaptic terminal. An important clue was revealed by chance when Katz and colleagues noticed small changes in the membrane potential in a muscle fiber when they were *not* stimulating the nerve. These responses appeared to occur randomly, and they tended to always be about the same magnitude (Figure 4A). They referred to these as *spontaneous miniature EPPs* (mini EPPs). To understand better the significance of these events, Katz and colleagues then bathed the nerve–muscle preparation in a solution containing very low concentration of Ca^{2+}. The reason for this is that under normal concentrations of Ca^{2+},

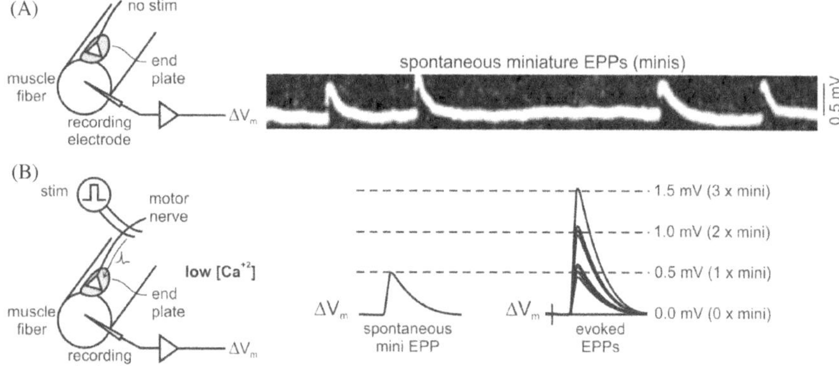

Figure 4.   Discovery of quantal transmission. (A) When not stimulating the nerve but while recording from the end-plate zone of a muscle fiber, small, spontaneously occurring changes in membrane potential (EPPs) were recorded that all tended to have about the same amplitude. (B) In a low [Ca^{2+}] bathing solution, repeatedly stimulating the motor nerve evoked small EPPs, after a small delay. These responses had amplitudes that varied randomly but were more or less integer multiples of the spontaneous miniature EPPs. These findings led Katz and colleagues to conclude that neurotransmitters are released in fixed packets called quanta. (Tracing in [A] adapted from Fatt and Katz [1952].)

activation of the nerve causes a huge EPP (~50 to 70 mV depolarization) that invariably triggers an AP in the muscle fiber. Therefore, to isolate the changes in membrane potential due to synaptic transmission from those associated with the AP, a low Ca^{2+} solution reduces the magnitude of the EPP below the threshold for activating voltage-gated Na^+ channels (and APs) in the muscle fiber.

Under these conditions, when the nerve was stimulated (Figure 4B), oftentimes the response to stimulation, and after a small delay, was an EPP with an amplitude nearly identical to that of a spontaneous miniature EPP, that is, about 0.5 mV. In other trials, the response was sometimes larger, about 1.0 mV. More rarely, the evoked response was about 1.5 mV. And on some occasions when stimulating the nerve, no response was detected. These different magnitudes of responses occurred more or less in random order. When all the responses were superimposed onto one another (Figure 4B), one could see that the amplitudes of the evoked EPPs were integer multiples of that of the spontaneous miniature EPP. This led Katz to correctly propose that *neurotransmitters are released in fixed*

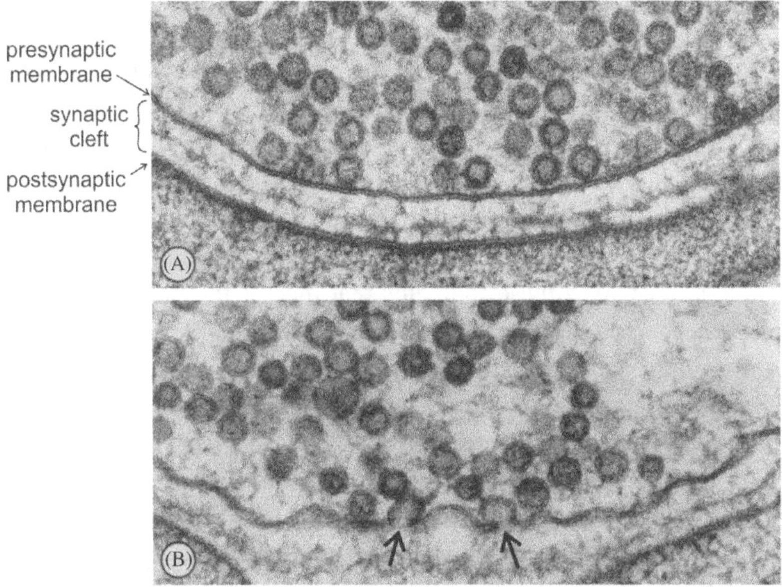

Figure 5.   (A) Electron micrograph of unstimulated frog NMJ. Circular bodies near the presynaptic membrane are vesicles filled with the neurotransmitter, Ach. (B) Upon stimulation, some of the vesicles merge with the presynaptic membrane (see Ω-shaped profiles in presynaptic membrane, arrows) to release their contents into the synaptic cleft. Vesicles are the physical basis of quantal transmission. (Adapted from Heuser and Reese [1981].)

packets, which he called "**quanta**" with enough neurotransmitter in each quantum to cause about a 0.5 mV change in membrane potential. As such, when an AP arrived in the presynaptic terminal, and under low [Ca^{2+}] conditions, it was as though a dice was rolled and either one, two, or three (or no) quanta were released.

Later, the physical basis of quanta was revealed with the use of electron microscopy. As shown in Figure 5A, the presynaptic terminal contains small spherical bodies (~40 nm in diameter) known as vesicles. The vesicles are containers filled with neurotransmitters. Upon stimulation of the presynaptic terminal, some of the vesicles that are already sitting in close proximity to the presynaptic membrane merge with the membrane (arrows, Figure 5B) to release their contents into the small *extracellular space* (the **synaptic cleft**) *separating the pre- and postsynaptic membranes at the synapse.*

Exocytosis

The mechanisms by which Ca^{2+} entry into the presynaptic terminal induces vesicles to disgorge their neurotransmitter contents into the synaptic cleft are complex. In brief, protein filaments in the presynaptic membrane latch onto vesicles situated close to the membrane. The Ca^{2+} that enters into the presynaptic terminal through voltage-gated Ca^{2+} channels binds to sites on these filaments. Ca^{2+} binding then drives a conformational change in these filaments that merges the membranes of the vesicle and the presynaptic terminal and then pulls the fused membrane apart forming a pore into the extracellular space. The contents of the vesicle are then expelled into the synaptic cleft. The set of *molecular mechanisms by which synaptic vesicles release their neurotransmitter contents into the synaptic cleft* is referred to as **exocytosis**.

One mystery that has not been entirely resolved is the functional significance, if any, of the spontaneous release of quanta (as shown in Figure 4A). Such unprovoked and sporadic release of neurotransmitters seems to be a feature of many types of synapses, not just the NMJ. One possibility is that such spontaneous release provides a chemical signal to maintain the clustering and localization of postsynaptic ligand-gated receptors in the neighborhood of the presynaptic terminal. Indeed, artificially blocking synaptic transmission can lead to the dispersal of receptors away from the synaptic zone within a period of hours (Akaaboune *et al.* 1999).

Quantitative Aspects of Synaptic Transmission

Another fundamental question about synaptic transmission is how many postsynaptic receptors are activated by the release of a quantum of neurotransmitter? This question can be addressed through the use of patch-clamp methods to calculate the approximate change in membrane potential (from the resting potential) caused by the opening of one ligand-gated channel at an excitatory synapse. These estimates reveal a figure of about 0.25×10^{-3} mV. Given that one quantum of neurotransmitter leads to ~0.5 mV depolarization, one can divide this quantal change in potential by the change in potential associated with the opening of one channel to obtain a rough estimate of the number of channels involved, namely:

$$number\ of\ channels\ per\ quantum = \frac{0.5\,mV/quantum}{0.25 \times 10^{-3}\,mV/channel}$$

$$= 2{,}000\frac{channels}{quantum}.$$

In other words, each package (quantum, vesicle) has enough molecules of neurotransmitter to simultaneously activate about ~2,000 receptors on the postsynaptic membrane.

Another important question relates to the number of quanta typically released at a synapse. The answer to this question depends on the specific synapse. For example, the synapse at the NMJ is highly unusual in that ~100 to 200 quanta are released for every AP that enters the NMJ. To understand why this is, let's examine the anatomy of an NMJ. Figure 6A shows multiple branches of a single motor axon, each terminating with an

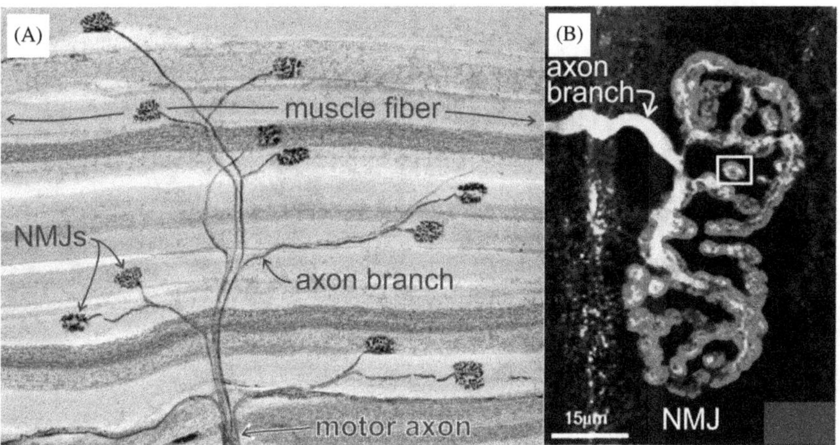

Figure 6.   (A) Branches of a motor axon terminating with elaborate NMJ on individual skeletal muscle fibers. (B) High magnification of one NMJ showing multiple presynaptic swellings (boutons), one of which is highlighted in the white box. ([A] from David G. Ward wardd@mjc.edu; [B] adapted from Keller-Peck *et al.* [2001].)

elaborate process (the NMJ) on different muscle fibers. Under higher magnification (Figure 6B), the presynaptic apparatus of a single NMJ can be seen as an extensive array of many little swellings (the presynaptic terminals or synaptic boutons), one of which is indicated in the white box in Figure 6B. Each of these terminals, in turn, may possess multiple sites for the release of neurotransmitters.

The ultrastructure of a couple of release sites at the NMJ is depicted schematically in Figure 7. Synaptic vesicles containing the neurotransmitter Ach are clustered in small groups near aggregations of voltage-gated Ca^{2+} channels. These "active zones" are positioned across from inward folds in the postsynaptic membrane of the muscle fiber. Found on the crests of these folds are thousands of ligand-gated channels—the nicotinic Ach (nAch) receptors. As we shall discuss later, when these channels bind to Ach, they open briefly to primarily enable Na^+ ions to flow into the muscle fiber to depolarize the muscle fiber locally at the end-plate zone.

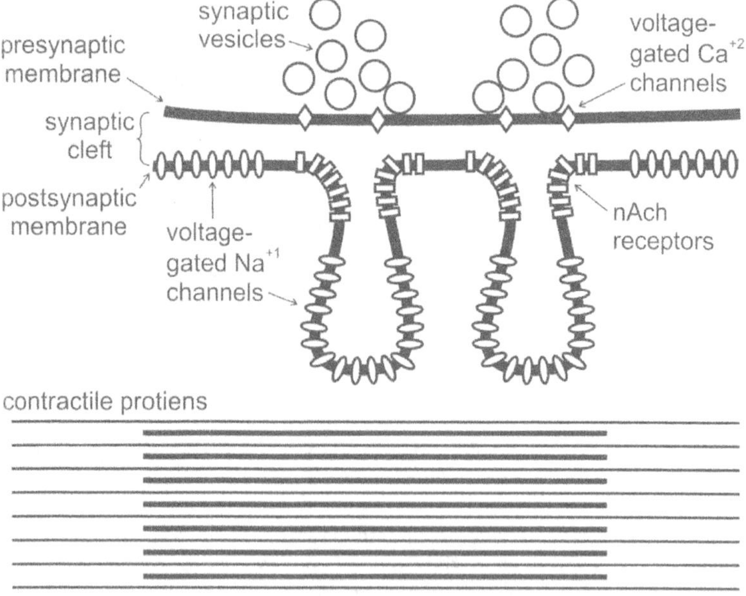

Figure 7.   Schematic diagram showing the ultrastructure of release sites at an NMJ.

At a single release site, the number of quanta expelled for each AP entering into the NMJ is probabilistic (i.e., a roll of the dice) and could be one, two, three, or none, with one being perhaps the most common. This effect gets multiplied by a few release sites per terminal and by multiple terminals at a single NMJ. As such the total number of quanta released at the NMJ can vary from AP to AP somewhere between 100 and 200 quanta.

Let's use the low-end value of 100 quanta released during an AP to estimate the magnitude of the associated EPP. We can (as a first approximation) simply multiply the number of quanta (q) released by the change in membrane potential (ΔV_m) associated with the release of a single quantum to determine the EPP:

$$EPP = \#q \times \frac{\Delta V_m}{q} = 100\ q \times \frac{0.5\,mV}{q} = 50\,mV.$$

This minimal value of an EPP is still well above that needed to cross the threshold (~15 mV) for igniting an AP in the muscle fiber.

Indeed, adjacent to the ligand-gated channels, in the folds of the postsynaptic membrane, are high densities of voltage-gated Na^+ channels (see Figure 7). These Na^+ channels are more or less equivalent to the spike-initiating zone in neurons. Yet, there is no need for decaying electrotonic conduction from postsynaptic receptors at distant synapses (as there is for dendritic synapses) to this spike-initiating zone: here the synapse and the spike-initiating zones are colocalized. This, along with the large number of quanta released, ensures a postsynaptic potential of more than sufficient magnitude to always instigate an AP at the end-plate zone. The AP is then propagated, up to a few centimeters in both directions away from the centrally located NMJ, along the muscle fiber by voltage-gated Na^+ (and K^+) channels, in a process not unlike conduction in unmyelinated axons. The large voltage change associated with the muscle fiber AP serves as the trigger to release Ca^{2+} from the sarcoplasmic reticulum, which in turn sets in motion the interactions among the contractile proteins to cause muscle contraction.

Diseases of Neuromuscular Transmission

There are a host of diseases that selectively impair different components of the NMJ, leading to weakness, fatigue, and paralysis (Wood & Slater, 2001). For example, in the *presynaptic* terminal (see Figure 7), there are diseases that (1) cause the degeneration of the voltage-gated Ca^{2+} channels (*Lambert–Eaton myasthenic syndrome*), (2) reduce the size of the vesicles (*congenital myasthenic syndrome with episodic apnea*), and (3) impair exocytosis, blocking neurotransmitter release altogether (*botulism*). Interestingly, the paralytic nature of the botulinum toxin has been deployed clinically to treat hyperexcitable muscle, such as that which occurs in certain dystonias (sustained contractions of muscles), spasticity in cerebral palsy, and perhaps more dubiously, the sustained contraction of facial muscles contributing to facial wrinkles. For diseases that affect the *postsynaptic* side of the NMJ, the most well-known is *myasthenia gravis*—an autoimmune disorder that leads to the breakdown and reduction in the number of nAch receptors in the postsynaptic membrane. All of these diseases cause reductions in the EPP, often to a level below the threshold for generating an AP, leading to the failure of muscle contraction.

Neurotransmitter Release in the Central Nervous System

A great deal was learned about synaptic transmission by studying the accessible NMJ. But do the principles of quantal release identified at the NMJ also hold for synapses in the central nervous system (CNS)? Extensive work following that of Katz and his colleagues largely confirmed the quantal nature of synaptic transmission in the CNS. However, the number of quanta released at CNS synapses is typically far fewer than at the NMJ. Commonly, the number of quanta released at synapses in the mammalian CNS is only one or two (Redman 1990). However, there are exceptions, particularly at the synaptic connections along ascending sensory pathways, where the number of quanta released can be many times higher (e.g., Meyer *et al.* 2001).

With only one or two quanta of neurotransmitter released at a typical central synapse, this will give rise to a local postsynaptic potential (i.e. immediately across from the presynaptic terminal) of only ~0.5 to 1 mV. Furthermore, because neuronal synapses are typically located out on the dendritic tree, the magnitude of the synaptic potentials detected at the spike-initiating zone will be much smaller (a fraction of a millivolt) because of the loss in amplitude with distance associated with electrotonic conduction (see Figure 10, Chapter 5). This means that neurons usually require synaptic input from hundreds of other neurons in order to fire (as will be discussed Chapter 7).

Direct and Indirect Gating of Postsynaptic Channels

Before addressing the mechanisms by which binding of neurotransmitter ligands to postsynaptic receptors leads to the opening of ion channels and a change in membrane potential in the postsynaptic cell, it is important to point out that there are two general categories of processes by which this takes place: **direct gating** and **indirect gating** of ion channels. In direct gating (Figure 8A), the receptor and ion channel are in one package. In indirect gating (Figure 8B), the receptor system for the neurotransmitter ligand and the ion channels are in different locations. In this case, the

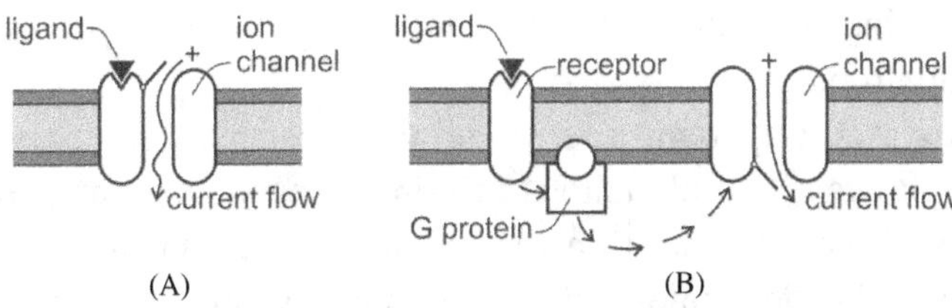

Figure 8.   Direct and indirect gating of ion channels. (A) In direct gating, a ligand binds to a receptor site on the ion channel, leading to a conformational change in the channel molecule that opens the pore through which ions flow. This type of gating is fast and is also referred to as **ionotropic**. (B) In indirect gating, ligand binding to a receptor molecule activates a G-protein, which in turn, instigates a metabolic cascade involving second messenger molecules that ultimately gate ion channels. This type of gating is slow and is also called **metabotropic**.

binding of the ligand to the receptor activates G-proteins that sets off a cascade of metabolic events involving second messengers that eventually gate multiple ion channels located away from the receptor. This type of postsynaptic receptor is sometimes referred to as **metabotropic**, *meaning that it works by instigating a metabolic cascade leading to the opening of ion channels*. On the other hand, the receptors involved in direct gating are often referred to as **ionotropic**, *meaning that they operate by directly instigating ionic current.*

Ionotropic (directly gated) transmission is fast, occurring in the time scale of milliseconds. Metabotropic (indirectly gated) transmission is slow, operating on the time scale of hundreds of milliseconds, seconds, minutes, and even longer. Directly gated transmission is crucial for moment-by-moment processing of information and production of behavior by the nervous system. Indirectly gated transmission oftentimes operates to globally change the functional state of part of the nervous system for relatively long periods of time. For example, if someone insults you, you may have a persistent feeling of anger despite that the stimulus (the insult) is no longer present—and may even remain so after the person has apologized. It is likely that in this situation, metabotropic receptors are activated by the stimulus (the insult) that pushed an emotional circuit into a new state. Because of the long-lasting nature of these receptors, it simply takes a long time for their activity to dissipate and return the circuit to a basal state before feelings of anger die out. So, the next time someone accuses you of retaining your anger much longer than is warranted, you can blame your metabotropic receptors.

While it is important to realize that metabotropic transmission plays a significant and ubiquitous role in the nervous system, for most of this book, we will focus on the ionotropic mechanisms of synaptic transmission. As such, unless otherwise stated, synaptic transmission will be assumed to be directly gated.

Excitatory Postsynaptic Potentials

Let's now examine what takes place in the postsynaptic receptors at *excitatory* synapses (like the nAch receptor at the NMJ) when they bind neurotransmitters released from the presynaptic terminal. Specifically, we are interested to know which ions pass through these ligand-gated channels when opened. Here we are in for a surprise—these channels are more or less equally permeable to both Na^+ and K^+ ions. At first glance, this arrangement may seem counterproductive: increasing the permeability to Na^+ will tend to depolarize the membrane (pushing the membrane potential toward the equilibrium potential for Na^+, $E_{Na}^+ = +55$ mV) whereas increasing permeability to K^+ will tend to hyperpolarize the membrane (drive membrane potential toward $E_K^+ = -75$ mV). How does this arrangement end up being an effective means to depolarize the membrane?

To address that question, let's take a look at the chemical and electrical forces acting on Na^+ and K^+ ions to drive them through these channels at different levels of membrane potential. The experimental arrangement is like that shown in Figure 9A—a microelectrode is inserted to record the postsynaptic potential near an excitatory synapse in response to an AP invading the presynaptic terminal. In addition, a second electrode is inserted into the postsynaptic cell through which different steady intensities of current are injected. Current injection serves to set the membrane potential to various levels when APs arrive.

Figure 9B shows the electrical (F_E) and chemical (F_C) forces acting on Na^+ and K^+ for each of the several levels of membrane potential. Although this may look complicated, keeping track of the forces is relatively straightforward if we proceed step-by-step (as we did in Chapter 3, Figure 7). Let's begin at the equilibrium potential for K^+, -75 mV (bottom Figure 9B). We know that the electrical and chemical forces acting on K^+ are equal and opposite at this membrane potential. Also, we know that the chemical force acting on K^+ is to drive it from high to low concentration, namely from inside to outside the cell. Because the chemical force normally does not change, note that the chemical force vector for K^+ is the same for all levels of membrane potential depicted in Figure 9B.

Recall from Chapter 3 that the electrical force changes in direct proportion to the membrane potential. In addition, the electrical force acting on a K^+ ion is *identical* to that on a Na^+ ion because they both possess +1 proton of charge and are both acted upon by the same membrane charge. Therefore, you should note in Figure 9B that the electrical force at -75 mV is the same for both Na^+ and K^+. Indeed, if you look across all levels

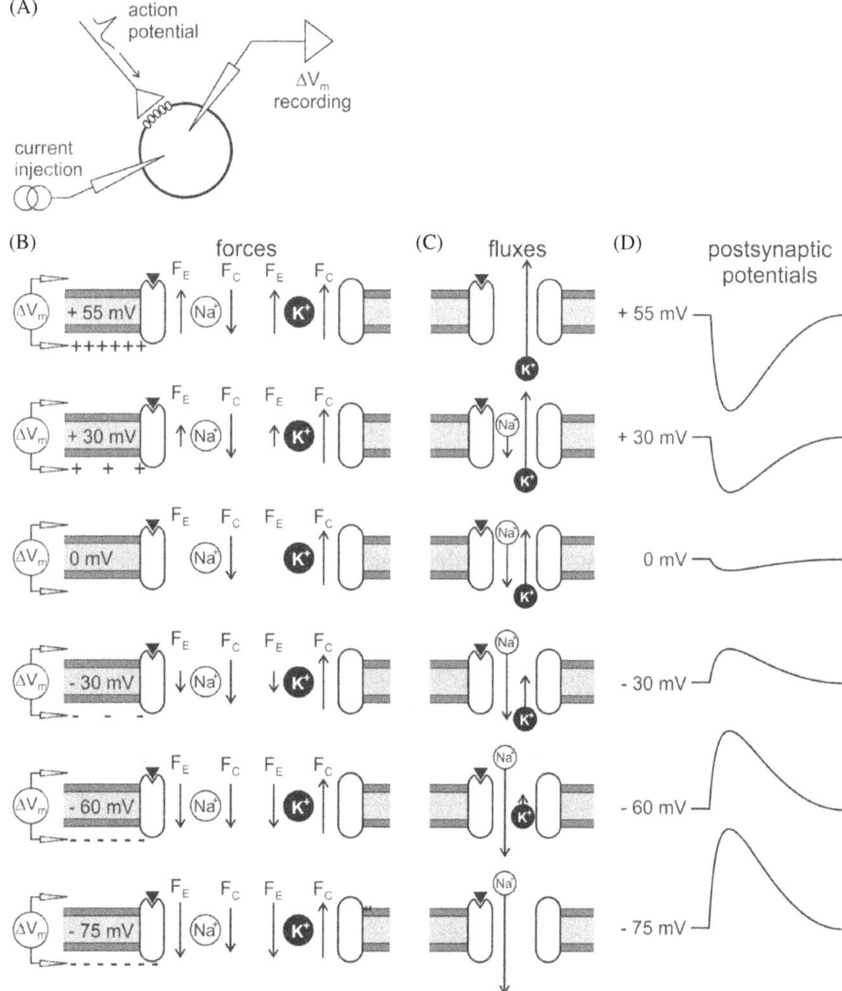

Figure 9.   (A) Experimental arrangement used to investigate ionic currents through the excitatory synapse. Steady current injection is used to bias membrane potential to different levels. Recording electrode near synapse in postsynaptic cell is used to record the change in membrane potential (ΔV_m) superimposed on biased membrane potential in response to the entry of AP into the presynaptic terminal. (B) Electrical (F_E) and chemical (F_C) forces acting on Na$^+$ and K$^+$ ions in ligand-gated channels that are equally permeable to both at different levels of membrane potential. (C) Flux of Na$^+$ and K$^+$ ions through an open channel at different membrane potential levels. (D) Associated change in membrane potential superimposed on different levels of membrane potential. The reversal potential (membrane potential at which net ionic current changes direction from inward to outward) would occur at about −10 mV.

of membrane potential in Figure 9B, you will see that the electrical force is always the same for both Na^+ and K^+.

Returning to the −75 mV level in Figure 9B, how do we get the chemical force for Na^+? If we go to the membrane potential associated with the equilibrium potential for Na^+, namely +55 mV, we know that the electrical and chemical forces are equal and opposite to one another. We also know that at +55 mV, the electrical force is to drive Na^+ out of the cell with a magnitude directly proportional to the membrane potential and that the chemical force for Na^+ is to enter the cell. Because the chemical force does not change, the chemical force vector at +55 mV is duplicated for every other membrane potential level shown in Figure 9B.

Now that we have accounted for all the forces acting on Na^+ and K^+ at −75 mV, let's estimate the flux of those ions through the opened ligand-gated channels. Again, from Chapter 3, recall that the flux for each ion can be estimated from the equation:

$$Flux = (F_C + F_E) \times P.$$

Unlike the case for the leak channels that dictate the resting membrane potential, here the ligand-gated channels at excitatory synapses are equally permeable to both Na^+ and K^+. Therefore, the permeability, P, in the flux equation can be assigned the same relative value of 1.0 for both Na^+ and K^+. As a consequence, the flux can be independently determined for both Na^+ and K^+ as simply the sum of their chemical (F_C) and electrical (F_E) forces at each membrane potential.

At −75 mV, the sum of F_C and F_E for K^+ is zero. Therefore, no flux of K^+ is shown at −75 mV in Figure 9C. On the other hand, the influx of Na^+ is large at −75 mV because of the large electrical and chemical forces both serving to drive Na^+ into the cell. Therefore, when ligand-gated channels at excitatory synapses open and if the membrane potential is at −75 mV, the large influx of positively charged Na^+ ions will cause a significant depolarization of the postsynaptic cell (Figure 9D).

At −60 mV (close to the resting potential of many neurons), the electrical forces for both Na^+ and K^+ are modestly reduced from what they were at −75 mV (Figure 9B). This slightly reduces the magnitude of the Na^+ influx compared to that at −75 mV (Figure 9C). K^+ is no longer in equilibrium, with F_C slightly larger than F_E. This leads to a small outward flux of K^+. As such, the *net* flux of positively charged ions through these ligand-gated channels at −60 mV is slightly less than at −75 mV. Therefore, the postsynaptic depolarization, while significant, is slightly less at −60 mV than at −75 mV (Figure 9D).

At −30 mV, the electrical forces are exactly half that at −60 mV (Figure 9B). As such, the influx of Na^+ is reduced while the efflux of K^+ increases (Figure 9C). Consequently, the net influx of positive charge is strongly reduced at −30 mV compared to at −60 mV, and the associated postsynaptic potential is similarly reduced (Figure 9D).

At 0 mV, the electrical forces are zero. Therefore, the only forces operating are chemical forces (Figure 9B). The chemical force for K^+ is larger than that for Na^+. Consequently, at 0 mV, there will be a net *efflux* of positive ions (Figure 9C). This in turn will cause the membrane potential to slightly *hyperpolarize* if these channels open when the membrane potential is at 0 mV (Figure 9D).

At increasingly positive membrane potentials (e.g., +30 and +55 mV), the electrical forces become progressively stronger to drive Na^+ and K^+ out of the cell. At +30 mV, the electrical force partially counteracts the chemical force driving Na^+ into the cell, whereas the chemical and electrical forces cooperate to drive K^+ out of the cell. This leads to a modestly large net efflux of positive charge (Figure 9C), causing a strong hyperpolarization (Figure 9D). At +55 mV, there is no flux of Na^+ and a large efflux of K^+ (Figure 9C) due to the cooperation of chemical and large electrical forces. This will cause the membrane potential to be driven strongly in the hyperpolarizing direction (Figure 9D).

When one looks across the family of postsynaptic potentials for the different levels of membrane potential in Figure 9D, one can see that for the most negative membrane potential, the depolarizing postsynaptic potential is the greatest. As the membrane potential becomes less negative, the associated postsynaptic potential becomes smaller. At 0 mV, opening the same set of ligand-gated channels leads to a slight hyperpolarization. As the membrane potential becomes more positive, the postsynaptic potentials become progressively stronger to hyperpolarize the membrane. Indeed, there is a membrane potential (~−10 mV) at which the influx of Na^+ perfectly matches the efflux of K^+. If the membrane is at this potential when an AP triggers the release of neurotransmitters, no change in membrane potential will be detected. This level of *membrane potential at which ion flux through a set of channels switches from net inward to net outward is referred to as the* **reversal potential**. Furthermore, if there are enough of these ion channels open and if they stay open for a relatively long time period, then the membrane potential will be driven toward this reversal potential from any other membrane potential. This is not really different from the concept of the *steady-state potential* discussed in Chapter 4 (e.g., Figure 1) except that in this case, only one set of channels (permeable to both Na$^+$ and K$^+$) is involved, whereas in Chapter 4, different sets of channels were involved.

Now, let's return to the question posed at the outset of this section: how can ligand-gated channels that are permeable to both Na$^+$ and K$^+$ be effective at depolarizing the membrane? The answer is that most of the time, the membrane potential of neurons and muscle fibers sit at quite negative values, in the vicinity of the resting potential (~−60 mV). As such, activation of excitatory synapses will drive the membrane potential in the direction of the reversal potential (slightly less than 0 mV), effectively causing the membrane to depolarize. This means of depolarizing the membrane is used at most excitatory synapses in the central nervous system.

Inhibitory Postsynaptic Potentials

Let's now examine the ionic mechanisms that operate at inhibitory synapses that tend to suppress activity in neurons. We will use the same experimental arrangement as shown for the excitatory synapse in Figure 9A. Namely, the change in membrane potential is recorded in a postsynaptic neuron in response to an AP entering the presynaptic terminal of an inhibitory synapse when the membrane potential has been biased to different levels with steady current injection.

Here, the situation is somewhat simpler than for excitatory synapses in that the ligand-gated channels at inhibitory synapses are permeable only to Cl$^-$ ions. Recall from Chapter 3 that the equilibrium potential for Cl$^-$ is about −60 mV, which is close to the resting potential for most neurons. So, let's start there. At −60 mV in Figure 10A, the chemical force driving Cl$^-$ into the cell is balanced by the electrical force pushing Cl$^-$ out.

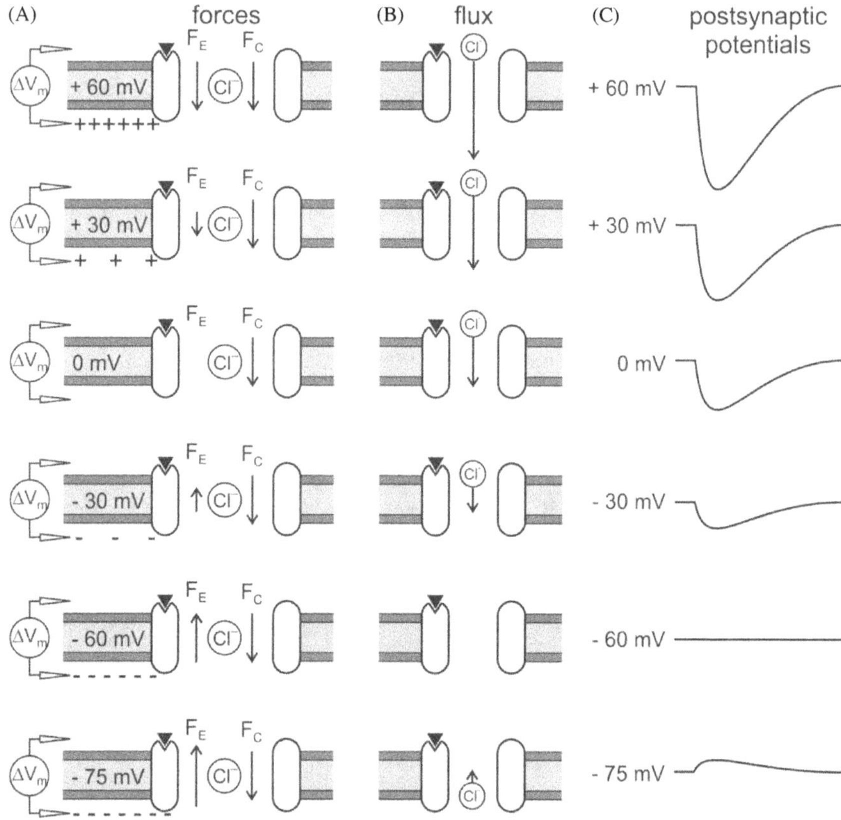

Figure 10.   Ionic mechanisms acting at a ligand-gated inhibitory synapse. (A) Electrical (F_E) and chemical (F_C) forces acting on Cl⁻ ions at different levels of membrane potential. (B) Flux of Cl⁻ through an open channel at different membrane potential levels. (C) Associated change in membrane potential superimposed on different levels of membrane potential. The reversal potential is at –60 mV, equivalent to the equilibrium potential for Cl⁻.

As such, there is no Cl⁻ flux (Figure 10B) and no change in membrane potential (Figure 10C). At –75 mV, the additional negative charge on the membrane increases the electrical force (Figure 10A), whereas the chemical force remains the same. This leads to a small net force to drive Cl⁻ out of the neuron (Figure 10B). This will cause the membrane to become less negative, that is, to *depolarize* slightly (Figure 10C). On the other hand, at holding potentials increasingly depolarized relative to the resting potential, Cl⁻ influx progressively increases (Figure 10B), causing *hyperpolarizing* postsynaptic potentials to also become larger (Figure 10C).

The *reversal potential* of inhibitory synapses is the same as the *equilibrium potential* for Cl⁻, which also is close to the *resting potential*. Perhaps the most surprising aspect of this state of affairs is that opening ligand-gated channels at inhibitory synapses when the neuron is sitting at its resting potential may cause no detectable change in membrane potential. So why is this even referred to as an inhibitory synapse? Keep in mind that as the postsynaptic membrane becomes more permeable to Cl⁻ through activation of inhibitory synapses, the membrane potential will be more strongly pulled toward −60 mV, effectively preventing the membrane from being depolarized to threshold. As such, there is a kind of competition between excitatory and inhibitory synapses. Excitatory synapses act to depolarize the membrane potential away from the resting potential toward 0 mV, whereas inhibitory synapses counteract that action by driving the membrane potential back to the resting potential.

Summary

Let's now summarize the basic steps involved in synaptic transmission using the schematic diagram shown in Figure 11. (**1**) An AP invades the presynaptic terminal. The large depolarization associated with the AP then (**2**) opens voltage-gated Ca^{2+} channels in the presynaptic membrane near the active zones. (**3**) Ca^{2+} enters the presynaptic terminal, which in turn, (**4**) triggers the process of exocytosis that causes synaptic vesicles, containing a few thousand molecules of neurotransmitters each, to merge with the presynaptic membrane and dump their contents into the synaptic cleft. The total number of vesicles that are released for each AP that enters the presynaptic terminal is probabilistic and also depends on the type of synapse. For example, ~100 vesicles (the quanta) may be released simultaneously at the NMJ whereas only one vesicle on average may be released at a typical synapse in the CNS. (**5**) The neurotransmitter released from the presynaptic terminal diffuses across the synaptic cleft and then (**6**) binds to ligand-gated channels in the postsynaptic membrane. Each vesicle of

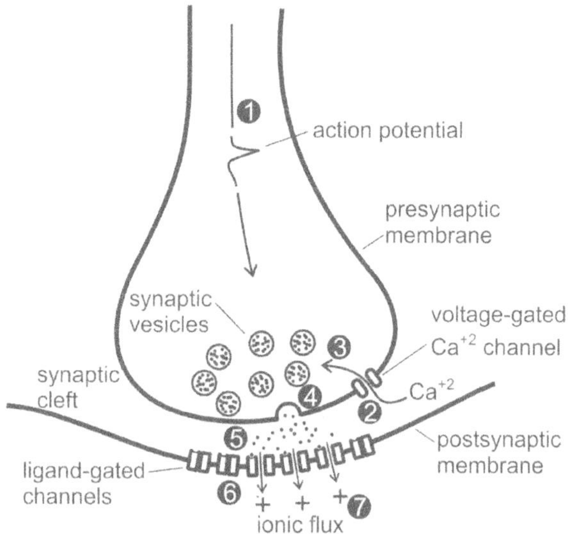

Figure 11.   Steps involved in synaptic transmission. (1) An AP enters the presynaptic terminal, (2) activating voltage-gated Ca^{2+} channels that (3) trigger the influx of Ca^{2+}, which (4) instigates exocytosis and the release of neurotransmitters into the synaptic cleft. (5) Neurotransmitters diffuse across the synaptic cleft to (6) bind to and activate ligand-gated channels enabling (7) an ionic flux across the postsynaptic membrane.

neurotransmitters may cause the simultaneous opening of a few thousand ligand-gated channels. The opening of the ligand-gated channels leads to **(7)** an ionic flux that changes the membrane potential of the postsynaptic cell. At excitatory synapses, the ligand-gated channels are permeable to both Na^+ and K^+. At (typical) negative levels of membrane potential, this leads to more Na^+ influx than K^+ efflux, causing the postsynaptic membrane to depolarize. Such a depolarization is referred to as an excitatory postsynaptic potential (EPSP) in neurons, and an EPP in muscle fibers. At inhibitory synapses, the ligand-gated channels are permeable to Cl^-. The increased permeability of the membrane to Cl^- pulls the membrane potential toward E_{Cl}^- ($\sim$$-60$ mV). If the membrane is depolarized above E_{Cl}^- when an AP arrives into the presynaptic terminal, the influx of Cl^- will drive the membrane in the hyperpolarizing direction. Such a change in membrane potential is called an inhibitory postsynaptic potential (IPSP).

References

Akaaboune M, Culican SM, Turney SG & Lichtman JW (1999). Rapid and reversible effects of activity on acetylcholine receptor density at the neuromuscular junction in vivo. *Science* **286**, 503–507.

Dieterich DC & Kreutz MR (2016). Proteomics of the synapse—A quantitative approach to neuronal plasticity. *Molecular and Cellular Proteomics* **15**, 368–381.

Fatt P & Katz B (1952). Spontaneous subthreshold activity at motor nerve endings. *Journal of Physiology* **117**, 109–128.

Heuser JE & Reese TS (1981). Structural changes after transmitter release at the frog neuromuscular junction. *Journal of Cell Biology* **88**, 564–580.

Katz B (1971). Nobel lecture: Quantal mechanism of neural transmitter release. *Science* **173**, 123–126.

Keller-Peck CR, Feng G, Sanes JR, Yan Q, Lichtman JW & Snider WD (2001). Glial cell line-derived neurotrophic factor administration in postnatal life results in motor unit enlargement and continuous synaptic remodeling at the neuromuscular junction. *Journal of Neuroscience* **21**, 6136–6146.

Meyer AC, Neher E & Schneggenburger R (2001). Estimation of quantal size and number of functional active zones at the Calyx of held synapse by nonstationary EPSC variance analysis. *Journal of Neuroscience* **21**, 7889–7900.

Redman S (1990). Quantal analysis of synaptic potentials in neurons of the central nervous system. *Physiological Reviews* **70**, 165–198.

Wood SJ & Slater CR (2001). Safety factor at the neuromuscular junction. *Progress in Neurobiology* **64**, 393–429.

Chapter 7

Synaptic Transmitters, Plasticity, and Integration

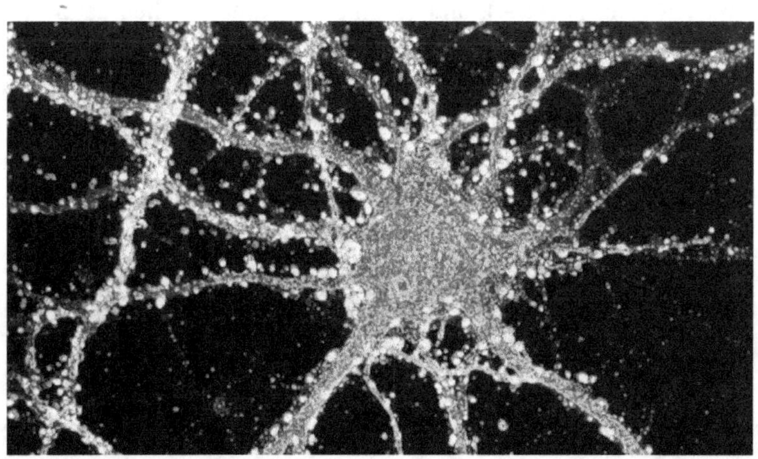

Glutamate synaptic contacts on soma and proximal dendrites of a hippocampal neuron. (With permission from Ferreira et al. [2015].)

In Chapter 6, we discussed the mechanisms by which synaptic transmission takes place. In this chapter, we address the types of *neurotransmitters* found at synapses, how synapses can be modified (*plasticity*), and how neurons process synaptic information from many different sources (*integration*).

Neurotransmitters

There are just a handful of key neurotransmitters that operate at directly gated synapses in the peripheral and central nervous systems (keep in mind, there are many more neurotransmitters that act at indirectly gated synapses). Table 1 provides an overview of these transmitters. Acetylcholine (Ach), as we have discussed, acts at nicotinic receptors in the neuromuscular junction. Ach and nicotinic receptors are also found at the peripheral ganglia (part of the autonomic nervous system) and throughout the central nervous system (CNS). As discussed in Chapter 6, the ion channels gated by Ach are permeable to both Na^+ and K^+, leading to depolarization (excitation) of the postsynaptic cell.

Within the CNS itself, there are the three "Gs": glutamate, gamma-aminobutyric acid (GABA), and glycine. Glutamate, when acting at the α-amino-3-hydroxy-5-methyl-4-isoxazolepropionic acid (AMPA) receptors, operates very similarly to Ach at nicotinic receptors. These receptors are called AMPA because this chemical selectively opens these channels (i.e., as an exogenous agonist) in a way that mimics the action of endogenous glutamate. These ligand-gated channels gate both Na^+ and K^+, leading to depolarization of the postsynaptic membrane under most circumstances. The glutamate–AMPA receptor system is the most prevalent excitatory synapse in the CNS.

Table 1.   Main neurotransmitters at directly gated synapses.

Neurotransmitter	Receptor	Ion(s) gated	Action	Comments
Ach	Nicotinic	Na^+, K^+	excitation	At neuromuscular junction, peripheral autonomic ganglia, & CNS
Glutamate	AMPA	Na^+, K^+	excitation	Main excitatory neurotransmitter-receptor system in CNS
	NMDA	Na^+, K^+, Ca^{+2}	excitation	- Often co-localized with AMPA receptors - Both ligand-gated AND voltage-gated - Important in learning and memory
GABA	GABA$_A$	Cl^-	inhibition	Main inhibitory neurotransmitter-receptor system in CNS
Glycine	Glycine	Cl^-	inhibition	Found primarily in spinal cord and brainstem

Glutamate can also bind to N-methyl-D-aspartate (NMDA) receptors at directly gated synapses. (Like AMPA, these receptors are named for the specific exogenous agonist that mimics the action of glutamate.) NMDA receptors are often colocalized with AMPA receptors at a single synapse. The NMDA receptor is highly unusual in that it is *both* ligand-gated and voltage-gated. In other words, opening NMDA channels requires both the binding of the ligand glutamate *and* substantial depolarization of the postsynaptic membrane. This is a door that has two locks needing two keys. When opened, in addition to Na^+ and K^+, this channel is also permeable to Ca^{2+}. As such, NMDA channel opening leads to depolarization of the postsynaptic membrane. More importantly, as we shall see, this intriguing channel plays a key role in learning and memory.

GABA acting at $GABA_A$ receptors represents the main inhibitory synaptic system in the CNS. (There are other GABA receptors, such as $GABA_B$ and $GABA_C$ that mainly act as metabotropic receptors.) GABA ion channels are permeable to Cl^- when open. Therefore, they will counteract the depolarizing action of excitatory synapses and tend to pull the membrane potential toward the equilibrium potential for Cl^- (which is close to the resting potential). There are a number of drugs, such as barbiturates, that serve as agonists at GABA receptors. In general, these drugs boost inhibition across the CNS to produce calming, relaxing effects. As such, they are widely used to treat anxiety disorders, insomnia, and to prevent seizures. At higher doses, they can induce general anesthesia. These drugs, however, can be highly addictive and they are dangerous because they can cause lack of consciousness and cessation of activity in neural circuits such as those that control breathing.

Glycine, acting at the simply called glycine receptor, works in almost an identical way to GABA at the $GABA_A$ receptor. It is distinguished from the GABA system in that is mostly found in the spinal cord and the brainstem. Strychnine, a highly toxic poison, acts as an *antagonist* to the glycine receptor. Strychnine-mediated removal of inhibition in the spinal cord and brainstem unleashes severe convulsions, including those of the respiratory muscles, which eventually prevent breathing and cause asphyxia.

Synaptic Plasticity

In the 1940s, the Canadian psychologist Donald Hebb articulated theoretical ideas as to how connections among groups of neurons might be shaped to promote learning and memory. His idea was that excitatory synaptic connections among neurons that are active at the same time become stronger (i.e., cause greater depolarization) whereas synaptic connections among neurons that are active at different times are weakened. This postulate has been simplified into the easy-to-remember aphorism: "*neurons that fire together, wire together.*"

At the heart of this prescient idea was the principle that synaptic connections are not static. Rather, many synapses are **plastic**—meaning that the *efficacy of synaptic connections can be modified for long periods of time in response to appropriate conditions*. In materials, for example, a plastic object takes on a particular shape under sufficient pressure and heat applied during fabrication. For the most part, that shape is enduring in response to everyday stresses and strains. However, if enough heat or pressure is applied, the object can take on a new lasting shape (think of an unfortunate frisbee left on a hot stove). In Hebb's notion of synaptic plasticity, the shaping conditions have to do with the *coactivity* of neurons.

But why would strengthening of synaptic connections among those neurons that fire together serve the process of learning? To address this, let's consider connections among a group of neurons shown in Figure 1A. Neuron Z (representing a particular set of neurons) is part of a motor pathway that ultimately gives rise to a reflex contraction that lifts the lower limb. Neuron Z (like most neurons) receives many synaptic inputs of varying strengths. Symbolically, the potency of a synapse is indicated by the size of the presynaptic terminal (even though the size of a synapse do not necessarily vary as a function of their synaptic strength). Neuron X (representing another set of neurons) makes potent excitatory connections to postsynaptic Neuron Z. Let's say that Neuron X gets its input from pain receptors in the skin of the foot.

Neuron Y, on the other hand, has very weak synaptic connections to Neuron Z. Let's assume that Neuron Y is part of the auditory sensory pathway. They have strong connections to other neurons in the auditory system. However, some of their axonal branches found their way to Neuron Z during early development. Such apparent "mis-wiring" is

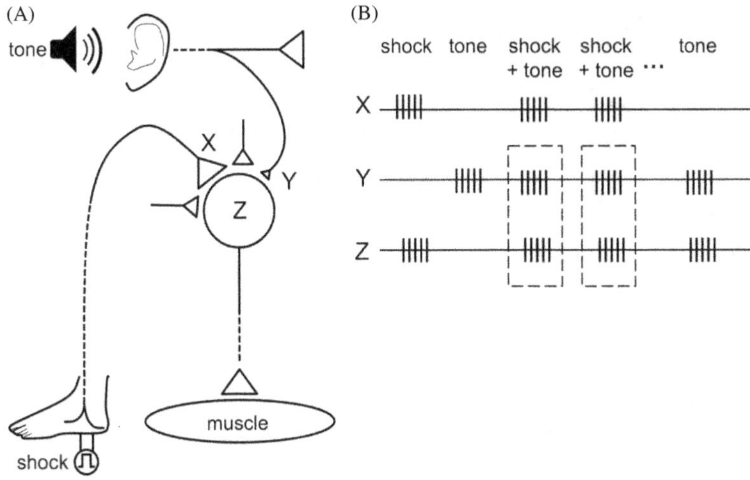

Figure 1.   (A) Schematic representation of a neural circuit that can "learn" based on Hebbian synaptic plasticity. Neuron Z is part of a reflex pathway that causes the foot to withdraw from noxious stimuli. Neuron Z receives many synaptic inputs; input from pain pathway X is potent whereas the input from auditory pathway Y is initially weak. (B) Electrical stimulation (shock) to the foot strongly excites pathway X (vertical lines indicate action potentials), which strongly excites Neuron Z to elicit reflex withdrawal of foot. An auditory stimulus (tone) alone has no detectable effect on Neuron Z. Pairing the timing of the shock with the tone (shock + tone) leads to simultaneous activity in Neuron Y and Neuron Z (dashed rectangles). According to Hebb's postulate, such coincident activity will strengthen Neuron Y's synapse onto Neuron Z. If repeated sufficiently, in theory, Neuron Y's input alone could become strong enough to drive Neuron Z and provoke a withdrawal of the foot. As such, the circuit has "learned" to associate a tone with a painful stimulus.

indeed widespread in the CNS and appears partly due to promiscuous connectivity among neurons during development (neurons "hooking up" indiscriminately with many partners). Many of these "inappropriate" connections are pruned away during the maturation process but many remain physically in place, albeit with greatly weakened synaptic effects. *These weak (and sometimes entirely impotent or "silent" synapses (Kerchner & Nicoll 2008) are often referred to as* **"latent" synaptic connections**.

Now if one delivers an electrical shock to the pathway including Neuron X, spiking the activity in Neuron X will drive the activity in Neuron Z because of X's potent synaptic connections to Z ("shock"; Figure 1B). Activity in the Neuron Z pathway, in turn, will elicit an immediate behavioral response—withdrawing the foot away from the noxious stimulus. On the other hand, playing a sound will evoke spiking activity in Neuron Y but this will not drive activity in Neuron Z because of Neuron Y's weak synaptic connection to Neuron Z ("tone"; Figure 1B). If one pairs the shock with the sound ("shock + tone"; Figure 1B), the activity in Neuron X will drive Neuron Z, and Neuron Y's activity (driven by the tone) is "artificially" paired with Z (highlighted inside the dashed boxes; Figure 1B). If done repeatedly, then according to Hebb's postulate, Neuron Y's connection to Neuron Z should get stronger. Indeed, it could become strong enough such that a tone alone (activating Neuron Y) elicits spiking in Z to trigger the withdrawal response. As such, the circuit has learned to associate an otherwise innocuous tone with a painful stimulus.

In order for Hebb's rule to be enacted at a synapse, synapses must have "knowledge" of when both the pre- and postsynaptic neurons are active at the same time (i.e., "firing together"). How can that be possible? Remarkably, there exists a molecule at individual synapses that serves to detect simultaneous activity in both the pre- and postsynaptic neurons. That molecule is the NMDA receptor.

As mentioned previously, the NMDA channel is both ligand-gated and voltage-gated. As such, it requires two signals to open (Figure 2): the

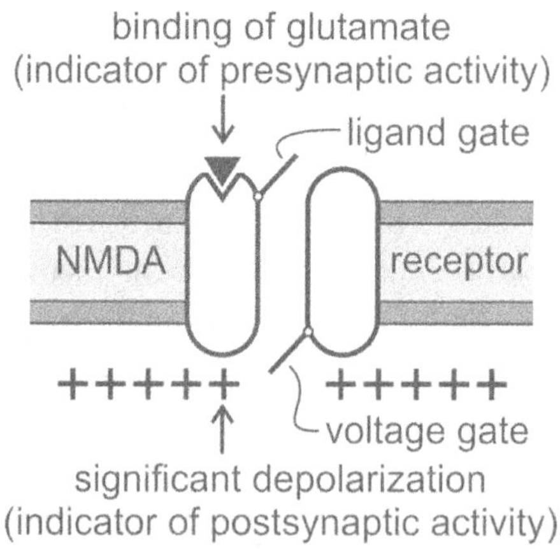

Figure 2.   NMDA receptor—molecular coincidence detector. Opening of the channel requires simultaneous binding of the ligand glutamate (indicates presynaptic neuron is active) and strong membrane depolarization (indicates postsynaptic neuron is active).

binding of glutamate and significant depolarization. The binding of the ligand glutamate is an indicator that the presynaptic neuron is active and releasing glutamate from its presynaptic terminal. Strong depolarization of the postsynaptic neuron typically occurs when many excitatory synaptic inputs from other neurons are simultaneously active and have driven the postsynaptic neuron above the threshold for spiking. When these conditions are met ("neurons firing together"), NMDA channels open. But what is it about NMDA channels opening that leads to a change in synaptic strength?

Remember that NMDA receptor channels are permeable not only to Na^+ and K^+ (like other excitatory synapses) but also to Ca^{2+}. The local influx of Ca^{2+} through NMDA channels is the trigger for the long-lasting change in the strength of the synapse. To understand how this works, let's consider the change in membrane potential in response to a single action potential entering a glutamatergic synapse that has not yet undergone synaptic strengthening (Figure 3A). Furthermore, let's assume that in this instance, the postsynaptic cell is not depolarized but sitting at its resting potential.

The postsynaptic membrane at such excitatory synapses typically expresses both AMPA and NMDA receptors. The binding of glutamate to AMPA receptors will open their channels leading to a small influx of positive charge (carried by Na^+ ions). NMDA receptor channels, however, will not open despite the binding of glutamate to the receptor because the membrane potential is not sufficiently depolarized to open the voltage gate. Consequently, the change in membrane potential (ΔV_m) detected locally at the postsynaptic site will be modest.

Now, let's assume that the postsynaptic neuron is strongly depolarized due to the action of many other synapses (not shown) when an action potential arrives at the presynaptic terminal of our synapse of interest (Figure 3B). This is a case when the two neurons are active together. As before, the AMPA receptors will open in response to binding glutamate released from the presynaptic neuron, causing a small ionic flux and local depolarization. However, in this case, the NMDA receptor will also open because its two conditions for activation are met: the ligand is bound to the receptor and the postsynaptic membrane is highly depolarized. This will cause Ca^{2+} to enter through the channel due to the high concentration gradient acting on Ca^{2+}.

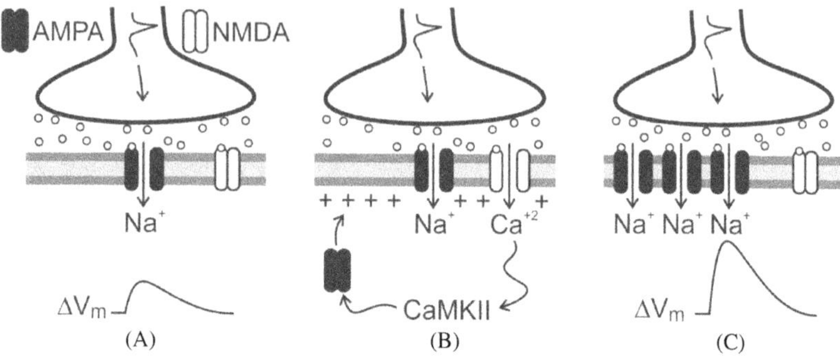

Figure 3.   NMDA receptor role in mediating plasticity at an excitatory synapse. Release of glutamate (small white circles) upon entry of action potential into the presynaptic terminal. Glutamate binds to both AMPA and NMDA receptors in the postsynaptic membrane. (A) The postsynaptic neuron is not active and accordingly, the membrane is not depolarized. Therefore, only AMPA receptor channels will open, leading to a small Na^+ influx and the associated small change in membrane potential (ΔV_m) locally in the postsynaptic neuron. (B) If the postsynaptic neuron is active (and the membrane depolarized), when glutamate binds to receptors, NMDA receptors will also open. Calcium entry through the NMDA channels activates a process involving calcium-calmodulin-dependent protein kinase II (CaMKII) that promotes the local insertion of more AMPA receptors into the postsynaptic membrane. (C) Subsequently, if the postsynaptic cell is again inactive (like in [A]) when an action potential enters the presynaptic terminal, glutamate will activate more AMPA receptors, leading to an overall increase in Na^+ flux, and an increased change in membrane potential (i.e., a "strengthened" synapse).

Calcium, in turn, will activate a local intracellular cascade mediated by the substance calcium-calmodulin-dependent protein kinase II (CaMKII). An important outcome of this cascade is that it causes the insertion of more AMPA receptors at the synapse (Malenka & Nicoll 1999).

As a consequence, if we now return to the original situation, and stimulate the presynaptic neuron while the postsynaptic neuron is at its resting potential (Figure 3C), the release of glutamate will now activate more AMPA receptors, leading to a greater ionic flux and a larger depolarization of the postsynaptic membrane. In essence, the potency of the synapse has been strengthened by the physical addition of more AMPA receptors. And, as long as these AMPA receptors remain in place (and they can for long periods of time), this synapse will provide strong depolarization of the postsynaptic neuron. Indeed, recent evidence has clearly demonstrated long-lasting increases in AMPA receptor insertion at synapses on motor cortical neurons involved in the learning of a new motor skill (Roth *et al.* 2020). It should also be said that if the presynaptic neuron starts to fire out of step with its postsynaptic neuron, this process can be reversed leading to fewer AMPA receptors and weakened synaptic connections (Rioult-Pedotti *et al.* 2000).

Synaptic Integration

A typical neuron has an elaborate dendritic tree (Figure 4A) that receives synaptic inputs of many varieties from thousands of other neurons (Figure 4B).

Depending on the type of neuron, the number of synaptic contacts can vary widely from a handful to hundreds of thousands. For example, granule cells in the cerebellum receive only about four synaptic inputs. Some relay neurons in sensory pathways may receive a few hundred synapses of which only one to four are excitatory. Pyramidal neurons in the cerebral cortex have about 10,000 synaptic contacts whereas spinal motor neurons have about 50,000. The neurons with the greatest number of synapses are the Purkinje cells of the cerebellum with >200,000 synapses. As a rough figure, a representative neuron probably possesses 10,000 to 30,000 synaptic contacts.

As such, a typical neuron is an impressive information-processing machine. It continuously takes in tremendous quantities of data through parallel synaptic channels (Figure 4C). These data are processed moment by moment and transformed into reliable, coded messages that are then communicated to other neurons. This *operation of transforming synaptic input into a spiking output by a neuron* is referred to as **synaptic integration**. In many respects, synaptic integration is the basis for the remarkable computational power of the nervous system and the brain. To begin to understand this process, let's consider how information is transferred at just one or a few synaptic contacts.

As discussed previously, the entry of an action potential into a presynaptic terminal provokes the release of neurotransmitters that activates ligand-gated channels (Figure 5A). This triggers a brief ionic current across the membrane of the target cell, leading to a local change in

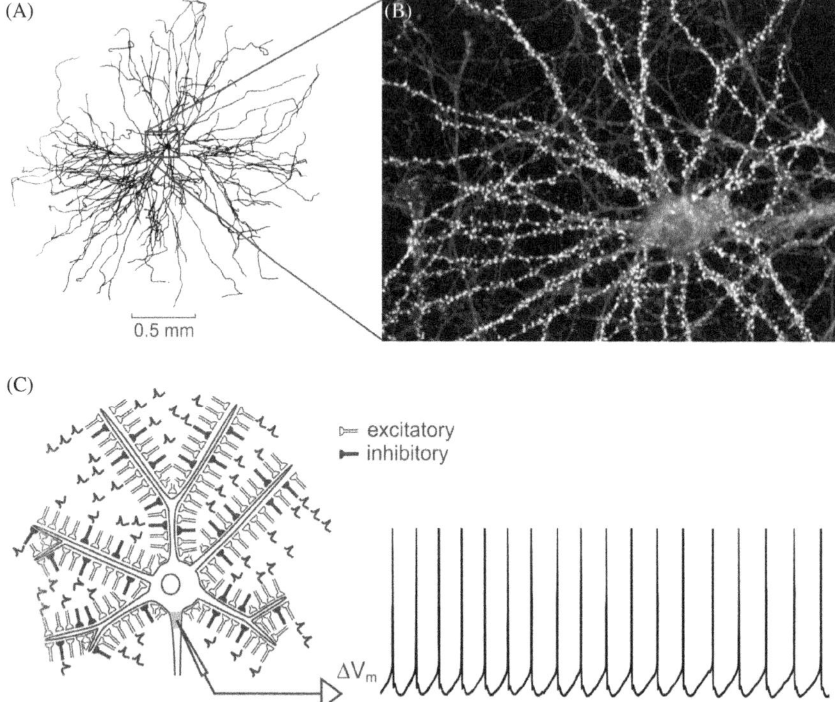

Figure 4.   (A) Extensive dendritic arbor of a motor neuron. (B) Synaptic contacts (bright spots) shown on the magnified image of dendrites. (C) A typical neuron has thousands of synaptic contacts of different types. Some are excitatory and some inhibitory. At any moment, a subset of these synapses may be active (indicated by icons of action potentials entering into presynaptic terminals). The net synaptic current delivered to the spike-initiating zone from these active synapses is transformed into a change in membrane potential (ΔV_m). If ΔV_m is above the threshold, then a sequence of action is generated whose frequency is proportional to the net synaptic current. This process of converting synaptic inputs into frequency-coded outputs that are then delivered to other cells is referred to as synaptic integration. ([A] Adapted from Cullheim *et al.* [1987]. [B] From Kennedy Lab, Cal Tech; http://www.its.caltech.edu/~mbklab/neurons.html. [C] Intracellular recording of motor neuron, from the author's laboratory.)

membrane potential. This influx of current is then propagated, in a largely passive (electrotonic) way, throughout the neuron. Some of it eventually makes its way to the spike-initiating zone where it can be detected as a small, subthreshold change in membrane potential. Such unitary

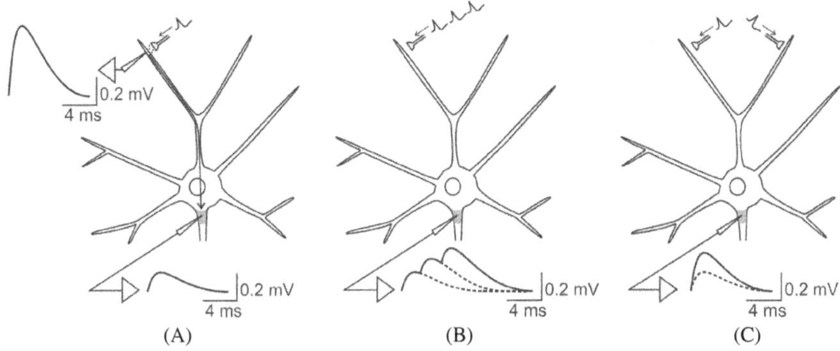

Figure 5.   Basic mechanisms of synaptic integration. (A) The entry of action potential triggers the release of neurotransmitters from the presynaptic terminal. This provokes a brief ionic current across the postsynaptic membrane and causes a local change in the membrane potential. Only a fraction of the original ionic current makes its way to the spike-initiating zone (long arrow) leading to a small PSP. (B) A sequence of action potentials arriving at a single synapse can cause the individual PSPs to add up over time. This is referred to as **temporal summation**. (C) The individual PSPs associated with action potentials arriving at different spatial locations on the dendritic tree sum at the spike-initiating zone. This is referred to as **spatial summation**.

postsynaptic potentials (PSPs), and in this case, an excitatory PSP (EPSP), represent the currency of synaptic integration.

There are a couple of ways by which these unitary responses can add up to drive the membrane potential at the spike-initiating zone toward spike threshold. First, the arrival of a sequence of action potentials at a given synapse will cause an associated sequence of PSPs, one for each action potential at the spike-initiating zone (Figure 5B). If the time between each PSP is briefer than the duration of the PSPs, then the unitary responses partially "stack" upon one another to increase the overall change in membrane potential. Such *changes in membrane potential due to PSPs adding up over time* is referred to as **temporal summation**.

Second, synaptic inputs arriving at different locations on the dendritic tree will each cause their own PSP that can sum at the spike-initiating zone (Figure 5C). The *addition of individual PSPs arriving from different spatial locations* is referred to as **spatial summation**. The rules for this synaptic "arithmetic" are, for the most part, relatively straightforward and in many

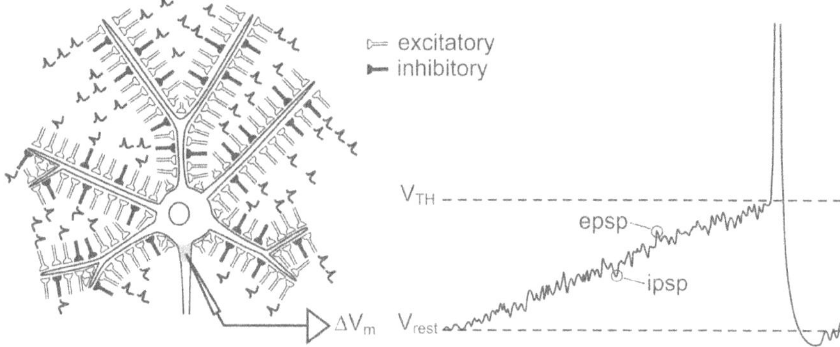

Figure 6.   Schematic showing individual neurons receiving many synaptic inputs (both excitatory and inhibitory). The spike-initiating zone sums these inputs over time (temporal summation) and from the many different locations (spatial summation). This process of synaptic integration typically involves many small PSPs that drives the membrane potential toward the threshold for generating action potentials (right side of figure). Example effects on the membrane potential of single excitatory and inhibitory PSPs are highlighted in the circles.

cases practically linear (i.e., 0.1 mV EPSP from synapse A + 0.1 mV EPSP from synapse B = 0.2 mV total EPSP) although there can be exceptions.

Regardless, the process of synaptic integration typically involves both temporal and spatial summation of hundreds of synaptic inputs to drive the membrane potential of the spike-initiating zone toward threshold (Figure 6). Keep in mind that inhibitory inputs also operate to counteract the depolarizing action of the excitatory inputs. For example, the small upward changes in membrane potential shown in Figure 6 might be associated with unitary EPSPs from individual synapses whereas downward deflections might represent the action of unitary inhibitory PSPs (IPSPs). At any moment, therefore, the total current delivered to the spike-initiating zone can be considered the algebraic sum of the currents (excitatory and inhibitory) delivered by all of the active synapses. This net current is then transformed into a change in membrane potential at the spike-initiating zone, largely dictated by Ohm's law ($\Delta V = I \times R$). If sufficient current is delivered to drive the membrane potential above the threshold, the neuron spikes. The magnitude of the net current above that needed to reach the threshold determines the rate of spiking (see Chapter 4, Figure 3). The rate of spiking represents a coded message sent to other neurons (or muscle fibers) indicating the intensity of the net (i.e., the *integrated*) synaptic current received by a neuron at any moment. Such *rate coding* is one of the main mechanisms of conveying information throughout the nervous system.

The Problem of Synapse Location

One riddle of synaptic integration has to do with the enormous range of distances that synaptic inputs must travel in order to affect a change in membrane potential at the spike-initiating zone. For example, consider the influence of synaptic input on the spike-initiating zone from a synapse located near the termination of the dendritic tree (greatly foreshortened in the schematic diagram in Figure 7A). The *local* change in membrane potential associated with transmitter release at this synapse might be in the order of 0.5 mV. However, because of the relatively long distance between the synapse and the spike-initiating zone, and because of the inherent losses in signal with distance associated with electrotonic conduction, the magnitude of the EPSP at the spike-initiating zone could be quite small— let's say in this case 0.2 mV.

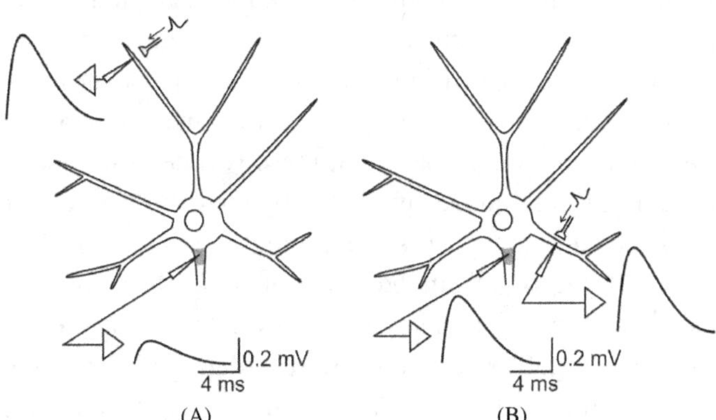

Figure 7.   (A) EPSP at the spike-initiating zone will be small for a synapse located on a distal dendrite compared to that (B) for a synapse located close to the spike-initiating zone.

For a synapse located near the soma (Figure 7B), the local change in membrane potential may be practically the same as for a distant synapse. However, because of the much shorter distance, the magnitude of the EPSP at the spike-initiating zone will be substantially larger (say 0.4 mV) than that of the distant synapse. Keeping this in mind, let's consider a neuron as a miniature government, with the parliament or congress located at the spike-initiating zone. Some members always "vote" yes (excitatory synapse) while others always vote "no" (inhibitory synapses, not unlike some members of actual governments). Moreover, the votes of the members whose homes are close to the site of decision-making count much more than those that live far away. Indeed, with large dendritic arbors (e.g., see Figure 4A), some evidence indicates that synapses beyond about 0.5 to 0.75 mm from the soma would have negligible influence on the spike-initiating zone (Williams & Stuart 2002). Given this, then why would the nervous system go to the trouble to build such expansive dendritic systems if many synaptic contacts on the dendrites would have little effect on synaptic integration?

This is a question that has often been neglected but can present significant problems to theories about information processing in the brain. Some resolution to this conundrum, however, was provided in an important set of studies by Jeffrey Magee and colleagues (2000). In these technically difficult studies, the investigators first injected current pulses of fixed amplitude directly into dendrites located at distal and proximal sites relative to the soma in pyramidal neurons of the hippocampus (Figure 8A). A microelectrode placed into the soma (i.e., adjacent to the spike-initiating zone) detected the change in membrane potential associated with the same current being injected at these two dendritic locations. As shown in Figure 8B, and just as predicted by the cable model, the amplitude of the detected potential was a decaying function of the distance of the site of current injection from the soma, such that the response from the proximal site was substantially larger than from the distal site.

Then the investigators removed the stimulating electrodes from the dendrites and stimulated the axons making synaptic contacts at the proximal and distal locations. Remarkably, the detected membrane potential response at the soma was practically the same for both the

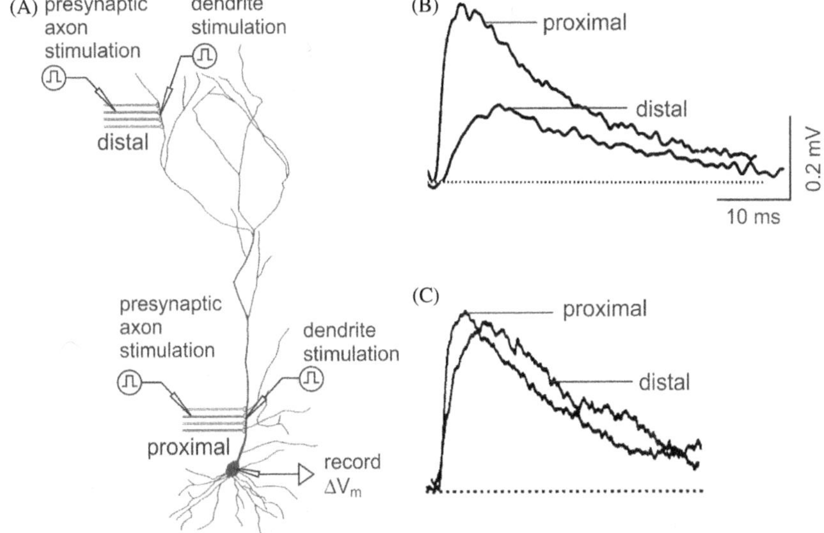

Figure 8.   Demonstration that synapses may compensate for disadvantaged distal location. (A) Arrangement for recording in hippocampal pyramidal neurons. Fixed amplitude current pulses were first delivered intra-dendritically at distal and proximal locations on the dendritic tree. Stimuli were then delivered to presynaptic axons at distal and proximal locations to provoke action potential input and synaptic transmission. The evoked change in membrane potential (ΔV_m) was recorded in response to the two types of stimulation (intra-dendritically and axonally) and from the two locations. (B) As predicted by the cable model, the magnitude of the evoked membrane potential was largest for intra-dendritic current injection at a location close to the soma (proximal). (C) When presynaptic axons were stimulated, however, there was practically no difference in the magnitude of the response for distal versus proximal synaptic sites. (Adapted, from Magee [2000].)

proximal and distal synapses (Figure 8C). A similar finding had been reported much earlier by another group of investigators for synaptic contacts onto motor neurons but where synapse location could only be estimated (Iansek & Redman 1973). Collectively, these findings suggest that some mechanism(s) compensate for the disadvantaged location of the distal synapses.

But what could those mechanisms be? Figure 9 shows some of the possibilities by which distal synapses could compensate for their handicapped positions relative to proximal synapses. In the presynaptic

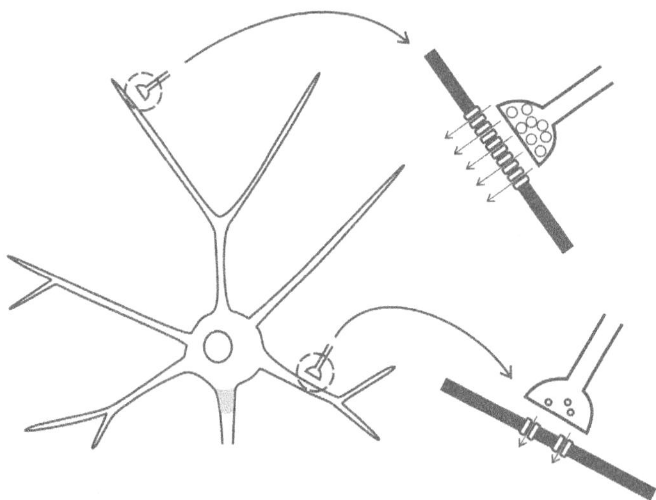

Figure 9. Possible mechanism of compensation for distal synapses. Presynaptically, distal synapses (top right) might have larger synaptic vesicles or more synaptic vesicles with greater numbers of quanta released compared to proximal synapses (bottom right). On the postsynaptic membrane, ligand-gated channels on proximal synapses might have higher conductance (longer arrows) or might have more ligand-gated channels compared to proximal synapses. Any of these factors will lead to an increased synaptic current at distal synapses.

terminal, it could be that more quanta are released or that the amount of neurotransmitter per synaptic vesicle is larger at distal compared to proximal synapses. The problem with this possibility is that the presynaptic neuron would need to "know" where on the dendritic tree of another neuron it had made a synaptic contact in order to adjust transmitter release properties accordingly.

As such, it seems more likely that the compensation takes place on the postsynaptic membrane. It could be that the conductance of ligand-gated channels at distal sites is higher than that at proximal sites (indicated by the length of the arrows in Figure 9) or that there are simply more ligand-gated channels available at distal synapses. Indeed, there is some experimental evidence supporting the latter of these possibilities (Alvarez *et al.*

1997). Regardless, any of these pre- or postsynaptic adaptations would serve to increase the magnitude of the ionic current delivered at distal synapses. As a consequence, the larger amount of current entering distal synapses will help equalize the current delivered to the spike-initiating zone given the greater losses associated with longer electrotonic conduction distances for these synapses. In this way, the synaptic government becomes more democratic.

Summary

The main neurotransmitters acting at directly gated synapses include Ach (in both peripheral and central nervous systems), glutamate, GABA, and glycine. At excitatory synapses, the ions gated by binding of ligand to receptor (nicotinic receptors for Ach and AMPA receptors for glutamate) are primarily Na^+ and K^+ whereas it is Cl^- for inhibitory synapses (GABA and glycine).

As predicted by Hebb, synapses are modifiable (plastic) based on the degree of coactivity in the presynaptic and postsynaptic neurons. The detectors of coincident activity in pre- and postsynaptic neurons are the glutamate NMDA receptors. These channels open when glutamate is available (due to activity in presynaptic neuron) and binds to the receptor, and when the membrane is strongly depolarized (due to activity in the postsynaptic neuron). The influx of Ca^{2+} through these channels triggers the insertion of more AMPA receptors in the synapse's postsynaptic membrane. This leads to a long-lasting increase in the ionic flux at the modified synapse, enhancing its capacity to depolarize the postsynaptic neuron.

A typical neuron requires temporal and spatial summation of hundreds of synaptic inputs for its spike-initiating zone to be brought to the threshold. Such synaptic integration is the main mechanism by which individual neurons process information coming from other neurons. However, synapses located far out on the dendritic tree have an inherent limitation in communicating (and influencing) the spike-initiating zone. Such synapses may partially compensate for this disadvantage by mechanisms that enhance synaptic current delivered at more distant locations.

References

Alvarez FJ, Dewey DE, Harrington DA & Fyffe REW (1997). Cell-type specific organization of glycine receptor clusters in the mammalian spinal cord. *Journal of Comparative Neurology* **379**, 150–169.

Cullheim S, Fleshman JW, Glenn LL & Burke RE (1987). Three-dimensional architecture of dendritic trees in type-identified alpha-motoneurons. *Journal of Comparative Neurology* **255**, 82–96.

Ferreira JS, Schmidt J, Rio P, Águas R, Rooyakkers A, Li KW, Smit AB, Craig AM & Carvalho AL (2015). GluN2B-containing NMDA receptors regulate AMPA receptor traffic through anchoring of the synaptic proteasome. *Journal of Neuroscience* **35**, 8462–8479.

Iansek R & Redman SJ (1973). The amplitude, time course and charge of unitary excitatory post-synaptic potentials evoked in spinal motoneurone dendrites. *Journal of Physiology* **234**, 665–688.

Kerchner GA & Nicoll RA (2008). Silent synapses and the emergence of a post-synaptic mechanism for LTP. *Nature Reviews Neuroscience* **9**, 813–825.

Magee JC (2000). Dendritic integration of excitatory synaptic input. *Nature Reviews Neuroscience* **1**, 181–190.

Malenka RC & Nicoll RA (1999). Long-term potentiation—A decade of progress? *Science* **285**, 1870–1874.

Rioult-Pedotti MS, Friedman D & Donoghue JP (2000). Learning-induced LTP in neocortex. *Science* **290**, 533–536.

Roth RH, Cudmore RH, Tan HL, Hong I, Zhang Y & Huganir RL (2020). Cortical synaptic AMPA receptor plasticity during motor learning. *Neuron* **105**, 895–908.e5.

Williams SR & Stuart GJ (2002). Dependence of EPSP efficacy on synapse location in neocortical pyramidal neurons. *Science* **295**, 1907–1910.

Part 2

Somatosensory System

Chapter 8

General Aspects of Sensory Processing

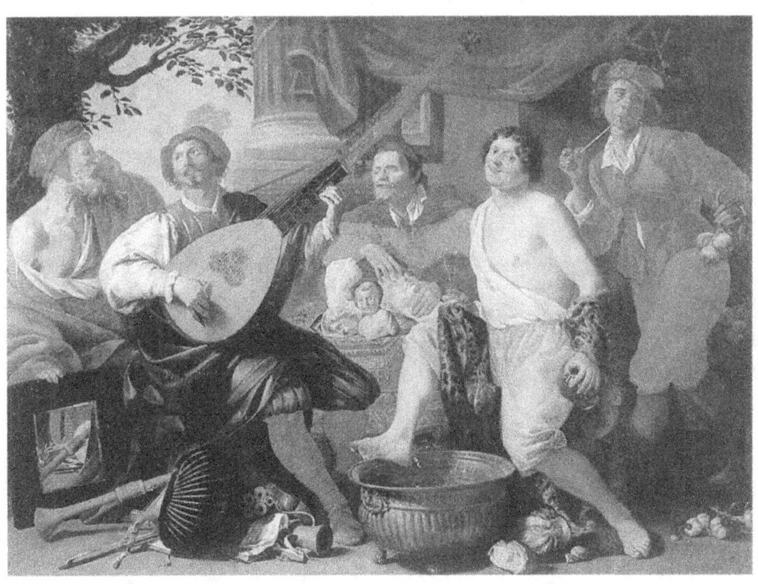

Allegory of the Five Senses, Theador Rombouts, 1632

One of the main functions of the nervous system is to act on information obtained from the outside environment. Specialized cells have evolved for receiving such information. These include the primary sensory neurons responsible for sight, hearing, taste, smell, touch, and temperature.

In addition, there are primary sensory neurons that provide awareness of the positions of body parts and that sense the internal state of the body.

Most external and internal signals are detected by just four main classes of primary sensory neurons. These neurons are also referred to as **receptors** (not to be confused with molecular receptors) based on the signals they respond to. These are the (1) **mechanoreceptors**—responsive to *mechanical signals*, (2) **chemoreceptors**—responsive to *chemical signals*, (3) **photoreceptors**—responsive to *light*, and (4) **thermoreceptors**—responsive to *temperature*. In all cases, the specific stimulus alters the permeability of ion channels in the membrane of the receptor neuron. It should be noted that the terms **primary sensory neuron**, **first-order neuron, receptor neuron**, and **receptor** are all used interchangeably to refer to these neurons that are the gateway to the nervous system.

Somatosensory System

The **somatosensory** system literally means the *"body sense," and largely involves sensations arising from the skin, body wall, tendons, muscles,* and *joints.* Somatosensation is a general term that encompasses a few subdivisions. These include the **tactile** sense—sense of touch, **thermoception**—sense of temperature, **nociception**—sense of pain, and **proprioception**—sense of position and movement of body parts. In addition, **visceroception** or **interoception**—the senses arising from internal organs, is also a form of somatosensation but will not be addressed here. The somatosensory system is emphasized in this book over other sensory systems because it is the system most intimately linked to the control of movement. Furthermore, the somatosensory system is relatively straightforward to understand. As such, it provides a good framework to learn principles of sensory processing that generally apply across the other sensory systems.

Sensory Transduction

Sensory receptor neurons receive physical signals and convert them into biological signals. The process by which this occurs is referred to as

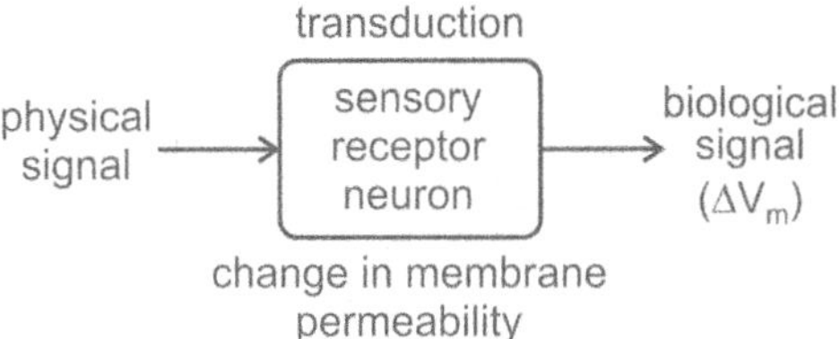

Figure 1.   Physical signals (such as light, sound, pressure, temperature, chemicals) are converted (transduced) by sensory receptor neurons into a biological signal, namely a change in the membrane potential (ΔV_m). The transduction process involves a change in the permeability of the membrane to certain ions caused by opening or closing ion channels.

sensory **transduction** (Figure 1). Regardless of the sensory system, the biological signal that is the outcome of the transduction process is a change in membrane potential in the receptor neuron. This occurs as a consequence of the physical signal (light, temperature, chemicals, pressure, etc.) inducing a change in the permeability of the receptor neuron membrane to certain ions caused by the opening (or closing) of ion channels. This can occur in a variety of ways. For example, mechanical pressure applied to tactile receptors causes the opening of specialized channels equally permeable to Na^+ and K^+ leading to depolarization (Coste *et al.* 2010). In contrast, light absorbed by specialized pigments in photoreceptors of the retina triggers a biochemical cascade that *reduces* the number of open Na^+ channels, leading to decreased depolarization in photoreceptors. In the auditory system, sound pressure waves cause the mechanical opening of K^+ channels leading to rapid changes in the membrane potential of receptor neurons of the cochlea in the inner ear.

Receptor Potential

The *generic term for a change in membrane potential associated with sensory transduction* is the **receptor potential**. Let's consider the genesis of the receptor potential in a somatosensory neuron. First, however, we need to briefly address the anatomy of a typical receptor neuron in the somatosensory system. As shown in Figure 2, the layout is different than that of a typical neuron. For example, there are no dendrites (nor are

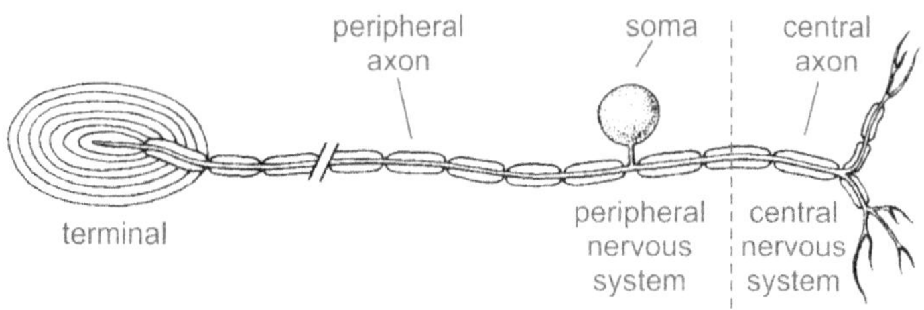

Figure 2.   Morphology of a typical primary sensory neuron of the somatosensory system. (Adapted from Kandel *et al.* 2012.)

dendrites found in receptor neurons of other sensory systems). Instead, there is a specialized apparatus for taking in information from the environment. This apparatus is referred to interchangeably as the **terminal, end organ**, or the **receptor**. This terminology is somewhat confusing because, despite the names, this region is not where signaling ends but rather where signaling begins.

Emerging directly from the terminal is the axon. The axon runs within a nerve of the peripheral nervous system that, at some point, enters the spinal cord or the brainstem (dashed vertical line, Figure 2). At that point, the axon is now within the central nervous system. The soma sits off to the side and is attached to the axon by a little stalk not far from the location where the axon enters the central nervous system. As such, action potentials simply pass by the soma as they traverse along the axon. Critically, the soma, containing the genetic material and important organelles to keep the neuron alive, resides in a ganglion (collection of cell bodies in the peripheral nervous system) that is protected within the bony structure of the vertebral column. If the soma was out near the terminal, it could be readily damaged by day-to-day injuries sustained by our skin, muscles, joints, and tendons. Such damage would quickly lead to the demise of these critical neurons.

Figure 3 shows a schematic diagram of a typical primary sensory neuron of the somatosensory system. A microelectrode placed in the terminal detects changes in membrane potential associated with the transduction process—the so-called receptor potential. A weak stimulus (arrow 1, Figure 3) causes the activation of relatively few ion channels in the membrane of the terminal. The associated receptor potential, therefore, is also relatively weak. The ionic current entering the terminal is

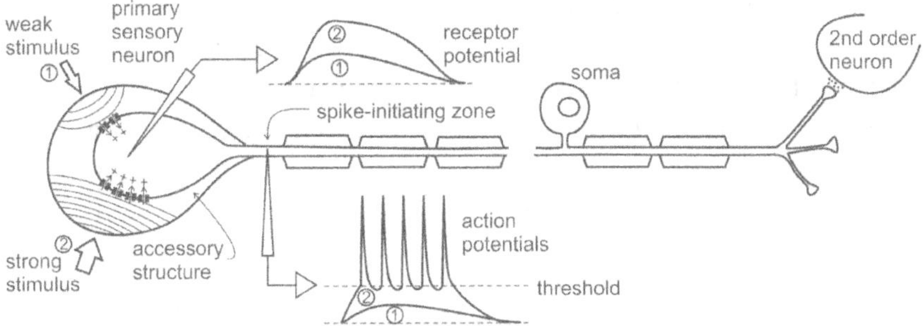

Figure 3.   Genesis of the receptor potential in a typical primary sensory neuron of the somatosensory system. A weak stimulus (arrow 1) activates relatively few channels in the receptor membrane, leading to a small ionic current. A microelectrode in the terminal detects this locally as a small change in potential—the receptor potential. A stronger stimulus (arrow 2) activates proportionately more ion channels, leading to a greater ionic flux and a greater receptor potential. Ionic currents associated with receptor potentials decay with distance as they are conveyed electrotonically to the spike-initiating zone. In the case of the weak stimulus (1), the change in potential at the spike-initiating zone is below the threshold, so no action potentials are produced, and no signal is delivered. For a stronger stimulus (2), the change in potential is above the spike threshold, leading to the instigation of action potentials with a frequency proportional to the magnitude of the receptor potential. These action potentials are sent along the axon into the central nervous system to produce excitatory postsynaptic potentials in the target second-order neurons. The accessory structure serves as an interface between the receptor membrane and the external environment, and can modify the characteristics of the external signal that is delivered to the ion channels that underlie sensory transduction.

conducted passively (and with decay) to the spike-initiating zone near where the axon emerges from the terminal. In this case (weak stimulus 1), the magnitude of the potential at the spike-initiating zone is below the spike threshold, and therefore no signal is communicated further along the axon.

If a stronger stimulus is applied (arrow 2, Figure 3), then proportionately more channels are activated, leading to a larger ionic current and a larger receptor potential. The passive conduction of this current causes a larger depolarization at the spike-initiating zone compared to the weak stimulus. In this case, the depolarization is above the threshold, and a sequence of action potentials is generated. The frequency of the action potentials is proportional to the magnitude of the conducted receptor potential above the threshold. These action potentials are then propagated along the axon, past the soma, and into the central nervous system to trigger the release of neurotransmitters and the excitation of second-order neurons. In virtually all cases, regardless of sensory system, primary sensory neurons make excitatory connections onto their target, the second-order neurons (an exception is found for certain synaptic connections in the retina).

Accessory Structure

In Figure 3, the physical stimulus is shown applied not to the receptor membrane but to a surrounding entity called the **accessory structure**. The accessory structure serves as a kind of *mechanical filter or buffer through which physical signals are transmitted to the receptor membrane*. As such, the accessory structure alters the characteristics of the physical signals that actually influence the ion channels responsible for sensory transduction. An accessory structure can enhance certain attributes of the physical signal while suppressing others. Indeed, the existence of a wide range of receptors in the somatosensory system is largely due to differences in the types of accessory structures associated with specific receptor types. Yet not all sensory receptor neurons possess accessory structures—those that don't are generally referred to as having **free nerve endings**.

Spike-Frequency Adaptation

Most sensory receptor neurons exhibit a *decline in firing rate in response to a sustained stimulus*. This reduction in firing rate is referred to as **spike-frequency adaptation** (or simply **adaptation**). There are two main patterns of adaptation: slow and rapid. As shown in Figure 4A, **slowly adapting receptors** exhibit a *gradual decline in the firing rate over time* during a constant stimulus. Rapidly adapting receptors (Figure 4B), on the other hand, respond in a very unusual way during a sustained stimulus: firing occurs primarily only at the onset and removal of the stimulus. Indeed, a key characteristic of **rapidly adapting receptors** is that they *respond only when the stimulus is changing*. Therefore, during the entire

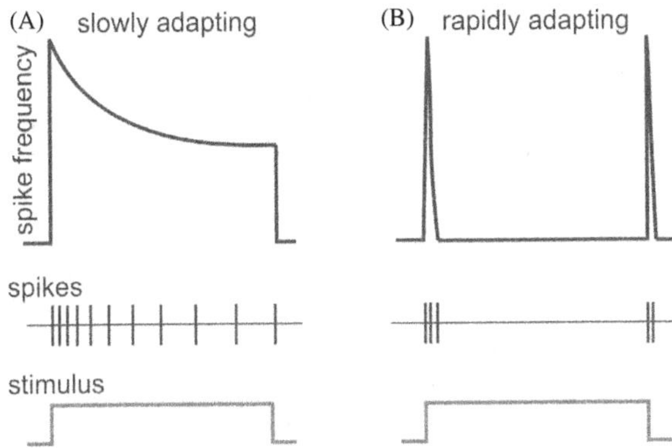

Figure 4.   Firing rate responses to a sustained, constant stimulus in (A) slowly adapting and (B) rapidly adapting sensory receptors.

period even when a strong (but unchanging) stimulus is applied, these sensory receptor neurons tend to be silent.

Adaptation is a key feature used to classify different types of sensory receptor neurons. The mechanisms underlying slow and rapid adaptation are not completely understood and likely vary from one type of receptor neuron to another. For example, adaptation could be due to (1) the *inactivation* of the ion channels responsible for sensory transduction, (2) the progressive *activation* of K^+ channels that tend to counteract the depolarizing action of the sensory transduction, or (3) the influence of the *accessory structure*. Regardless, spike-frequency adaptation can be partially responsible for the changing perception of the intensity of a stimulus. For example, when you jump into the cool water of a swimming pool, you may first experience an intense awareness of cold. However, if you continue to swim, the intensity of the cold sensation gradually abates, that is, you get "used to it." This change in perception of cold in the face of unchanging water temperature is due in part to the adaptation of certain types of thermoreceptors in your skin.

Sensation versus Perception

In the previous section, the terms "sensation" and "perception" were used colloquially and interchangeably. It can be helpful, however, to apply more rigor to the definition of these terms when considering how sensory information is processed. As such, we will use the term **sensation** to refer to the *basic recognition that a stimulus has been applied*. For example, a sensation might refer simply to the awareness that something is touching your finger. **Perception**, on the other hand, is a more complex process and typically *involves integration and interpretation of multiple sensations, with links to memory*. For example, if your eyes are closed and someone places a cold beverage can into your hand, you sense the weight of the object with certain types of receptors, the smooth texture of the can is detected by another set of receptors, the shape of the can is inferred from the receptors that signal the orientation of the fingers grasping the can, the coolness in the object is detected with the thermoreceptors in the skin of the fingers, and so on. From these basic *sensations*, an overall representation is put together giving rise to the *perception* that the thing in your hand is a beverage can. Your ability to formulate such a perception is also partly dependent on your prior knowledge and experience (memory) of such objects. As we shall see, different brain structures underlie sensations and perceptions. It should also be said that the definitions of sensation and perception outlined above may not be universally agreed upon but will be useful in the context of this book.

Dimensions of Sensation

For even the most basic sensation, the nervous system swiftly extracts different kinds of information about the stimulus. These *basic attributes of a sensation* are referred to as the **dimensions of sensation**. These include the **modality**—referring to the *type of sensation*. For example, is the stimulus a touch sensation, a thermal sensation, a painful sensation, or the sensation associated with the movement of a body part? It is the "what." Another attribute that is immediately extracted is the *site of stimulus application*, referred to as **localization**. Was the stimulus applied to the finger, the back of the neck, or the arm? Obviously, this is the "where." And third, we detect the strength of the stimulus, namely its **intensity**. It is the "how much." The dimensions of sensation are the building blocks of sensory processing. What follows is a brief exploration of the mechanisms by which the nervous system extracts these different pieces of information about a stimulus.

Modality

For some time, there were two competing theories about how the nervous system identifies the type of stimulus applied, that is, the *modality*. One is called the **labeled line theory**. This theory is intuitively appealing. It simply proposes that *different kinds of sensory receptors respond preferentially to specific types of stimuli—and that the responses to different stimuli are processed along separate pathways in the nervous system.* Modality, therefore, depends on *which* sensory receptors (and associated pathways) are activated. Because each sensory receptor can convey only a single modality, its axon (the "line") theoretically could be "tagged" as that associated with a particular modality—that is, a "labeled line" (Figure 5). This is no different in principle from how an electrician might label each wire in an electrical cable of a house: that wire goes to the lights in the kitchen, this wire goes to the air-conditioning system, this one supplies the outlets in the living room, and so on. In the nervous system, the cable can be a peripheral nerve, and the wires would be individual axons arising from various sensory receptors. If a particular line is activated, then the individual will sense that specific modality.

The other theory is called the **pattern theory**. It proposes that *individual pathways can convey information about different modalities based*

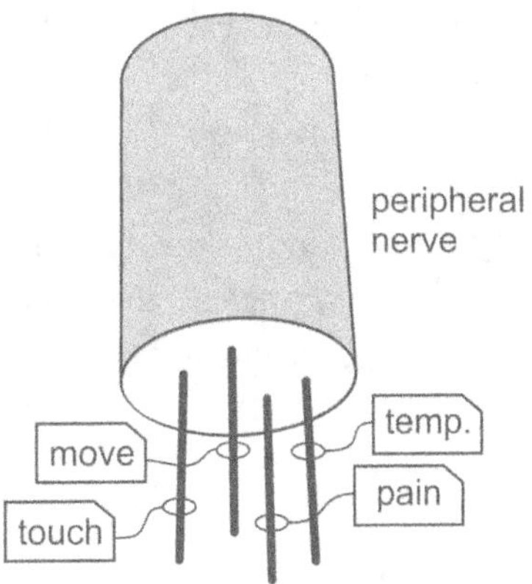

Figure 5.   Labeled line theory. Each sensory receptor responds preferentially to a specific type of stimulus. The axon (line) from each receptor type in a peripheral nerve could be labeled with tags representing the type of sensation perceived when that line is activated.

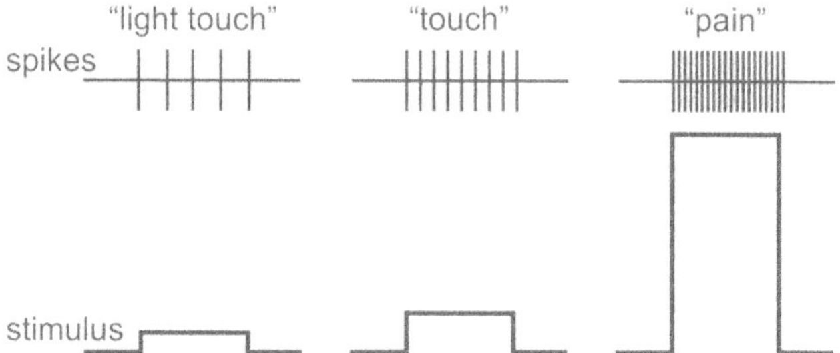

Figure 6.   Pattern theory. The pattern (frequency) of action potentials dictates which modality is perceived. A weak touch stimulus provokes low-frequency action potentials and is perceived as a light touch. A modest intensity stimulus generates a higher-frequency train of action potentials and is perceived simply as a touch. A very strong stimulus produces a high frequency of action potentials and is perceived as pain.

on the pattern (or frequency) of action potentials set up in the pathway. A particular role of the pattern theory has been ascribed to how touch sensations are distinguished from painful ones. For example, under the pattern theory of coding modality, light pressure applied to the skin would cause a low firing rate of receptor neurons, which would then be interpreted by the brain as a gentle touch (Figure 6). Moderate pressure would lead to higher firing rates and a perception of stronger touch. Intense pressure that could potentially lead to tissue damage would trigger very high firing rates in the receptor neurons. These high firing rates would now be interpreted as a painful stimulus.

Experimental evidence (discussed in Chapter 9) quite convincingly demonstrated that the labeled line theory is the most probable explanation as to how the nervous system distinguishes touch from pain; indeed, how most modalities are encoded. Nevertheless, there may be some role for the pattern of action potentials in distinguishing some sub-modalities from one another (as will also be discussed).

Localization

Our knowledge about where a stimulus has been applied derives largely from the topographic organization of the somatosensory system. **Topographic organization** refers to the *preservation of the relative spatial* *locations of the sensory receptors in the periphery as sensory signals are conveyed along ascending pathways.* Namely, there is a systematic "mapping" (i.e., topography) of peripheral receptor locations onto higher brain structures.

This can be readily understood by considering, for example, the spatial locations of tactile receptors supplying the thumb, index finger, and middle finger (Figure 7). The receptors in the skin of the index finger are

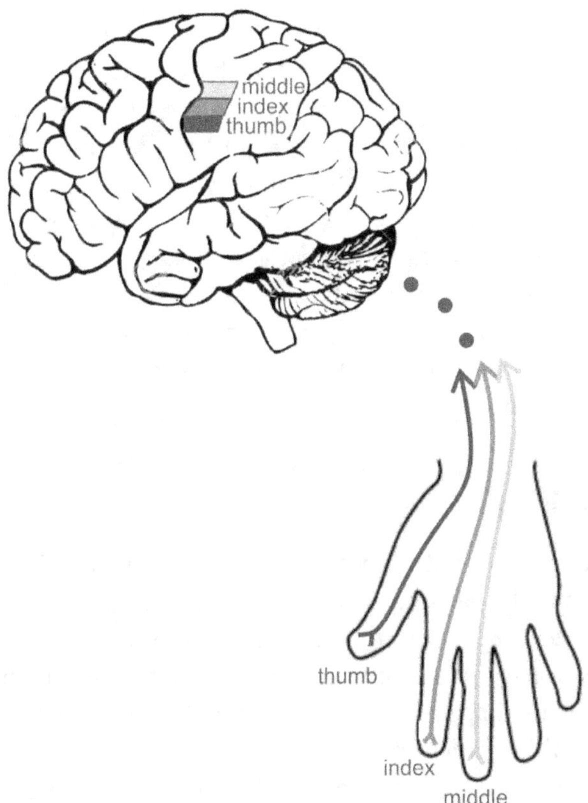

Figure 7.   Topographic organization. The relative locations of sensory receptors in the periphery (e.g., those supplying the skin of the thumb, index, and middle fingers) are maintained and mapped onto higher brain structures. For example, in the somatosensory cortex, the region representing the index finger is physically situated between those regions representing the thumb and middle finger, replicating the relative spatial configuration of those body parts.

physically located between the receptors supplying the skin of the thumb and those innervating the skin of the middle finger. The signals arising from the activation of those receptors are processed along a pathway involving a series of structures in the central nervous system that culminates in the somatosensory cortex of the brain (Figure 7). At each of these processing stations, the neurons processing and conveying information about touch to the index finger are physically located between those neurons representing the thumb and those representing the middle finger (as shown schematically in Figure 7 for the somatosensory cortex). As such, information about where the stimulus was applied to the body is indicated by the location of the neurons activated by the stimulus. Such *topographic organization within the somatosensory system* is sometimes referred to as **somatotopy**. There are equivalent types of topographic organization for other sensory systems. For example, some of the brain structures responsible for conveying and processing visual information are spatially organized based on the locations of the photoreceptors in the retina, referred to as "retinotopic" organization. In the auditory system, it is not the spatial location of sounds but their pitch (i.e., their "tone") that is spatially represented in different auditory brain regions. This is referred to as a "tonotopic" organization.

Receptive Field

A critical concept related to localization is the receptive field (RF) of a sensory neuron. The **RF** simply refers to the *spatial location within which a stimulus causes a neuron to fire*. Figure 8A shows schematically an array of RFs for tactile receptor neurons in the skin on the back of the hand. Touch stimuli applied within the highlighted RF will be detected as action potentials recorded from the axon of the sensory receptor neuron. Figure 8B shows the locations and sizes of actual RFs recorded from a few tactile receptor neurons supplying the palmar skin of the human hand.

Overlap

One interesting aspect of the organization of RFs is that they typically **overlap**. Namely, *the territory of a given sensory neuron's RF is partially*

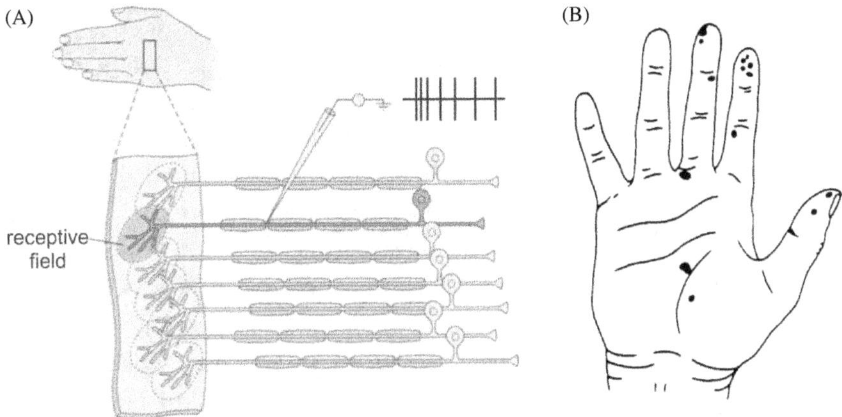

Figure 8.   (A) Overlapping RFs of tactile receptors on the back of the hand. Touch stimuli applied within a neuron's RF will cause it to fire. (B) Actual RFs of a subset of tactile receptors recorded from the human hand. ([A] Adapted from Kandel *et al.* [2012]; [B] from Johansson and Vallbo [1983].)

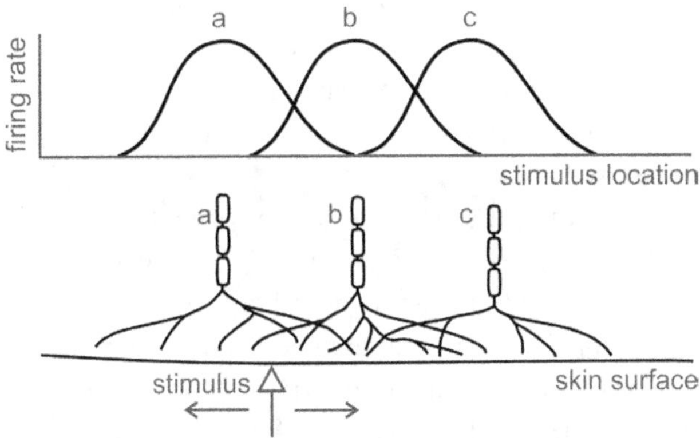

Figure 9.   Firing rate profiles and RFs for three neighboring neurons. As a fixed amplitude stimulus is applied closer to the center of the RF of a given neuron, the firing rate increases. Also, RFs can exhibit substantial overlap. (Adapted from Brown [1989].)

shared with other neurons. This is shown schematically for an array of three neighboring tactile receptor neurons in Figure 9. The firing rate responses to the same mechanical stimulus applied to different skin locations are also shown in the upper part of Figure 9. Obviously, if the touch location is outside (to the far left or right) of any of the RFs, no firing rates are detected. When the stimulus is presented to the leftmost edge of the RF for *neuron a*, then a low firing rate response is recorded in *neuron a*. As the same stimulus is applied to slightly more rightward locations within the RF of *neuron a*, the firing rates become higher. If the stimulus is applied near the center of the RF for *neuron a*, then the firing rate is maximal. Applying the stimulus to locations progressively to the right of the center of the RF leads to a decrease in the recorded firing rates in *neuron a*. Overall, this gives rise to a more or less symmetric, bell-shaped profile of firing rate for different locations within the neuron's RF. This type of profile is similar for *neuron b* and *neuron c*. Note, however, that before the stimulus is beyond the boundaries of the RF of one neuron, neighboring neurons begin to be activated; namely, the RFs overlap.

At first glance, this overlap might seem a trivial outcome of the nervous system "coloring outside the lines" when laying down sensory nerve endings in the periphery. Indeed, biomedical engineers, who are developing sensory arrays in the coverings of prosthetic hands, tile the sensors such that each pixel-like sensor is exclusively responsible for a separate small patch of the artificial skin, thereby avoiding the apparent sloppiness of natural receptor overlap. Yet, it turns out that overlap in the RFs in biological systems is a clever design feature that actually improves precision in sensory processing.

To understand this, let's first consider a case where there is no overlap (Figure 10A). Each receptor neuron's RF is clearly delineated and is separate from the neighbors. Now, let's identify the response of these neurons to a mechanical stimulus applied to two different locations on the skin. Site 1 is on the left side of the RF of *neuron b* and causes a firing rate in *neuron b* of 10 impulses/s (imp/s). Site 2 is on the right side of the RF of *neuron b* and also causes a firing rate of 10 imp/s. This equivalence in firing rate is due to the symmetry in the firing rate profiles for individual receptor neurons. In both cases, the only information delivered into the central nervous system is that *neuron b* fired at 10 imp/s. As such, there would be no way for the nervous system to distinguish the location of the stimulus at sites 1 and 2—they would "feel" the same. It should be kept in mind that the distance between sites 1 and 2 could be substantial—indeed, the RFs of some sensory receptors can be centimeters in diameter.

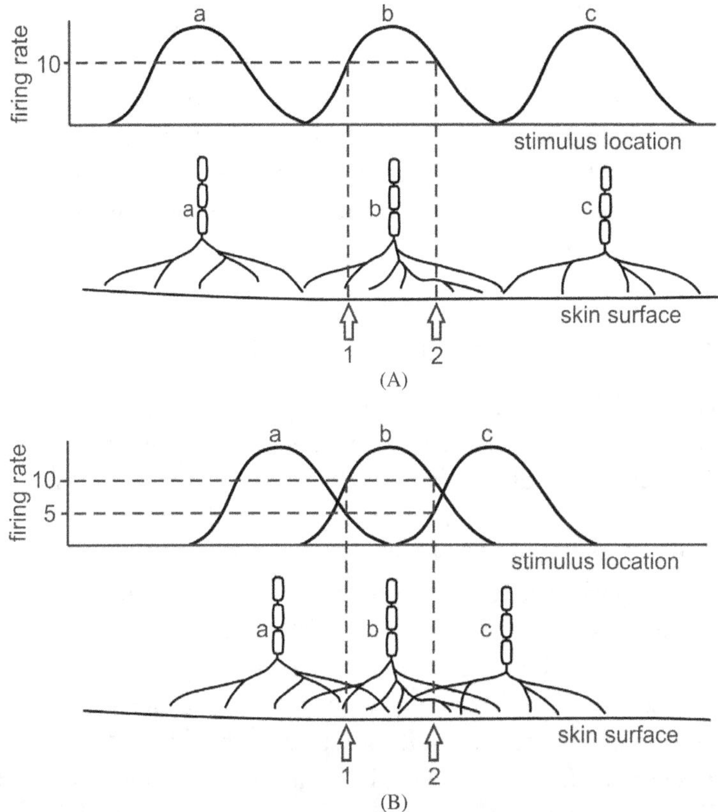

Figure 10.   Importance of receptive-field overlap. (A) No overlap in RFs. Stimulus at location 1 would cause *neuron b* to fire at 10 imp/s as would the stimulus at location 2. Therefore, stimulus location is ambiguous. (B) Overlap of RFs. Stimulus at location 1 causes *neuron b* to fire at 10 imp/s and *neuron a* to fire at 5 imp/s. Stimulus at location 2 causes *neuron b* to fire at 10 imp/s and *neuron c* to fire at 5 imp/s. Therefore, the neural code is unique and distinguishable for the two locations.

Figure 10B shows the responses to the stimulus at the same locations but now the RFs overlap. The stimulus at site 1 causes *neuron b* to fire at 10 imp/s (as before) and also causes *neuron a* to fire at 5 imps/s. When the stimulus is applied at site 2, *neuron b* fires 10 imp/s and *neuron c* 5 imp/s. As such, there is a unique and distinguishable code for each location: site 1 = *neuron b* at 10 imp/s AND *neuron a* at 5 imp/s; site 2 = *neuron b* at 10 imp/s AND *neuron c* at 5 imp/s. The central nervous system interprets these codes that are based on the activities of more than one neuron (sometimes called a population code) to identify where the stimulus was applied. Indeed, at *every* location along the span of skin shown in Figure 10B, there will be a unique neural code of stimulus location. This improvement in the ability to specify the location of a stimulus derives from overlapping the RFs. Indeed, such a strategy is implemented in a number of ways for a variety of sensory systems.

Receptive Fields in Higher-Order Neurons

The concept of RFs not only applies to primary sensory receptors but also to the higher-order neurons they communicate with. Figure 11 shows a simplified schematic of an array of first-order (receptor) neurons, the second-order neurons they project to, and the third-order neurons that receive input from the second-order neurons. First, consider the response to a stimulus applied near the center of the RF for primary sensory *neuron c.* If above the threshold, the stimulus will trigger a sequence of action potentials (arrow 1) that ascend along *neuron c*'s axon. Within the central nervous system, axons typically give off many branches (only two are shown in Figure 11 for simplicity), with each branch usually targeting different neurons. It should be noted that at such branch points, the number of action potentials set up in each daughter branch is equal to the total number of action potentials entering the branch point. For example, if 10 action potentials enter the branch point, then 10 action potentials would be delivered along both the left and right branches of the axon of *neuron c.* In this way, the same information is conveyed to all the postsynaptic neurons. The *process by which the same information is delivered to multiple targets through branching of axons* is referred to as **divergence.**

The flip side of divergence is **convergence.** This term indicates that *a given higher-order neuron receives input from multiple sources.* In other words, multiple neurons send input that focuses upon a particular neuron. For example, in Figure 11, action potentials set up in *neuron c* **diverges** to act on *neurons e* and *f.* Conversely, *neuron e* receives **converging** input from lower-order *neurons b* and *c.*

One consequence of such divergence and convergence is that higher-order neurons tend to have larger RFs than lower-order neurons. As shown

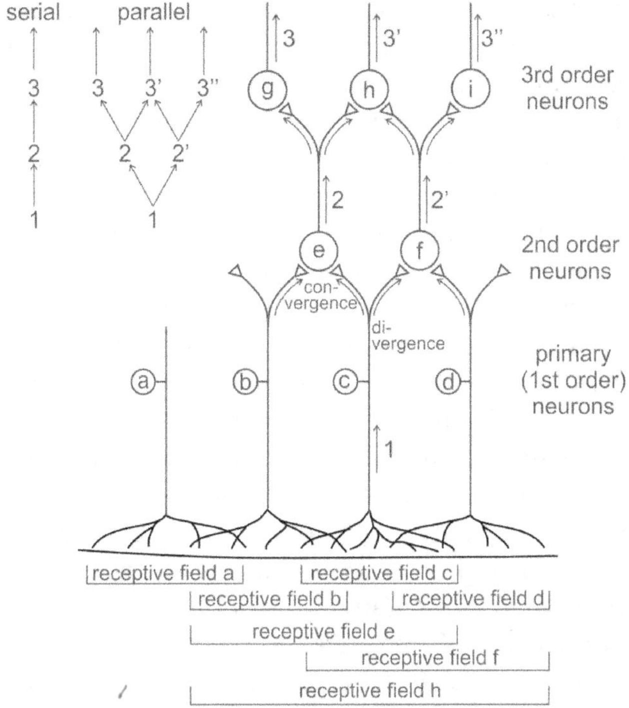

Figure 11.   Axons from first-order neurons (*a, b, c, d*) diverge to contact multiple second-order neurons (e.g., *e* and *f*). Second-order neurons diverge to contact multiple third-order neurons (e.g., *g, h*, and *i*). A given higher-order neuron (e.g., *neuron e*) receives converging input from multiple lower-order neurons. As a consequence of this divergence and convergence, RFs are more expansive for higher-order neurons. The delivery of information along a sequence of progressively higher-order neurons (arrow 1, arrow 2, arrow 3) is referred to as serial processing (inset upper left). Divergence of connections means that the same information may be processed along multiple paths at the same time, referred to as parallel processing.

in Figure 11, the RF of the second-order *neuron e* encompasses that of the first-order *neurons b* and *c* and as such has a larger RF than the first-order neurons. Likewise, the second-order *neuron f* has a RF that includes the RFs of first-order *neurons c* and *d*. The RF of the third-order *neuron h* encompasses the RFs of second-order *neurons e* and *f*, and therefore, has the largest RF of all the neurons shown.

It should be recognized that an individual neuron, in such an array of sensory neurons, can "know" only if a stimulus has been applied to its RF.

It has no information as to where within the RF the stimulus was delivered. As a consequence, at higher levels in a sensory pathway, individual neurons have broader, and as such, blurrier information about stimulus location. However, when information from multiple neurons is put together (as discussed earlier in terms of a population code for RF overlap), more precise localization can occur.

The *conveyance of information from lower-order to progressively higher-order neurons means that there will be a temporal sequence of processing steps* (first-order neurons, then second order, then third, etc.) referred to as **serial processing**. This is depicted in Figure 11, for example, by activity in *neuron c* (arrow 1) then being processed and advanced by *neuron e* (arrow 2), and then that information being processed and advanced by *neuron g* (arrow 3). At the same time, and as a consequence of divergence, *information is processed and delivered along multiple pathways* referred to as **parallel processing**. Therefore, information about a touch stimulus applied to the RF of *neuron c* (arrow 1) is passed on to second-order *neurons e* and *f* (arrows 2 and 2′), which is then passed on to third-order *neurons g, h,* and *i* (arrows 3, 3′, and 3″).

Keep in mind, Figure 11 is a simplified schematic. In reality, information about a single stimulus may be carried along numerous pathways at the same time (instead of just a few as shown in Figure 11), with the number of pathways increasing at higher levels in the sensory hierarchy. Such parallel processing means that information about a stimulus can be richly represented across a large population of neurons with each pathway encoding slightly different aspects of the stimulus. From a clinical perspective, such parallel processing is important. Namely, if there is damage to one pathway, there remain other parallel routes by which information can be delivered and processed. This effect is most pronounced at the highest levels of the nervous system—within the cerebral cortex, with the greatest extent of parallel pathways. Consequently, individuals with damage or lesions to circumscribed regions of the cortex may exhibit surprisingly minor (or even undetectable) long-lasting deficits.

Acuity

Another important aspect of localization is *how precisely one can identify where a stimulus has been applied*, referred to as **acuity**. In the

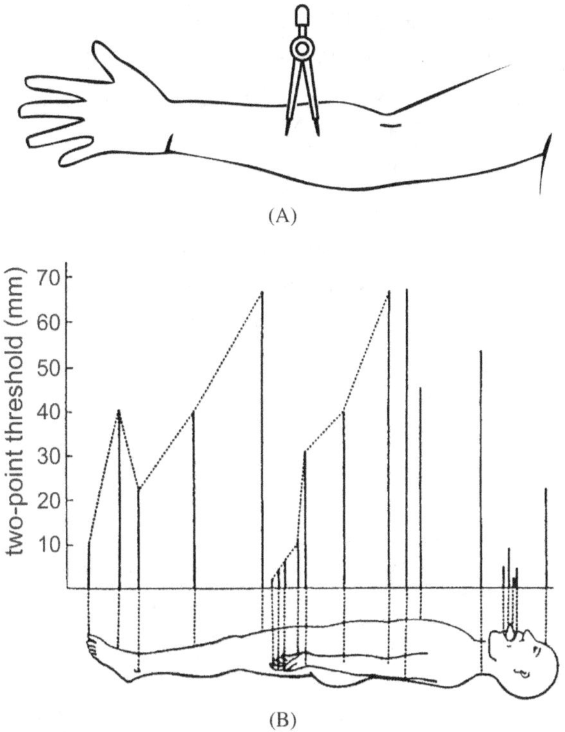

Figure 12.   Two-point threshold. (A) One or two probes of a caliper are touched to a region of the skin and the subject reports whether they feel one or two stimuli. This is repeated for progressively narrower spacing between the probes. The minimum distance at which the subject consistently and accurately reports two stimuli when indeed two stimuli were delivered is the two-point threshold. (B) Map of two-point thresholds across the body surface. Small values of the two-point threshold indicate high spatial acuity. ([B] Adapted from Weinstein [1968]).

somatosensory system, acuity varies considerably over the body surface. One approach used to assess acuity for tactile stimuli is called the two-point threshold method. With the subject's eyes closed, either one or two points of a pair of calipers are randomly applied to a site on the skin, and the subject is asked to report whether they felt one or two stimuli (Figure 12A). The experimenter progressively reduces the spacing between the two points until the subject can no longer distinguish one from two points. The *minimum distance at which a subject accurately reports feeling two stimuli when indeed two stimuli are delivered* is deemed the **two-point threshold**. Figure 12B shows the outcome of two-point threshold testing over the body surface. Note that on the fingertips and around the mouth, two points can be accurately detected when only a few *millimeters* apart. On the other hand, when applied to the upper leg, upper arm, or back, stimuli have to be several *centimeters* apart before subjects can correctly distinguish two stimuli from one.

What can account for such widely different levels of acuity as indicated in the two-point threshold map? There are a number of different mechanisms that interact to shape acuity. Some of these are depicted schematically in Figure 13. Large open circles are meant to represent RFs

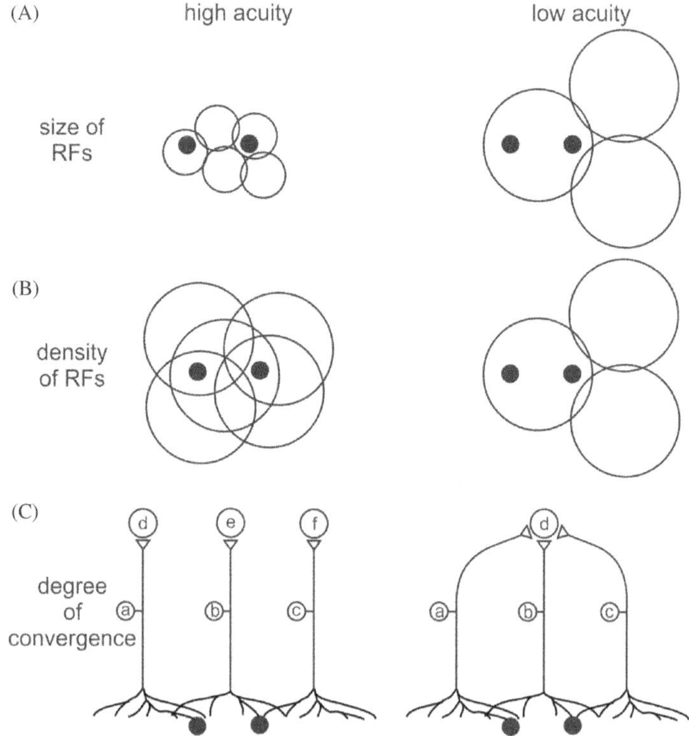

Figure 13.   Schematic indicating factors that affect acuity. In (A) and (B), open circles indicate a planar projection of the RFs of first-order neurons on the surface of the skin. Filled small circles indicate locations where stimuli are applied to the skin. (A) High acuity is associated with small RFs. (B) High acuity is associated with high density of receptors. (C) High acuity associated with low degree of convergence onto higher-order neurons.

of individual first-order neurons projected onto the skin surface. Small, filled circles indicate two different locations where stimuli might be applied to the skin, first at one location and then at the other. The question is whether a person would be able to distinguish stimuli applied to these two locations. For example, Figure 13A shows how the **size of RFs** affect acuity. The left side shows a site with small RFs whereas the right side shows a site with larger RFs. With small RFs, the two stimuli activate different sets of receptors. Therefore, different (and distinguishable) neural signals would be set up for stimuli applied to the two locations. In the case of large RFs, the two stimuli would activate the same primary sensory neuron. As such, there would be no way to distinguish one location from the other.

Another important mechanism affecting acuity is the **density of receptors**. The schematic shown in Figure 13B show two cases: high density of receptors on the left and low density of receptors on the right. In both cases, the sizes of the RFs are the same. In the case of the high density of receptors, the leftmost stimulus would activate a particular array of neurons, say *neurons a, b*, and *c* whereas the rightmost stimulus would activate a different array of neurons, say *a, d*, and *e*. As such, different neural populations are activated by the stimulus applied to the two locations and therefore the two stimulus sites should be distinguishable. In the case of low density of receptors (right side, Figure 13B), the two stimulus locations might simply activate the same neuron, and therefore the stimuli at the two locations would not be distinguishable.

A third important factor influencing acuity has to do with the degree of **convergence** onto higher-order neurons. The diagrams depicted in Figure 13C show simplified representations of the connections between primary sensory neurons and their second-order neurons. The left side shows a situation of very low convergence with each primary sensory neuron targeting only one higher-order neuron. The right side shows a case of high convergence with all three lower-order neurons converging onto a single second-order neuron. In the case of low convergence, the leftmost stimulus activates primary sensory *neurons a* and *b*, which in turn activate higher-order *neurons d* and *e*. The rightmost stimulus activates primary sensory *neurons b* and *c*, which excite higher-order *neurons e* and *f*. Consequently, stimuli applied to those two locations are distinguishable because different populations of higher-order neurons are activated. Under the high convergence situation (right side, Figure 13C), stimuli applied at both locations causes the same higher-order *neuron d* to be activated. Therefore, the same neural signal is advanced from the second-order neuron in response to stimuli applied to the two different locations. As such, the locations of the two stimuli will not be distinguishable—namely the acuity will be poor.

A fourth and very intriguing mechanism that affects acuity is referred to as **surround or lateral inhibition**. This mechanism refers to a specific pattern of connections among neurons at second-order levels and higher. To give the bottom line first, **acuity is enhanced with an increased degree of surround inhibition**. But what exactly do we mean by surround inhibition and how does it improve acuity? To answer these questions, let's begin by first describing the phenomenon associated with surround inhibition.

Surround Inhibition

Figure 14 shows an experiment from the 1950s during which Vernon Mountcastle and colleagues were characterizing RFs in the somatosensory cortex of monkeys. A microelectrode placed in the cortex recorded action potentials of single neurons during the application of tactile stimuli (Figure 14A). In the example shown, the RF of the recorded neuron was a relatively large area on the forearm (dotted region, Figure 14B). This large RF is consistent with the idea that at higher levels of sensory processing, the RFs of individual neurons are large. The neuron recorded in this instance would have been at least fourth order or higher.

While applying touch stimuli to the RF of the neuron, it was discovered that *simultaneous touch to regions surrounding the RF caused a marked inhibition of the firing* of the neuron. The shaded region neighboring the RF in Figure 14B indicates this so-called **inhibitory surround**. Figure 14C shows the firing rate of the neuron during touch to the RF and then to the inhibitory surround. The top line drawn above the firing rate response indicates when the stimulus was delivered to the RF. The lower line indicates when a touch stimulus was applied to the inhibitory surround. When first touching just within the RF (starting at about 4 s), the

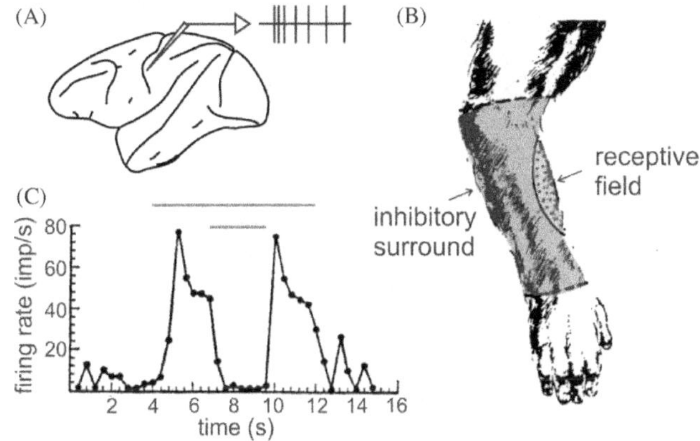

Figure 14.   Evidence for surround inhibition. (A) Recording of single neuron in monkey somatosensory cortex. (B) RF (dotted area) and inhibitory surround (shaded area) for neuron recorded in monkey somatosensory cortex. (C) Firing rate response to touch in RF (upper horizontal line) and simultaneous touch in the inhibitory surround (lower horizontal line). (Adapted from Mountcastle and Powell [1959].)

neuron increased its spiking rate up to ~75 imp/s. The firing rate then slowly dropped off, perhaps due to spike-frequency adaptation. Then beginning at about 7 s into the record, touch was simultaneously applied to the inhibitory surround. This caused a strong suppression of firing of the neuron during the entire time the inhibitory surround was touched. At about 10 s, the touch to the inhibitory surround was removed, and the firing rate of the neuron sprung back to a high firing rate followed by a slow reduction in rate—similar to what was seen upon the original application of the stimulus to the RF. Then at around 12 s, touch to the RF was removed and the firing rate of the neuron decreased back to its background level.

Importantly, when the investigators placed their recording electrode in different locations in the somatosensory cortex, a similar pattern was found—RFs of neurons were encompassed by a surrounding region that caused inhibition. It was also discovered that such an arrangement was evident at lower levels of processing, at second- and third-order neurons. Furthermore, inhibitory surround is not just a phenomenon of the somatosensory system but is also a feature of other sensory systems. Clearly the nervous system dedicates substantial processing to implement inhibitory

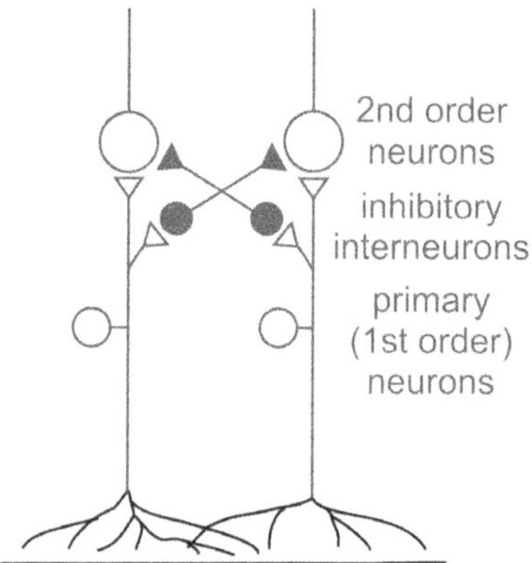

Figure 15.   Basic circuit underlying surround inhibition. Open symbols denote excitatory neurons and synapses, filled symbols denote inhibitory neurons and synapses. First-order neurons, in addition to exciting second-order neurons, excite inhibitory interneurons that suppress the neighboring second-order neurons.

surround—but why? To address that question, it is important to first understand the neural circuitry that accounts for surround inhibition.

The basic circuit that can account for surround inhibition is depicted in Figure 15. In this diagram, individual primary sensory neurons project to and excite their own second-order projection neurons. The axons of the primary sensory neurons, however, also diverge to make synaptic contact onto local inhibitory interneurons. The inhibitory interneurons synapse onto and tend to suppress activity in the neighboring second-order projection neurons. (*Note*: Throughout this book, filled circles and triangles represent inhibitory neurons and their synaptic terminals, whereas open circles and triangles indicate excitatory neurons and their terminals.) This arrangement is complementary: if a primary sensory neuron inhibits (via its inhibitory interneurons) the second-order projection neurons of its neighbors, then its projection neuron can receive more or less equivalent inhibition from the neighboring neurons.

For example, let's assume we are recording the spiking activity of the second-order neuron on the left. If we apply a stimulus to the center of the RF of its primary sensory neuron, then we should detect significant activity in this neuron. Now, while we maintain the stimulus in its RF, we simultaneously touch the RF of the neighboring primary sensory neuron.

This second touch will excite the second-order projection neuron on the right. In addition, this second touch will activate the local inhibitory interneuron to suppress activity in the second-order neuron that we are recording from. This pattern of responses is similar to that depicted for the neuron recorded in the somatosensory cortex shown in Figure 14C.

Of course, the second-order neuron depicted in Figure 15 not only receives inhibition from the neighbor on the right but also from neighbors on left (not shown), and neighbors that would be into the page and out of the page. Furthermore, the inhibition that a higher-order neuron receives is not necessarily only from its immediate neighbors but could be farther afield. A more realistic (although still simplified) diagram is shown in Figure 16. The middle second-order neuron receives converging excitation from a set of primary sensory neurons with overlapping RFs. As such, the RF of the highlighted second-order neuron encompasses the RFs of the inner set of primary sensory neurons. The primary sensory neurons with RFs surrounding that set each project to and excite their own second-order neurons, only two of which are shown (on the left and on the right). Furthermore, each of the primary sensory neurons in the surrounding area, when activated, will excite inhibitory interneurons that target and diminish the activity of the middle second-order neuron. Therefore, the RF of

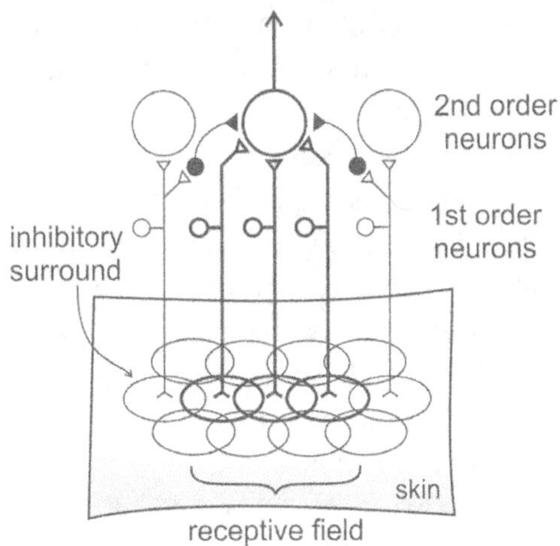

Figure 16.   Schematic depicting RF and surround inhibition for a given second-order neuron.

the second-order neuron is literally surrounded by a band of neurons that can suppress its activity. For simplicity, the connections to inhibitory interneurons from the primary sensory neurons making up the indicated RF are not shown in Figure 16. Finally, it is important to point out that the type of circuitry shown in Figure 16 can also be found at connections between second- and third-order neurons and between third- and fourth-order neurons.

Now that we understand the circuitry that underlies surround inhibition, how is it useful in sensory processing? To gain insight into that question, let's consider two situations, one in which there is no surround inhibition, and one in which surround inhibition is in place. Figure 17A shows the simplest case for two neighboring primary tactile neurons and the second-order neurons they project to with no surround inhibition. A touch stimulus using a cotton swab applied closer to the center of the receptive of *neuron a* and then to *neuron b* will cause *a* to fire at a higher rate than *b*. To have some numbers with which to carry out some simple arithmetic, let's say *neuron a* fires at 10 imp/s and *neuron b* at 6 imp/s in response to the stimulus that is applied for 1 s.

Let's assume that the connections between the primary and second-order neurons are very potent; indeed, so strong that each action potential delivered by a first-order neuron triggers a corresponding action potential in the second-order neuron. Given what was discussed in Chapter 7 about synaptic integration, that might seem unrealistic. Yet, there is clear evidence that such 1-for-1 synaptic transmission can take place in somatosensory (Gynther *et al.* 1995, Vallbo 1995) and other sensory pathways (e.g., Futai *et al.* 2001). Consequently, in our example, second-order *neurons a′* and *b′* will discharge at 10 and 6 imp/s, respectively. We will assume that this pattern of activity is ultimately conveyed to the cerebral cortex. The cerebral cortex is the seat of conscious awareness—like a little person in your brain who is observing and interpreting what is taking place based on the signals it receives. In this case, it receives 10 imp/s on the line associated with the RF of *neuron a* and 6 imp/s on the line related to the RF of *neuron b*. This represents a 67% difference in firing rates on these two paths (Figure 17B). Therefore, the intensity of activities

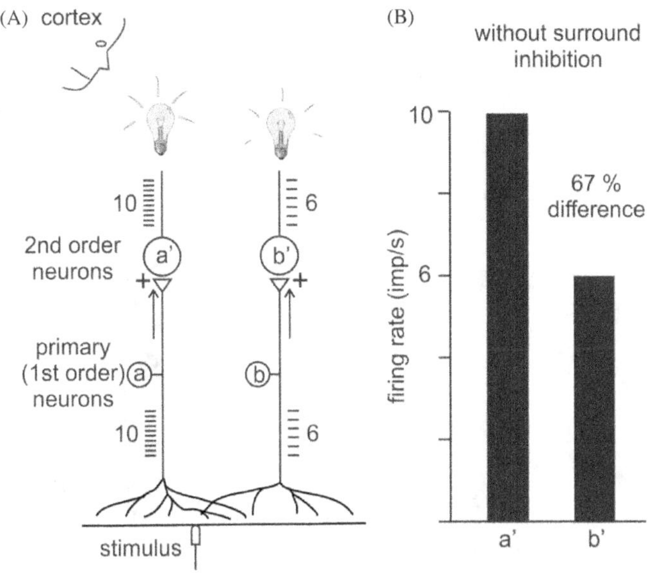

Figure 17.   Effect of surround inhibition. (A) A simple circuit without surround inhibition. A 1-s touch stimulus causes the first-order *neuron a* to fire 10 impulses and *neuron b* to fire six. The excitatory synapses onto the second-order neurons are potent, causing the second-order *neurons a′ and b′* to fire 1-for-1. As such, (B) the firing rates of *a′* and *b′* are 10 and 6 impulses/s, respectively—a 67% difference. This information is eventually conveyed to the cerebral cortex, which uses it to ascertain the location of the stimulus. (C) The circuit including surround inhibition. Activity in first-order *neuron a* strongly excites second-order *neuron a′* and also excites the inhibitory interneuron. The strength of this synapse is such that two arriving impulses are needed to evoke one impulse in the inhibitory neuron. As such a total of five impulses are conveyed to the neighboring second-order *neuron b′*. Each of these inhibitory events extinguishes an impulse that otherwise would have been set up in the second-order neuron. The same principles hold for the first-order *neuron b*. As such, its six impulses will set up three impulses on its inhibitory neuron, which are then delivered to the second-order *neuron a′*. Therefore, the output of *neuron a′* will be 10 − 3 = 7 impulses, whereas *neuron b′* will be 6 − 5 = 1 impulse. This represents (D) a 600% difference in the firing rates conveyed to the cortex. This amplification of the differences in firing rates across these two pathways enables better localization of the stimulus to pathway *a*.

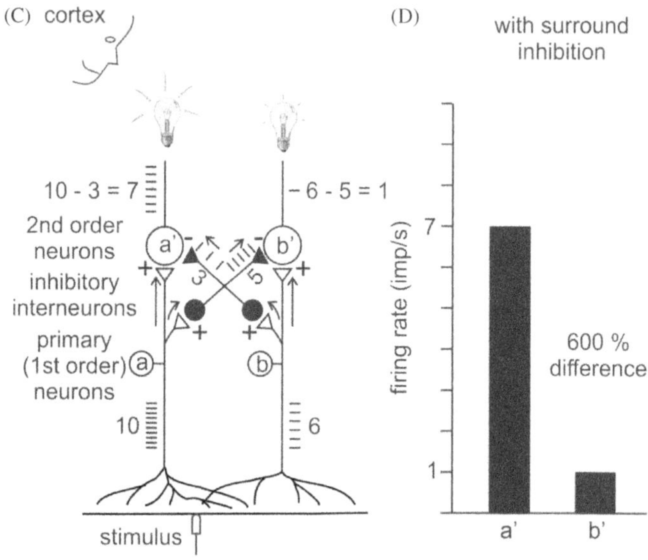

Figure 17.   (*Continued*)

(the "lighting up") of the associated cortical regions will only be modestly different—making the task of determining where precisely the stimulus is located somewhat blurry for the little person in your brain.

Now, let's include the circuitry underlying surround inhibition into this system (Figure 17C). The connections between primary sensory neurons and their second-order neurons are the same as before. However, each primary sensory neuron now has an axon branch to excite an inhibitory interneuron that acts to suppress activity in the neighboring second-order neuron. The potency of the synaptic connection of primary sensory neurons to inhibitory interneurons is typically weaker than that to the second-order projection neurons. For simplicity, therefore, let's assume that temporal summation of two presynaptic action potentials is needed to drive the postsynaptic potential in the inhibitory interneuron above the threshold to generate one action potential, that is, a 2-for-1 synapse (two action potentials "in" yield one action potential "out"). In that case, the inhibitory interneuron receiving 10 imp/s from *neuron a* will discharge at 5 imp/s whereas the inhibitory interneuron receiving 6 imp/s from *neuron b* will generate 3 imp/s.

Let's also assume that the synaptic connections between the inhibitory interneurons and the second-order neurons are strong. Indeed, let's assume that every synaptic input delivered by an inhibitory interneuron is sufficient to eliminate an action potential that otherwise would have been set up in the second-order neuron. We can think of this as a 1-to-minus-1 synapse. If we now perform schematic arithmetic and simply sum up the effects of the excitatory and inhibitory inputs onto the second-order neurons, we will find that the output of *neuron a'* will be 10 imp/s – 3 imp/s = 7 imp/s. Likewise, the output of *neuron b'* will be 6 imp/s – 5 imp/s = 1 imp/s. The difference in the activities on these two pathways is now 600% (Figure 17D). This makes the task of interpreting where the stimulus is located much easier for the cortex. In a nutshell, **surround inhibition** *amplifies differences in the activities of neighboring neurons as a way to enhance acuity.*

To better appreciate the function of surround inhibition, let's take a look at a couple of other examples. Figure 18 shows the case for two points of high pressure delivered simultaneously to the skin (not unlike what happens during the two-point threshold test). Figure 18A shows the responses when there is no surround inhibition. The bumps on the probe when pressed into the skin will lead to high pressure exerted on the RFs of the primary sensory *neurons a* and *c*. Because of RF overlap, primary sensory *neuron b* will detect some of the pressure applied by both the bumps on its right and left sides. Furthermore, the flat region of the probe between the two raised regions may also contact the skin but with less pressure than that under the two bumps. Consequently, the overall activity of *neuron b* will only be slightly less than that of *neurons a* and *c*. In the case of no surround inhibition, those activities would be passed on to their second-order neurons, *a'*, *b'*, and *c'*. The plot at the top of Figure 18A shows the profile of firing rates across the array of second-order neurons. This plot shows two high-firing-rate regions but with a middle region just about as high. When this information is presented to the cerebral cortex, it may be difficult to determine if there were two points of pressure or one broad region of pressure.

Figure 18B shows the same situation but now with surround inhibition included. Second-order *neuron a'* receives strong excitation from primary

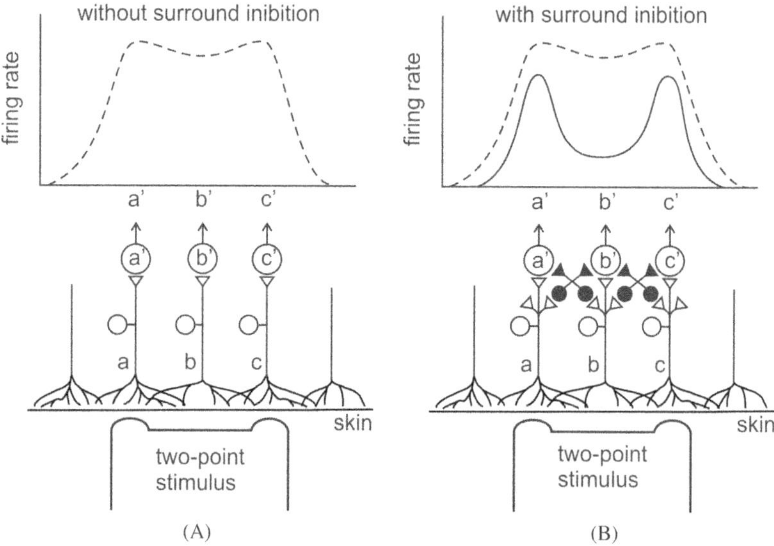

Figure 18.   Effect of surround inhibition in distinguishing two points of stimulation. (A) Two-point stimulus is pressed into the skin that activates first- and second-order neurons with no surround inhibition. Above: firing rate profile (dashed line) of second-order *neurons a′, b′*, and *c′* in response to application of the two-point stimulus. Little difference in firing rate is seen across the population of second-order neurons. (B) First- and second-order neurons with surround inhibition mediated by inhibitory interneurons. Above: firing rate profile (solid line) of second-order neurons in response to two-point stimulus in the case of surround inhibition. While the firing rates of all second-order neurons are reduced with surround inhibition compared to without such inhibition (dashed line), the differences in firing rates across the population are amplified to produce two clear peaks of firing rate. (Adapted from Brown [1989].)

sensory *neuron a* but also receives inhibition from the interneuron activated by primary sensory *neuron b*. Therefore, its activity is less than that without surround inhibition. The situation is the same for second-order *neuron c′*. Second-order *neuron b′* is excited by its primary sensory *neuron b* but receives a double dose of inhibition from interneurons activated by the neighboring *neurons a* and *c*. Therefore, *neuron b′*'s firing rate will be pulled down much more than that of *neurons a′* and *c′*. The overall firing rate profile presented to the cortex, therefore, is one with two distinct peaks of activity separated by a region of low activity. Such a profile could be more readily interpreted as two points of pressure rather than one.

Another important function of surround inhibition is to enhance the ability to detect edges of objects. This is particularly well established in the visual system where slight changes in luminesce within a visual scene are heightened to increase the ability to identify the outline of objects. In the somatosensory system, surround inhibition can greatly facilitate the ability to detect small transitions in pressure; for example, when detecting the edges of keys on a keyboard when touch typing. Figure 19 shows, for example, a region of the skin of a fingertip about to contact the edge of a flat thin object—say a piece of paper sitting on a tabletop. The RFs of primary sensory *neurons a, b,* and *c* will be in contact with the tabletop whereas those of *d, e,* and *f* will be in contact with the piece of paper when the finger is pressed down onto the surface. The raised region of the paper will lead to slightly greater pressures applied to the RFs of *neurons d, e,*

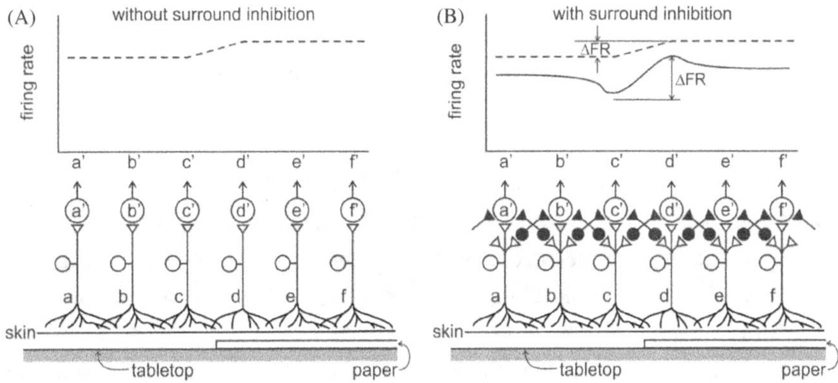

Figure 19.   Effect of surround inhibition on edge detection. (A) Below: First- and second-order neurons without surround inhibition. Skin is pressed down onto tabletop spanning the edge of a piece of paper. Above: Firing rate profile (dashed line) of second-order *neurons a′–f′* in response to the skin pressed onto tabletop and paper. Little difference in firing rate is seen across the population of second-order neurons. (B) Below: First- and second-order neurons with surround inhibition mediated by inhibitory interneurons. Above: Firing rate profile (solid line) of second-order neurons in response to edge stimulus in the case of surround inhibition. While the firing rates of all second-order neurons are reduced with surround inhibition compared to without such inhibition (dashed line), the differences in firing rate (DFR) between the neighboring second-order neurons on either side of the edge (*c′* and *d′*) are magnified with surround inhibition. (Adapted with permission from Brown [1989].)

and *f* compared to *a*, *b*, and *c*. Without surround inhibition (Figure 19A), this would lead to only slight differences in firing rates across the array of higher-order neurons. This would make it difficult for the cortex to discern if the surface in contact with the skin is uniform or whether there is a transition between two surfaces (i.e., an edge).

Figure 19B depicts the same situation but with surround inhibition included. Let's first consider the case of higher-order *neuron c'*. It receives modest excitation from its lower-order *neuron c*. At the same time, it receives modest inhibition from the interneuron activated by *b* on the left and stronger inhibition by the interneuron activated by *d* on its right. As such, the firing rate of the second-order *neuron c'* is reduced from what it would be without surround inhibition. The second-order *neuron b'* is similarly excited by its lower-order *neuron b*. Yet *neuron b'* receives only modest inhibition from the neighboring neurons on its left (*neuron a*) and right (*neuron c*). This means that the firing rate of *neuron b'* is not reduced as much by surround inhibition than that for *neuron c'*. This situation will be the same for *neuron a'* and the entire array of second-order neurons with RFs to the left of *neuron a* (not shown).

Let's now consider the high-pressure side and begin with the second-order *neuron e'*. This neuron is strongly excited by its lower-order *neuron e*. It also receives strong inhibition arising from interneurons on both the left and right driven by lower-order *neurons d* and *f*. Therefore, the firing rate of *neuron e'* will be markedly reduced from what it would be without surround inhibition. This is also the case for *neuron f'* and the array of the second-order neurons to its right (not shown). If we now jump back to the higher-order *neuron d'*, like it's neighbors to the right, it receives strong excitation from its lower-order *neuron d*. Yet it receives strong inhibition only from the interneuron to its right (driven by primary *neuron e*). Inhibition from the left interneuron will only be moderate because its primary *neuron c* is only modestly activated since it is on the low-pressure side. Consequently, the firing rate of the second-order *neuron d'* will be reduced less than that of its neighbors to the right with surround inhibition. Across the entire array of neurons, the firing rate profile with surround inhibition is such that the firing rate is lowest immediately at the transition to the low-pressure side and greatest immediately at the transition to the high-pressure side. This means that the difference in firing rate (ΔFR) between the neighboring higher-order neurons on either side of the transition are magnified with surround inhibition (compared to that without surround inhibition; top, Figure 19B). This facilitates the perception of a transition (i.e., an edge) at this location.

In all three examples described above (Figures 17, 18, and 19), the overall effect of surround inhibition was to reduce the firing rates of all neurons involved compared to that without surround inhibition. However, the degree of the inhibition was not uniform. The net effect was to amplify differences in firing rate across neighboring neurons that receive slightly different inputs. It is these *differences* in activities of neighboring neurons that the cerebral cortex attends to. Indeed, when the activities across an array of neurons are uniform, the cortex tends to "ignore" that input as being unimportant. Moreover, the effect of surround inhibition can even partially distort reality. In the case of edge detection (Figure 19), the situation without surround inhibition most accurately reflects the reality of the stimulus, namely, that there was only a small change in pressure on the skin between regions in contact with the paper and the tabletop. Yet the firing rate profile provided with lateral inhibition was distorted, indicating higher pressure than elsewhere just at the transition onto the paper and lower pressure than elsewhere just at the transition to the tabletop.

Such distortions caused by surround inhibition are the basis of a number of illusions in the visual system. This also occurs in the somatosensory system. For example, the pressure exerted on the skin under the heel is relatively uniform when standing. Therefore, even though a large array of tactile neurons in the heel are activated, because of its uniformity, that sensory information is largely ignored by the cortex. However, if there is a small pebble in the shoe, this will cause some variation in the pressure distribution across the heel and lead to slight differences in the firing rates of the primary sensory neurons with receptors in the heel. These differences become amplified with surround inhibition, which will prompt immediate attention of the cortex to the inputs coming from the heel— indeed, it may be difficult to ignore. When removing the pebble from the shoe, the size of the pebble is often smaller than imagined given the amplified (and distorting) effect of surround inhibition.

Intensity

As discussed above, topographic organization, RFs, acuity, and surround inhibition are all features of the dimension of sensation associated with localization. Another dimension of sensation is that of **intensity**, that is, *how strong is the applied stimulus*. As discussed in Chapter 3, one of the main mechanisms by which neurons represent (encode) the magnitude of depolarizing current is **rate coding**, namely, *the frequency of action potentials generated by a neuron is proportional to the strength of the excitation received*. Indeed, rate coding is a main mechanism used by primary sensory neurons to convey information to the central nervous system about stimulus intensity. As shown in Figure 3, the greater the stimulus strength, the more ion channels in the receptor membrane are activated, leading to a larger change in membrane potential, which then causes a higher rate of action potentials to be emitted from the spike-initiating zone of the primary sensory neuron.

An example of such rate coding in a tactile primary sensory neuron is shown in Figure 20 from the work of Mountcastle and colleagues. A small probe was controlled to touch and indent the skin of the fingertip of a monkey by precise amounts on each trial. Each trial lasted 0.6 s and the magnitude of the indentation increased for each trial. Figure 20A shows example recordings from the axon of a slowly adapting tactile neuron in response to these incrementing steps of tactile stimuli (from 300 to 1,440 µm) applied to its RF. For each trial, the average firing rate was calculated. This was done over many trials, each with slightly different magnitudes of skin indentation. The firing rate was then plotted as a function of the stimulus strength (i.e., amount of skin indentation) across all the trials. As seen in Figure 20B, the firing rate is a near-linear function of stimulus strength. This means that a given change in stimulus strength is represented as a proportionate change in the firing rate of the primary sensory neuron. The cerebral cortex interprets these variations in the firing rate as changes in the sensed intensity of the stimulus.

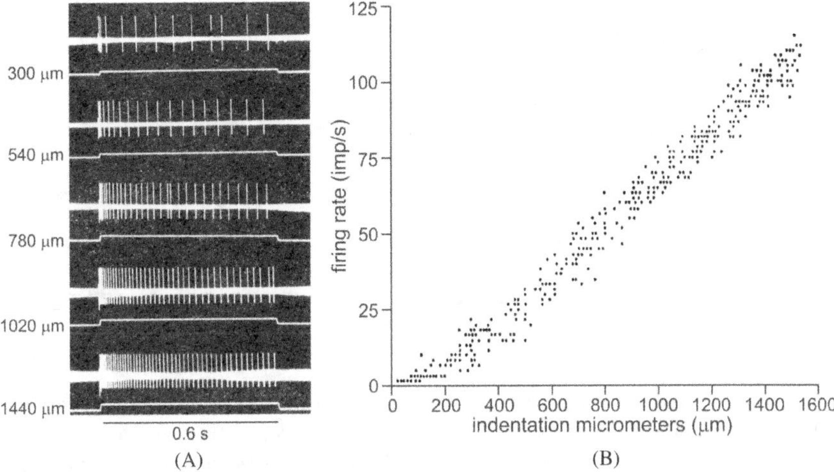

Figure 20.   (A) Example recordings from the axon of a slowly adapting tactile receptor in the fingertip of monkey in response to increasing levels of skin indentation by a small probe. For each pair of traces, the lower trace indicates the displacement of the stimulus probe. The upper trace shows the recorded action potentials. (B) Firing rate recorded from axon of single tactile receptor in response to many trials with varying degrees of skin indentation. (Adapted from Mountcastle *et al.* 1966.)

It should be said, however, that for many primary sensory neurons, the firing rate begins to level off for higher stimulus strengths (e.g., Knibestöl & Vallbo 1980). How, then, can the cerebral cortex accurately discern the intensity of a stronger stimuli if the firing rates of the primary sensory neurons fail to increase in proportion to the stimulus strength? One way that this is accomplished is through the *activation of more sensory receptor neurons*, called **recruitment**. Figure 21 shows schematically the process of recruitment. Figure 21A shows a small wedge applied to the finger to indent the skin to different extents. The wedge is positioned over the RF of *neuron a*. The RFs of two other neurons, *b* and *c*, are also shown. In response to the weakest stimulus, the skin is gently indented just in the vicinity of *neuron a*'s RF. As a consequence, only *neuron a* will discharge, and at a low rate. If the stimulus is increased, this will lead to greater indentation of the skin in the area of neuron *a*'s RF and an increased firing rate. In addition, the skin in which *neuron b*'s RF resides may now get slightly distorted, causing *neuron b* to start firing (i.e., to be recruited).

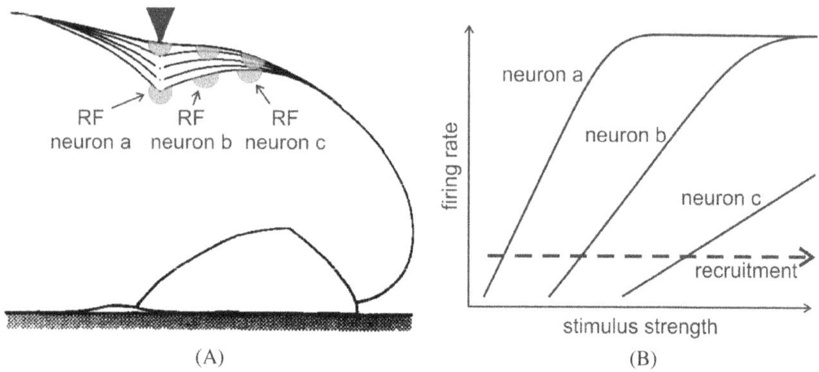

Figure 21.   Intensity encoding by recruitment. (A) Small wedge applied to the skin of the fingertip indents it to different extents. The RF of *neuron a* is directly under the wedge and its skin gets distorted to the greatest degree. With increasing indentation, the skin encompassing the RFs of *neurons b* and *c* also gets distorted (but to lesser degrees than *neuron a*), eventually causing them to be activated. For a given level of indentation, the firing rates will tend to be the largest for *neuron a*, less in *neuron b*, and the least in *neuron c*. (B) Plot of firing rates of *neurons a*, *b*, and *c* with increased indentation (stimulus strength). With increasing stimulus strength, the firing rate increases more or less linearly for an individual neuron but levels off at high rates. In addition, with increasing stimulus strength, progressively more neurons are activated referred to as recruitment. (Panel A adapted from Srinivasan [1989].)

At even stronger indentations, the skin containing neurons with RFs even farther afield, like *neuron c*, may start to be distorted and now cause those neurons to be recruited. As such, with stronger stimuli, there will be an expanding field of neurons that get recruited by the stimulus.

Figure 21B shows a schematic diagram representing the firing rates of *neurons a*, *b*, and *c* for different stimulus strengths. As the stimulus strength increases, individual neurons (like *neuron a*) increase their firing rate. That firing rate may begin to plateau at higher levels. In parallel, more neurons are recruited. Consequently, the total number of action potentials delivered to the central nervous system multiplies as more neurons are recruited, which continues to escalate with stronger stimuli. Presumably, neurons in the cerebral cortex integrate the entire barrage of action potentials delivered from the periphery to form a representation of the overall intensity of the applied stimulus.

Summary

Ion channels embedded in the membranes of primary sensory neurons transduce physical signals (mechanical, thermal, chemical, light) into a change in membrane potential. If large enough, the change in membrane potential elicits action potentials that are transmitted into the central nervous system. In response to sustained stimuli, the firing rates of most primary sensory neurons adapt (i.e., decrease slowly or rapidly), which can be partially responsible for the reduced awareness of a stimulus over time. The basic recognition that a stimulus has been applied is referred to as a sensation. There are three main dimensions of sensation: modality, localization, and intensity. Modality, namely, the type of sensation, is distinguished based on the type of sensory receptor neurons activated, referred to as a labeled line. Localization (i.e., where the stimulus was applied) is discerned based on the topographic organization of brain structures that process input from different regions of the periphery. The precision with which one can identify where a stimulus has been applied (called acuity) depends on four factors: the size of RFs, the density of RFs, the degree of convergence onto higher-order neurons, and the extent of surround inhibition. Surround inhibition refers to a type of neural circuitry that serves to magnify the differences in the firing rates of neighboring neurons that receive slightly different inputs. Finally, the intensity of a stimulus is represented by the firing rates (rate coding) and number of primary sensory neurons activated (recruitment) by a stimulus.

References

Brown AC (1989). Introduction to sensory mechanisms. In: Patton HD, Fuchs AF, Hille B, Scher AM & Steiner R (eds.) Textbook of Physiology: Excitable Cells and Neurophysiology (Volume 1), WB Saunders: Philadelphia, pp. 306.

Coste B, Mathur J, Schmidt M, Earley TJ, Ranade S, Petrus MJ, Dubin AE & Patapoutian A (2010). Piezo1 and Piezo2 are essential components of distinct mechanically activated cation channels. *Science* **330**, 55–60.

Futai K, Okada M, Matsuyama K & Takahashi T (2001). High-fidelity transmission acquired via a developmental decrease in NMDA receptor expression at an auditory synapse. *Journal of Neuroscience* **21**, 3342–3349.

Gynther BD, Vickery RM & Rowe MJ (1995). Transmission characteristics for the 1:1 linkage between slowly adapting type II fibers and their cuneate target neurons in cat. *Experimental Brain Research* **105**, 67–75.

Johansson RS & Vallbo ÅB (1983). Tactile sensory coding in the glabrous skin of the human hand. *Trends in Neurosciences* **6**, 27–32.

Knibestöl M & Vallbo ÅB (1980). Intensity of sensation related to activity of slowly adapting mechanoreceptive units in the human hand. *Journal of Physiology* **300**, 251–267.

Mountcastle VB & Powell TP (1959). Neural mechanisms subserving cutaneous sensibility, with special reference to the role of afferent inhibition in sensory perception and discrimination. *Bulletin of the Johns Hopkins Hospital* **105**, 201–232.

Mountcastle VB, Talbot WH & Kornhuber HH (1966). The neural transformation of mechanical stimuli delivered to the monkey's hand. In: De Feuck AVS & Knight J (eds.), Touch, Heat and Pain: Ciba Foundation Symposium, JA Churchill: London, pp. 325–344.

Srinivasan MA (1989). Surface deflection of primate fingertip under line load. *Journal of Biomechanics* **22**, 343–349.

Vallbo ÅB (1995). Single-afferent neurons and somatic sensation in humans. In: Gazzaniga MS (ed.), The Cognitive Neurosciences, MIT Press: Cambridge, MA, pp. 237–252.

Weinstein S (1968). Intensive and extensive aspects of tactile sensitivity as a function of body part, sex and laterality. In: Kenshalo D (ed.), The Skin Senses, Charles C Thomas: Springfield, IL, pp. 195–222.

Chapter 9

Somatosensory Receptors

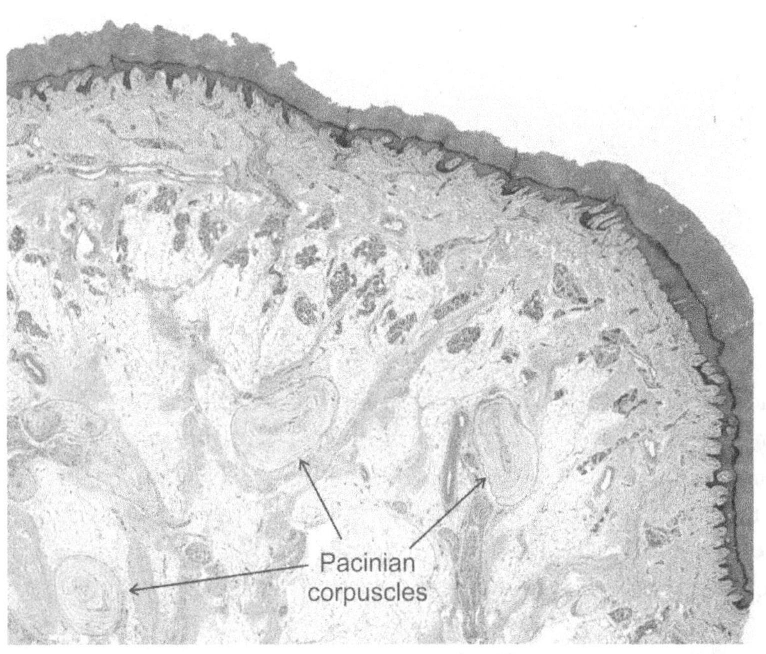

Micrograph of human skin showing Pacinian corpuscles. They resemble a sliced onion due to the concentric membranes and fluid spaces that serve as the accessory structure surrounding a central receptor membrane. The Pacinian corpuscle is a tactile receptor that detects vibration. (Adapted from www.sciencephoto.com.)

In Chapter 8, we discussed some general principles of sensory processing. In this chapter, we will describe the operations of the various peripheral receptors in the **somatosensory** system, including **tactile, thermal, nociceptive**, and **proprioceptive** receptors. Before going forward with this survey of receptors, however, we need to first briefly discuss the nomenclature of different types of axons that innervate somatosensory receptors.

Nerves and Axons

Axons that convey information from sensory receptors are carried in peripheral nerves. In humans, peripheral nerves have a wide range of sizes, with diameters ranging from a couple of millimeters up to ~20 mm for the large sciatic nerve. Often the cross-sectional shape of a nerve is more oval than circular, with typical diameters for the wide axis of 5 to 7 mm. The nerve itself is not simply a collection of axons. As shown in Figure 1A, nerves are complex structures containing a great deal of connective tissue needed to protect the delicate axons and to furnish strength to the nerve. The *axons themselves are bundled into little cables* called **fascicles**, several of which are shown in Figure 1A. The *connective tissue support surrounding the fascicles* is called the **epineurium**. Each fascicle may contain a few thousand tightly packed axons (Figure 1B). Typical fascicles contain sensory axons (sending information into the central nervous system), motor axons (sending signals to muscles), as well as axons of the autonomic nervous system. Both unmyelinated and myelinated axons are found within a fascicle (Figure 1C). Indeed, depending on the nerve, unmyelinated axons can outnumber myelinated axons by as much as fourfold (Figure 1D). Unmyelinated axons have the smallest diameters while myelinated axons have a wide range of larger diameters (Figure 1D).

---→

Figure 1.   (Figure on facing page) Morphology of a peripheral nerve. (A) Reconstruction of a short segment of a human peripheral nerve showing several fascicles (longitudinal bundles of axons) embedded in connective tissue epineurium. (B) Cross-section of a single fascicle of a human sural nerve. Only myelinated axons are stained. (C) Electron micrograph showing a myelinated axon and several unmyelinated axons. (D) Histogram showing a number of axons of different diameters from fascicles of a human sural nerve. Thin bars indicate unmyelinated axons, thick bars are myelinated axons. ([A] Adapted from Sunderland [1978]; [B] and [D] adapted from Ochoa and Mair [1969]; [C] from SciencePhotoLibrary, www.sciencephoto.com.)

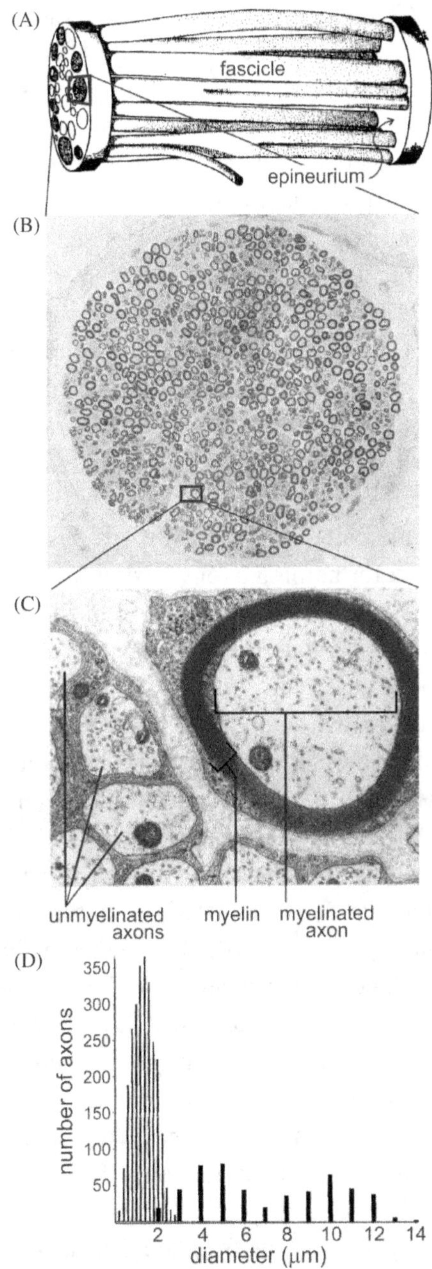
(A)
fascicle
epineurium
(B)
(C)
unmyelinated
axons
myelin
myelinated
axon
(D)
number of axons
350
300
250
200
150
100
50
2 4 6 8 10 12 14
diameter (μm)

As discussed in Chapter 5, axon diameter and the presence (or not) of myelin markedly affects the conduction velocity of action potentials along the axon. Different types of sensory receptors possess axons with a specific range of diameters. In addition, axons of some sensory receptors have myelin whereas others do not. Therefore, each type of sensory receptor will conduct action potentials within a particular range of velocities. Indeed, the identification of different classes of sensory receptors in neurophysiology experiments often relies on the measurements of axonal conduction velocity. For convenience, naming systems have been developed to keep track of the ranges of conduction velocities associated with axons of various diameters and myelinization. In the somatosensory system, two separate nomenclatures developed in parallel: one for sensory axons arising primarily from muscle, joints, and tendons, and another for sensory axons arising from the skin.

Figure 2 shows the categorization of axons based on these two systems. The system used for naming axons arising from the muscle (as well as joints and tendons) uses a Roman numeral designation. Type I axons have the largest diameter and are heavily myelinated. As such they conduct very rapidly, indeed they can convey action potentials above 100 m/s. Certain proprioceptors (as we shall discuss later in this chapter) have Type I axons—indeed, these are some of the fastest conducting axons in the body. Type II axons are somewhat smaller in diameter with less myelin. Typical conduction speeds for these axons are ~50 m/s. Type III axons are quite small in diameter and are only lightly myelinated. As such, they conduct action potentials relatively slowly—a typical value would be about 15 m/s. And lastly, Type IV axons have the smallest diameters and no myelin. Their conduction speeds are very slow, indeed, as slow as 0.5 m/s. That is 200 times slower than a typical Type I axons.

The naming system for axons arising *from the skin* (also referred to as **cutaneous**) uses a combination of Latin and Greek letters. The largest diameter cutaneous axons, called Aβ, have diameters and conduction velocities more or less in the same range as Type II axons for muscle. Various forms of tactile receptors possess Aβ axons. Aδ axons of the skin are similar to Type III axons arising from the muscle, with small diameters and light myelinization, and as such conduct slowly. Example receptors having Aδ axons are certain nociceptors and thermoreceptors. And lastly, the thinnest axons with no myelin arising from the skin are called C fibers.

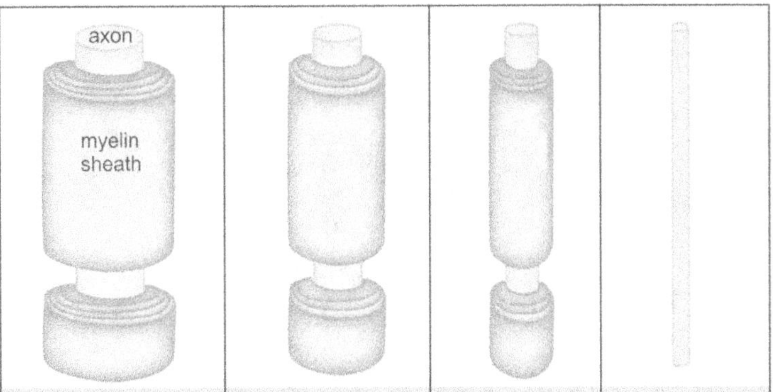

axon				
muscle	I	II	III	IV
skin		Aβ	Aδ	C
diameter (μm)	13 - 20	6 - 12	2 - 5	0.2 - 2
speed (m/s)	80 - 120	35 - 75	5 - 30	0.5 - 2
example receptors	proprioceptors	tactile	pain temperature	pain temperature

Figure 2.   Naming system for axons arising from muscle (as well as joints and tendons) use Roman numerals I, II, III, and IV. Type I conduct action potentials the fastest and Type IV the slowest. The naming system for axons arising from skin receptors use a combination of Latin and Greek letters: Aβ, Aδ, and C. The largest diameter axons from the skin (Aβ) are equivalent in size and conduction velocity to that of Type II axons from muscle. C fibers are the thinnest axons with no myelin and conduct very slowly. (Adapted from Kandel *et al.* [2012] and Rajan and Clarke, https://www.alexandriarepository.org/syllabus/topic-2-nerve-function-module-3-propagating-the-action-potential/11622/   Monash University.)

Nociceptors and thermoreceptors have these very slowly conducting axons, as we shall discuss.

Tactile Receptors

The somatosensory receptors responsible for the *sense of touch* are collectively called **tactile receptors**. There are four main types found in the

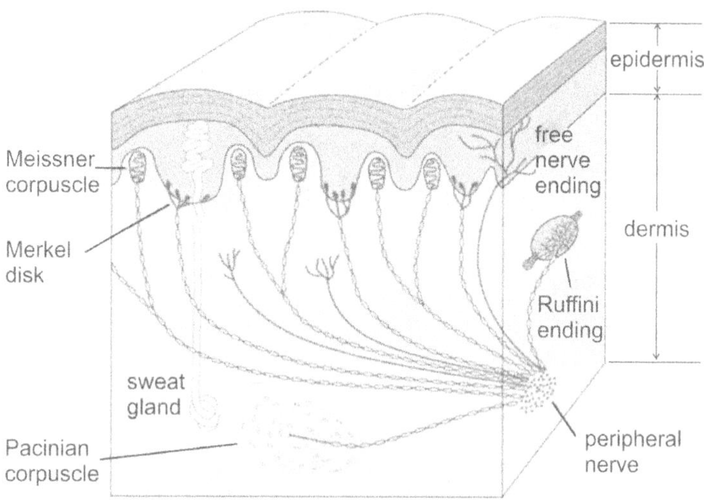

Figure 3.   Small segment of human glabrous (non-hairy) skin showing tactile receptors. Axons from various receptors eventually are collected into a peripheral nerve for the delivery of sensory information to the central nervous system. (Adapted from Kandel *et al.* [2012].)

glabrous (*non-hairy*) skin. (There are additional tactile receptors found at the base of hair follicles that won't be discussed here.) All four types are supplied by the fastest conducting axon that arises from the skin, the **Aβ axon**. One type, the **Meissner corpuscles**, is found close to the skin surface, just below the epidermal layer (Figure 3). In general, the closer a receptor is to the skin surface, the smaller its receptive field. As such, Meissner corpuscles tend to have *small receptive fields*. The **corpuscle** refers to the accessory structure, which is essentially **a fluid-filled bag**. Such corpuscles endow receptors with *rapidly adapting* firing rate responses. As we shall discuss later, these features (small receptive field and rapidly adapting responses) make Meissner corpuscles ideally suited to detect the *texture* of objects touched by the skin.

A second type of tactile receptor that sits close to the skin surface is the **Merkel-disk** receptors (Figure 3). The disk refers to a specialized accessory structure associated with these sensory endings. Because they sit close to the skin surface, they also tend to have *small receptive fields*.

These receptors have *slowly adapting* firing rate responses. Overall, Merkel-disk receptors are well-suited to detect the touch *pressure* applied to the skin. Indeed, the tactile receptor recorded in Figure 20 of Chapter 8 has characteristics consistent with that of a Merkel-disk receptor.

Another type of receptor that sits deeper in the skin is the **Ruffini ending** (Figure 3). Because of its deeper location, its *receptive field tends to be large*. The Ruffini ending has an elongated connective tissue capsule as its accessory structure. These receptors have a *slowly adapting* response. Moreover, these receptors are sensitive to the elongation of the capsule along its long axis but not perpendicular to it. Consequently, these receptors are sensitive to *skin stretch* in a certain direction. For example, when one splays their fingers, the sense of tightness that arises from the webbing at the base of the fingers is likely conveyed by activation of Ruffini endings.

The fourth major type of tactile receptor is the **Pacinian corpuscles**. They sit very deep in the skin (Figure 3) and sometimes well below the skin. Because of their deep location, Pacinian corpuscles tend to have extremely *large receptive fields*. The corpuscle itself is relatively huge (~1 to 1.5 mm in diameter) and can be seen without the aid of a microscope (see image at the frontispiece of this chapter). The corpuscle (the accessory structure) consists of concentric layers of elastic membranes separated by fluid-filled regions. Such an elaborate corpuscle (as discussed later) makes these receptors very *rapidly adapting*. Overall, Pacinian corpuscles are exquisitely sensitive to *vibration*. For example, if you place one hand on a tabletop and then gently tap elsewhere on the table surface with your other hand, the vibrations that you feel with the hand on the tabletop are most likely due to Pacinian corpuscles. Keep in mind that the magnitude of the physical oscillations set up in the tabletop by the tapping are extraordinarily minuscule—yet you sense them with relative clarity. This speaks to the awesome sensitivity of the Pacinian corpuscle. Interestingly, predators, such as cats, have a great number of Pacinian corpuscles found in the mesentery of the abdomen. It is thought that while lounging with their bellies in contact with the ground, Pacinian corpuscles can detect and alert the predator of movements of little creatures (and possible lunch) in their vicinity based on the tiny vibrations set up through the ground.

Summary of Tactile Receptors

As a quick summary, Merkel-disk and Meissner corpuscle receptors both reside near the skin margin (all starting with the letter *m*) and therefore have small receptive fields. Ruffini endings and Pacinian corpuscles are situated deeper and therefore have large receptive fields. Meissner and Pacinian endings have corpuscles as their accessory structures, and therefore are rapidly adapting. Receptors without corpuscles (Merkel-disk and Ruffini endings) are slowly adapting. All four tactile receptors have myelinated Aβ axons.

These main features are depicting graphically in a two-dimensional matrix in Figure 4. One dimension is for the size of the receptive field (small or large) and the other is for the type of adaptation (slow or fast). Receptors with small receptive fields are placed in the top row whereas those with large receptive fields in the bottom row. Note the exceptionally large receptive fields for the example Pacinian corpuscles in Figure 4. Also, for the Ruffini endings, arrows are shown along with the receptive fields to indicate the direction of skin stretch that the receptor primarily responded to. Action potential responses to sustained stimuli are shown below the pictures of receptive fields for each receptor type: fast adapting (i.e., only responding when the stimulus is changing) for the corpuscles (Meissner and Pacinian) and slowly adapting for the non-corpuscle receptors (Merkel-disk and Ruffini). The information represented in this type of matrix is important for the identification of specific receptors based on axonal recordings in animals and humans where it is not possible to have direct knowledge of the receptor type.

Texture Coding

As mentioned above, the broad submodalities associated with each tactile receptor are *texture* for Meissner corpuscle, *pressure* for Merkel-disks, skin *stretch* for Ruffini endings, and *vibration* for Pacinian corpuscles. While the encoding of the latter three submodalities seems reasonably straightforward, how would a receptor respond to and encode a more obscure parameter like texture? Keep in mind that Meissner corpuscles are rapidly adapting. As such, if you simply pressed your fingertips down

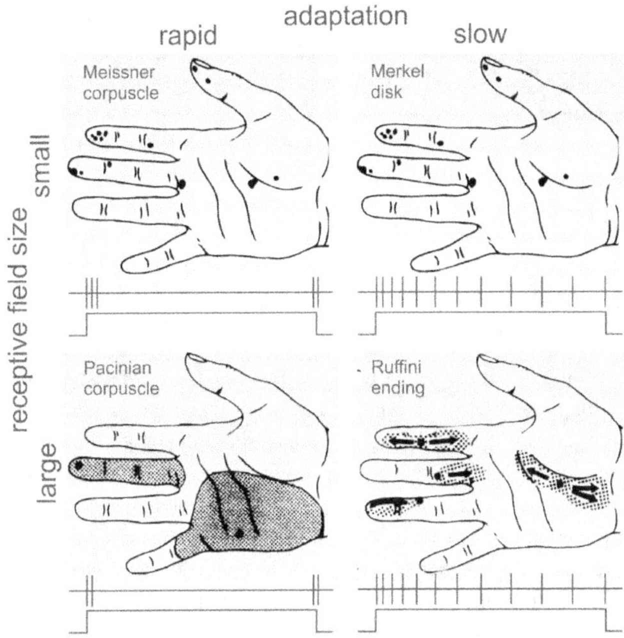

Figure 4.   Tactile receptors can be classified based on their receptive field size and firing rate adaptation. Receptors with small receptive fields (black dots) include the Meissner corpuscles and Merkel-disk receptors. Receptors with large receptive fields (gray areas) include Pacinian corpuscles and Ruffini endings. The arrows on the receptive fields of the Ruffini endings indicate the direction of skin stretch that the receptor best responded to. Rapidly adapting receptors (Meissner and Pacinian corpuscles) generate action potentials (vertical ticks) only at the onset and removal of a sustained stimulus (lower trace). Slowly adapting receptors (Merkel-disk and Ruffini endings) exhibit a gradual decline in the firing rate during sustained stimuli. (Adapted from Johansson and Vallbo [1983].)

onto objects of various textures, the Meissner corpuscles would swiftly stop firing, and provide little information about the object touched. Indeed, when one wants to discern the texture of an object, we *move* our fingertips across the surface of the object.

How does such movement of the skin across a surface provide information about texture? When we move the skin across a surface, Meissner corpuscles will fire on each little rise in the surface because the pressure will slightly increase when encountering these small transitions. Because we normally move our fingertips across a surface with a relatively

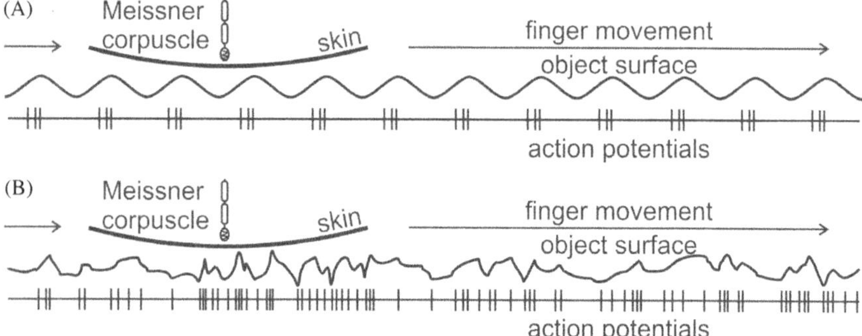

Figure 5.   Encoding of texture by Meissner corpuscles. (A) A Meissner corpuscle in the skin of a fingertip pressed into and swept at a constant speed across a fabric with a regular weave, like a corduroy. Each small rise in the material will slightly increase the pressure on the Meissner corpuscle, causing it to fire. The consistent pattern in the fabric will provoke a regular pattern of action potentials set up by the Meissner corpuscle. (B) When sweeping the finger across a material with an irregular rough surface, like sandpaper, the pattern of action potentials generated by the Meissner corpuscle will also be irregular. These differences in the patterns of action potentials are used to discern the texture of an object.

constant speed when detecting texture, this will generate a temporal *pattern* of action potentials that represents the characteristics of the texture. For example, when sweeping a finger across a fabric with a regular weave, like a narrow corduroy, Meissner corpuscles will fire at consistent intervals associated with each undulation in the material (Figure 5A). On the other hand, when moving the finger across a material that has a more irregular, rough surface, like sandpaper, the pattern of activity set up in the Meissner corpuscles will be irregular (Figure 5B). These variations in firing patterns are perceived by the cerebral cortex as differences in texture. As such, this represents one example of the pattern theory (see Chapter 8) likely used by the nervous system to distinguish one submodality (type of texture) from another.

Corpuscles and Rapid Adaptation

One issue that we have not addressed is how does a corpuscle, like that associated with a Meissner or Pacinian corpuscle, give rise to a rapidly adapting response. Remember that rapid adaptation means that the receptor only generates action potentials when the physical signal is changing. Pacinian corpuscles are very sensitive to vibrations (as are Meissner corpuscles) because vibrations are by definition continuously changing signals. Indeed, a Pacinian corpuscle will spike on each rising phase of a minuscule oscillatory mechanical signal (displacements <1 μm) with near-perfect fidelity up to very high frequencies (>500 cycles/s; Pawson *et al.,* 2009).

Because of the large physical size of Pacinian corpuscles, they can be dissected out of the skin and kept alive in a bath of physiological saline solution. In experiments carried out by Lowenstein and colleagues in the 1960s, intracellular recordings were made near the spike-initiating zone of the axon emerging from the corpuscle (Figure 6A). Changes in membrane potential were then recorded in response to precisely controlled, brief, and gentle touches of the outer capsule of the Pacinian corpuscle with a stimulus probe. With the corpuscle intact, increasing the strength of very brief stimuli (<1 ms in duration) led to progressively greater degrees of membrane depolarization until threshold was crossed and an action potential was generated (Figure 6B). Interestingly, when the same stimuli were applied directly to the receptor membrane after the corpuscle had been dissected away, the responses were virtually the same (Figure 6C).

Lowenstein and colleagues then delivered much longer stimuli but at a strength below that needed to evoke an action potential. This was done so as to not contaminate the recording of the receptor potential associated with a sensory transduction with that associated with an action potential. When such longer-duration stimuli were applied to the intact corpuscle (Figure 6D), two brief peaks of depolarization occurred—one at the stimulus onset and one at the removal of the stimulus. Between these two peaks, there was virtually no excess depolarization despite the stimulus being maintained over the entire time period. On the other hand, when this longer-duration stimulus was applied to the receptor denuded of the corpuscle, an entirely different response was recorded (Figure 6E). In this case, the membrane was depolarized throughout the application of the stimulus and the depolarization gradually decayed over the course of the stimulus. This response is very similar to what one would expect of a slowly adapting receptor. Therefore, this experiment clearly showed that

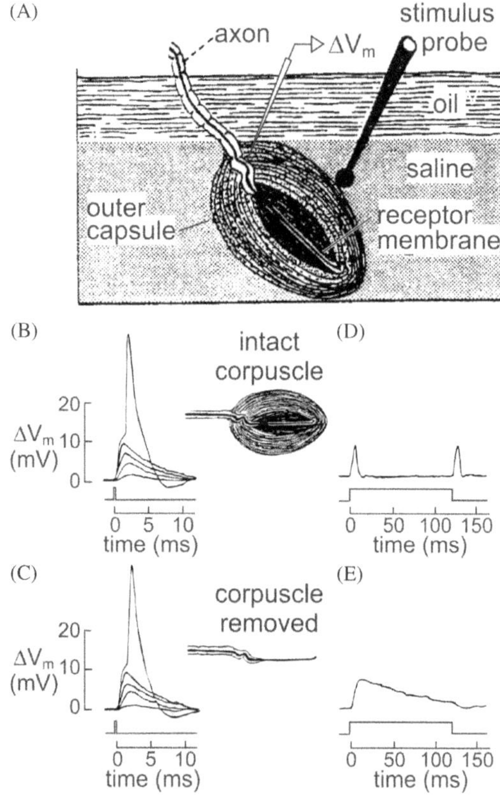

Figure 6.   Influence of corpuscle on the receptor potential of a Pacinian corpuscle. (A) Dissected Pacinian corpuscle placed in physiological saline solution. Change in membrane potential (ΔV_m) recorded with a microelectrode placed in the initial region of an axon. A stimulus probe was used to apply brief, minuscule indentations to the outer capsule of the corpuscle. (B) Changes in membrane potential recorded in response to progressively stronger stimuli of very brief duration (<1 ms duration). The strongest stimulus evoked an action potential. (C) Same as (B) but applied to the receptor membrane after the corpuscle had been dissected. (D) Change in membrane potential in response to long duration stimulus (>100 ms) applied to an intact corpuscle with a strength below that needed to trigger an action potential. Two clear peaks of depolarization seen at the outset and on removal of the stimulus. (E) Same as in (D) but applied to the receptor membrane after the corpuscle has been removed. Stimulus now causes long-lasting but decaying depolarization. Therefore, the corpuscle causes the rapidly adapting response seen in (D). (Adapted with permission from Detwiler [1989], based on Loewenstein and Mendelson [1965].)

the accessory structure (the corpuscle) is responsible for the rapidly adapting response normally observed in these receptors.

Of course, the next question is how does the corpuscle cause such a rapidly adapting response? Although the mechanisms are complex, one can appreciate how the corpuscle might endow a rapidly adapting response by considering the simplified representation in Figure 7. The Pacinian corpuscle consists of concentric layers of elastic membranes separated by fluid with a highly sensitive receptor membrane located in the interior. A gentle touch by a probe to the outer capsule will transmit fluid pressure to the interior where it will distort the receptor membrane that, in turn, will provoke the opening of mechanically gated ion channels to depolarize the membrane. Because of the fluid-filled laminae and the associated

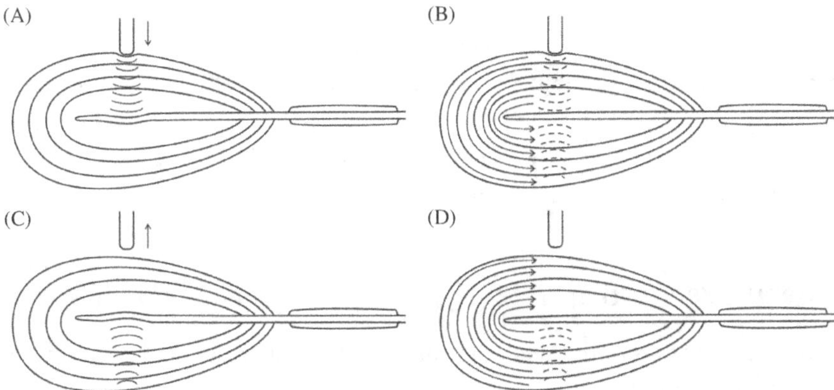

Figure 7.   Mechanism of rapidly adapting response in Pacinian corpuscle. (A) Application of a stimulus probe to the capsule of a Pacinian corpuscle causes a brief localized increase in fluid pressure below the probe, which distorts the receptor membrane. This distortion causes the opening of mechanically gated ion channels leading to depolarization. (B) Maintenance of the stimulus quickly leads to redistribution and equalization of fluid pressure, thereby, restoring the receptor membrane to its original configuration and deactivation of mechanically gated channels. (C) Quick release of stimulus probe briefly causes the pressure above the membrane to be less than that below, causing upward deflection of the membrane, opening of mechanically gated channels, and depolarization. (D) After the removal of the stimulus, pressure again quickly redistributes, restoring the membrane to its resting configuration and membrane potential.

viscoelastic properties of the corpuscle, pressure will rapidly redistribute throughout the corpuscle (Figure 7B), such that the downward pressure will be balanced by upward pressure. This will restore the membrane to its original shape, causing the mechanically gated channels to close, and the membrane to return to the resting potential. As long as the stimulus probe is held in place (i.e., a sustained stimulus), there will be virtually no distortion of the receptor membrane and no depolarization.

When the stimulus is rapidly removed (Figure 7C), the pressure immediately above the receptor membrane will, for just a moment, be less than that below. This leads to a distortion of the membrane in the opposite direction to that when the stimulus was first applied. The bending of the membrane will again cause the opening of mechanically gated channels and lead to depolarization. As before, the pressure quickly equilibrates in this fluid-filled system and the receptor membrane restores to its original configuration and the membrane potential returns to rest (Figure 7D). This process is not that different from pushing down on a water-filled balloon. When you press down, the pressure rapidly equilibrates. When you quickly release it, the balloon jiggles briefly. That jiggling would serve to momentarily displace a membrane at the center of the balloon.

Thermoreceptors

Temperature is a continuous environmental variable. As such, one might speculate that temperature is encoded by thermoreceptors in the same way that slowly adapting mechanoreceptors encode pressure—by increasing firing rate in proportion to increases in stimulus strength (i.e., temperature). Interestingly, however, nature has developed a different means for detecting temperature. As shown in Figure 8, there are two separate classes of thermoreceptors, cold and warm. As implied by their names, cold receptors respond most vigorously to cooler temperatures, whereas warm receptors respond to hotter temperatures. Both types of thermoreceptors have **free nerve endings** with no accessory structures. **Cold receptors** give rise to thinly myelinated **Aδ axons** that conduct action potentials slowly, whereas **warm receptors** are supplied primarily by the very slowly conducting unmyelinated **C fibers**. The ion channels that mediate temperature transduction have only recently been discovered.

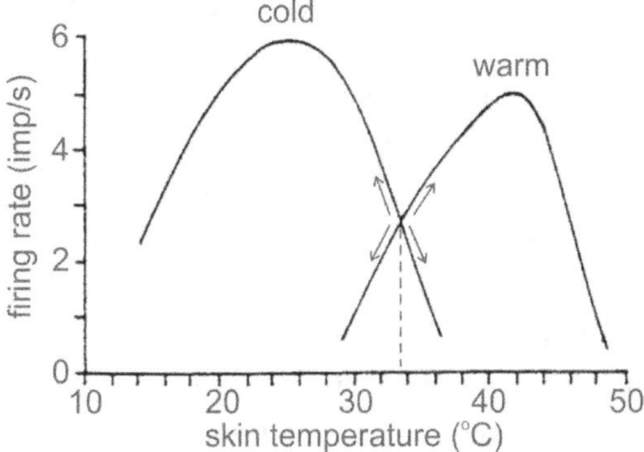

Figure 8.   Thermoreceptors. Firing rate responses of a cold and warm thermoreceptor. At ~34 °C (dashed vertical line), the skin temperature humans feel as neutral temperature, the firing rates of cold and warm are about the same. Increasing the temperature from that level causes a steep increase in the firing of warm receptors and concomitant decrease in the firing rate of cold receptors (right arrows). Decreasing the temperature from thermoneutral causes a steep increase in cold and a decline in warm receptors. (Adapted from Brown [1989].)

Different types of these so-called transient receptor protein (TRP) channels are gated at different temperature ranges (Dhaka *et al.*, 2006). Interestingly, those channels that respond to cool temperatures (and that serve as the transducers in cold receptors) also are gated by the chemical menthol. Similarly, the TRP ions channel that respond to warm temperatures (and are the transducers in warm receptors) are also gated by the chemical capsaicin, the active ingredient in hot chili peppers.

Like tactile receptors, the highest firing rates are generated at the temperature that is in the center of its temperature "receptive field" (Figure 8). The firing rate then falls off for temperatures on either side of that temperature. Because of this symmetry of firing rate responses, there will be ambiguity in identifying temperature based exclusively on the activity of a single class of thermoreceptors. For example, the peak firing rate occurs around 25 °C for cold receptors. Note, however, that for temperatures of about 18 or 32 °C, the firing rates would be about the same (~4 imp/s) for the cold receptors. To help avoid this ambiguity, the temperature receptive fields for cold and warm receptors overlap, just as we discussed for touch receptors in Chapter 8. As such, there is a unique population code to represent each temperature across the range of temperatures typically encountered. At the extremes of cold or warm, where firing rates start to fall off for cold receptors (on the left of Figure 8) and for warm receptors at high temperatures (on the right of Figure 8), certain types of pain receptors (not shown) begin to be activated. Activation of these nociceptors gives rise to the uncomfortable sensations associated with extreme cold and extreme heat.

The *skin* temperature that humans report as being "neutral" is about 34 °C. Think of lukewarm bathwater that feels neither warm nor cold. That temperature (vertical dashed line, Figure 8) is close to that which causes cold and warm receptors to discharge with similar firing rates. A slight increase in temperature from that level will simultaneously cause warm receptors to increase and cold receptors to decrease their firing rates (right set of arrows). That combination of changes will be perceived as an increase in warmth. Likewise, a slight reduction in temperature from thermoneutral will cause the cold receptors to increase and warm receptors to decrease their firing rates (left set of arrows). That combination will be interpreted as an increased sense of cold.

Nociceptors

Based on his experiments at the outset of the 20th century, future Nobel laureate Charles Sherrington hypothesized there must exist a certain class of *primary sensory neurons that have high thresholds, and that are activated only with damaging or potentially damaging stimuli.* Activation of these sensory neurons would trigger withdrawal responses and the perception of pain. These responses would serve a protective role to remove the affected body part from the offending stimulus and to safeguard an injury from further insults in order to facilitate wound healing. Sherrington called these sensory receptors **nociceptors**, from the same root word for noxious.

Indeed, as predicted by Sherrington, there is such a class of sensory neurons. Figure 9 is a plot showing the cumulative number of cutaneous sensory neurons having various mechanical thresholds (i.e., minimum pressure just needed to cause the receptor neuron to fire). Tactile receptors all had very low thresholds. On the other hand, nociceptors required

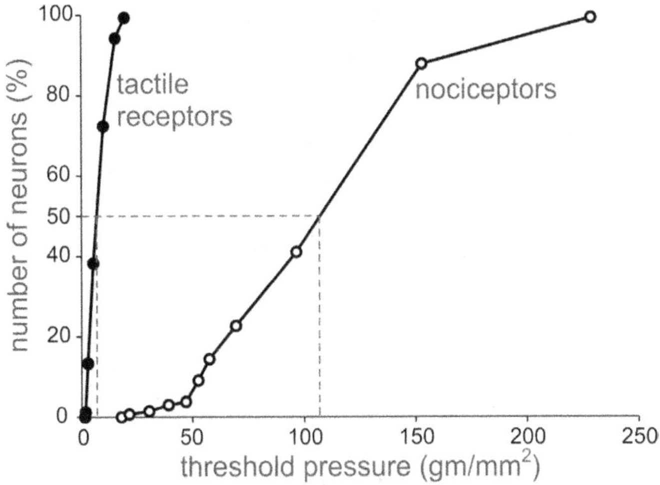

Figure 9.   Cumulative histogram showing the proportion of neurons recorded having different mechanical thresholds. Recordings made from axons supplying the palmar skin in monkeys. All tactile neurons had thresholds less than 20 gm/mm^2, and 50% had threshold <7 gm/mm^2. Nociceptors had much higher thresholds with some requiring as high as 230 gm/mm^2 to be activated and 50% with thresholds <108 gm/mm^2. (Adapted from Georgopoulos [1976].)

substantially greater mechanical pressure to activate them. For example, 50% of tactile receptors (dashed horizontal line, Figure 7) had thresholds of <7 gm/mm^2 (left vertical dashed line) whereas 50% of the nociceptors had thresholds of <108 gm/mm^2 (right vertical dashed line). This means that nociceptors required, on average, about 15 times higher mechanical pressure just to get them to start to fire as compared to tactile receptors. Such high thresholds are in keeping with Sherrington's original idea of nociceptors.

Like thermoreceptors, nociceptors do not have accessory structures surrounding the receptor membrane, and as such are referred to as having **free nerve endings**. Also, like thermoreceptors, two types of axons emerge from the free nerve endings of nociceptors: **Aδ** and **C-fibers**. Some nociceptors respond to intense mechanical signals, others to extreme temperatures, and some to particular irritant chemicals. In addition, some types of *nociceptors respond to all three types of stimuli* and are referred to as **polymodal nociceptors**. Polymodal nociceptors typically are those associated with C-fibers. Figure 10 shows action potentials recorded from such a polymodal nociceptor in response to noxious mechanical, thermal, and chemical stimuli. Nociceptors are found in most tissues. If the tissue is a muscle, joint, or tendon, then the axons that supply those nociceptors are referred to as Type III and IV rather than as Aδ and C (see Figure 2). For example, the progressive discomfort associated with intense exercise is due to the activation of chemosensitive nociceptors in the muscle. Interestingly, the brain itself does not have nociceptors. This means that neurosurgeons can perform brain surgery in awake patients using only local anesthetics for the scalp and skull.

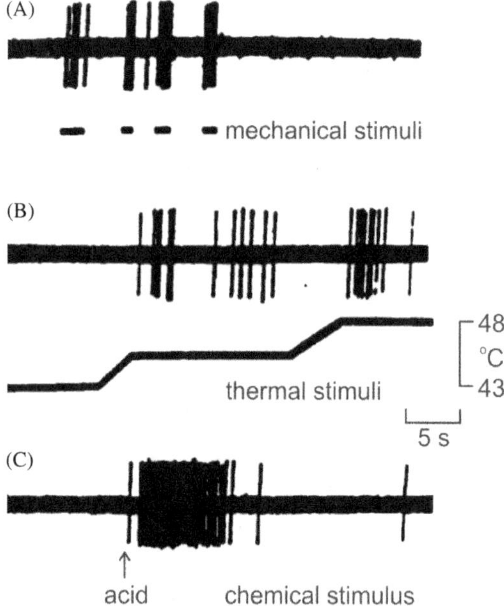

Figure 10.   Action potentials generated in a polymodal nociceptor in response to (A) mechanical, (B) thermal, and (C) chemical stimuli. Recordings were made from a C-fiber axon (conduction velocity of ~1 m/s) in a nerve supplying the cornea of an anesthetized cat. In (A), four bouts of mechanical stimulation (horizontal bars, forces not recorded) are shown. In (B), a thermode was applied to the receptive field and the temperature was increased in 2° C steps that each lasted 15 s. In (C), 10 mM acetic acid was applied to the receptive field with a pipette. (Adapted with permission from Belmonte *et al.* 1991.)

Similar to thermoreceptors with two types of receptors (cold and warm), there are two general types of nociceptors that give rise to different perceptual qualities of pain. One type is innervated by Aδ (or Type III) axons, which conduct action potentials at ~15 m/s. When activated, *these nociceptors give rise to sharp, stabbing, immediate pain.* This is often referred to as **first pain**. The other type is innervated by thin, unmyelinated C-fiber (or Type IV) axons, which conduct action potentials very slowly (indeed can be <1 m/s). These nociceptors provoke *delayed, dull, achy, throbbing,* and *persistent pain.* This is often called **second pain**. Both types of nociceptors typically are activated simultaneously in response to an abrupt insult, for example, inadvertently hitting a finger with a hammer or spraining an ankle. Because of the differences in conduction velocities and conveyance of their activities to the brain, the perceptions associated with the activation of the two types of nociceptors are distinguishable. For example, it could take a full 2 s for action potentials conveyed along C-fibers to travel from the foot to the brain. Experiments using anesthetics to selectively block C-fibers or Aδ axons have clearly shown the specific involvement of the two nociceptor types for each type of pain (e.g., Mackenzie *et al.* 1975). Blockade of C-fibers eliminated long-lasting, delayed second pain, whereas blockade of Aδ axons eliminated the sharp, immediate first pain.

Microneurography

A contentious debate about the nature of pain signaling continued through the latter part of the 20th century. One group of investigators argued that the perception of pain comes about by the pattern (and rates) of firing arising from a wide array of peripheral sensory neurons. This idea was directly tied to the pattern theory of modality encoding (discussed in Chapter 8). The other group asserted that pain arises when specific classes of neurons are activated (nociceptors) independent of their pattern of firing—consistent with the labeled line theory. This debate was largely put to rest with the development of a new experimental method called **microneurography** by a group of investigators in Sweden (see Vallbo 2018). As shown in Figure 11, this *method entails the insertion of a* *microelectrode through the skin and into a peripheral nerve fascicle to record the activity of single axons in an awake human subject.*

Once the microelectrode is situated within the nerve, the experimenter makes fine manual adjustments to the microelectrode position until clear action potentials are detected from an axon. The next task for the experimenter is to determine what type of receptor the recorded axon belongs to. Based on the nerve, the experimenter knows the general vicinity of the body supplied by the nerve. Figure 11 shows the microelectrode in the median nerve that supplies the palmar skin, muscles, and joints of the thumb side of the hand. As such, the experimenter can brush that region of the skin (to activate tactile receptors), move the joints (to activate proprioceptors), or apply heat or cold (to activate thermoreceptors). In addition, the experimenter could apply noxious stimuli, like pinching the skin. When one of those stimuli leads to activation of the recorded axon, the general category of the sensory receptor can be established. Then, the experimenter performs additional tests to identify the specific type of receptor within that category. For example, in Figure 11, the receptor is identified to be a tactile receptor having a low mechanical threshold and small receptive field on the index finger. A small receptive field indicates

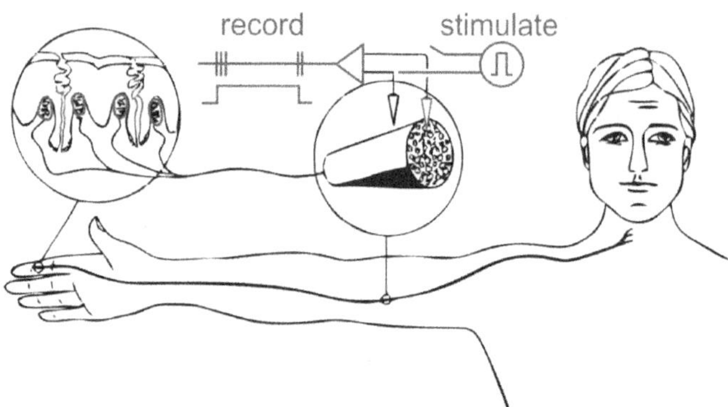

Figure 11.   Microneurography. A thin microelectrode inserted into a peripheral nerve of an awake human subject can be used to record action potentials from a single sensory axon. The receptive field is indicated as a small circle on the index finger. The response to a sustained stimulus is shown as rapidly adapting. This suggests that the recorded axon arises from a Meissner corpuscle (inset). The same axon can be stimulated, and the subject is asked to report the evoked sensation. (Adapted from Shepherd [1988].)

that the receptor is either a Meissner corpuscle or a Merkel-disk ending. If application of a sustained mechanical stimulus leads to firing only at the onset and removal of the stimulus (Figure 11), the probable identity of the receptor is a Meissner corpuscle.

One of the powerful features of this method is that the recording electrode can then be connected to a stimulator to precisely activate the now-identified axon to produce a designated pattern of action potentials. While recording from the axon is like doing a wiretap to listen in on a phone conversation that the sensory receptor is having with the central nervous system, stimulating the axon provides the experimenter the ability to place a call themselves. Because this is done in an awake human subject, the subject can report to the experimenter what they felt in response to the axon being stimulated. Such information typically would be impossible to obtain in non-human experiments. Usually, when stimulating the axon, the subjects report a sensation as arising from the same location as the previously identified receptive field obtained while recording from the axon. In the case of the Meissner corpuscle depicted in Figure 11, stimulation would provoke the sensation of tapping or buzzing restricted to the region indicated by the small circle on the finger. Crucially, when stimulating such an axon at progressively higher frequencies, subjects reported that while the intensity of the sensation increased, it never converted to a painful sensation. Likewise, when stimulating an axon arising from a nociceptor, even low frequencies of stimulation were perceived as painful and the intensity of the pain increased with higher frequencies. These findings were direct evidence against the notion of the pattern theory of pain perception and strong proof for the existence of labeled lines (Torebjörk *et al.*, 1987).

Poor Acuity and Referred Pain

In general, pain has relatively poor acuity, particularly that associated with C-fiber-mediated second pain. For example, if you have a toothache, it is sometimes difficult to indicate to a dentist precisely which tooth is the source of the pain. The reasons for this are many, including relatively large receptive fields, low densities of receptors, modest levels of surround inhibition, and a high degree of convergence onto higher-order neurons for nociceptors (see Figure 13 in Chapter 8).

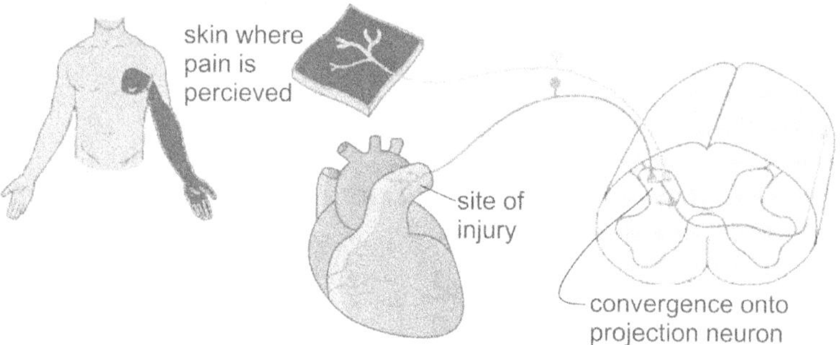

Figure 12.   Referred pain. Activation of nociceptors due to injury in tissues like in the heart excites second-order projection neurons. These second-order neurons also receive converging input from nociceptors in other tissues like those found in the arm and pectoral region. Consequently, when tissue is damaged, like during a heart attack, the individual perceives the pain as arising from their arm and chest rather than from the actual site of the injury. (Adapted from Kandel *et al.* [2012].)

Indeed, in some instances, the high degree of convergence can lead to misidentification of the site of pain. Such misidentification is called **referred pain**, that is, the *pain is "referred" to a location different from its source*. The most notorious referred pain is that associated with a heart attack. As shown in Figure 12, during a heart attack, people often report severe pain arising from their left arm and the pectoralis region. This is because chemically sensitive nociceptors in the vasculature of the heart that detect a disrupted metabolic environment associated with obstructed blood flow, project onto and activate the same second-order neurons that receive a nociceptive input from the arm and chest. Because the lifetime experience of the individual associated with activation of these second-order neurons has been related to strong stimuli delivered to the arm and chest, the person perceives the pain as arising from those structures, not the heart.

Hereditary Insensitivity to Pain

The treatment of pain represents one of the major clinical challenges of our time. It should be said, however, that pain is not just a source of misery and discomfort to be eliminated as quickly as possible by any means. While it might seem an idyllic state not to have to experience pain, rare hereditary diseases that cause nociceptors not to develop highlight the importance of the pain system. Afflicted individuals have no perception of pain, yet their tactile and other senses are intact. As a consequence, they continuously injure themselves and then do nothing to protect the injuries. They often break bones, sustain burns, scar their corneas, and mangle their fingers, toes, and tongue without being aware of it (Zhang *et al.*, 2016). These injuries often lead to serious infections (the patients don't feel the discomfort of infection), which oftentimes can only be treated with amputations. As such, these individuals have severely impaired health and require constant vigilance to prevent injuries.

Proprioceptors

The last major subdivision of the somatosensory system is **proprioception**, which underlies our *awareness of the location and movement of our body parts*. The term proprioception (another term coined by Sherrington) literally means sense of self. A number of different types of proprioceptors have evolved for sensing various aspects of body position and movement. In some respects, however, proprioception is a kind of "hidden" sense that is often taken for granted. Part of the reason for this is that it is very difficult to recognize the crucial role that proprioception plays in our lives because it is not readily possible to "turn off" proprioception. In contrast, one can simply close their eyes to get some idea of what blindness would be like or plug their ears to understand deafness.

Muscle Spindle

The most complex of all somatosensory receptors is the muscle spindle. In a nutshell, the **muscle spindle** *detects the length and speed of lengthening of the muscle* within which it is embedded. As shown in Figure 13, it is composed of several parts. The spindle is enclosed in a connective tissue capsule. This capsule has a shape that is tapered on both ends. Early anatomists referred to it as being shaped like a spindle—a tapered wooden

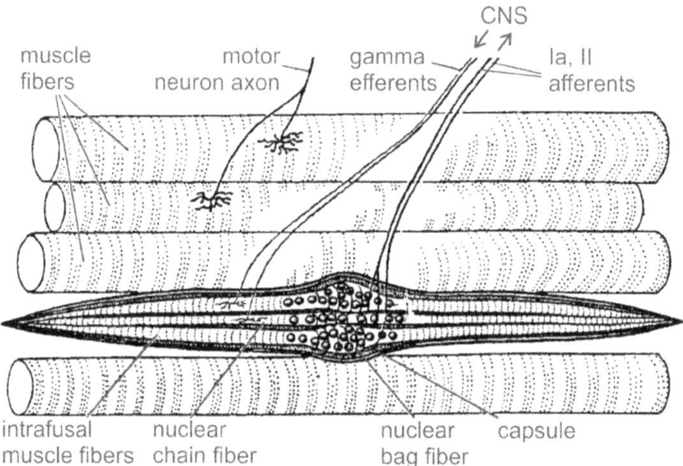

Figure 13.   The muscle spindle is a fusiform, encapsulated structure situated in parallel with the fibers making up the muscle. It contains approximately six thin muscle fibers called intrafusal fibers. There are two types of intrafusal fibers, nuclear bag and nuclear chain fibers. Sensory receptors spiral around the central region of the intrafusal fibers and give rise to two axons, Ia and II. These afferents send action potentials to the central nervous system (CNS). The intrafusal fibers receive input from the CNS via gamma efferent axons. (Adapted with permission from Nicholls *et al.* [1992].)

stick used to wind wool into thread. The general morphological term for such *tapered shapes* is **fusiform**. The spindle runs in parallel with the muscle fibers. In some cases, muscle spindles, like muscle fibers, attach to the tendons at the ends of the muscle. In other cases, the spindle terminates into a connective tissue bundle that incorporates into the connective tissue surrounding muscle fibers, which then ultimately merges into the tendon. Regardless, the diagram in Figure 13 is greatly foreshortened. Keep in mind that tendon-to-tendon length can be several centimeters while the diameter of a muscle spindle is typically less than 100 μm. This means that the actual length of a muscle spindle combined with its connections to tendons would be on the order of 1,000 times greater than its diameter. Typical single human muscles have approximately 20 to 400 muscle spindles distributed throughout them, with the number of spindles increasing with the size of the muscle (Banks 2006).

Within the fusiform capsule are found a handful of small-diameter muscle fibers. These *diminutive fibers within the muscle spindle* are called

intrafusal muscle fibers (i.e., inside the fusiform capsule). These muscle fibers are unusual in that, in the central region, they lose most of the contractile material. This central region is instead filled with nuclei and fluid. Based on the arrangement of the nuclei in this central region, two types of intrafusal muscle fibers are distinguished. In one, the *nuclei in the central region are aligned in series* and are referred to as **nuclear chain fibers** (Figure 13). In the other, *the nuclei are bunched together in a cluster* and are called **nuclear bag fibers**.

It is within this central region that muscle spindle receptors wrap around the intrafusal muscle fibers. There are two types of axons that emerge from the central region. One type has a myelinated axon with a very large diameter (indeed, one of the largest in the body), and therefore is categorized as Type I axon. These axons conduct action potentials very rapidly. To distinguish it from another Type I axon arising from a different kind of muscle receptor (discussed later), it is referred to as the **Ia axon**. The other myelinated axon that emerges from the muscle spindle has a smaller diameter and conducts action potentials somewhat more slowly. It is a **Type II axon**.

Lastly, there are thin, myelinated axons that make synaptic contact with the intrafusal muscle fibers to cause them to contract. These axons arise from small neurons in the central nervous system called **gamma motor neurons**. Their axons are therefore called **gamma axons**. These axons form neuromuscular junctions on the intrafusual fibers on both sides of the central region (only shown on one side in Figure 13). Finally, it is crucial to note the direction of signaling amongst these axons. Gamma *axons send signals out of (exiting) the central nervous system*, and such axons are generally referred to as **efferents**. On the other hand, the Type Ia and II *axons send information toward (approaching) the central nervous system* and are called **afferents**.

Muscle Spindle Function

Now that we have discussed the general structure of the muscle spindle, let's turn our attention to how it works and what information it provides to the central nervous system. To do this, let's consider a schematic diagram of just the central region containing one nuclear bag and one nuclear chain fiber (Figure 14). The **Type II** axon arises from a spiral-shaped

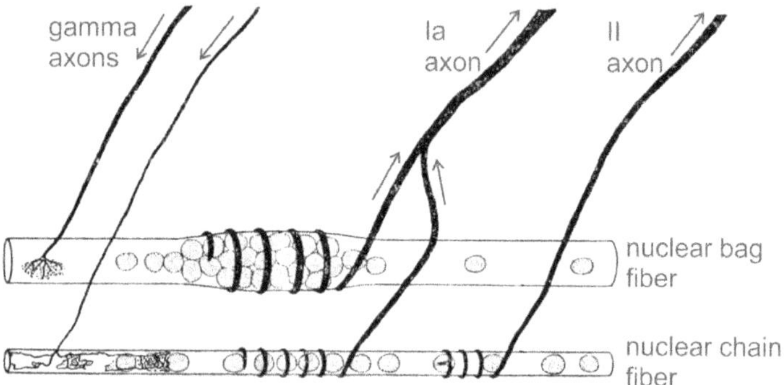

Figure 14.   Innervation of muscle spindle. Type II axon has spiral-shaped receptors on nuclear chain fibers. Ia axon has spiral receptors on both nuclear chain and nuclear bag fibers. Intrafusal fibers receive efferent innervation from gamma axons. (Adapted from Matthews [1964].)

ending on the nuclear chain fiber (Boyd 1962), which serves as the receptor membrane. This spiral adheres to the nuclear chain fiber. As the nuclear chain fiber gets stretched, the spiral also gets extended, like a little spring. This distortion of the spiral causes opening of mechanically gated channels and depolarization of the receptor membrane. The greater the degree of the stretch, the greater the receptor depolarization, and higher the frequency of action potentials generated on the Type II axon. Keep in mind that the muscle spindle is in parallel with the muscle fibers of the muscle and is tied directly or indirectly to tendons on both ends. Therefore, the muscle spindle will change length in the same way as the muscle. As a consequence, the Type II afferent provides a continuous report to the central nervous system of the length of the muscle based on its firing rate.

The **Ia axon** has a more complicated configuration. One branch of the Ia axon encircles the nuclear chain fiber with a spiral receptor more or less equivalent to that formed by the Type II axon. As such, like the Type II axon, *that branch of the Ia axon signals the length of the muscle.* The other branch of the Ia axon ends in a receptor that spirals around the nuclear bag fiber. This ending on the bag (like a corpuscle) has a rapidly adapting response not unlike that for Meissner or Pacinian corpuscles. As such, *the receptor on the nuclear bag fiber will only respond when the* *length is changing* and ceases when the length is not changing. Furthermore, the firing rate of the Ia axon branch from the nuclear bag fiber increases with *rate of length change*, that is, with the velocity of stretch (*Note*: the activity on this branch ceases during muscle *shortening*). What ultimately is conveyed by the Ia axon to the central nervous system is more or less the summation of the signals arising from the two branches of the nuclear chain and nuclear bag fibers.

To better understand the nature of signaling by Ia and II axons, let's consider the firing rates generated by both in response to a ramp stretch of a muscle (Figure 15). When the muscle is initially held at a short length, the firing rate on the Type II axon is low. As the muscle is lengthened, the firing rate of the Type II axon progressively increases and then reaches a new high steady level when the muscle is held at the long length. As such, the firing rate of the Type II axon faithfully indicates the length of the muscle at any moment.

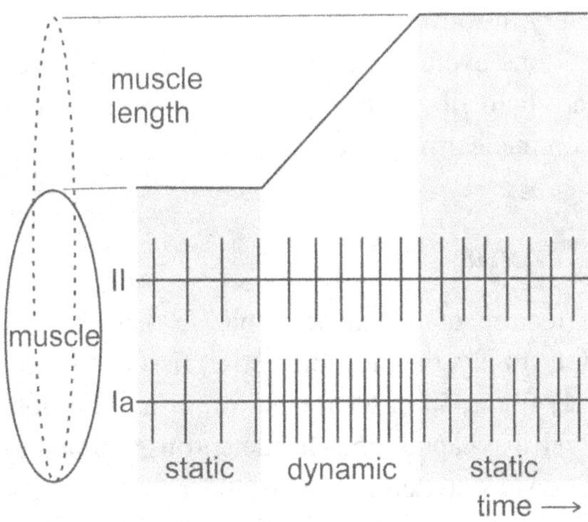

Figure 15.   Schematic depicting firing on muscle spindle Type II and Ia axons during a ramp stretch of a muscle. The firing rate on Type II axon is proportional to the length of muscle. For the Ia axon, during the hold phases (static), the firing rate is similar to that of the Type II axon (due to their endings on nuclear chain fibers). During the stretch (dynamic), activation of the Ia receptor on nuclear bag fibers adds to that arising from nuclear chain fibers to give an increased firing rate that is proportional to the speed of the stretch. (Adapted from Matthews [1964].)

If we now look at the firing of the Ia axon, during periods when the muscle length is held constant (labeled "static" in Figure 15), its firing is similar to that on the Type II axon. That is because when the muscle is not changing length, the ending of the Ia axon on the nuclear bag fiber is quiescent. Therefore, the only signal that is sent to the central nervous system by the Ia axon during those periods is that associated with its receptor on the nuclear chain fiber, just like that of the Type II axon. However, during the period of lengthening (labeled "dynamic"), the receptor on the nuclear bag fiber comes to life. The activity arising from the receptor on the nuclear bag fiber will combine with the activity arising from the nuclear chain fiber to yield a high firing rate during the dynamic phase. The faster the speed of lengthening, the greater the contribution of the nuclear bag fiber, and the higher the firing rate during the lengthening phase. Overall, the Ia axon provides two types of information: the length of the muscle under static conditions (via the nuclear chain fiber) and the speed of lengthening during dynamic conditions (via the nuclear bag fiber). It remains a mystery, however, as to why nature didn't simply create two separate "lines": one exclusively to indicate the muscle length (receptor only on nuclear chain fibers) and one exclusively to indicate the speed (receptor only on nuclear bag fibers).

Gamma Efferents

It is a notable feature of the muscle spindle that the sensory–receptor apparatus is not simply tied to connective tissue on either end but to intrafusal muscle fibers. In order for intrafusal muscle fibers to contract, they need to receive synaptic input from neurons (gamma motor neurons) in the central nervous system. Why would nature go to the trouble to incorporate the complexities of contractile material and its required innervation into this sensory organ? There have been several theories proposed as to the role of the intrafusal muscle fibers and its drive from gamma motor neurons. Perhaps *one function is simply to take up the slack in the connections of the muscle spindle to enable signaling over a wide range of possible muscle lengths.*

To illustrate this idea, consider first a nuclear chain fiber of a muscle spindle without intrafusal fibers but instead attached by long, passive,

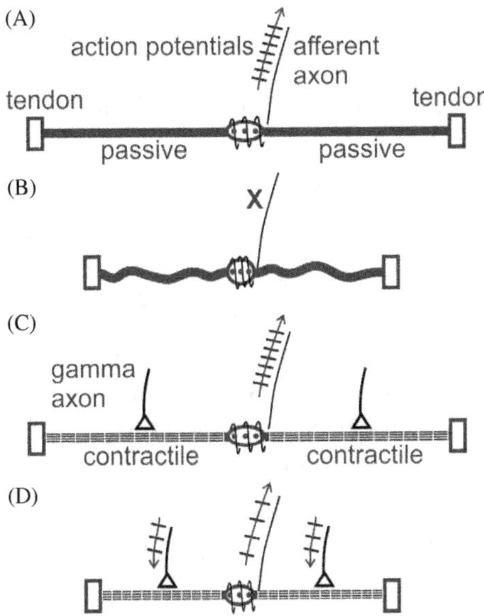

Figure 16.   Function of gamma drive to intrafusal muscle fibers. (A) Nuclear chain fiber of muscle spindle without intrafusal muscle fibers that are connected to tendons (rectangles) on either end by passive connective tissue. At long lengths, the spiral receptor would be stretched leading to activity on the afferent axon. (B) At shorter lengths, the passive linkages would go slack, eliminating the tension on the spiral receptor, and loss of signaling. (C) Passive connection is replaced with contractile material of the intrafusal muscle fiber. At long lengths, passive tension in the intrafusal muscle fiber may be sufficient to stretch the spiral receptor and generate activity on the afferent. (D) When the muscle shortens, activity on gamma axons causes the intrafusal muscle fibers to contract, thereby maintaining some tension on the spiral receptor and signaling on the afferent axon.

connective tissue strands to the tendons on either end (Figure 16A). At the long muscle length, the spiral receptor in the central portion is stretched, leading to the production of action potentials on the afferent. If, however, the muscle is shortened (Figure 16B), the connective tissue linkages will readily become slack, and thereby provide no tension to extend the centrally located receptor. As such, signaling from the muscle spindle would cease after only a small degree of shortening. Keep in mind that connective tissue can only change length by a relatively small amount before going slack whereas skeletal muscle has an enormous capacity to change its length while still producing tension.

In Figure 16C, the connective tissue linkages are replaced with intrafusal muscle fibers. At long lengths, the passive properties of the intrafusal muscle fibers will exert tension on the coiled receptor at the center of the spindle, leading to activation of the afferent. Now, let's assume that the neural drive from the motor neurons causes the muscle to shorten. In parallel, similar commands are sent to the intrafusal muscle fibers through the gamma axons. That gamma activity will cause some degree of shortening in the intrafusal fibers, contributing to some level of tension exerted upon the receptor and activity on the afferent. In this way, signaling from the muscle spindle is maintained over much of the range of length changes in the muscle. Nevertheless, there still remain open questions as to how the central nervous system controls the gamma drive to the intrafusal fibers such that the read-out of the afferent accurately represents the length and rate of length change of the muscle.

Golgi Tendon Organ

Another (and simpler) proprioceptor is the Golgi tendon organ (named for its discoverer, Camillo Golgi). The **Golgi tendon organ** is a *muscle force sensor*. It is situated at the junction between muscle fibers and tendon (Figure 17). This "in-series" arrangement is like links in a chain, where the tensile force is the same for every link in the chain. As such, the Golgi tendon organ experiences the same tensile forces as the muscle fibers attached to it. The receptor endings of the Golgi tendon organ weave between collagen fibers enveloped within a capsule. The axon that emerges from the capsule is a large-diameter, myelinated axon of the Type I variety. To distinguish it from the Type I axon arising from the muscle spindle, it is called the **Ib axon**. A typical muscle will have approximately 20 to 80 Golgi tendon organs, each connected to a different slip of tendon or aponeurosis (fascia sheet that attaches some muscles to bone).

As force develops in the muscle fibers, that tension pulls the collagen fibers within the capsule taut, squeezing the receptor endings of the Golgi tendon organ that are entwined within the collagen fibers (inset, Figure 17). That distortion serves as the stimulus to open mechanically gated channels in the membrane to depolarize the receptor. As such, the **Golgi tendon organ** is exquisitely *sensitive to the contractile force*

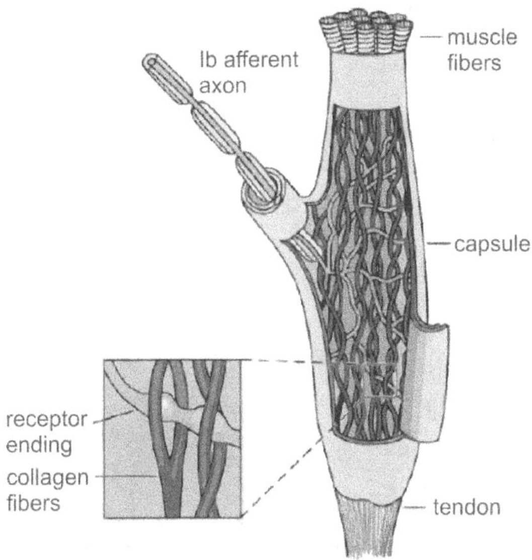

Figure 17.   The Golgi tendon organ is an encapsulated structure found at the junction between a set of muscle fibers and the small segment of the tendon. The sensory receptor endings weave between collagen fibers that connect the muscle fibers to the tendon. As force develops in the muscle, the collagen fibers become taut and compress the receptor endings. That compression leads to the opening of mechanically gated channels, depolarization of the receptor membrane, and instigation of action potentials on the Ib axon that emerges from the Golgi tendon organ. As such, the Golgi tendon organ signals the contractile force developed in muscle. (Adapted from Kandel *et al.* [2012].)

developed in muscle. This is highlighted in Figure 18, which shows the firing rate recorded from the Ib axon at many different levels of muscle force. There are two important features depicted in Figure 18 that are typical of most Golgi tendon organs. First, Golgi tendon organs respond to even the gentlest of muscle contractions. This finding dispels one of the old ideas that Golgi tendon organs only become active at high forces to trigger reflexes that cause muscle contraction to cease, thereby protecting the muscle from damage. Second, the firing rate of Golgi tendon organs is a remarkably linear function of the contractile force over a wide range of forces. As such, rate coding by Golgi tendon organs provides a high-fidelity signal to the central nervous system about the intensity of muscle contraction. Therefore, for example, when we hold various objects in our

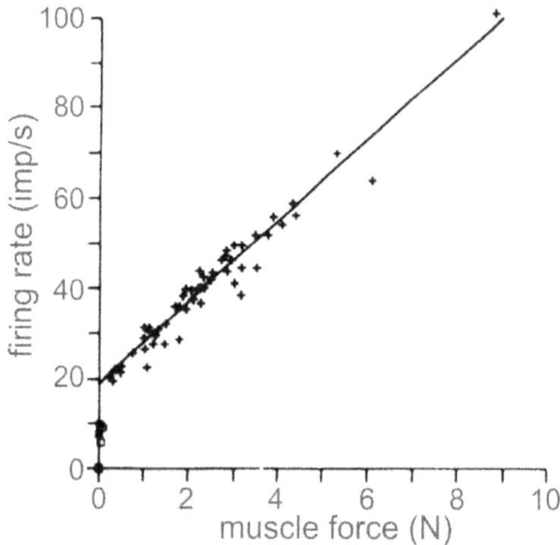

Figure 18.   The firing rate response of a single Ib axon from a Golgi tendon organ recorded at different levels of muscle contraction force. Each symbol indicates the average firing rate recorded during a steady-force contraction. The relation between the firing rate and force is highly linear. Also, the Golgi tendon organ responds even to the lowest levels of force produced by the muscle. (Adapted from Crago *et al.* [1982].)

hands (from a pencil to a bowling ball), we accurately gauge the weights of those objects due to muscle forces developed (and the precise readout by the Golgi tendon organ) to support the weight of the object against gravity.

Joint Receptors

The tissues surrounding a joint, namely, the articular surfaces, the joint capsule, and the ligaments, are richly invested with a host of sensory receptors collectively referred to as **joint receptors** (Figure 19). This array of sensory receptors gives rise to the entire spectrum of axon diameters, from **Type I to Type IV**. Most joint receptors have a slowly adapting firing rate response. Importantly, *joint receptors only become active near the extremes of the joint range of motion* (Burgess & Clark 1969). Figure 20 depicts the general firing rate response to changes in joint angle for joint receptors. As the joint approaches its most flexed position (small joint angles), some joint receptors begin to fire, and the firing rate

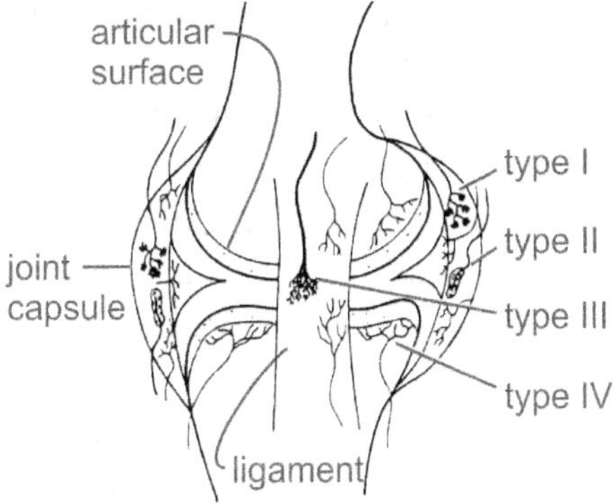

Figure 19.   Schematic of a joint indicating the joint capsule, ligaments, and articular surface richly innervated by a variety of sensory receptors that give rise to axon Types I–IV. These sensory receptors are collectively referred to as joint receptors. (Adapted from Shepherd [1988].)

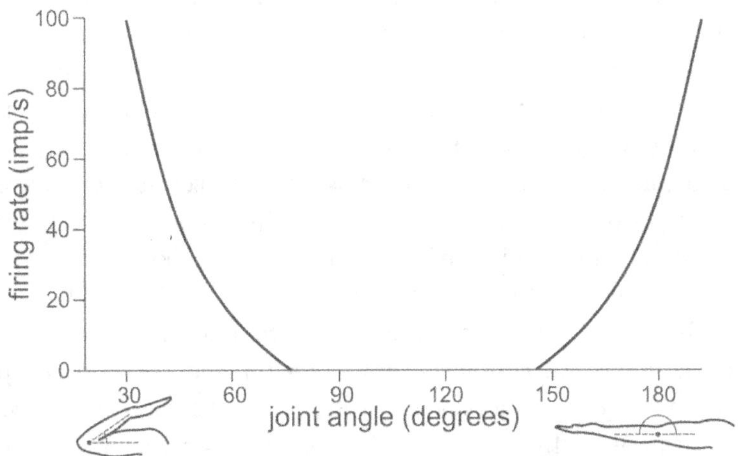

Figure 20.   General firing rate responses of joint receptors to change in joint angle. Different sets of receptors are active when the joint is in flexion versus extension. Joint receptors usually are active only near the extremes of the joint range of motion. The firing rate tends to accelerate as the joint is moved toward the extremes. (Based on data from Grigg and Greenspan [1977].)

increases as the joint is pushed further into flexion. At the other extreme, a different set of receptors is activated as the joint approaches full extension. Because the receptor endings are embedded in the various tissues surrounding the joint, as those tissues become stretched at one joint extreme or the other, the receptor endings are also put under strain. This leads to the opening of mechanically gated channels, depolarization of the receptor membrane, and generation of action potentials.

Joint receptors may serve as a kind of limit detector to signal the central nervous system that a joint is approaching the end of its range of motion. This information may be important to prevent joint damage from hyperflexion or hyperextension. As such, should joint receptors be considered as a kind of nociceptor (i.e., high-threshold receptors activated only with damaging or potentially damaging stimuli) rather than as proprioceptors (detectors of position and movement of body parts)?

To partially address this question, we can perform a simple experiment. Slowly flex your own elbow until you can flex it no more. While doing this, pay attention to the sensations arising from the elbow region. As you advance closer to the fully flexed position, you will probably first start to perceive some increasing sense of tightness, stretch, and compression in different regions surrounding the elbow. These sensations typically are not painful and become stronger as you advance farther. However, when you get quite close to the fully flexed position, you will start to perceive some sense of discomfort arising from the elbow region that can become more intense if you try to push the joint much beyond that which it normally moves. The same type of sensation occurs when you fully extend the elbow. So how can we account for both the proprioceptive (increasing awareness of joint angle) and nociceptive (feelings of discomfort) senses arising from this one class of sensory receptors? The most likely explanation is that both types of sensory receptors exist among the joint receptor class. Those that are activated before the position of the joint becomes painful are proprioceptors with Type I and II axons. Whereas, those receptors that become activated at more extreme joint angles and that trigger the sense of discomfort are nociceptors having Type III and IV axons.

To illustrate the proprioceptive role of joint receptors, Figure 21 shows a microneurographic recording made of a joint receptor afferent

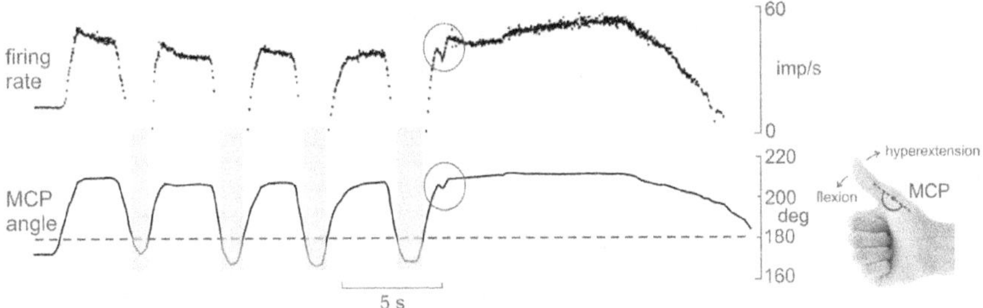

Figure 21.   Microneurographic recording of the firing rate of a joint receptor afferent supplying the MCP joint in the thumb of a human subject. Joint angle (lower trace) was detected with a small device attached to the back of the MCP joint. The experimenter slowly rotated the joint while the firing rate (top trace) of the receptor afferent was recorded. At joint angles of approximately >180° (joint angles above the dashed horizontal line), the firing rate provided an accurate representation of the joint angle. Even small changes in joint angle (circle in MCP angle trace) were clearly encoded in the firing rate of the receptor (circle in firing rate trace). The firing ceased, however, for joint angles flexed more than ~180° (gray bars). (From the author's laboratory.)

supplying the metacarpophalangeal (MCP) joint at the base of the thumb in a human. The experimenter slowly rotated the joint out near the full extension, and the joint angle was recorded with a small device affixed to the back of the MCP joint (lower trace, Figure 21). In most people, this joint can be hyperextended beyond 180° without discomfort, as was the case for this subject.

The firing rate of the joint receptor (top trace, Figure 21) generally reproduced joint angle with remarkable fidelity in the hyperextended range (MCP angles above the dashed horizontal line, Figure 21). Even a very small change in the direction of joint rotation (indicated by the small circle in Figure 21) was clearly mimicked and even amplified in the firing rate of the joint receptor. The slightly exaggerated firing rate responses at the most extended positions were likely due to the nonlinear responses of joint receptors to change in angle (see Figure 20). This means that the change in firing rate increases in greater proportion than the change in joint angle as a joint is moved toward the extremes. On the other hand, when the joint was flexed to angles less than ~180° (gray bars in Figure 21), the receptor stopped firing all together. As such, this joint receptor signaled joint angle with good accuracy at extended positions that were not associated with discomfort. Therefore, this joint receptor would seem to clearly qualify as a proprioceptor.

Ruffini Endings

One type of somatosensory receptor that has a kind of dual personality is the **Ruffini ending**. As discussed under tactile receptors, Ruffini endings are found in the skin, are innervated by Aβ axons, have large receptive fields, are slowly adapting, and can respond to skin stretch. It is the responsiveness to skin stretch that provides the Ruffini ending with proprioceptive capabilities. When we move most joints, the skin on one side of the joint will become stretched for movements in one direction, and the skin on the other side of the joint becomes stretched for movements in the opposite direction. Ruffini endings found in the skin surrounding joints, therefore, can respond to this skin stretch and provide information about the joint angle.

Figure 22A shows the firing rate response of a tactile afferent to a sustained touch applied to the center of its large receptive field on the back of a human hand (Figure 22B) using microneurography. The firing rate exhibited a slowly adapting profile. Therefore, given its large receptive field and slowly adapting response, the most likely type of receptor associated with this recording was a Ruffini ending. Furthermore, when the investigators manually stretched that region of the skin along the long axis of the receptive field, the afferent fired vigorously.

The investigators then asked the subject to slowly flex and extend the MCP joint at the base of the index finger while they recorded the firing of the afferent. As the subject flexed the joint, the skin on the back of the hand became stretched, and this led to increased firing of the Ruffini ending afferent (Figure 22C). When the subject extended the finger back toward its original configuration (and the stretch of skin on the back of the hand lessened), the firing of the Ruffini ending afferent diminished. Therefore, the firing rate of the Ruffini ending changed systematically with change in joint angle (via the degree of skin stretch). As such, Ruffini endings can provide proprioceptive information to the central nervous system.

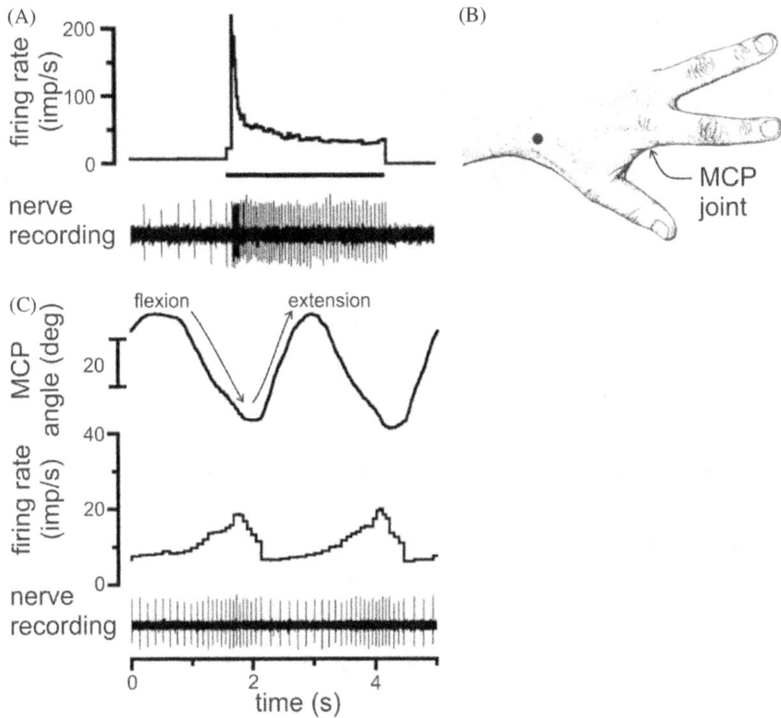

Figure 22.   (A) Discharge of a Ruffini ending afferent in response to sustained application of a touch stimulus (horizontal line) applied to (B) the center of the receptive field (dot) on the back of the hand of a human subject. (C) When the subject flexed the MCP joint, the skin on the back of the hand stretched, increasing the firing rate of the receptor. When the MCP joint was extended, skin stretch lessened, and firing rate decreased. Therefore, Ruffini ending activity can provide information about joint angle. (Adapted from Edin and Abbs [1991].)

Which Receptors Underlie Joint Position Sense?

Since before Sherrington's time, there has been a somewhat tortuous debate as to which receptors are responsible for our sense of joint angle and limb orientation (see Matthews 1982). Sherrington made a strong argument at the beginning of the 20th century that muscle receptors (i.e., muscle spindles) must be most important for this function. Muscle spindles respond to the length of muscle, and muscles change length when joint angles change. Therefore, muscle spindles would seem well suited to encode joint angles. Somewhat inexplicably, in the late 1950s, the influential Vernon Mountcastle rejected Sherrington's idea and suggested that joint receptors, rather than muscle spindles, were the key receptor encoding joint angle sense. However, the finding in the late 1960s (like that in Figure 20) that joint receptors respond primarily at the extremes of the joint range of motion, yet joint angles in the middle of the range can readily be perceived, swung the debate again in favor of muscle spindles. Indeed, it was subsequently shown that vibrating a muscle tendon (a potent stimulus to muscle spindle receptors, particularly those supplied by the Ia afferent) in human subjects caused an illusion that the associated joint was rotating when indeed it was not (Goodwin *et al.*, 1972). Incredibly, when blindfolded subjects flexed their elbow to touch their nose with their fingers and the biceps tendon was vibrated, the illusion of the elbow joint extending led subjects (like Pinocchio) to perceive their noses were elongating (Lackner 1988).

Despite this strong evidence, a host of clever experiments using local anesthesia and other manipulations to selectively remove the contribution of individual classes of receptors, demonstrated that muscle spindles, joint afferents, and skin receptors all contribute in varying ways to the sense of joint position (Proske & Gandevia 2012). To get some idea of how a collection of sensory receptors might work together, let's consider just muscle spindle and joint afferent contributions to joint angle changes at the elbow (Figure 23). When the joint is at very flexed angles (e.g., ~30°), the flexion joint receptors will respond with high firing rates. Likewise, in this joint configuration, the triceps muscle is elongated. Therefore, muscle spindles afferents within the triceps will discharge at high rates. The biceps, however, is in a very shortened position. As such, firing rates of biceps muscle spindles will be low. Now, as the joint moves from a flexed toward a midrange position, the firing rate of the flexion joint receptor will diminish rapidly and then cease to fire. At the same time, the triceps spindle activity will also decay but not as steeply as for the joint receptor. Furthermore, muscle spindle activity arising from the biceps will progressively increase. Finally, as the movement continues to the fully extended position, extension joint receptors will begin to fire, triceps muscle spindle activity will further decrease as the triceps

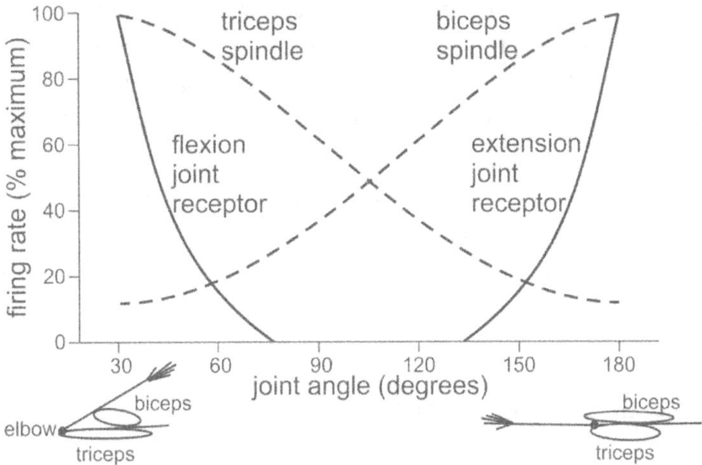

Figure 23.   Schematic showing joint afferent (solid lines) and muscle spindle (dashed lines) responses to different angles of the elbow joint. At very flexed (small) angles, flexion joint receptor activity would be high. The triceps muscle would be elongated at flexed angles leading to high firing rates in triceps muscle spindles whereas the biceps would be short with low activity in its muscle spindles. Moving the joint into the midrange will cause flexion joint receptors to stop firing, triceps spindle afferents to reduce firing, and biceps spindle afferents to increase their firing. Movement toward full extension will cause extension joint afferents to become active, biceps spindle afferents to continue to increase their firing and triceps spindle afferent activity to diminish. From this collective activity, there is a unique neural code for each joint position.

continues to shorten, and biceps muscle spindle activity will increase as the biceps is lengthened.

Collectively, there will be a unique neural code arising from this population of receptors associated with every joint position. In the midrange, the code is carried primarily by the combination of triceps and biceps muscle spindles. Beyond the midrange, joint receptors provide additional information. Furthermore, although not shown, the activities of the Ruffini endings in the skin surrounding the elbow will also furnish firing rate data about the joint angle. Presumably, this code, distributed over the activities of multiple receptors, is brought together and interpreted in regions of the cerebral cortex that impart the perception of joint angle.

Indeed, this kind of integration likely occurs across multiple joints in a limb. For example, when playing the piano (with eyes closed), our mental representation of the positions of our fingers is that of the fingertips, not the angles of the individual joints in the fingers, wrist, elbow, and shoulder that actually dictate the locations of the fingertips. Indeed, neurophysiological experiments have demonstrated that certain brain areas integrate signals arising from an enormous set of proprioceptors distributed across an entire limb to indicate the position of the endpoint (e.g., the fingertip) independent of the individual angles of the joints of the limb (Bosco *et al.*, 2000).

Absence of Proprioception

As mentioned at the outset of this section on proprioception, it is difficult to recognize the importance of proprioception because we cannot "turn it off." In addition, there are very few clinical disorders associated with impaired proprioception. One such case, however, was documented in a poignant book by Jonathan Cole (1995). An otherwise healthy 19-year-old man developed a disease that destroyed the large-diameter sensory axons (Type I, II, and Aβ) in his peripheral nerves. As such, he effectively lost proprioceptive and tactile senses from the neck down. He was unable to stand, walk, or even control his limbs to do simple tasks like feeding himself. Yet, he was not paralyzed in the classical sense because motor pathways and motor axons were unaffected, and his muscles could be made to contract. He just could not *control* the activation of his muscles. Consequently, this selective loss of sensations from muscles, joints, tendons, and skin was devastating, leaving him bedridden and completely dependent on others for his care. Doctors indicated that there was nothing that could be done for him. Remarkably, however, over a period of years and on his own, he tenaciously developed a number of clever "tricks" using vision and extreme mental effort to enable him to regain the ability to walk and perform simple motor tasks. However, if the lights were turned off while he was standing, he would collapse onto the floor. This case highlights the inextricable link between the somatosensory system (and in particular, the proprioceptive system) and the motor system. This important matter will be further discussed in later chapters.

Summary

In this chapter, we have examined the diverse array of sensory receptors that underlie our body sense—the somatosensory receptors. There are four main types of these receptors (tactile, thermal, nociceptive, and proprioceptive), and each category has its own subset of receptors that encode various kinds of information (see Table 1). In the following chapter, we will take a short interlude to outline the basics of neuroanatomy before describing how information from these receptors is conveyed and processed in the brain.

Table 1.   Summary of somatosensory receptors.

Tactile

Receptor	Receptive Field	Adaptation	Axon	Sub-modality
Merkel disk	Small	Slow	Aβ	Touch pressure
Meissner corpuscle	Small	Fast	Aβ	Texture
Ruffini ending	Large	Slow	Aβ	Skin stretch
Pacinian corpuscle	Large	Fast	Aβ	Vibration

Thermal

Receptor	Axon	Sub-modality
Cold (free nerve ending)	Aδ	Coolness
Warm (free nerve ending)	C-fiber	Warmth

Nociceptive

Receptor	Axon	Sub-modality
1st pain (free nerve ending)	Aδ	Fast, sharp, stabbing pain
2nd pain (free nerve ending)	C-fiber	Slow, achy, persistent pain

Proprioceptive

Receptor	Axon(s)	Sub-Modality
Muscle spindle		
Nuclear chain fiber	Ia, II	Muscle length
Nuclear bag fiber	Ia	Speed of muscle stretch
Golgi tendon organ	Ib	Muscle contraction force
Joint receptors	I, II, III, IV	Joint angle (extremes)
Ruffini ending	Aβ	Joint angle (skin stretch)

References

Banks RW (2006). An allometric analysis of the number of muscle spindles in mammalian skeletal muscles. *Journal of Anatomy* **208**, 753–768.

Belmonte C, Gallar J, Pozo MA & Rebollo I (1991). Excitation by irritant chemical substances of sensory afferent units in the cat's cornea. *Journal of Physiology* **437**, 709–725.

Bosco G, Poppele RE & Eian J (2000). Reference frames for spinal proprioception: limb endpoint based or joint-level based? *Journal of Neurophysiology* **83**, 2931–2945.

Boyd IA (1962). The structure and innervation of the nuclear bag muscle fibre system and the nuclear chain muscle fibre system in mammalian muscle spindles. *Proceedings of the Royal Society of London Series B* **245**: 81–136.

Brown AC (1989). Introduction to sensory mechanisms. In: Patton HD, Fuchs AF, Hille B, Scher AM & Steiner R (eds.) Textbook of Physiology: Excitable Cells and Neurophysiology, (Volume 1), WB Saunders: Philadelphia, pp. 306.

Burgess PR & Clark FJ (1969). Characteristics of knee joint receptors in the cat. *Journal of Physiology* **203**, 317–335.

Cole J (1995). Pride and a Daily Marathon, Bradford Book, MIT Press: Cambridge, Massachusetts.

Crago PE, Houk JC & Rymer WZ (1982). Sampling of total muscle force by tendon organs. *Journal of Neurophysiology* **47**, 1069–1083.

Detwiler PB (1989). Sensory transduction. In: Patton HD, Fuchs AF, Hille B, Scher AM & Steiner R (eds.) Textbook of Physiology: Excitable Cells and Neurophysiology (Volume 1), WB Saunders: Philadelphia, pp. 114.

Dhaka A, Viswanath V & Patapoutian A (2006). TRP ion channels and temperature sensation. *Annual Review of Neuroscience* **29**, 135–161.

Edin BB & Abbs JH (1991). Finger movement responses of cutaneous mechanoreceptors in the dorsal skin of the human hand. *Journal of Neurophysiology* **65**, 657–670.

Georgopoulos AP (1976). Functional properties of primary afferent units probably related to pain mechanisms in primate glabrous skin. *Journal of Neurophysiology* **39**, 71–83.

Goodwin GM, McCloskey DI & Matthews PB (1972). Proprioceptive illusions induced by muscle vibration: Contribution by muscle spindles to perception? *Science* **175**, 1382–1384.

Grigg P & Greenspan BJ (1977). Response of primate joint afferent neurons to mechanical stimulation of knee joint. *Journal of Neurophysiology* **40**, 1–8.

Johansson RS & Vallbo ÅB (1983). Tactile sensory coding in the glabrous skin of the human hand. *Trends in Neurosciences* **6**, 27–32.

Kandel ER, Schwartz JH, Jessell TM, Siegelbaum SA & Hudspeth AJ (2012). Principles of Neural Science (5th Edition). McGraw-Hill: New York.

Lackner JR (1988). Some proprioceptive influences on the perceptual representation of body shape and orientation. *Brain* **111 (Pt 2)**, 281–297.

Loewenstein WR & Mendelson M (1965). Components of receptor adaptation in a Pacinian corpuscle. *Journal of Physiology* **177**, 377–397.

Mackenzie RA, Burke D, Skuse NF & Lethlean AK (1975). Fibre function and perception during cutaneous nerve block. *Journal of Neurology, Neurosurgery, and Psychiatry* **38**, 865–873.

Matthews PB (1964). Muscle spindles and their motor control. *Physiological Reviews* **44**, 219–288.

Matthews PB (1982). Where does Sherrington's 'muscular sense' originate? Muscles, joints, corollary discharges? *Annual Review of Neuroscience* **5**, 189–218.

Nicholls JG, Martin AR, & Wallace BG (1992). From Neuron to Brain (3rd Edition). Sinauer Associates: Sunderland MA.

Ochoa J & Mair WG (1969). The normal sural nerve in man. I. Ultrastructure and numbers of fibres and cells. *Acta Neuropathologica* **13**, 197–216.

Pawson L, Checkosky CM, Pack AK & Bolanowski SJ (2009). Mesenteric and tactile Pacinian corpuscles are anatomically and physiologically comparable. *Somatosensory & Motor Research* **25**, 194–206.

Proske U & Gandevia SC (2012). The proprioceptive senses: their roles in signaling body shape, body position and movement, and muscle force. *Physiological Reviews* **92**, 1651–1697.

Shepherd GM (1988). Neurobiology (2nd Edition). Oxford University Press: Oxford.

Sunderland S (1978). Nerve and Nerve Injuries (2nd Edition). Churchill Livingstone: London.

Torebjörk HE, Vallbo ÅB & Ochoa JL (1987). Intraneural microstimulation in man. Its relation to specificity of tactile sensations. *Brain* **110 (Pt 6)**, 1509–1529.

Vallbo ÅB (2018). Microneurography: How it started and how it works. *Journal of Neurophysiology* **120**, 1415–1427.

Zhang S, Malik Sharif S, Chen Y-C, Valente EM, Ahmed M, Sheridan E, Bennett C & Woods G (2016). Clinical features for diagnosis and management of patients with PRDM12 congenital insensitivity to pain. *Journal of Medical Genetics* **53**, 533–535.

Chapter 10

Basic Neuroanatomy

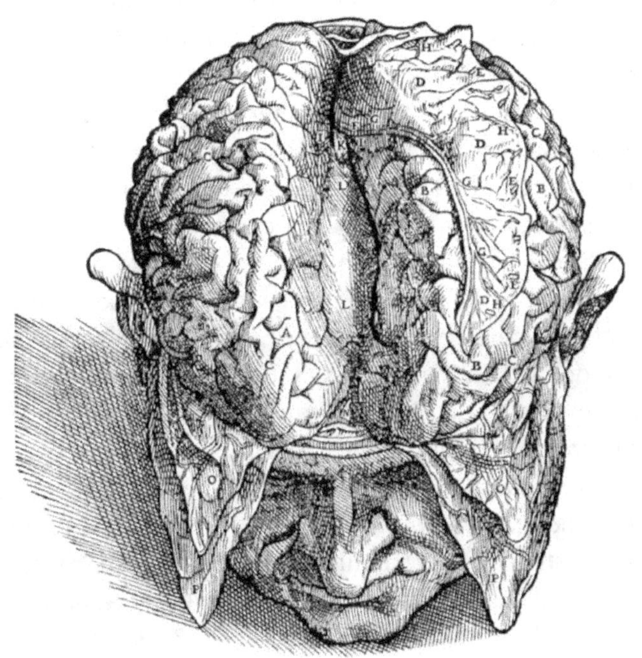

Dissection of the human brain, by the 16th-century anatomist Andreas Vesalius (from De Humani Corporis Fabrica, *1544).*

The naming system for structures within the nervous system is not always consistent and can vary from one literature source to another. For example, the primary motor cortex is referred to interchangeably as M1, area 4, or F1. Furthermore, from a modern perspective, the names for many brain structures may seem bewildering (e.g., zona incerta, nucleus ambiguous, and raphe obscurus, just to name a few). Yet, these Latin names were logically based on what early neuroanatomists observed in brain dissections (and were not invented just to torture students). In this brief survey, only key neuroanatomical terms and structures will be described. Other neuroanatomical information will be added in context when we describe specific neurophysiological functions in later chapters.

As mentioned in Chapter 1, the two main subdivisions of the nervous system are the **central nervous system (CNS)**, which includes *the brain and the spinal cord*, and the **peripheral nervous system (PNS)**, which includes *neurons and nerves outside of the CNS*. As the first organizational level, *clusters of neurons within the CNS that have similar functions* are referred to as **nuclei**, whereas *clusters of such neurons in the PNS* are generally referred to as **ganglia**. The *axon bundles in the CNS that connect one structure to another* are typically referred to as **tracts** or **pathways**. One convention that is often used to name such tracts is that the *first half of the name indicates the site of origin* and the *second half of the name indicates the destination* of the tract. For example, the spinothalamic tract refers to a set of axons that project from the spinal cord to the thalamus (a structure at the center of the brain). Likewise, the corticospinal tract refers to a bundle of axons that project from the cerebral cortex to the spinal cord.

"Navigation" within the nervous system is facilitated by the concept of a reference axis—just like the arrow pointing north on geographic maps. The neuroanatomical *reference axis* (the **neuroaxis**) is the long axis that runs *longitudinally from head to tail through the center of the CNS* (Figure 1A). The *direction of the neuroaxis pointing toward the nose* is referred to as **rostral** (from the Latin word for beak; also, "rostral" rhymes with "nostril") whereas the direction pointing *toward the tail* is referred to as **caudal** (from the Latin word for tail). The *direction perpendicular to the neuroaxis and pointing toward the back* is **dorsal**, whereas the *perpendicular direction to the neuroaxis but pointing toward the front* is **ventral**. The *direction perpendicular to the neuroaxis but pointing to the side* is **lateral** whereas the direction *pointing from the side toward the midline* is **medial.**

Keep in mind that the neuroaxis is not a rigid rod but bends as the CNS bends. As such, if the little creature shown in Figure 1A got up and

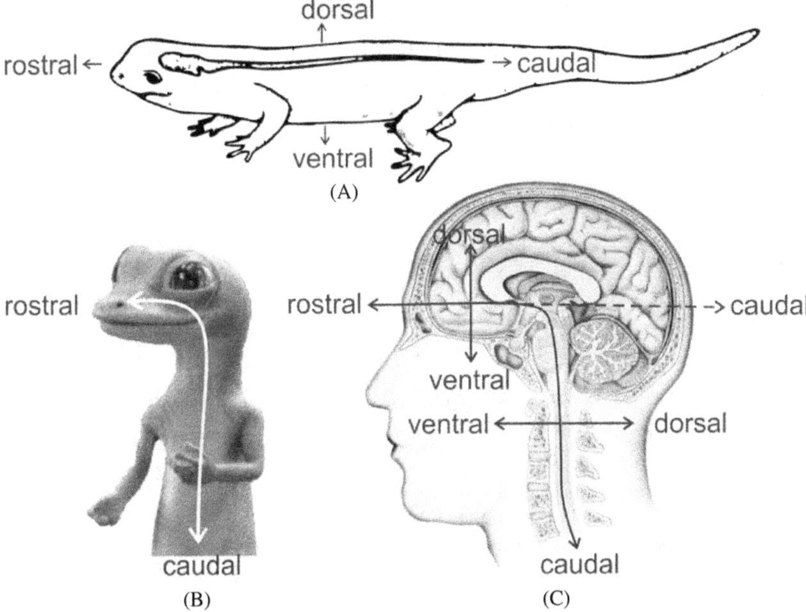

Figure 1.   Reference axis for neuroanatomy. (A) The neuroaxis runs from head to tail. Toward the nose is caudal whereas toward the tail is caudal. Perpendicular to the neuroaxis and toward the back is dorsal while toward the front is ventral. (B) The neuroaxis is flexible and can bend. (C) The human brain has permanent flexure of neuroaxis. In the brainstem and spinal cord, the neuroaxis is vertical whereas above the brainstem the neuroaxis runs horizontally. ([A] Adapted from Kandel *et al.* [2012]; [B] from Geico, and [C] from iStock.com.)

walked around on its hind legs, it would need to bend its head forward to be able to see where it is going (Figure 1B). This would cause the neuroaxis (the reference frame for neuroanatomy) to have a ~90° bend. Indeed, the evolution of humans (and some nonhuman primates) toward an upright stance and bipedal walking has led to a permanent flexion in our neuroaxis (Figure 1C). This means that in the spinal cord, rostral points vertically toward the top of the head. In the brain, however, after the bend of the neuroaxis has occurred (the specific location will be described later), rostral now points horizontally toward the nose and caudal toward the back of the head. In the spinal cord (and the lower part of the brain) dorsal points to the back and ventral toward the front of the body (i.e., perpendicular to the neuroaxis at that point). Yet in the upper brain, dorsal points to the top of the head and ventral toward the jaw. Understanding the layout of the neuroaxis and the associated directional terms is crucial for making sense of the relative orientations of structures in the nervous system.

Spinal Cord

The caudal portion of the CNS is the spinal cord and it runs from the base of the skull to the upper lumbar vertebrae. There is a *repeating and bilaterally symmetric anatomical configuration* found at each of the 31 different levels (or **segments**) along the length of the spinal cord. Figure 2 shows one such segment. On the dorsal surface of the spinal cord, a set of rootlets penetrate the spinal cord that emerge from a single bundle called the dorsal root. The **dorsal root** serves as the *entry point into the spinal cord and carries the afferent axons from the somatosensory receptor*

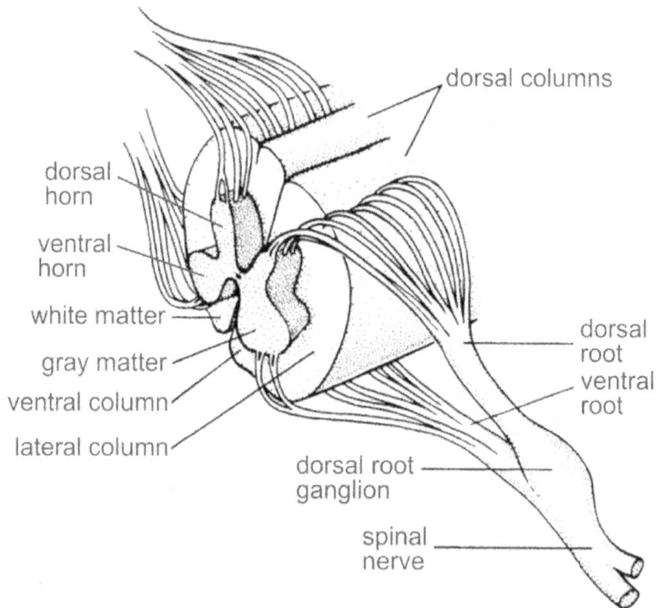

Figure 2.   Anatomy of the spinal cord. (Adapted from Kandel *et al.* [2012].)

neurons that we discussed in Chapter 9 into the CNS. If you recall, these primary sensory neurons have their *cell bodies situated off to the side of the axon and are located within a swelling of the dorsal root* called the **dorsal root ganglion**. On the ventral side, a number of rootlets emerge from the spinal segment that coalesce into a bundle called the ventral root. The **ventral root** serves as the *exit path from the CNS and carries the efferent axons of motor neurons* (whose cell bodies are in the spinal cord) toward their peripheral targets. The two roots join together (at a site still within the protective housing of the vertebral column) to form a spinal nerve that then emerges from the vertebral column.

In the interior of the spinal cord is a butterfly-shaped structure that is the gray matter of the spinal cord. **Gray matter** refers to parts of the CNS largely made up of *neuron cell bodies, dendrites,* and *synaptic connections.* As such, the gray matter is the site of neural interactions and information processing. The parts of the *gray matter wings pointing toward the back* are called the **dorsal horns** whereas the *wings pointing to the front of the body* are called the **ventral horns**. Surrounding the gray matter is the white matter. **White matter** is *mostly composed of axons*, many of which have myelin. Myelin has a whitish appearance, hence the name white matter. The *white matter of the spinal cord* is divided into three main **columns** (sometimes called **funiculi**) that carry axons up and down the spinal cord. On the dorsal surface, between the midline and the dorsal roots is a wedge of white matter called the **dorsal column**. Along the lateral side of the spinal cord, between the dorsal and ventral roots, is the **lateral column**. And on the ventral side of the spinal cord, between the ventral roots and the midline is the **ventral column**. We will discuss later the kinds of information carried by the axons in these different columns. As a general point, the configuration of the spinal cord with the gray matter on the inside and the white matter on the outside is just opposite to that found in the cerebrum where the gray matter is on the outside and the white matter is on the inside.

Brain

As a starting point for examining the anatomy of the brain, let's begin by just inspecting the surface structures. Figure 3A shows a top down (dorsal) view of the brain surface. In this image, the nose would be at the top

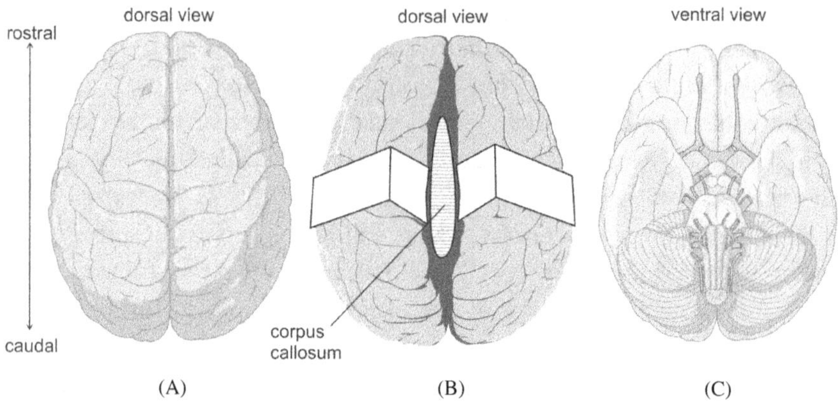

Figure 3.   Dorsal (A, B) and ventral (C) views of surface structures of the brain. (Created with BioRender.com.)

of the figure (in the rostral direction) and the back of the head would be at the bottom (in the caudal direction). Most of what is seen from this view is the folded cerebral cortex. The *groove between the two hemispheres* is called the **longitudinal** (or **interhemispheric**) *fissure*. If the two hemispheres are gently separated (Figure 3B), then one can see a massive body of white matter deep in the brain (also see Vesalius's dissection of the brain at frontispiece of this chapter). This mass of white matter has hundreds of millions of axons that interconnect the two hemispheres and is called the **corpus callosum**. If the brain is flipped over (Figure 3C) and examined from the underside (i.e., a ventral view), several rather complex structures are apparent that are not evident from the dorsal view.

Figure 4A shows a lateral view of the brain (with the nose to the left and the back of the head to the right), which mostly shows folded cerebral cortex. If the lobe of the brain that is closest to the ear is gently pulled down (Figure 4B), *a hidden (or "insulated") part of the cerebral cortex* is exposed. This region is called the **insula** (from the Latin word for island). And lastly, if we cut the brain into two halves by slicing down through the longitudinal fissure and then examine the cut face (Figure 4C), this medial view exposes several important brain structures. Indeed, we will use this view in Figure 5 to identify those structures.

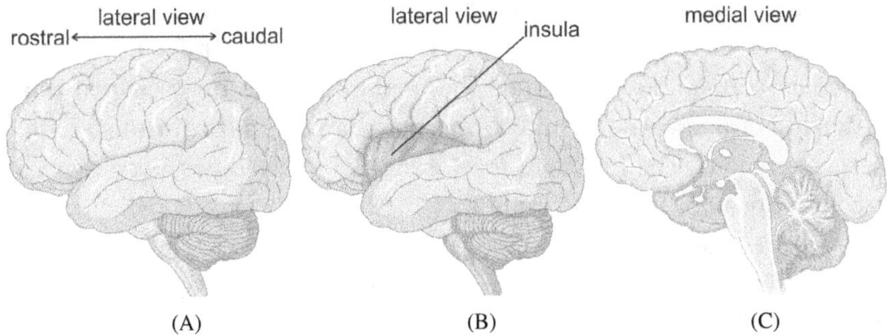

Figure 4.   Lateral (A, B) and medial (C) views of surface structures of the brain. (Created with BioRender.com.)

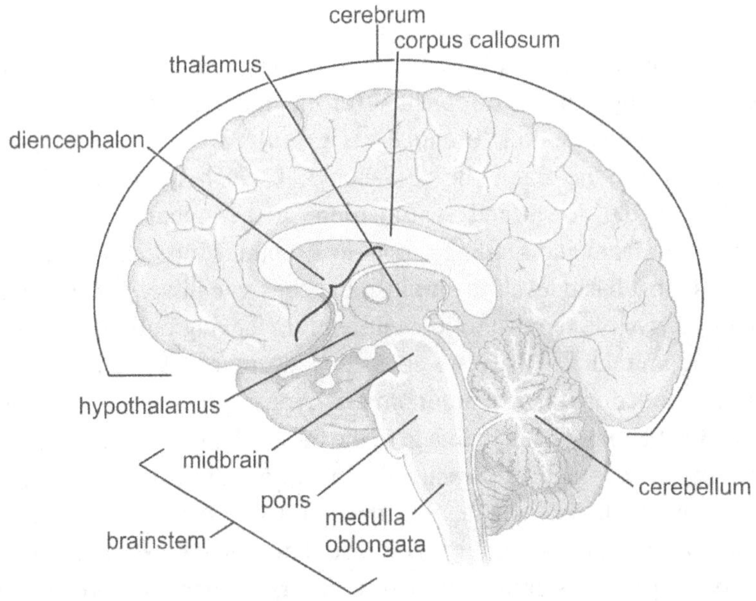

Figure 5.   Key structures of the human brain. (Created by BioRender.com.)

As seen in Figure 5, at the transition from the spinal cord to the brain upon entering the skull is a stalk-like structure called the **medulla oblongata**. Medulla means "marrow" and oblongata means "extension." In ancient times, the spinal cord was considered the bone marrow of the vertebral column and therefore, the medulla oblongata represented the extension of that marrow into the brain. Immediately rostral to the medulla oblongata (oftentimes just called the medulla) is the belly-shaped **pons** (Latin for bridge). And rostral to the pons is the **midbrain** (also called mesencephalon). The midbrain may seem like a misnomer given that this structure does not sit in the middle of the human brain. Its name derives from its precursor as the middle of three main entities during embryonic brain development (rhombencephalon, mesencephalon, and prosencephalon).

Collectively, the *medulla oblongata*, *the pons*, and *the midbrain* make up the **brainstem**. The brainstem is easily the most complex part of the brain. It contains a large array of nuclei involved in sensory processing and motor functions. Importantly, the brainstem also holds a host of crucial components of the autonomic nervous system, for example, those that regulate breathing and cardiovascular function. In addition, some structures in the brainstem are responsible for maintaining the conscious state of the cerebral cortex—and if damaged, it results in coma. The brainstem also gives rise to the cranial nerves—some of which are more or less the equivalent of the dorsal and ventral roots of the spinal cord, receiving sensory input from and sending output to structures in the head and neck.

At its most basic level, the brainstem keeps you alive. Indeed, an animal can survive the removal of the entire brain leaving only the brainstem intact. The animal will have no conscious awareness, but the basic life-sustaining functions of the autonomic nervous system will continue to operate. On the other hand, damage to the brainstem often results in death. When emergency medical personnel shine a light in the eye of an unconscious individual, they are testing the pupil constriction reflex that is mediated by brainstem circuitry. This test, therefore, quickly evaluates the integrity of the brainstem and provides a coarse indication of the severity of the injury.

It is just above the midbrain that the flexure of the neuroaxis occurs (see Figure 1C). As such, the neuroaxis runs almost horizontally above the brainstem, with rostral pointing toward the nose and caudal toward the back of the head. The next structure encountered above the brainstem is the **thalamus** (Figure 5). There are two egg-shaped thalami, one on each side. The thalamus is a remarkable structure that *serves as the gateway to* *the cerebral cortex*. Virtually all sensory information (apart from that associated with the sense of smell—olfaction) and information from other brain structures are processed in the thalamus before being forwarded to the cerebral cortex. Sitting just below (i.e., ventral) and slightly rostral (toward the nose) to the thalamus is the aptly named **hypothalamus**. The hypothalamus, like the brainstem, houses many nuclei that are *involved in a wide array of crucial functions, including regulation of circadian rhythms, thermoregulation, sexual and reproductive behaviors, cardiovascular control, and control of food intake*. Together, the thalamus and the hypothalamus constitute an anatomical entity called the **diencephalon**, which literally means the "between brain." It is called so because it is situated between the "low" brain (the brain stem) and the "high" brain (the cerebrum).

The **cerebrum** is made up of two cerebral hemispheres. Each hemisphere possesses an *outer, folded layer of gray matter, a few millimeters thick*, called the **cerebral cortex**. Below the cerebral cortex is a massive array of white matter (not visible in Figure 5). In addition, deep in the interior of each cerebral hemisphere are a collection of nuclei (also not visible in Figure 5). As mentioned earlier, the enormous white matter track that interconnects the two cerebral hemispheres, the **corpus callosum**, can be clearly seen in the medial section of the brain in Figure 5. The last major structure in the brain, the **cerebellum** (the "little brain"), hangs like a piece of fruit off the dorsal side of the brainstem. The cerebellum has a prominent role in the control of movement and will be discussed in depth in a later chapter.

The cerebral cortex represents that highest level of processing in the brain. It is the site that gives rise to cognition, conscious awareness, reasoning, sensory perception, and voluntary behaviors. Compared to other animals, humans have a massive cerebral cortex. The human cerebral cortex (both hemispheres) has a surface area of about 2,000 cm^2 (Van Essen *et al.* 2018), approximately the same surface area as a 50-cm (20-inch) diameter pizza. In comparison, the surface area of the cerebral cortex in the large domestic dog is only about one-twentieth that of humans (Grewal *et al.* 2020) despite a body weight of about one-fourth that of humans. In order to fit the large cerebral cortex within the confines of a reasonably sized skull, the human cortex (and that of some nonhuman

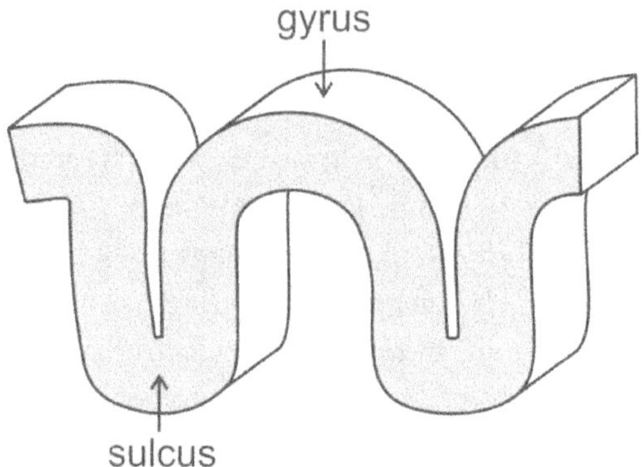

Figure 6.   The cerebral cortex in humans has many folds that increase the surface area. The inward folds are called sulci (singular—sulcus) and the ridges between the sulci are called gyri (singular—gyrus).

primates) has many folds that greatly increase its surface area. The *inward folds are called* **sulci** (sulcus is the singular form; think of "sulking"—being down in the dumps) whereas the *raised ridges between the sulci* are called the **gyri** (gyrus is the singular form, meaning ring or circle in Greek; Figure 6).

Some sulci are more or less consistent from one individual to another and can demark functional subdivisions in the brain. Major sulci separate the cerebral cortex into four main sectors—the lobes (Figure 7A). The **central sulcus** is situated about halfway between the most rostral and most caudal ends of the cortex and serves as the boundary between the **frontal** and the **parietal lobes**. The **lateral sulcus,** situated on the side of the brain, separates the ventrally positioned **temporal lobe** from the more dorsally situated frontal and parietal lobes. The most caudal part of the cerebral cortex is the **occipital lobe**. The sulcus that distinguishes the occipital lobe from the parietal lobe (the **parietooccipital sulcus**) is not visible on the lateral surface of the brain but rather on the medial surface (Figure 7B).

In Chapter 11, we will use this anatomical information to examine the pathways by which information set up in the first-order neurons of the somatosensory system is conveyed to the cerebral cortex and the types of processing that takes place along the way.

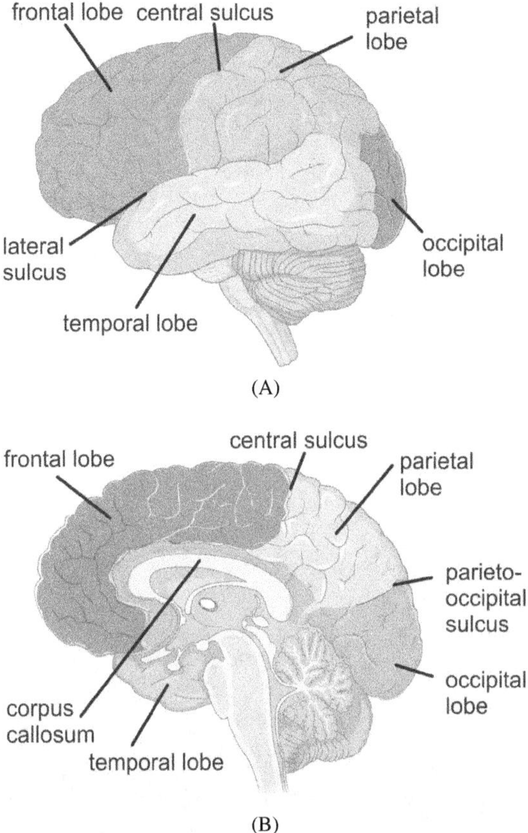

Figure 7.   Lobes of the cerebral cortex and associated major sulci seen on (A) the lateral view and (B) on the medial view of the brain. (Created using BioRender.com.)

References

Grewal JS *et al.* (2020). Brain gyrification in wild and domestic canids: Has domestication changed the gyrification index in domestic dogs? *Journal of Comparative Neurology* **528**, 3209–3228.

Kandel ER, Schwartz JH, Jessell TM, Siegelbaum SA & Hudspeth AJ (2012). Principles of Neural Science (5th Edition). McGraw-Hill.

Van Essen DC, Donahue CJ & Glasser MF (2018). Development and evolution of cerebral and cerebellar cortex. *Brain Behavior and Evolution* **91**, 158–169.

Chapter 11

Somatosensory Pathways

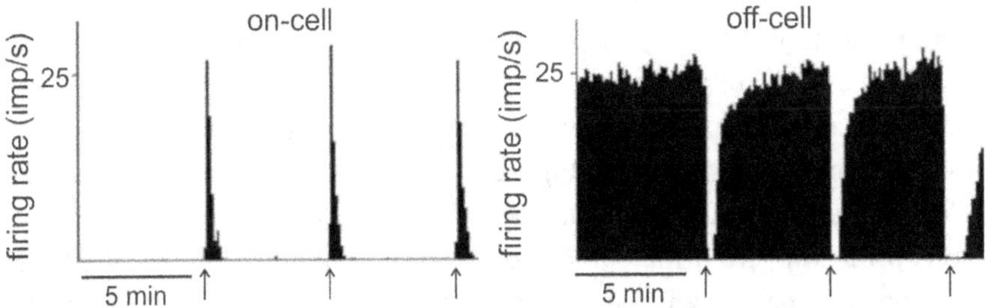

Firing rates of a pain on-cell (left) and a pain off-cell (right) recorded in the rat brainstem. These descending neurons contact the second-order projection neurons of the pain pathway in the spinal cord. On-cell activity facilitates (i.e., turns pain "on"), whereas off-cell activity inhibits (i.e., turns pain "off") the pain pathway. The arrows indicate times when the rat's tail was placed in hot water and it flicked its tail as a nociceptive response. In such cases, on-cell activity increased and off-cell activity decreased. (Adapted from Lane et al. [2004].)

Now with some basic neuroanatomy under our belt, we can better understand the pathways by which signals originating in the primary sensory neurons of the somatosensory system are conveyed to the cerebral cortex. Figure 1 is a schematic that depicts those pathways. In the top part of the figure, the viewpoint is standing behind someone and with X-ray vision one can see the central nervous system to about the level of the ears. In the lower part of Figure 1, the spinal cord is sectioned horizontally with the cut face of the cross-section expanded and shown with dorsal at the top and ventral at the bottom. The dorsal root is shown only on the left side and no ventral roots are depicted.

There are two separate pathways by which somatosensory information reaches the cortex. One pathway carries information from nociceptors
and thermoreceptors whose axons are all small-diameter axons (Aδ, C, III,
IV). The other pathway delivers information from tactile receptors and
proprioceptors whose axons are large-diameter axons (Aδ, I, II). Let's
begin with the pathway arising from nociceptive and thermal afferents. As
discussed before, all the somatosensory afferents have their cell bodies
located in the dorsal root ganglion (Figure 1, bottom). As such, this is the
location of the first-order (1°) neurons in this pathway. Upon entering the
spinal cord at a particular segment via the dorsal root, these small-diameter
axons immediately make synaptic contact with the second-order neurons
in the dorsal horn of the spinal cord. These second-order projection neurons then send their axons to the opposite side of the spinal cord to enter
the lateral column of white matter. These axons then ascend all the way up
the spinal cord, through the brainstem, and ultimately terminate on third-
order neurons in the thalamus (Figure 1, top). This bundle of second-order
axons is thereby referred to as the **spinothalamic pathway**—namely,
axons *projecting from the spinal cord to the thalamus*. Indeed, the term
spinothalamic pathway is the general term used to refer to this somatosensory pathway conveying pain and temperature information. The third-
order neurons in this pathway project from the thalamus to synapse on
fourth-order neurons in the insula. As such, the insula is one of the main
cortical areas that underlies the perception of pain and temperature.

The pathway conveying tactile and proprioceptive information (via
large-diameter afferents) also has its first-order neurons in the dorsal root
ganglion (Figure 1, bottom). These axons, upon entry into the spinal cord
through the dorsal roots, immediately enter into the large white matter
tract called the dorsal column on the same side of the spinal cord. From
here, these first-order axons ascend all the way up to the medulla oblongata of the brainstem where they make contact with the second-order
neurons in a set of nuclei called the **dorsal column nuclei**. As such, for
example, the axons from tactile sensory receptors in the big toe will travel,
without break, all the way to the brain. Therefore, such single neurons can
have axons almost as long as full body height. The general term used for
this *somatosensory pathway carrying tactile and proprioceptive information* is the **dorsal column pathway**. The second-order neurons in the

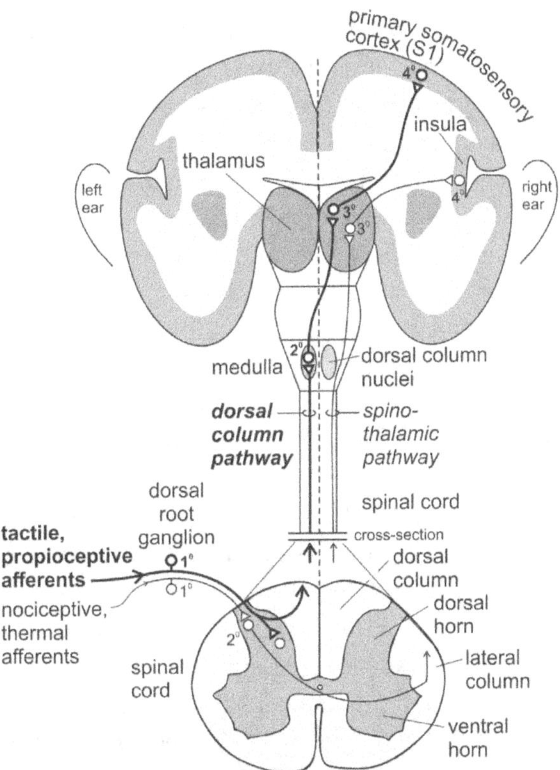

Figure 1.   Somatosensory pathways. The spinothalamic pathway carries information aris-ing on small-diameter nociceptive and thermal afferents. The first-order (1°) neurons have their somas in the dorsal root ganglion. These neurons synapse on 2° neurons in the dorsal horn of the spinal cord. The axons of the 2° neurons cross the midline to ascend in the lateral column of the spinal cord. These axons pass through the brainstem to synapse on the 3° neurons in the thalamus, which then project to the 4° neurons in the insula. Large-diameter tactile and proprioceptive afferents have their 1° neurons in the dorsal root gan-glion. Their axons ascend all the way to the medulla oblongata in the dorsal column of the spinal cord on the same side. There they synapse on the 2° neurons in the dorsal column nuclei. The axons of the 2° neurons cross the midline to synapse on the 3° neurons in the thalamus, which then project to the 4° neurons in the primary somatosensory cortex (SI).

dorsal column nuclei send axons that cross the midline and ascend to synapse on the third-order neurons in a different part of the thalamus than for the spinothalamic pathway. (The white matter tract carrying axons that cross over from the dorsal column nuclei on one side to the thalamus on the other is called the medial lemniscus—where lemniscus means "ribbon.") The third-order neurons in the thalamus then project to the fourth-order neurons in the **primary somatosensory cortex** of the parietal lobe of the cerebrum. The general term used to describe *sensory cortices that directly receive information from the thalamus* is "**primary cortex**." Primary cortices are then abbreviated to indicate the associated modality, for example, primary somatosensory cortex (SI), primary visual cortex (V1), and primary auditory cortex (A1). Interestingly, the part of the insula that serves as the primary cortex for thermal and pain information does not follow this convention.

Note that both pathways cross over from one side of the body to the other. As such, cortical processing is on the opposite side of the body from the site of stimulation. For example, touch to the left hand is processed in the right SI. Also, it should be pointed out that these diagrams only show the main projection pathways. There are, however, a large number of *axon branches* (called **collaterals**) *that innervate structures other than that targeted by the main axon branches.* For example, the first- order axons of proprioceptive and tactile afferents have collaterals that contact local interneurons within the spinal cord (Figure 1, bottom). These spinal cord connections are largely involved in mediating certain types of reflexes (discussed in a later chapter). Similarly, the second-order neurons of the spinothalamic pathway give off collaterals to innervate structures in the brainstem (Kevetter & Willis 1983). Furthermore, there are some pathways that convey somatosensory information that are not depicted. For example, proprioceptive afferents from the legs contact second-order projection neurons within the spinal cord instead of ascending in the dorsal column all the way to the medulla. The axons of these second-order neurons are then carried in the lateral and not the dorsal column. These axons then make synaptic contact onto third-order neurons in a small region of the medulla called nucleus Z (Mackel & Miyashita 1993). From nucleus Z, neurons then project first to the thalamus and then to the primary somatosensory cortex.

Nevertheless, the spinothalamic (for pain and temperature) and dorsal column pathways (for touch and proprioception) represent the main routes by which somatosensory signals reach the brain. Note that for each of these two pathways, there are two intervening structures between the primary sensory neuron in the periphery and the cerebral cortex: the spinal dorsal horn neurons and the thalamus for the spinothalamic pathway, and the dorsal column nuclei and the thalamus for the dorsal column pathway. The generic term used for such intervening structures is **relay nucleus** or simply **relay**. In many respects, however, this term can be easily misconstrued. It seems to imply that the main function of such structures is to pass on information received from lower-order neurons to the next station with good fidelity, like the passing of a baton in a relay race. But if that were the case, then why not simply have axons project directly from the periphery to the cortex? As mentioned earlier, there already exist axons that run from the toe to the brainstem—extending them a couple of more centimeters to reach the cerebral cortex would not impose any signaling challenges for the axons.

The reason for such intervening structures is that they provide critical sites for the signals to be processed before reaching the cortex. As such, perhaps a more appropriate term for such structures (although not as concise as "relay") would be "processing station." Indeed, it is important to recognize that in most instances, the signals that exit from a processing station are different from what enters. As we will discuss in the following sections, certain aspects of transmitted signals can be amplified in one situation or suppressed in another.

Gate Control of Pain

As one example of the type of processing that takes place at a station in the spinothalamic pathway, let's consider the neurons of the dorsal horn in the spinal cord that receive nociceptive signals. It seems reasonable to believe that perception of pain is an unalterable consequence of activating nociceptors in the periphery, whose signals reach the cerebral cortex without modification. Yet this is not always the case. One form of pain signal modification is referred to as **gate control** by which *activity in the second-order projection neurons of the spinothalamic pathway are reduced or suppressed altogether (i.e., "gated") by activity on nonnociceptive sensory afferents.*

Figure 2 shows a simplified schematic that represents such gate control. Small-diameter nociceptive afferents make synaptic contact onto

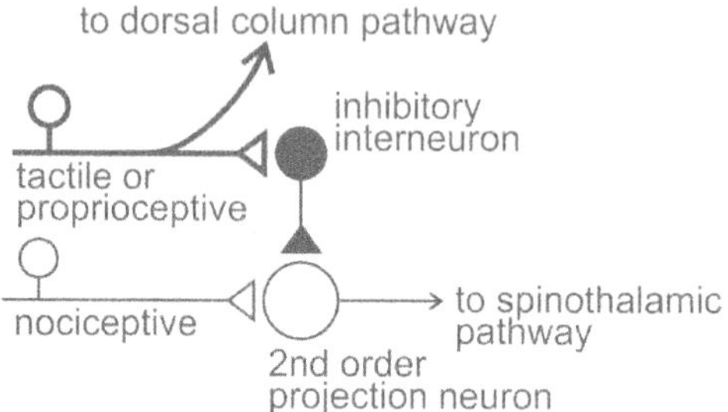

Figure 2.   Gate control. Activity of second-order projection neurons of the spinothalamic pathway that receive input from nociceptive afferents can be suppressed by inhibitory interneurons in the dorsal horn of the spinal cord. These inhibitory interneurons receive excitatory input from tactile or proprioceptive afferents.

second-order projection neurons that carry pain information to the brain via the spinothalamic pathway (Figure 2, bottom). Interestingly, large-diameter tactile and proprioceptive afferents, in addition to ascending in the dorsal column, give off collaterals to target inhibitory interneurons in the dorsal horn of the spinal cord (Figure 2, top). These inhibitory interneurons synapse on the second-order projection neurons of the nociceptive pathway. As such, when activated, these inhibitory interneurons can partially suppress (i.e., "gate") nociceptive signaling and thereby lessen the intensity of the perceived pain. For example, in response to a sprained wrist, individuals will often rub the skin surrounding the wrist. This rubbing action activates large-diameter tactile afferents that can relieve, to some extent, the intense discomfort associated with the sprained wrist via gate control. Likewise, if someone hits their finger with a hammer, a typical immediate reaction is vigorous shaking of the hand and fingers. This shaking action activates large-diameter proprioceptive afferents that may also partially gate the second-order nociceptive neurons. Indeed, therapists have capitalized on gate control to treat pain by electrically stimulating the skin and muscles in the vicinity of a damaged area (e.g., that associated with a recent surgery). The electrical stimulation is of a moderate intensity such that it primarily activates large-diameter axons (tactile and proprioceptive but not nociceptive) which, in turn, tends to suppress activity on the second-order nociceptive neurons by activating the inhibitory interneurons.

Top-Down Modulation of Pain

Gate control of pain is sometimes referred to as **bottom-up modulation**. It is called this because *low-order* (in this case, first-order tactile and proprioceptive) neurons *modulate, via interneurons, the activity of higher-order projection neurons* (second-order projection neurons of the nociceptive pathway). Likewise, processing stations along both the spinothalamic and dorsal column pathways (as well as along pathways for other sensory modalities like vision and hearing) provide rich opportunities for *higher-order neurons to influence the activities of lower-order neurons* called **top-down modulation**.

An interesting and clinically relevant type of top-down modulation that targets second-order neurons in the pain pathway is shown in Figure 3. A key structure in this system is a nucleus found in the midbrain of the brainstem surrounding the aqueduct that connects the third and fourth ventricles of the brain. It is therefore called the periaqueductal gray matter (PAG; Figure 3). The PAG is involved in a host of autonomic functions and control of innate behaviors. In addition, there are neurons that project from the PAG to nuclei in the medulla oblongata. Some neurons in these nuclei of the medulla send axons down to the dorsal horn of the spinal cord to synapse on the second-order projection neurons of the pain pathway (Figure 3). These synapses are inhibitory and thereby can suppress pain signals sent to the brain (Ossipov *et al.* 2010). Indeed, the inhibitory action of this top-down pathway can be so potent as to eliminate the sense of pain altogether. For example, electrical stimulation of the PAG enabled surgery to be performed in rats without the need for anesthetics (Reynolds 1969).

But what role does this pathway play under natural circumstances? Activation of the descending neurons of the PAG seems to occur under periods of high stress and arousal. The brainstem nuclei that receive input from the PAG and that contribute to top-down modulation of the pain pathway are also those that lead to the release of neuromodulators such as noradrenaline and serotonin during stressful situations. Indeed, it is thought that the well-documented cases of individuals reporting little or no pain despite significant traumatic injuries, such as soldiers in battle, athletes injured during a competition, or car accident victims, can be

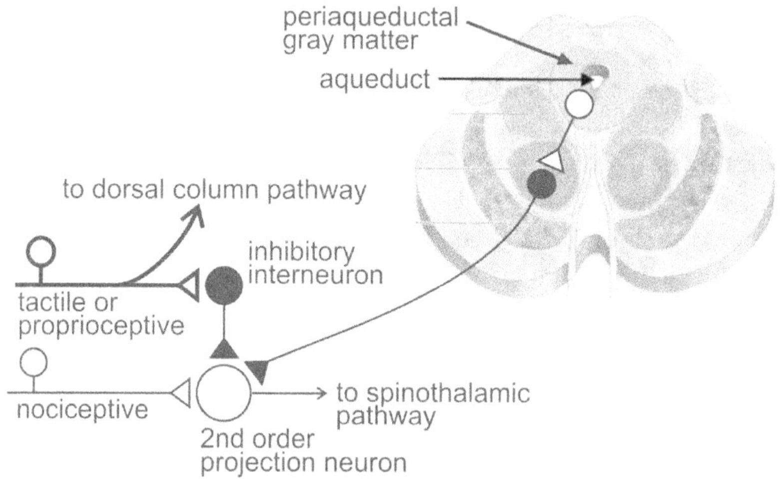

Figure 3.   Top-down modulation of pain. Under high stress or arousal, activation of neurons in the PAG in the midbrain can activate inhibitory neurons in nuclei of the medulla (actual location of these nuclei not shown). These neurons project to the dorsal horn of the spinal cord where they can suppress the activity on second-order neurons that convey pain information to the brain via the spinothalamic pathway.

accounted for by activation of the descending pathway shown in Figure 3. Of course, there is great clinical interest to harness the pain-relieving capacity of this in-built circuitry.

It should also be said that there is similar top-down modulation of the pain pathway that *enhances*, rather than suppresses, activities in the second-order projection neurons (not shown in Figure 3). This form of top-down modulation will amplify the perception of pain. Indeed, there are pain syndromes that are believed to be due to aberrant overactivity in these top-down excitatory pathways that can excite the second-order projection neurons of the spinothalamic tract in the absence of activity on the first-order nociceptors. In such cases, patients may feel excruciating and persistent pain when there is no actual injury. Such cases represent a vivid demonstration that what exits from a sensory processing station is not necessarily what enters from lower levels.

The figure at the beginning of this chapter shows recordings from brainstem neurons involved in both forms of top-down modulation of pain. One type (called "on cells" because they turn pain "on") serves to amplify pain signals. When a rat's tail was placed in hot water, these neurons fired strongly. The other type (called "off cells" because they turn pain "off") was active strongly when no nociceptive signal was present (preventing inadvertent activation of the pain pathway). When the tail was placed in hot water, the activity of this neuron ceased, removing the inhibitory "gate" and allowing the pain signal to ascend to the brain.

Topographic Organization in the Dorsal Column Nuclei

Lets' now consider the processing stations that are part of the dorsal column pathway: the dorsal column nuclei and the thalamus. If one makes a section through the caudal portion of the medulla oblongata (Figure 4A), three nuclei near the dorsal surface of the medulla are observed (Figure 4B) that are collectively referred to as the dorsal column nuclei (from medial to lateral these are called gracile, cuneate, and the trigeminal nuclei). Experiments carried out in cats demonstrate a clear topographic organization across the dorsal column nuclei. Figure 4C shows the classical neurophysiological approach to map topography in the brain (from Kruger *et al.* 1961). The little dots indicate the locations of neuron cell bodies in the dorsal column nuclei (determined by histology after the experiment was completed). The four vertical lines passing down through the dorsal column nuclei indicate tracts made by four successive microelectrode penetrations. The horizontal hatch marks along the electrode tract indicate sites where electrode advancement was halted and the activity of a neuron near the tip of the electrode was recorded in response to tactile or proprioceptive stimuli. The electrode trajectories and recoding sites are shown magnified in the lower part of the figure. In addition, for each recording site, a small figurine is shown indicating (in black) the location of the tactile receptive field for the neuron recorded at that site. In a few cases, the neuron did not respond to touch but to joint rotation. Such proprioceptive neurons are indicated with small arrows through the associated joint.

If we first focus on the leftmost (and most medial) tract in Figure 4C, all of the receptive fields recorded were on the hindlimb of the animal. Moreover, as the electrode penetrated deeper (i.e., more ventrally), the

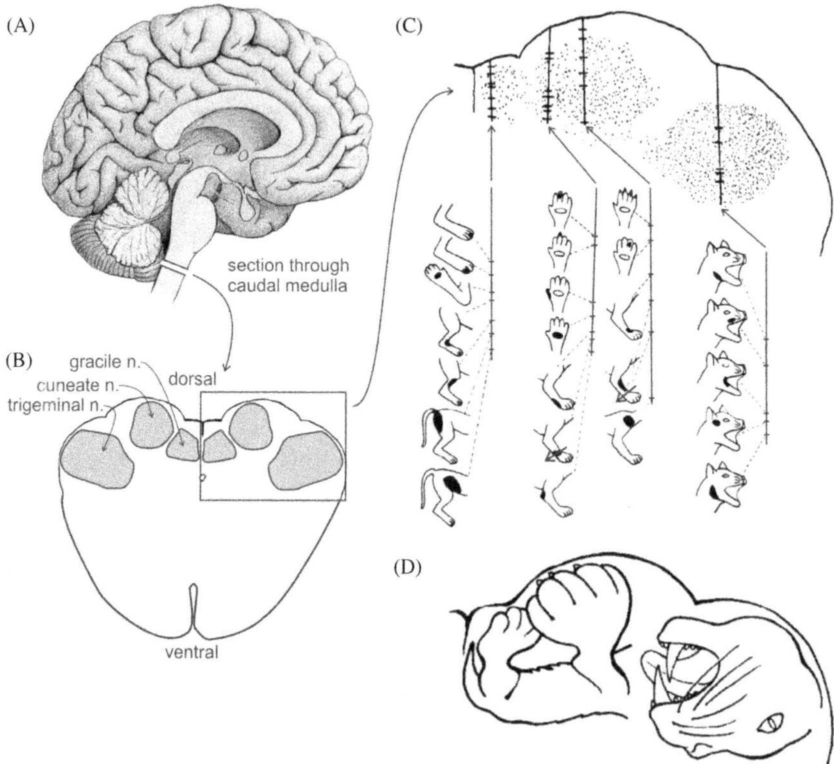

Figure 4.   Topographic organization of the dorsal column nuclei. (A) Medial view of the brain showing the level of a horizontal section through the caudal medulla oblongata that transects the dorsal column nuclei. (B) Cross-section of the caudal medulla showing the locations of the dorsal column nuclei (from medial to lateral: gracile, cuneate, and trigeminal). (C) Expanded view of the right dorsal region of cat caudal medulla. Small dots indicate the locations of cell bodies in the dorsal column nuclei. Vertical lines indicate electrode tracts. Horizontal marks are sites where individual neurons were recorded. The electrode tracts are shown on an expanded scale along with figurines depicting the receptive fields (black areas) of the recorded neurons at each recording site to tactile stimuli. Small arrows indicate neurons that responded to the rotation of the indicated joint (i.e., proprioceptive). (D) "Felinculus"—cartoon representation of the topographic organization in the dorsal column nuclei of the cat. ([C] and [D] adapted from Kruger *et al.* [1961].)

locations of the receptive fields were found to be further up the limb—from paw, to ankle, to knee, to hip, to flank. Also, note that the sizes of the receptive fields are quite small for the paw and becomes progressively larger as we move up the limb. The next two electrode tracts to the right of the most medial tract encountered neurons all with receptive fields in the forelimb. The spatial pattern is similar to that for the medial region representing the hindlimb: receptive fields move up the limb for neurons recorded at progressively more ventral locations. Also, the receptive fields are small for neurons representing the most distal parts of the limb (i.e., the paw) and become larger for neurons responsive to touch of the more proximal parts of the limb (i.e., the shoulder). For the most lateral tract through the dorsal column nuclei, all of the neurons encountered had receptive fields in the face and head. In this study, only about 15% of the neurons encountered in the dorsal column nuclei had proprioceptive responses. These neurons were comingled among neurons with tactile responses that had receptive fields close to the associated joint.

One way to present the outcome of experiments like these is to create a *schematic diagram that indicates the spatial (topographic) organization of the receptive fields projected onto the evaluated brain structure.* If this is done for areas in the human brain, it is referred to as a **homunculus**—literally "little person." Figure 4D shows such a schematic diagram based on the extensive mapping of the dorsal column nuclei in the cat, and as such should be called "felinculus." Importantly, in these diagrams, the relative sizes of the different body parts are scaled to the amount of brain area recorded with receptive fields for those body parts. As such, the homunculus (or felinculus) has a distorted shape. In Figure 4D, the fore-paw and face, in particular, are larger than more proximal body parts because of the high density of sensory receptors supplying those areas. This means that much more brain territory is needed to process the large number of sensory receptors arising from these parts of the body.

Thalamus

As mentioned previously, the **thalamus** is the *gateway to the cerebral cortex.* It is a bilateral egg-like structure that sits atop the brainstem.

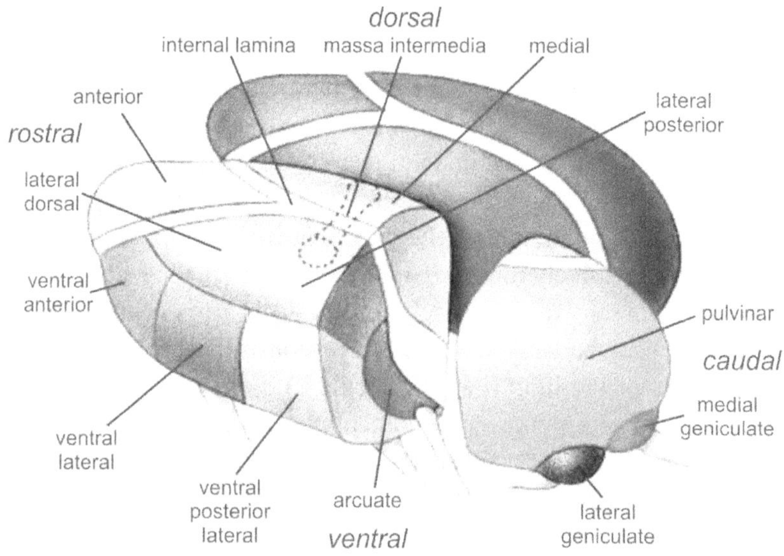

Figure 5.   The right and left thalami. The left thalamus shows some of the many nuclei and white matter tracts (internal lamina) that make up the thalamus.

Each thalamus is composed of multiple subnuclei (Figure 5) each of which processes different kinds of information destined for the cerebral cortex. Indeed, virtually all sensory information is processed in the thalamus before being delivered to the cortex. In addition, inputs to the cortex from other parts of the brain (e.g., from the cerebellum or from the deep nuclei in the cerebrum) must also pass through processing in the thalamus. As such, one can liken the thalamus to the stern secretary who sits outside the office of the chief executive officer: no one gets in to see the boss (i.e., the cortex) without first going through the secretary. Moreover, the secretary turns away many inquiring visitors because the boss is currently "in a meeting." It is as though the boss can only deal with a limited amount of information at a time. It is an important task of the thalamus, therefore, to seamlessly regulate what information gets through to the cortex while suppressing nonessential information. The knowledge as to what is and is not important at any moment derives from rich communication between the cortex and thalamus.

The nucleus of the thalamus that processes tactile and proprioceptive information (ventral posterior lateral [VPL]), like the dorsal column

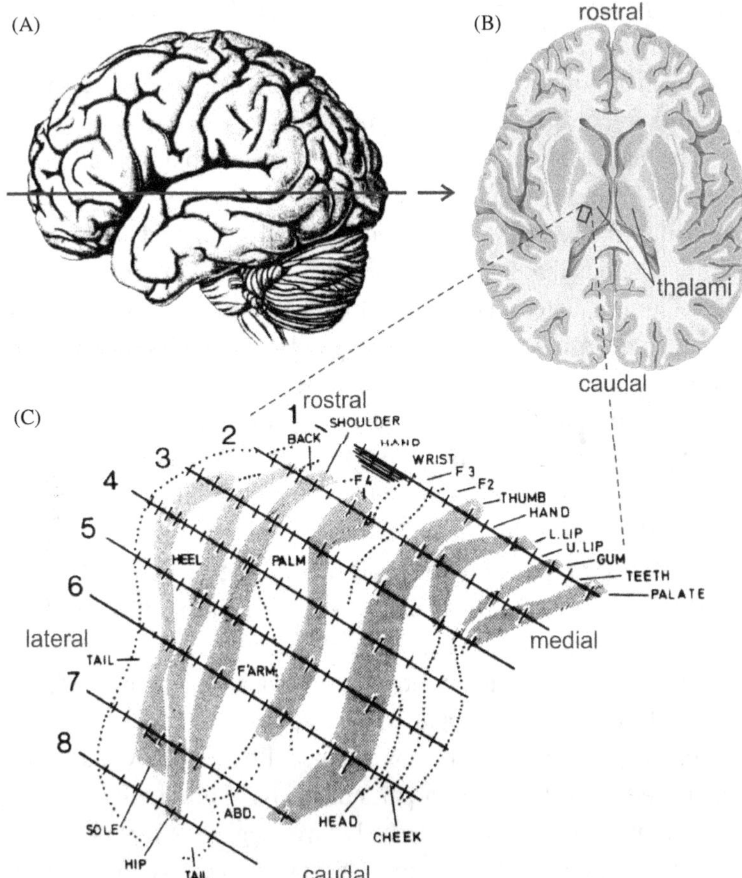

Figure 6.   Topographic organization of the VPL nucleus of the thalamus. (A) Lateral view of the brain showing a level of the horizontal section that passes through the thalamus. (B) Horizontal section of brain showing thalami and the approximate location of VPL (box) in the left thalamus. (C) Expanded view of the horizontal section through the left VPL in the thalamus of a monkey showing electrode tracts and sites of recording (hatch marks). White and hatched regions indicate receptive fields to tactile stimuli in those areas of the VPL ([C] from Phillips & Fuchs [1989], adapted from Jones [1985].)

nuclei, has a clear topographic organization. Figure 6A shows the location of a horizontal section of the brain that passes through the thalamus. Figure 6B shows a top-down view of the brain with such a horizontal section. The thalami can be seen near the midline, and the approximate location of the somatosensory nucleus of the left thalamus (VPL) is indicated in a box. Figure 4C shows a magnified view of that region of the thalamus from a monkey. It also shows the tracts of several electrode penetrations and recording locations (hatch marks) of neurons to tactile stimuli. The electrode trajectories are in the horizontal plane and run roughly at a 45° angle from the rostral–caudal axis.

The stripe-like regions (white and stippled areas) indicate those portions of this nucleus that had similar receptive fields. Moving from lateral to medial, the most lateral (white) region responded to touch in the monkey's tail. The next region (stippled) responded to touch in the sole of the foot, and the following region (white) to touch in the heel. The next region (stippled) had neurons that responded to touch in the hip area. No region is indicated with receptive fields in the leg because this experiment involved rather coarse sampling of the thalamus. As such, the small representation of the leg in the thalamus was simply missed. The next thin stripe (white) medial to the hip region is that for the skin of the back. Note that despite the large surface area of the skin of the back, its representation in the thalamus is not larger than that of the sole of the foot—a much smaller skin surface area but a region possessing a high density of sensory receptors and associated high acuity. The next most medial region (stippled) is for the shoulder. Then, moving medially, a large expanse of the thalamus is dedicated to different parts of the hand and individual fingers (Fs). For example, observe the relatively large region (stippled) dedicated to the skin of the thumb. Most of this region had receptive fields localized to the pad of the distal segment of the thumb. This brain representation of the thumb occupies an area at least double that dedicated to the back, again illustrating the importance of sensory receptor density in dictating the amount of brain real estate needed for processing input from high-acuity parts of the body. Lastly, the most medial and relatively large portion of this thalamic nucleus represents the face, head, and mouth.

Figure 7 shows a simplified schematic summarizing the topographic organization of the dorsal column pathway. Sensory axons arising from the right foot enter the spinal cord and ascend in the right dorsal column close to the midline. As axons enter the spinal cord from more rostral body parts (e.g., from the hand), they position themselves at progressively more lateral positions in the dorsal column. These topographically

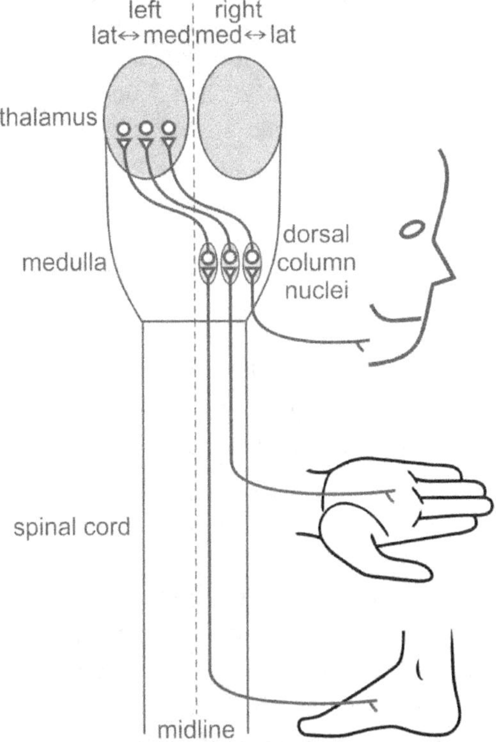

Figure 7.　Schematic representation of topographic organizations in dorsal column nuclei (DCN) and thalamus of the dorsal column pathway. Sensory afferents from the right side of the body (foot, hand) enter the right side of the spinal cord and ascend to the DCN in the right medulla. Inputs from the head enter directly into the brainstem. The most caudal parts of the body (e.g., foot) are represented most medially whereas the most rostral parts (e.g., head or face) are represented most laterally in the DCN. Axons from the right DCN sweep to the left thalamus. As such, the foot representation is found most laterally and the head most medially in the thalamus.

organized sensory axons then project onto congruently organized dorsal column nuclei, with the most caudal regions of the body (foot) represented most medially, and then most rostral body parts (face) represented laterally (also see Figure 4D). The second-order neurons of the dorsal column nuclei then send their axons across the midline to contact the neurons in the VPL nucleus of the left thalamus. These axons maintain the topography seen in the dorsal column nuclei. However, because they switch to the other side of the brain (Figure 7), the topographic organization of the recipient neurons in the thalamus have a mirror image to that in the dorsal column nuclei, namely, caudal body parts are represented laterally whereas the face and head are represented medially (also see Figure 6C).

Processing in the Dorsal Column Nuclei and the Thalamus

Like in the spinothalamic pathway, both bottom-up and top-down operations take place at processing stations of the dorsal column pathway. One major form of bottom-up processing in these regions that we have already discussed in detail (see Chapter 8) is surround inhibition. Recall that surround inhibition involves lower-order neurons that activate local inhibitory neurons to suppress the activities of neighboring higher-order projection neurons. The lower part of Figure 8 shows such bottom-up circuitry associated with lateral inhibition in the thalamus. A similar diagram could also have been drawn for the dorsal column nuclei.

Also indicated in Figure 8 is some circuitry associated with top-down modulation. Axons descending from neurons in the cerebral cortex act on local inhibitory interneurons to suppress the activity of neurons that project to the cortex from the thalamus. Similarly (but not shown in Figure 8), there are inputs from the cortex that excite neurons in the thalamus. Indeed, this top-down (cortically mediated) modulation of activity underlies the crucial gatekeeping function within the thalamus. The importance of this role can be appreciated by the relative numbers of these top-down projections: it has been estimated that there is 10-fold greater number of inputs from the sensory cortex to associated thalamic nuclei (top-down) than the sensory inputs to the thalamic nuclei (Briggs 2020; Sherman 2016).

At any moment, this top-down circuitry is responsible for gating out much of the sensory input that continuously bombards the thalamus while permitting only crucial information needed by the cortex at that instant. This *selective enabling of information flow for some signals but not others* is the basis of **attention**. Figure 9 shows an example recording of a tactile-responsive neuron in the primary somatosensory (SI) cortex of a monkey

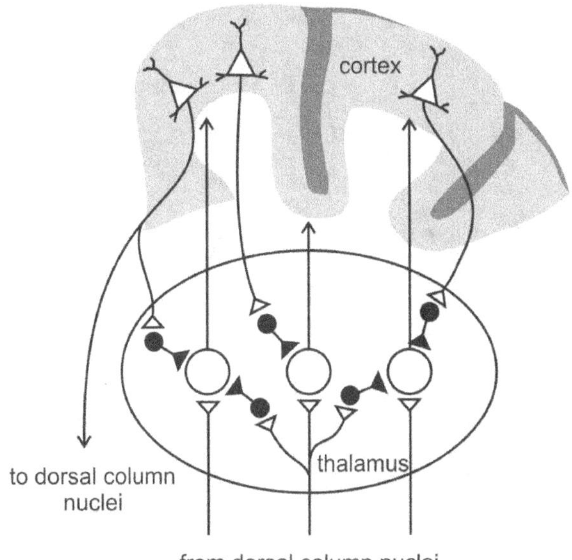

Figure 8.   Circuitry underlying some aspects of bottom-up and top-down modulation in the thalamus. Inputs from second-order neurons in the dorsal column nuclei project into the VPL nucleus of the thalamus. These inputs synapse on third-order neurons in the thalamus that project to the cerebral cortex. In addition, branches of the second-order neurons can activate local inhibitory interneurons to mediate surround inhibition—a form of bottom-up modulation. Pyramidal cells in the cerebral cortex send axons to the thalamus and dorsal column nuclei to activate local inhibitory interneurons that can gate the activity of projection neurons—a form of top-down modulation.

demonstrating such top-down gating associated with selective attention (from Hsiao *et al.* 1993). The monkey had been trained to perform two tasks: a tactile discrimination task and a visual task. In the tactile discrimination task, a set of separated raised letters on a rotating drum were scanned across the neuron's receptive field on the hand. When the raised letter being scanned across the skin matched the letter displayed on a computer screen in front of the monkey, the monkey was trained to pull a lever with the other hand to indicate a match. If done correctly, the monkey received a juice reward. In the visual task, three squares were displayed on a computer screen. When one of the squares was dimmed in intensity, the monkey was trained to pull the lever. If accomplished within

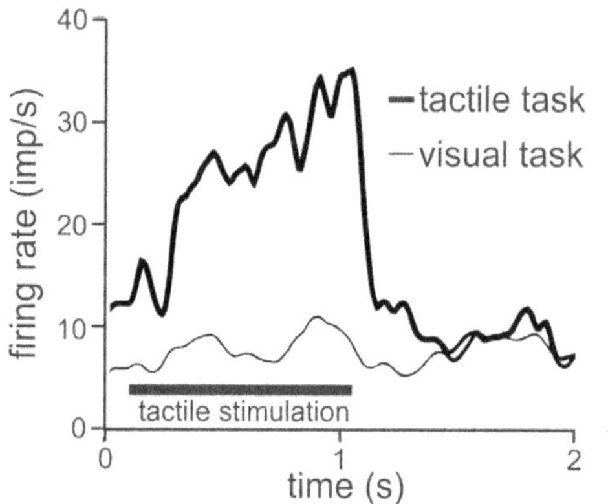

Figure 9.   Effects of attention on the firing rate of a neuron recorded in monkey primary somatosensory cortex. The monkey was trained to perform two tasks. In the tactile task, the monkey was required to identify the shapes of raised letters swept across the hand. In the visual task, the monkey needed to determine when a visual object dimmed in intensity. During the visual task, tactile stimuli continued to sweep across the hand. The firing rate was greatly reduced during the visual task compared to the tactile task even though tactile stimulation (indicated by black bar) was the same. (Adapted from Hsiao *et al.* [1993].)

a specified time window, the monkey received a juice reward. Importantly, during the visual task, the drum with the raised letters continued to scan across the skin of the hand. As seen in Figure 9, when the monkey performed the tactile task, the movement of a raised letter across the receptive field caused robust firing of the neuron in SI. However, when the identical stimulus was scanned across the hand during the visual task, there was virtually no response in the SI neuron above background levels. This indicates that the tactile information was gated out and not being relayed to the SI cortex during the task requiring visual attention.

Because the thalamus (in communication with the cortex) carries out this switch-boarding operation so seamlessly and briskly, we are "tricked" into believing that we have continuous access to all sensory inputs at all times. Yet some common experiences tell us otherwise. For example, when sitting in a coffee shop and engrossed in reading, one may gate out auditory signals arising from background music or conversations taking place at other tables. Likewise, while sitting and reading, tactile signals arising from the soles of the feet in contact with shoes are largely subdued in the thalamus. In such a situation, visual input specifically related to the text on the page or screen is the crucial information required by the cortex at that moment, and as such, the thalamus suppresses inputs from these other sensory modalities. An excellent demonstration of this gating action associated with focused attention can be found at https://www.youtube.com/watch?v=Ahg6qcgoay4 (or type *"test your awareness: do the test — YouTube"* into a browser search engine).

Summary

In this chapter, the pathways that convey somatosensory information to the cerebral cortex have been described. One pathway, called the spinothalamic pathway, carries information from nociceptive and thermal afferents. These small-diameter axons make synaptic contact onto second-order neurons in the dorsal horn of the spinal cord. The axons of these second-order neurons cross over to the other side of the spinal cord and ascend all the way to the thalamus to contact third-order neurons. Those third-order thalamic neurons project to fourth-order neurons in the insula giving rise to the conscious awareness of pain and temperature. The other pathway, called the dorsal column pathway, carries signals arising on large-diameter tactile and proprioceptive afferents. These axons ascend all the way to the medulla oblongata on the same side of the body to contact second-order neurons in the dorsal column nuclei. Axons of these neurons cross over to the other side of the brain to contact third-order neurons in the thalamus, which then project to fourth-order neurons in the primary somatosensory cortex. Each of these processing stations has a topographic organization. Importantly, these stations are not simple relays but sites where both bottom-up and top-down processing takes place that can markedly alter the signals that are forwarded to the next station. In Chapter 12, we will describe the organization of the cerebral cortex—the ultimate destination of these sensory signals.

References

Briggs F (2020). Role of feedback connections in central visual processing. *Annual Review of Vision Science* **6**, 313–334.

Hsiao SS, O'Shaughnessy DM & Johnson KO (1993). Effects of selective attention on spatial form processing in monkey primary and secondary somatosensory cortex. *Journal of Neurophysiology* **70**, 444–447.

Jones EG (1985). The Thalamus. Plenum Press: New York.

Kandel ER, Schwartz JH, Jessell TM, Siegelbaum SA & Hudspeth AJ (2012). Principles of Neural Science (5th Edition). McGraw-Hill.

Kevetter GA & Willis WD (1983). Collaterals of spinothalamic cells in the rat. *Journal of Comparative Neurology* **215**, 453–464.

Kruger L, Siminoff R & Witkovsky P (1961). Single neuron analysis of dorsal column nuclei and spinal nucleus of trigeminal in cat. *Journal of Neurophysiology* **24**, 333–349.

Lane DA, Tortorici V & Morgan MM (2004). Behavioral and electrophysiological evidence for tolerance to continuous morphine administration into the ventrolateral periaqueductal gray. *Neuroscience* **125**, 63–69.

Mackel R & Miyashita E (1993). Nucleus Z: A somatosensory relay to motor thalamus. *Journal of Neurophysiology* **69**, 1607–1620.

Ossipov MH, Dussor GO & Porreca F (2010). Central modulation of pain. *Journal of Clinical Investigation* **120**, 3779–3787.

Phillips JO & Fuchs AF (1989). Somatic sensation: Central processing. In: Patton HD, Fuchs AF, Hille B, Scher AM & Steiner R (eds.) Textbook of Physiology, (Volume 1, 21st Edition). WB Saunders: Philadelphia.

Purves D, Augustine GJ, Fitzpatrick D, Katz LC, LaMantia A-S, McNamara JO & Williams SM (2001). Neuroscience, (2nd Edition). Sinauer: Sunderland Massachusetts.

Reynolds DV (1969). Surgery in the rat during electrical analgesia induced by focal brain stimulation. *Science* **164**, 444–445.

Sherman SM (2016). Thalamus plays a central role in ongoing cortical functioning. *Nature Neuroscience* **19**, 533–541.

Chapter 12

Somatosensory Cortex

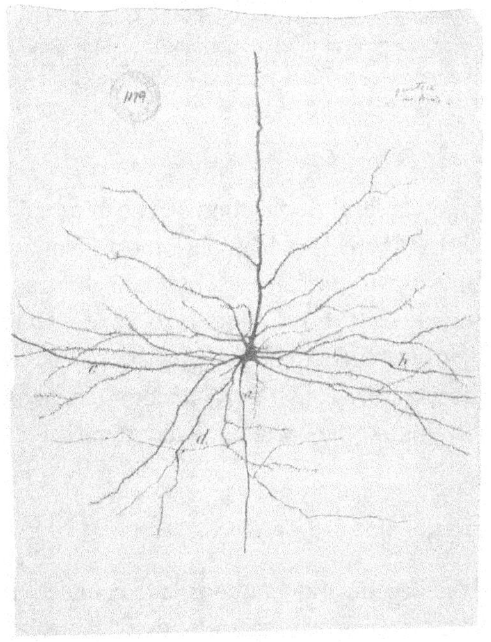

Pyramidal neuron of the cerebral cortex. Santigo Ramon y Calal, 1904 (from the Cajal Institute, Madrid).

The somatosensory cortex is the site that underlies conscious awareness and interpretation of somatosensory stimuli. Before describing its operations, it will be useful to outline the organization of the cerebral cortex in general. The cerebral cortex is a canopy of gray matter, ~2 to 4 mm thick,

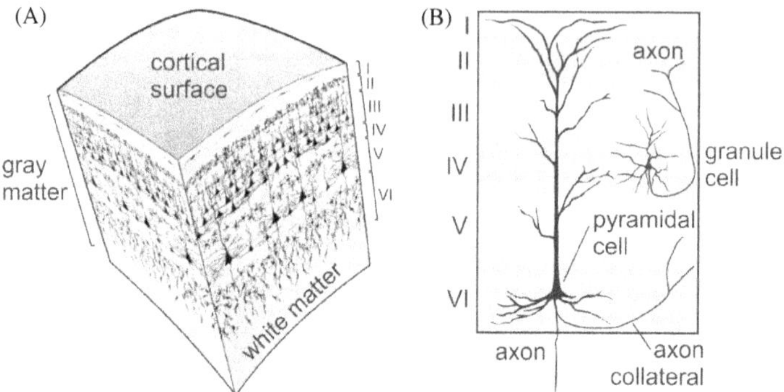

Figure 1.   (A) Schematic of a small cube of cerebral cortex depicting the six cortical layers and underlying white matter. (B) Two main types of cells in the cerebral cortex. Large pyramidal cells whose axons project to other parts of the brain. Small local interneurons, called granule cells that connect to other neurons in the immediate cortical vicinity. ([A] adapted from https://neuwritesd.org/.)

which envelopes the cerebral hemispheres. The cerebral cortex typically comprises six layers (Figure 1A). The outermost layer, layer I, possesses few cell bodies and mostly contains axons and the tips of dendrites of neurons located in deeper layers. Layers II to VI are densely packed with a wide array of neurons. Immediately below layer VI is white matter—a complex superhighway of axons interconnecting various regions of the cerebral cortex and linking the cortex to subcortical structures.

Cortical Layers

As a first view of the organization and intricate connectivity of the cortex, one can coarsely distinguish two main types of neurons in the cerebral cortex. One is the **pyramidal cells,** so called because the soma has a roughly pyramid shape (Figure 1B; also see the illustration at frontispiece of this chapter). These relatively large neurons have dendrites that extend from the base of the pyramid with a single dendritic trunk that reaches upward from the apex of the pyramid (and therefore are called apical dendrites) toward layer I. The axon emerges from the bottom of the pyramid to enter the white matter below the cortex. As such, the pyramidal cells are the output neurons of a region of the cortex. Axon collaterals of the pyramidal cells (Figure 1B), however, remain within the cortex to make synaptic connections with neurons in the local territory of the pyramidal cell. The other general type of neuron is the **granule cells**. These are small, local interneurons of many varieties that interconnect neurons into complex processing circuits within a small neighborhood of the cortex (Figure 1B). They are called granule cells because their small size makes them look grainy in histological preparations.

Different layers of the cortex possess different densities of pyramidal and granule cells. Furthermore, pyramidal cells have a wide range of sizes. In sensory cortices, layer IV has a high density of granule cells (Figure 2) with few pyramidal cells. This layer, sometimes referred to as the granule cell layer, is also the main recipient of input from the thalamus. The granule cells then make connections to neurons in the two layers above (II, III) and two layers below (V, VI) the granule cell layer

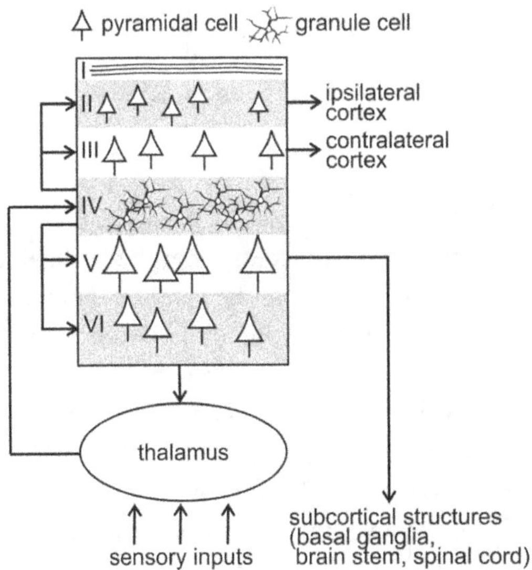

Figure 2. Schematic depicting main cell types and connectivity of different cortical layers. Layer I possess few neurons containing mostly axons and some apical dendrites. Layer IV is the main input layer and has a high density of granule cells. In primary sensory cortices, layer IV is the main recipient of inputs from the thalamus. Granule cells of layer IV project to neurons in layers II, III, V, and VI, the main output layers of the cortex with high densities of pyramidal cells. These layers tend to project to different cortical and subcortical targets.

(see arrows on the left side of Figure 2). These upper and lower layers possess high densities of pyramidal cells. The axons of the pyramidal cells in different layers tend to project to different targets. Many pyramidal cells in layer II project to other cortical regions on the same side of the brain (i.e., ipsilateral cortex) whereas the pyramidal cells in layer III send axons to the cortex on the other side (contralateral cortex) of the brain via the corpus callosum.

The axons of many layer V pyramidal cells leave the cortex altogether and project to a variety of subcortical targets (e.g., brain stem, spinal cord). Layer V pyramidal cells also tend to be large. Neurons with large somas often have large-diameter axons, and larger-diameter axons conduct action potentials more rapidly than thinner axons (see Chapter 5). Therefore, it seems reasonable to assume that layer V neurons tend to be large with fast-conducting axons to minimize delays in delivering action potentials to distant subcortical targets. Finally, many layer VI neurons project back to the thalamus (Figure 2). This forms the critical communication link between the cortex and thalamus that underlies top-down modulation of sensory signals (see Figure 8, Chapter 11).

Cortical Areas

There is a large variation in the thicknesses of the cortical layers and densities of cells in different layers across the cerebral cortex. In the early part of the 20th century, German neuroanatomist Korbinian Brodmann systematically and meticulously mapped these variations in the architecture of the cortical layers in both nonhuman primate and human brains. Figure 3A shows examples of early drawings made of histological sections made by contemporaries of Brodmann (Vogt & Vogt 1919) from four different parts of the human cerebral cortex. Based on such differences, Brodmann identified 43 different regions of the human cerebral cortex (Figure 3B). Somewhat confusingly, Brodmann numbered the cortical regions from 1 to 52 but nine numbers were not shown for the human brain. These "missing" areas were not identified in the human brain but were distinguishable in other primate species. Importantly, Brodmann speculated that the different cortical areas would possess distinctly

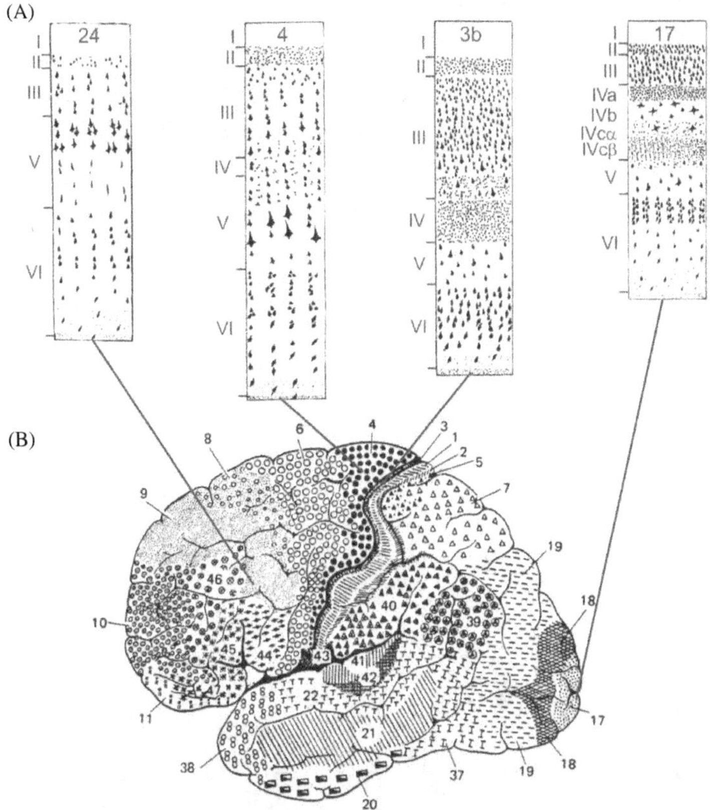

Figure 3.   (A) Drawings of cortical histological sections taken from different Brodmann's areas (indicated at the top of each section) highlighting variations in cell or layer architecture in different regions. (Adapted from Vogt & Vogt [1919].) (B) Drawing by Brodmann (1909) showing different regions of the cerebral cortex based on differences in cell densities and layer thicknesses. These regions are referred to as Brodmann's areas. Note that the section from Brodmann's area 24 in (A) resides on the medial surface of the cortex, and therefore is not visible on the lateral image of the brain.

different functions, an idea that was largely supported in later neurophysiological and imaging studies. While other investigators have identified many more cortical areas than 43 (Amunts & Zilles 2015), Brodmann's designations (Figure 3B) continue to serve as a kind of geographical map of the cerebral cortex.

Primary Somatosensory Cortex

The primary somatosensory cortex, SI (Figure 4A), consists of four parallel ribbons of cortex that run medial to lateral across the convexity of the cortex, just caudal to and within the central sulcus. These four regions, in

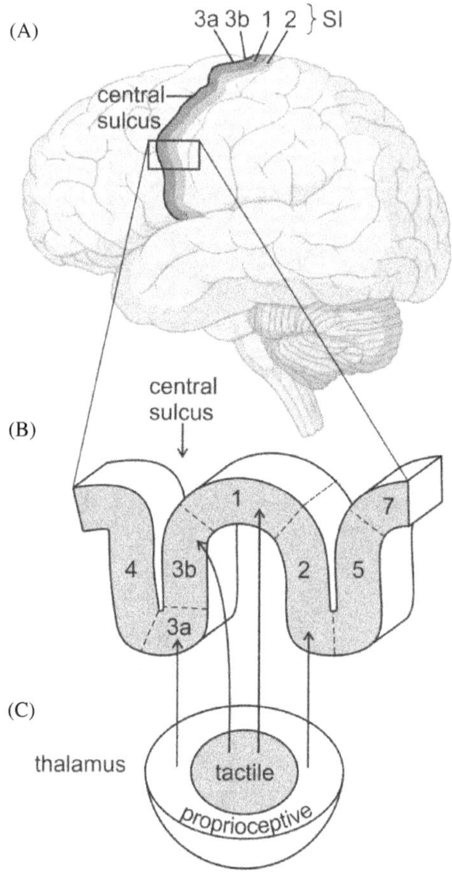

Figure 4.   (A) Four parallel regions of SI run across the cerebral convexity just caudal to the central sulcus. These are Brodmann's areas 3a, 3b (neither visible in the surface view of the brain), 1, and 2. (B) Section through the cortex spanning the central sulcus showing four divisions of SI (3a, 3b, 1, 2). Rostral to the central sulcus is area 4 (motor cortex). Caudal to area 2 are areas 5 (association cortex for somatosensation) and 7 (association cortex for vision). (C) The thalamic region that process proprioceptive signals projects mainly to areas 3a and 2, whereas the thalamic area that processes tactile signals projects to areas 3b and 1. ([A] made with BioRender.com.)

rostral to caudal order (Figure 4B), have Brodmann area designations 3a (deep in the central sulcus), 3b (along the posterior bank of the central sulcus), 1 (along the crest of the gyrus), and 2 along the anterior bank of the next sulcus.

Each of these subdivisions of SI process somewhat different aspects of somatosensory information partly due to different inputs from the thalamus. The subnuclei of the thalamus that receive proprioceptive and tactile information are arranged in a kind of core-and-shell configuration (Figure 4C). Proprioceptive inputs are mostly processed in the shell region and project primarily to the flanking areas of SI, namely Brodmann's areas 3a and 2. The core region receives tactile information, and primarily projects to the inner areas of SI, 3b, and 1 (Figures 4B and 4C). As such areas 3a and 2 are largely dedicated to processing proprioceptive information whereas 3b and 1 mostly handle tactile signals.

There is rich interconnectivity among the different subregions of SI. The dominant pattern of connections is shown in Figure 5. Area 3a sends extensive output connections to the other proprioceptive region, area 2.

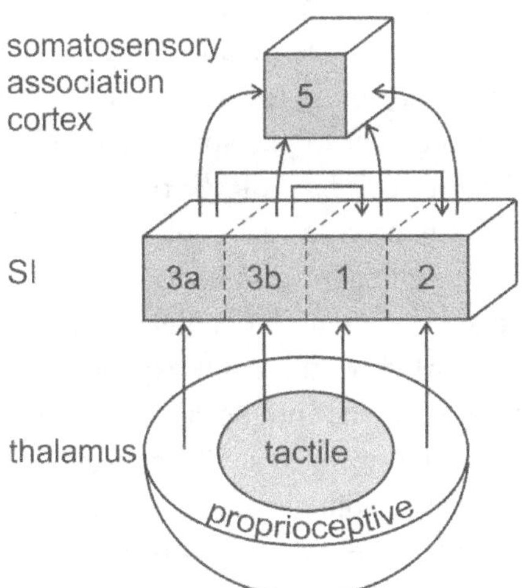

Figure 5.   Connectivity among somatosensory cortices. Proprioceptive inputs from the thalamus mainly target areas 3a and 2 of the SI, whereas tactile inputs project mainly areas 3b and 1. Output from area 3a projects to area 2, while projections from area 3b target area 1. All four divisions of SI send converging inputs to area 5, an association cortex for somatosensation.

Likewise, area 3b sends projections to the other tactile region, area 1. As such, areas 1 and 2 could be considered as higher in the hierarchy of somatosensory signal processing than 3a and 3b. Because areas 1 and 2 both receive input directly from the thalamus as well, they are considered "primary" sensory cortices. Finally, all four regions of SI send converging inputs to area 5 (Figure 5). Area 5, in the posterior parietal cortex, is considered an **association cortex**, namely, a *cortical area that ties together (i.e., associates) information from many other cortical regions needed for high-level processing and perception.* Another association cortex for somatosensation is called the secondary somatosensory cortex, SII (not shown in Figure 5) located ventral to SI in the ceiling of the lateral sulcus.

Given the connectivity depicted in Figure 5, we might expect receptive field properties and sizes to vary for different areas of SI. Keep in mind, that with ascension in the hierarchy of processing, receptive fields tend to expand (see Figure 11, Chapter 8). Consequently, receptive fields should be larger in areas 1 and 2 compared to areas 3a and 3b. Figure 6 shows examples of individual neurons recorded in each of the four regions of SI in the monkey brain. The neuron recorded in area 3a (Figure 6A) responded with spiking only to the rotation of the elbow joint. Figure 6B shows a neuron recorded in area 3b that responded in a sustained way only to touch in the distal segment of the middle finger. The tactile neuron recorded in area 1 (Figure 6C) had a large receptive field on the palm of the hand. Moreover, this neuron had a complex response property; namely, it was activated mainly when a touch stimulus was swept across the palm from the little (L) finger to the thumb (T) but not in the opposite direction. Finally, the neuron recorded from area 2 responded strongly to rotations of the joints at the bases of the middle, ring, and little fingers, and the wrist. When all these joints were rotated together, the spiking frequency was higher than when each joint was rotated individually. This implies that this neuron received converging inputs from several lower-order neurons (presumably including those from area 3a), each of which responded to movements of single joints. These example neural responses illustrate the expanded receptive fields in areas 1 and 2 compared to 3a and 3b. While the neurons depicted in Figure 6 mostly exhibited slowly adapting responses, some SI neurons have rapidly adapting spiking profiles.

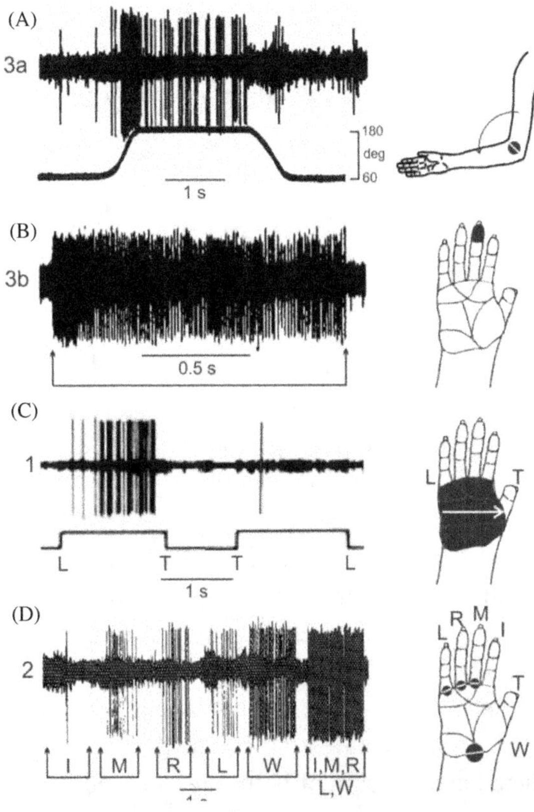

Figure 6.   Example spiking responses and receptive fields of neurons recorded in each of the four areas of monkey SI. Black circles bisected with a line indicate joint rotation that activated a neuron. Blackened regions on figurines indicate touch-receptive fields. (A) Proprioceptive neuron in area 3a responded when the elbow joint was extended. (B) A tactile neuron in area 3b responded only to touch of the distal segment of the middle finger. Arrows demark the time when the stimulus was applied. (C) Neuron in area 1 that responded to a tactile stimulus moved across the palm from the little (L) finger side to the thumb (T) but not in the opposite direction. (D) Neuron in area 2 that responded robustly to the rotations of joints at the bases of the middle (M), ring (R), little (L) fingers, and wrist (W) but not the index (I) finger. Activity was further increased when all joints were rotated together. ([A] and [D] adapted from Gardner [1988]; [B] from Paul *et al.* [1972]; [C] from Costanzo and Gardner [1980]. Figurines adapted from Gardner [1988] and Iwamura *et al.* [1993]; recordings in [B], [C], and [D] were concatenated from separate traces for illustration purposes.)

However, most SI neurons exhibit a composite of slowly and rapidly adapting responses, suggesting that they receive converging inputs originating from slowly and rapidly adapting primary sensory receptors (Delhaye *et al.* 2018).

Brodmann Area 5—Somatosensory Association Cortex

As shown in Figure 5, area 5 receives convergent input from all subdivisions of SI. Area 5 neurons, however, typically show weak or no responses to simple inputs such as touch to one part of the body or movement of one joint. Instead, these neurons require a complex and unique combination of tactile and proprioceptive inputs to cause them to fire. Furthermore, many area 5 neurons respond to input from both sides of the body—a feature rarely encountered in SI neurons. Such bilateral responses derive from extensive interhemispheric connections (via the corpus callosum) between area 5 on both sides of the brain and contralateral (as well as ipsilateral) projections from SI.

Figure 7A shows the receptive field of a neuron recorded in area 5 of a monkey. This neuron generated the greatest activity when both shoulders were adducted and the skin of both forearms and hands were in contact with one another. This neuron did not fire when the skin of the regions indicated were touched in isolation. It is as though this neuron signaled the situation of holding a large object between both arms, like that shown in Figure 7B.

As an association cortex, area 5 is not especially involved with the basic sensations arising from individual sensory receptors but with the interpretation of a given somatosensory situation. This function is vividly illustrated by the rare cases of patients with a stroke that selectively damaged area 5 but not SI. **Stroke** refers to *damage to a part of the brain when its blood supply has been interrupted by an occlusion in an artery (ischemic) or by the rupture of a blood vessel (hemorrhagic).* Such area 5 stroke patients have no deficits in touch threshold, two-point discrimination, or joint position sense (Knecht *et al.* 1996). However, when blindfolded and attempting to recognize

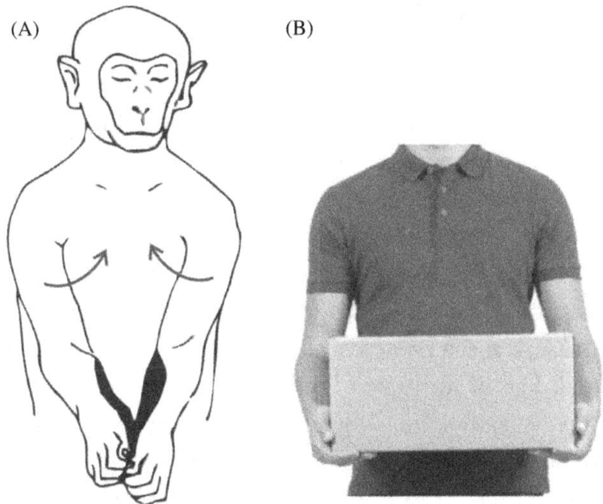

Figure 7.   (A) Response of neurons in area 5 of the monkey was enhanced by simultaneous adduction of both shoulders and contact of skin on inner forearms and hands. Such a complex set of inputs might arise when (B) holding an object in both arms. ([A] from Sakata *et al.* [1973].)

everyday objects (e.g., tennis ball, spoon, pencil, etc.) placed in their hand, they cannot do so. Instead, they report "I can feel it, but I have not the least idea what it is" (Head & Holmes, 1911). When shown the object, however, they readily recognize it.

Overall, association cortices, like area 5, integrate multiple simple sensations into holistic representations that underlie global sensory perceptions. For example, as mentioned in Chapter 8, consider the situation when someone places a cold beverage can into your hand when your eyes are closed. What "comes to mind" is a representation of a can. But how does your brain come to such an awareness? It must derive from an enormous set of sensory signals originating from a wide array of receptors in the hand. These include Meissner corpuscles in the skin of the fingertips that detect the smooth texture of the can, Merkel-disk receptors that signal the amount of pressure on each fingertip, and cold receptors indicating the coolness of the object in the hand. In addition, Golgi tendon organs in the hand, wrist, and elbow muscles signal the weight of the object indicated by the contraction forces needed to hold the object against gravity. The width and shape of the object are derived from a complex amalgam of activities in joint receptors, muscle spindles, and Ruffini endings associated with the configuration of the fingers while grasping the can. All these individual signals are ultimately processed in primary sensory cortices. Yet, unless prompted, we typically are not attentive to these individual signals (e.g., the angle of the middle joint of the index finger while grasping the object). Instead, we perceive the whole. It is the function of association cortices, like area 5, to put the pieces together into an overall representation. Given the complexity of this function, association cortices take up a great deal of territory in the cortex. Indeed, most of the human cerebral cortex is association cortex, whereas primary sensory cortices (i.e., those regions receiving extensive input directly from the thalamus) and the primary motor cortex are a much smaller fraction. Our understanding as to how association cortices stitch together the various pieces of information into a perceptual whole, however, remains rudimentary.

Topographic Organization of the Somatosensory Cortex

Like the subcortical processing stations along the dorsal column pathway (Chapter 11), SI has a systematic and detailed topographic organization. Indeed, the body map is replicated four times in the SI—one for each of the four subdivisions. Figure 8A shows six sites (labeled a to f) just caudal to the central sulcus where individual neurons in area 3B were recorded. The associated receptive fields to touch stimuli are shown in Figure 8B. The neurons recorded at the most lateral sites (a and b) had receptive fields on the face. The neuron recorded at the next most medial site c had a small receptive field on the tip of the index finger. The neuron at site d had a large receptive field on the flank above the lower limb. Most medially and near the interhemispheric fissure, the neurons recorded at sites e and f had receptive fields on the sole of the foot. From this coarse sampling, one can discern the topographic layout of the SI: moving lateral to medial (also ventral to dorsal), one encounters cortical regions dedicated to processing inputs from head, to hand, to foot.

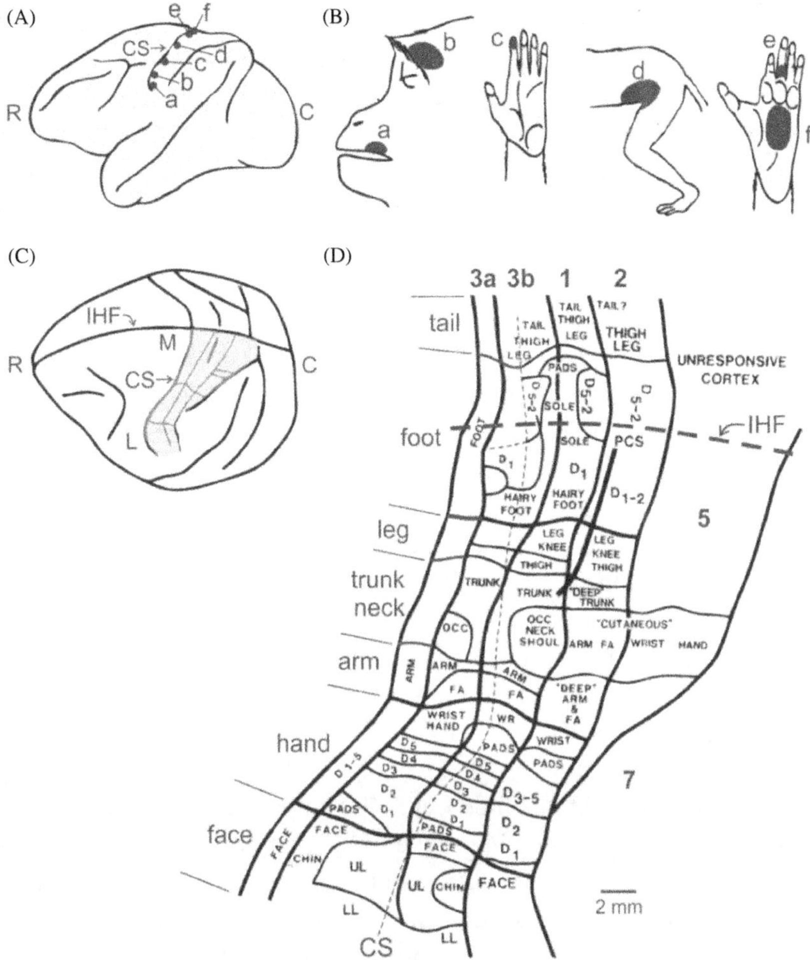

Figure 8.   Topographic organization of the somatosensory cortex. (A) Recording sites (a to f) of individual neurons in area 3b of a monkey's brain. (B) Tactile receptive fields associated with recording sites in (A). (C) Dorsal–lateral view of monkey brain with somatosensory cortex region highlighted in gray. (D) Expanded view of highlighted region in C showing receptive fields across the subdivisions of SI (areas 3a, 3b, 1, 2). Neurons in areas 3a and 2 responded primarily to joint rotations whereas neurons in areas 3b and 1 responded to touch. Area 5 was largely unresponsive to simple joint rotations or touch. R—rostral, C—caudal, M—medial, L—lateral, CS—central sulcus, IHF—interhemispheric fissure. ([A] and [B] adapted from Phillips & Fuchs [1989], [C] and [D] from Pons *et al.* [1985].)

Using a much more extensive sampling of neurons in the somatosensory cortex, fine-grain details of the topographic organization can be revealed. Figure 8C shows the region of the monkey's brain that was meticulously recorded in a grid-like pattern with thousands of individual microelectrode penetrations separated by ~0.25 mm. At each electrode site, the receptive field of a neuron was identified in the anesthetized monkey in response to simple tactile stimuli and joint rotations. Figure 8D shows the outcome of such recordings. Across the four subdivisions of SI, there are parallel representations of the body, with the face most lateral and foot or tail most medial. Area 3a is shown with little detail because it sits deep in the central sulcus (i.e., in the *fundus*) making it difficult to precisely access with microelectrodes, and therefore, it was only sparsely sampled. Areas 3a and 2 were mostly responsive to joint rotations (proprioceptive inputs—sometimes labeled as "deep stimuli" in Figure 8D) whereas areas 3b and 1 responded primarily to touch stimulation. Note that virtually no topographic information is indicated in area 5 because neurons in that region rarely respond to simple tactile or proprioceptive stimuli. Within the hand regions of areas 3B and 1, there are areas labeled D1 to D5, representing the five digits of the hand (D1 = thumb, D5 = little finger). These are consistently arranged—with the region dedicated to processing inputs from the skin of the thumb (D1) found most laterally and that associated with the little finger (D5) most medially. Furthermore, an even more detailed sampling of the hand region of area 3b (not shown in Figure 8) reveals separate subdivisions for the skin overlying each of the proximal, middle, and distal phalanges of the fingers. Overall, SI has an exquisitely detailed and systematic topographic organization, presumably facilitating the identification of the location and types of somatosensory stimuli applied to the body.

Topographic Organization of the Human Somatosensory Cortex

Of course, it is not possible to carry out the type of detailed mapping experiments as depicted in Figure 8 in human subjects. Nevertheless, much insight into the topographic organization of the human cerebral cortex was obtained by Wilder Penfield in the 1930s associated with new neurosurgical procedures he pioneered to treat intractable epilepsy. Penfield (a former trainee of Charles Sherrington) used focal electrical stimulation of the exposed brain in awake patients to identify the aberrant site that triggered seizures. Because there is typically no visible demarcation of these sites, systematic weak electrical stimulation was delivered with a small probe in small steps across the exposed cortex to find the location that induced seizures. Once identified, that region was excised — usually leading to marked improvement or a complete remedy of the seizures.

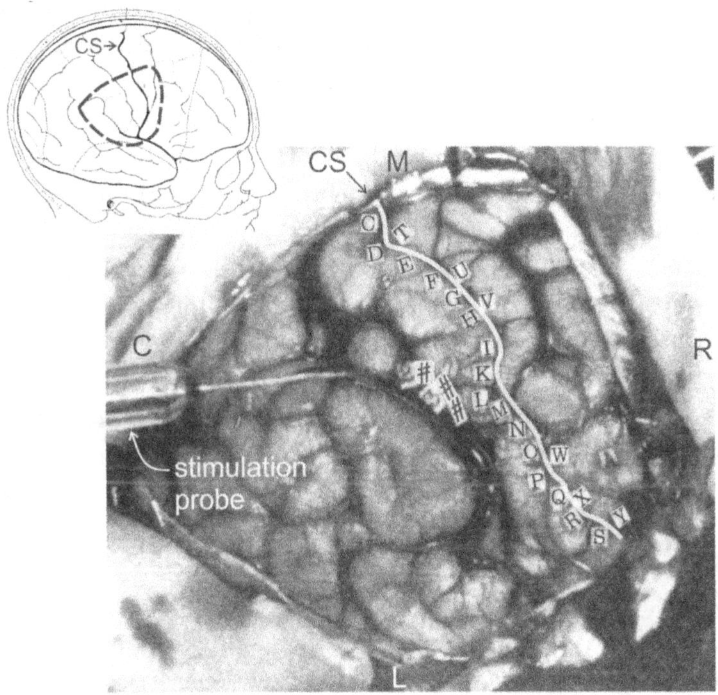

Figure 9. Photograph showing exposed cortex in a human epilepsy patient. The approximate region of the exposed cortex is indicated within the dashed area in the inset. Small paper tags indicate sites where electrical stimulation with a small probe evoked sensations or movements. Tags labeled with "#" symbols indicate sites that provoked seizures upon stimulation. CS—central sulcus, C—caudal, R—rostral, M—medial, L—lateral. (Adapted from Penfield and Bouldrey [1937].)

Keep in mind that the brain itself does not possess nociceptors—so these procedures could be carried out without causing pain to the subject. Moreover, because the patients were awake, they could inform the surgeon of what they perceived, providing important clues to the location and function of various brain regions.

Figure 9 shows a photograph taken from the brain of one of Penfield's neurosurgery patients, a 21-year-old woman. The exposed right cortex (dashed line area, inset in Figure 9) spanned regions mostly caudal to the central sulcus (CS), with the medial (dorsal) boundary about halfway down the length of the central sulcus. Most of the stimulation sites that evoked sensations were caudal to the central sulcus and are indicated by paper tags placed on the brain. The intrasurgical record of what the patient reported when stimulating at different sites is revealing (Penfield & Boldrey 1937). For the most part, the evoked percepts were nonpainful, tingling sensations on the left side. Beginning with site C, near the medial border of the exposed cortex and moving ventral-laterally along the caudal border of the central sulcus, the following was reported: "*C. Numbness left side above umbilicus, D. Sensation in right arm and hand, E. Sensation in hand and fingers, F. Sensation in ring and little finger, G. Sensation in same [ring and little] fingers. H. Same feeling in index and large fingers I. Sensation in index finger. K. Sensation in thumb. L. Sensation in thumb and toward index finger, but not in that finger. M. Sensation left side of face—numbness. N. Sensation in lower left lip O. [Sensation in] lower lip, left side. P. [Sensation in] upper and lower teeth and gums. Q. [Sensation in] left side of tongue and tip. R. [Sensation in] tip of tongue, left side. S. [Sensation in] back of left side of tongue.*"

When stimulating rostral to the central sulcus, the main outcome was some type of movement. For example, stimulating at sites beginning at the medial site T and working toward the lateral site Y, gave rise to the following: "*T. Marked flexion of forearm on arm. Repeated—no sensation. U. Inward rotation of hand and arm and slight flexion of fingers. V. Slight flexion of hand and fingers; no sensation. W. Mouth drawn to left and downward; no sensation. X. Tongue drawn downward and to left; no sensation. Y. Tongue drawn to left; movement of neck to left.*" Each of the stimulation sites marked with the symbol "#" provoked a seizure lasting about 1 minute. This region of the brain was then surgically excised to alleviate the seizures. Unfortunately, in this patient, the surgery failed to eliminate the seizures.

Penfield summarized these kinds of observations from hundreds of patients in a schematic diagram depicting the *spatial arrangement of the locations of perceived sensations projected onto the somatosensory cortex using a schematic representation of a little man* (i.e., a **homunculus**). As shown in Figure 10, there is a systematic progression of sensory fields from head to foot moving across the cerebral convexity from ventral–lateral to dorsal–medial. As encountered previously in the dorsal column nuclei and thalamus (Chapter 11), the relative extent of the cortical territory dedicated to processing information arising from the face and hands

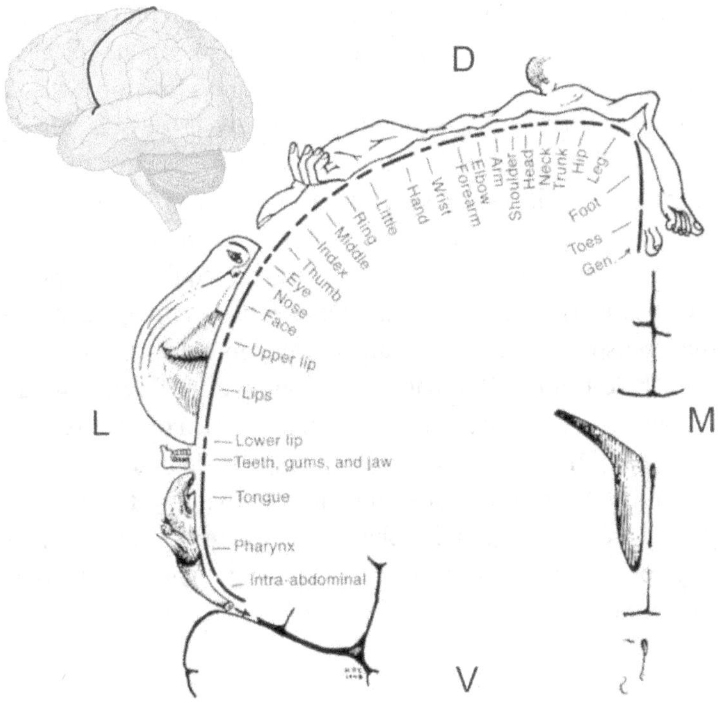

Figure 10.   Somatosensory homunculus. Schematic depicting locations of perceived sensations in response to electrical stimulation at different sites along the gyrus caudal to the central sulcus in the human brain. Inset shows the location of the gyrus on the lateral view of the brain. L—lateral, M—medial, D—dorsal, V—ventral. (Adapted from Penfield and Rasmussen [1950]).

is immense—reflecting the high density of primary sensory receptors, and associated high acuity, in those regions.

Summary

The cerebral cortex is the outer surface of the cerebral hemispheres and is responsible for a host of functions, including conscious awareness, high-level processing of sensory information, various cognitive functions, and voluntary movement. It typically comprises six layers, with each possessing different densities of pyramidal and granule cells. Across the expanse of the cerebral cortex, the thicknesses and cell densities of the layers vary, which Brodmann used to designate 43 distinct areas. SI comprises four parallel bands running medial–lateral across the cerebral convexity just caudal to the central sulcus. The outermost bands, areas 3a and 2 are mostly dedicated to processing proprioceptive information, whereas the innermost bands, areas 3b and 1 predominantly process tactile signals. Area 5, one of the association cortices for somatosensation, receives converging input from all four subdivisions (i.e., areas 3a, 3b, 1, 2) of the SI. Neurons in area 5 are mostly nonresponsive to simple somatosensory inputs. Instead, each neuron in area 5 seems to require a complex set of inputs. Collectively, area 5 (and other association cortices) assembles the individual sensory "pieces" into an overall representation of a sensory situation. There is a parallel mapping of the body surface across the four subdivisions of SI with clear-cut segregation between regions representing different parts of the body. Such detailed mapping facilitates the ability to readily identify the locations of stimuli applied to the body. In addition, as will be discussed in Chapter 13, changes in the topography of the somatosensory cortex under certain circumstances highlight the potential of the brain to reorganize.

References

Amunts K & Zilles K (2015). Architectonic mapping of the human brain beyond Brodmann. *Neuron* **88**, 1086–1107.

Brodmann, K (1909). Vergleichende Lokalisationslehre der Grosshirnrinde in ihren Prinzipien dargestellt auf Grund des Zellenbaues. Leipzig: Barth JA.

Costanzo RM & Gardner EP (1980). A quantitative analysis of responses of direction-sensitive neurons in somatosensory cortex of awake monkeys. *Journal of Neurophysiology* **43**, 1319–1341.

Delhaye BP, Long KH & Bensmaia SJ (2018). Neural basis of touch and proprioception in primate cortex. *Comprehensive Physiology* **8**, 1575–1602.

Gardner EP (1988). Somatosensory cortical mechanisms of feature detection in tactile and kinesthetic discrimination. *Canadian Journal of Physiology and Pharmacology* **66**, 439–454.

Head H & Holmes G (1911). Sensory disturbances from cerebral lesions. *Brain* **34**, 102–254.

Iwamura Y, Tanaka M, Sakamoto M & Hikosaka O (1993). Rostrocaudal gradients in the neuronal receptive field complexity in the finger region of the alert monkey's postcentral gyrus. *Experimental Brain Research* **92**, 360–368.

Knecht S, Kunesch E & Schnitzler A (1996). Parallel and serial processing of haptic information in man: Effects of parietal lesions on sensorimotor hand function. *Neuropsychologia* **34**, 669–687.

Paul RL, Merzenich M & Goodman H (1972). Representation of slowly and rapidly adapting cutaneous mechanoreceptors of the hand in Brodmann's areas 3 and 1 of Macaca mulatta. *Brain Research* **36**, 229–249.

Penfield W & Boldrey E (1937). Somatic motor and sensory representation in the cerebral cortex of man as studied by electrical stimulation. *Brain* **60**, 389–443.

Penfield W & Rasmussen T (1950). The cerebral cortex of man; a clinical study of localization of function.

Phillips JO & Fuchs AF (1989). Somatic sensation: Central processing. In: Patton HD, Fuchs AF, Hille B, Scher AM & Steiner R (eds.) Textbook of Physiology, Volume 1, Excitable Cells and Neurophysiology. WB Saunders: Philadelphia, pp. 336.

Sakata H, Takaoka Y, Kawarasaki A & Shibutani H (1973). Somatosensory properties of neurons in the superior parietal cortex (area 5) of the rhesus monkey. *Brain Research* **64**, 85–102.

Vogt C & Vogt O (1919). Allgemeine ergebnisse unserer hirnforschung, (Volume 21). Leipzig: Barth JA.

Chapter 13

Cortical Plasticity

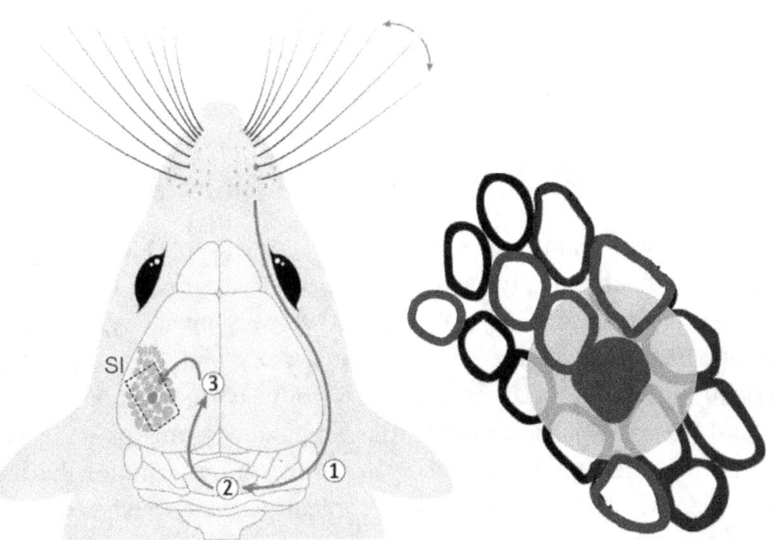

Plasticity of the barrel cortex. Sensory endings at the base of each whisker on the snout of a rodent respond to deflections of the whisker and project (1) to the dorsal column nuclei (DCN) (2), which conveys information to the thalamus (3) and then to the primary somatosensory (SI) cortex. This part of the rodent SI has distinct oval regions (called "barrels"), each of which responds to touch of a single whisker. If all the whiskers are removed except one (the one whose barrel is shown darker), then after a period, the receptive field of that whisker enlarges (gray region on the right, superimposed on the expanded view of barrel cortex) to encompass barrels previously dedicated to other whiskers. (left from Petersen [2019]; right adapted from Feldman and Brecht [2005]).

Up until relatively recently, it was thought that the adult brain could not change significantly how it was organized in response to a change in experience. In other words, once "wired up" early in development, changes in brain architecture could not take place. In an impressive series of studies carried out in the 1980s and 1990s, two groups of investigators (led by the Americans Michael Merzenich and Jon Kaas), however, clearly demonstrated that the brain is not static but can be extensively remodeled in adult animals depending on the extent of change in sensory input. Such reorganization of the cortex, referred to as cortical plasticity, has been studied most comprehensively in the somatosensory cortex. This is due, in part, to the clearly delineated and detailed topographic organization in the primary somatosensory cortex (as described in Chapter 12). Accordingly, if an intervention leads to a distinct change in topography, then some form of brain reorganization must have occurred.

Cortical Plasticity Mediated by Sensory Deprivation

There are two main modes by which cortical plasticity has been demonstrated: chronically depriving a part of the brain of its normal sensory input or chronically enhancing its sensory input. Experimentally, it is often easier to reduce or eliminate sensory input, for example, by surgically lesioning a particular sensory pathway. In addition, there are "natural" cases associated with injuries, amputations, or strokes that cause long-lasting interruption of sensory input to various parts of the brain. Consequently, we know more about cortical plasticity mediated by sensory deprivation than that associated with sensory enhancement.

Initial work related to cortical reorganization associated with sensory deprivation was done in monkeys whose primary somatosensory cortices had already been thoroughly mapped (e.g., see Figure 8, Chapter 12). To understand the nature of these experiments, it is first useful to briefly summarize the organization of the peripheral nerves that supply the hand. As shown in Figure 1, the median nerve carries sensory axons arising from the glabrous (non-hairy) skin on the thumb side (digit 1, D1) of the hand, the ulnar nerve carries sensory axons from the glabrous skin on the little finger (digit 5, D5) side of the hand, and the radial nerve has sensory axons from the back (dorsum) of the hand.

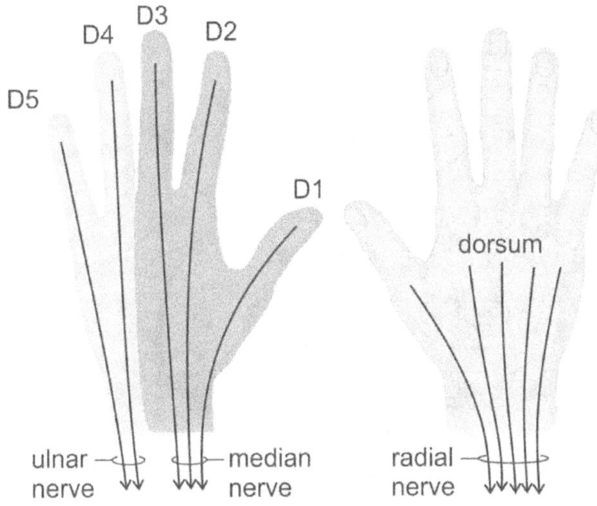

Figure 1.   Sensory innervation of the hand. Sensory axons from the glabrous skin of fingers on the little finger (D5) side of the palm of the hand are carried in the ulnar nerve, the median nerve carries the axons supplying the glabrous skin of the digits and palm on the thumb (D1) side of the hand, and the radial nerve carries axons arising from the back (dorsum) of the hand. (Created in BioRender.com.)

Figure 2 provides an overview of the changes in the topographic organization of area 3b of the somatosensory cortex in monkey in response to different types of lesions (from Kaas *et al.* 1997). Figure 2A shows a lateral view of a monkey brain with area 3b highlighted. Figure 2B shows an expanded view of the face and hand region of area 3b in the normal monkey. The face region is situated most laterally (and ventrally). The areas representing the skin of the digits of the hand are arranged systematically with the thumb (D1) most laterally and the little finger (D5) most medially. The palm of the hand is represented just caudal and somewhat medial to the finger representations. Small islands of cortex, indicated by the hatched regions, are those that represent the skin on the back of the hand.

When the median nerve was cut (Figure 2C), which supplies the skin of digits D1 to D3 and the palm on that side of the hand (see Figure 1), the associated regions of area 3b responded to touch of the back of the hand. This reorganization only took a few days. Remarkably, neurons that

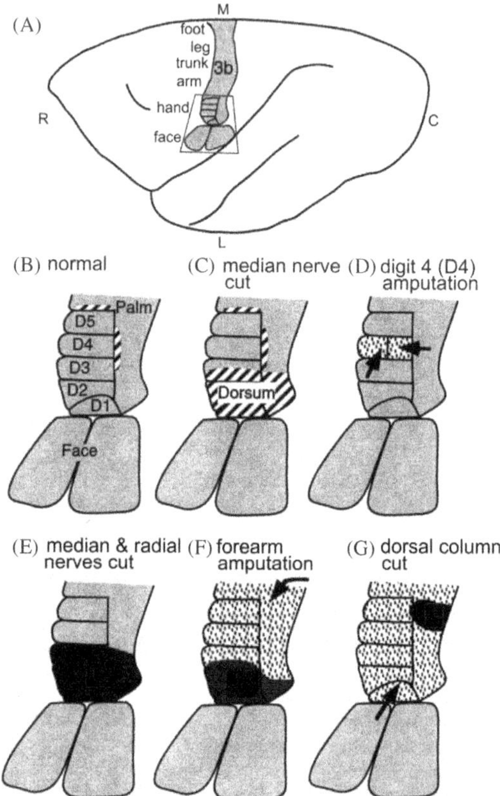

Figure 2.   Reorganization of the hand region of area 3b in response to different types of lesions. (A) Lateral view of owl monkey brain with area 3b highlighted. The region outlined in the box is that depicted in subsequent panels. M—medial, L—lateral, R—rostral, C—caudal. (B) Topographic organization of hand and face regions in area 3b of normal monkey. D1—thumb, D5—little finger. Hatched areas indicate regions with receptive fields on the back of the hand supplied by the radial nerve. (C) A few days following a lesion to the median nerve, touch to the skin of the dorsum of the hand activates the cortex that previously responded exclusively to touch of D1 to D3 and palm. (D) A few days following the amputation of D4 (ring finger), touch to the neighboring fingers and palm activates the cortex (arrows and stippled region) previously dedicated to D4. (E) If both median and radial nerves are cut, then D1 to D3, palm on the thumb side, and hand dorsum cortex go silent (black) in the short term. (F) Several months following forearm amputation, touch to the upper arm activates much of the cortex previously representing the hand. (G) Several months following a dorsal column lesion in the cervical spinal cord, touch to the face activates previous hand representation in area 3b. (Adapted from Kaas *et al.* [1997].)

for the entire lifetime of the animal responded exclusively to touch of the index finger (for example), were now activated by touch to the back of the hand. Similarly, in monkeys that had to have a finger amputated because of an injury (Figure 2D), the region of area 3b that previously was dedicated to that finger, responded to touch of neighboring fingers and the palm after a few days. (Also see equivalent reorganization in the barrel cortex of rodents shown at the outset of this chapter.)

In the case of the lesion of the median nerve (Figure 2C), note that the skin of the hand supplied by the radial nerve "takes over" the region of the cortex previously activated by skin innervated by the median nerve. But what happens if both the median and radial nerves are cut (Figure 2E)? In this case, there is a region of the cortex (shown in black) that is unresponsive (at least in the short term). After a period of several months following such a severe injury, however, such silent regions of the cortex can be reactivated by stimuli quite distant from the original sites of the receptive fields. For example, Figure 2F shows a case where a monkey had his hand and forearm amputated because of an injury. When the receptive fields were mapped months later, much of the previous hand and finger regions of area 3b were now activated by touch to the upper arm (arrow and stippled region, Figure 2F). Likewise, a monkey whose dorsal column was cut in the cervical region of the spinal cord (Figure 2G), largely eliminated somatosensory input from the leg, body, and arm to the brain (but not from the face). Many months later it was found that neurons in the hand and arm regions of area 3b could now be activated by touch to the face (Figure 2G).

A similar investigation was carried out in monkeys whose cervical dorsal roots had been severed years earlier. Such lesions eliminated sensory inputs from the entire arm and hand. In these animals, the complete primary somatosensory (SI) cortex (i.e., areas 3a, 3b, 1, 2) was mapped (like that shown in Figure 8, Chapter 12). Remarkably, the entire hand and arm regions of SI in normal animals (Figure 3A) now responded to stimuli applied to the face in the lesioned animal (Figure 3B).

Phantom Limb Sensations

An important question relates to what kind of perceptions arise in cases such as that shown in Figure 3B to touches (or movements) of the face:

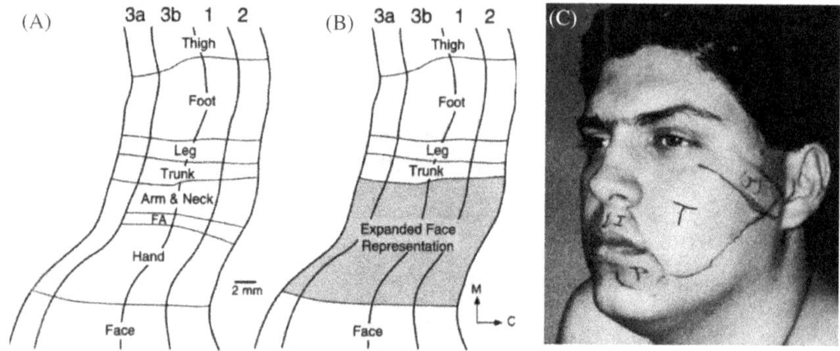

Figure 3.   (A) Topographic organization of the entire primary somatosensory (SI) cortex in a normal monkey. (B) Following long-standing (years) lesions of the dorsal roots supplying the upper limb in monkeys, hand and arm regions of normal SI cortex now responded to input delivered to the face (gray region). (C) Regions on the face of an upper arm amputee that provoked phantom limb sensations on the index finger (I), little finger (pinkie, P), thumb (T), and palm (G). M—medial, C—caudal. ([A], [B] from Kass *et al.* [1997]; [C] from Ramachandran [1993].)

are they felt on the face, on the hand, or both? Insight into this question has been gained through investigation into the perceptual experiences of humans who have had limbs amputated. A large percentage of amputees experience so-called **phantom limb sensations,** wherein *stimuli applied to one part of the body provoke sensory perceptions that seem to arise from the missing, "phantom" limb.* For example, Figure 3C shows areas drawn on the face of an arm amputee that when touched, in addition to the sensation arising from the face, triggered distinct sensations in different regions of the person's missing (i.e., phantom) hand. Large-scale reorganization of the somatosensory cortex, like that shown in Figure 3B, most probably accounts for these misperceptions. Of clinical importance, such phantom limb sensations are often accompanied by excruciating pain. Keep in mind that nociceptive regions of the spinal cord (such as in the dorsal horn) and brain (such as the insula) likely undergo massive reorganization in response to the elimination of normal pain signaling from the limb associated with an amputation. In ways not yet understood (nor readily treated), otherwise innocuous stimuli provoke severe discomfort referred to the missing limb.

Mechanisms Underlying Brain Reorganization

There are two main types of reorganization that occur when a brain region is deprived of sensory input—that associated with relatively small-scale reductions (like that following a finger amputation) and that associated with more massive deprivation of input (like that following amputation of an entire limb). That associated with "minor" loss of input occurs quickly (within a few days), typically with no misperceptions like phantom sensations. Conversely, brain reorganization following "major" loss of sensory input is slow, taking several months, and is often accompanied with misperceptions.

Different mechanisms are thought to underlie these two forms or reorganization. First, consider the case of minor sensory deprivation, for example, that associated with a lesion of the median nerve (like that shown in Figure 2C). Figure 4A shows a schematic representation of a neuron along the dorsal column pathway in the dorsal column nuclei (DCN). Under normal circumstances, this DCN neuron has a receptive field on the tip of the index finger. This neuron receives strong synaptic excitation from primary sensory neurons with tactile receptors in the skin of the index finger and axons carried in the median nerve to the dorsal column, which then project to the DCN. As discussed in Chapter 7, *many neurons also receive weak or ineffective synaptic inputs*, called **latent synapses**. As shown in Figure 4A, some of these latent inputs (shown symbolically to have small presynaptic terminals) likely arise from the radial nerve. Activation of these excitatory inputs has little impact on the postsynaptic neuron, partly because there are few AMPA receptors at those synapses on the postsynaptic membrane. In addition, it appears as though latent inputs can be actively suppressed by inhibitory interneurons that themselves are activated by the median nerve (Figure 4A).

When the median nerve is cut (Figure 4B), the DCN neuron no longer receives excitation from the median nerve. The inhibitory interneurons are also inactivated. Therefore, *latent inputs* from the radial nerve *undergo synaptic strengthening via synaptic plasticity (see Chapter 7) and are relieved of inhibition*. As such, they can now act to depolarize the postsynaptic neuron. This change in the source of effective synaptic input is referred to as **unmasking** of latent synaptic input (Biella & Sotgiu 1995;

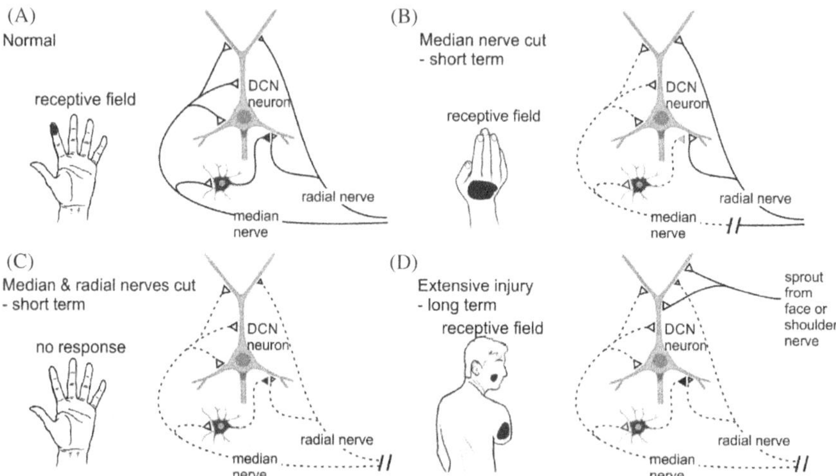

Figure 4.   Mechanisms of brain reorganization following minor and major deprivation of sensory input. (A) Schematic representation of neuron in DCN that receives tactile input from the median nerve and has its receptive field on the palmar surface of the index finger. This neuron also receives latent inputs arising from the radial nerve (supplying the back of the hand). The latent inputs are weak and may also receive tonic inhibition from interneurons (in black) that are driven by the median nerve. (B) Following the lesion of the median nerve, the DCN neuron loses its normal activation from the index finger. The suppression of latent inputs by inhibitory interneurons is relieved, unmasking latent inputs, which also undergo synaptic strengthening (depicted as increased size of the presynaptic terminal). Such changes can cause activation of the DCN neuron by touch to the back of the hand (and activation of the radial nerve) a few days after the median nerve lesion. (C) If both the median and radial nerves are cut, then all inputs, normal and latent, are eliminated, leading to the silencing of the DCN neuron. (D) After several months of elimination of inputs to a DCN neuron, like that due to arm amputation, sprouts of intact axons from distant sources can grow and make synaptic contact with the silenced neuron. These sprouts often arise from axons originating in the skin of the face or shoulder. Eventually, these synaptic contacts can be strengthened, and lead to activation of the DCN neuron (which previously responded only to touch of the tip of the index finger) by stimuli to the face or shoulder. The amputee then often perceives touch as arising simultaneously from the face or shoulder and the missing hand (i.e., a phantom sensation). (Adapted from Kaas *et al.* [1997].)

Wall 1977). Consequently, the receptive field of the DCN neuron will change from the tip of the index finger on the palmar side to the innervation field of the radial nerve on the back of the hand. These changes associated with a *minor* loss of sensory input take place relatively quickly (a few days). Interestingly, this form of reorganization usually does not lead to misperceptions. For example, a touch to the back of the hand, and activation of neurons that previously were responsive only to inputs from the index finger, is not perceived as a touch to the index finger but simply to the back of the hand. Perhaps this is because the activating inputs from the radial nerve are not entirely novel, and the dominant signaling is to intact perceptual circuits representing the back of the hand. Touch to the tip of the index finger, however, will not be perceived.

Now, if both the median and radial nerves are cut (Figure 4C), then the DCN neuron will lose both its normal and latent inputs. Consequently, in the face of this *major* loss of sensory input, such neurons will fall silent as no peripheral signals are available to activate them. However, over a period of months, such silenced neurons may release various **neurotrophic factors** (*small molecules involved in the development of the nervous system*) that attract synaptic input by promoting the outgrowth of intact, more distant axons (Figure 4D). It may take months for such axonal sprouts to make their way to the silenced neurons that beckon with neurotrophic signals. In the case of an arm amputation, intact axons from the skin of the shoulder or from the face eventually make synaptic contacts with neurons that were previously activated by axons arising, for example, from the tip of the index finger of the amputated arm. Such a major loss of sensory input and subsequent growth of axonal sprouts results in completely novel sensory inputs. Therefore, a neuron that previously had a receptive field on a finger now can have a receptive field on the hand or shoulder. This seems to "confuse" the brain as to where stimuli are delivered to the body, provoking misperceptions (i.e., phantom sensations).

Mechanisms Underlying Phantom Limb Sensations

There has been a vigorous debate as to the actual sites of brain reorganization that can account for phantom limb sensations. To understand this debate, consider the simplified schematic in Figure 5. Figure 5A shows the connectivity to the somatosensory cortex (SI) from the face and hand in the normal case. Primary sensory neurons project to the DCN, which communicate with the thalamus, which conveys information to the SI cortex. If the face is touched, a distinct region of the SI cortex is activated, leading to a tactile perception on the face. Likewise for the hand.

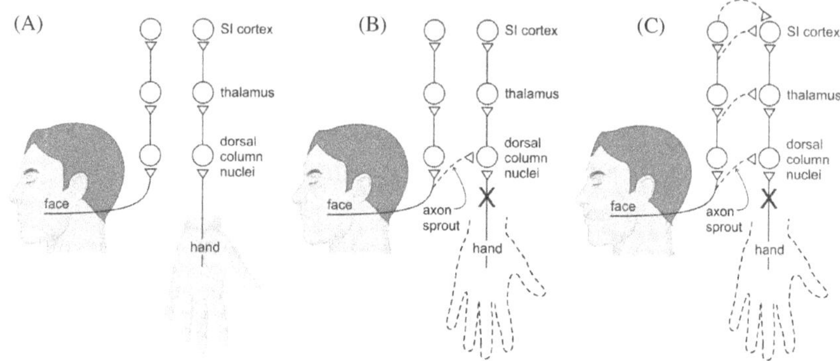

Figure 5.   Mechanisms of phantom limb sensation. (A) Schematic representation of parallel pathways conveying tactile input from face and hand to different regions of the DCN, thalamus, and primary somatosensory (SI) cortex. (B) Following amputation, all sensory input from the arm and hand are eliminated (X). This will cause the hand and arm regions of the DCN, thalamus, and SI cortex to go silent. With time, sprouts emerge from the face axons to make synaptic contact on the DCN neurons that previously conveyed information from the hand. When strengthened, these inputs can activate the hand pathway in response to touch of the face—leading to simultaneous sensations on the face and missing (phantom) hand. In this case, reorganization in the somatosensory cortex could arise due to changes that mainly occur in the brainstem (i.e., in the DCN). (C) Evaluation at other levels of the somatosensory pathway indicates substantial axonal sprouting at the thalamus and within the cortex underlying massive changes in the topographic organization associated with phantom limb sensations. (Made with BioRender.com.)

In the case of an amputated arm (Figure 5B), all sensory inputs from the arm are eliminated. Consequently, the associated hand and arm regions of the DCN, thalamus, and cortex go silent. Months following an arm amputation, primary sensory axons arising from the skin of the face develop axonal sprouts that grow into the hand and arm regions of the DCN (Jain *et al.* 2000). These sprouts make synaptic contact onto neurons that project to the thalamus (Figure 5B). Therefore, in theory, once those connections are established, touch to the face could lead to simultaneous activity of neurons in both the hand and face regions of the SI cortex, contributing to concurrent perceptions of touch to the face and missing hand.

Note that in this scenario, there is no "rewiring" in the cortex per se. A changed topographic organization in the SI cortex would be the consequence of altered connectivity at lower levels in the brainstem (i.e., the DCN). However, there is compelling evidence that sprouting of axons likely occurs at all levels of processing along the pathway (Figure 5C), including from cortical neurons of the intact region to cortical regions in the deprived area of SI (Florence *et al.* 1998). Collectively, these long-term adaptations to reduced sensory input associated with amputation could result in the activation of the deprived cortex and precipitation of phantom sensations.

Cortical Plasticity Mediated by Sensory Enhancement

The previous sections highlight the capacity of the brain to reorganize in response to a reduction in sensory input. Such changes have been shown to occur not only in the somatosensory cortex but also in other cortical regions (such as primary visual, auditory, and motor cortices). While sometimes this type of brain plasticity can be maladaptive (as in the case of phantom limb sensations), it can also underlie substantial recovery from injury or stroke—repurposing some parts of the brain to partially restore functions that might otherwise be lost (Nudo *et al.* 1996).

Cortical reorganization can also arise as a normal consequence of increased usage. For example, in professional violinists, brain imaging has shown an expanded representation of the fingers of the left hand (which are used to press the strings of the violin, involving great dexterity) compared to control subjects (Elbert *et al.* 1995). Such expansion of cortical representation with increased usage has also been directly demonstrated in monkeys (Jenkins *et al.* 1990). In these experiments, the topographic organization of the hand region of area 3b of monkeys was characterized by extensive recording of the tactile receptive fields of individual neurons throughout that area. The monkeys then underwent a period of training that involved the use of the tips of one or two fingers. Figure 6A shows the behavioral apparatus that was used in these experiments. The monkeys were first trained to touch the edge of a metal disk that emerged from a box to obtain a banana pellet reward. The duration over which the monkeys needed to maintain contact with the disk to obtain rewards was gradually increased to 15 s. Then, over a period of

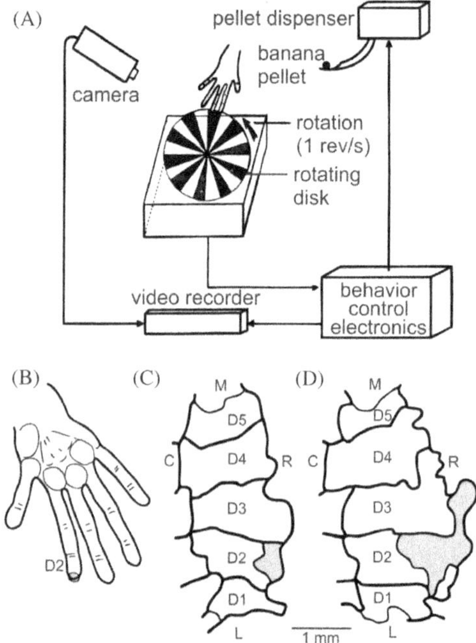

Figure 6.   Brain reorganization mediated by increased usage. (A) Setup used to promote long-term usage of skin at the tip of a finger. Monkeys were trained to hold the tip of their finger in contact with a textured rotating disk. If the finger remained in contact for 15 s, the monkey received a banana pellet reward. Monkeys were free to use this apparatus as much as they wished (1 to 2 hours/day). (B) Diagram of monkey hand showing receptive field location on D2 of an example neuron recorded in area 3B. (C) Topography of hand region of area 3b in the monkey before training. Gray region shows the area associated with touch to the tip of the index finger (D2). (D) Following 3 months of training, the area of cortex dedicated to the tip of the D2 (gray) greatly expanded—more than three times larger than that when the animal was untrained on this task. M—medial, L—lateral, C—caudal, R—rostral. (Adapted from Jenkins *et al.* [s1990].)

days, the box was moved farther and farther away from the monkey's cage, so that eventually, monkeys could only reach the disk with just the tips of the index or middle fingers (i.e., D2 or D3). Finally, to make the task even more challenging, the textured disk rotated so that monkeys needed to concentrate on how much pressure they applied to keep the finger in contact with the disk for the entire 15 s. The disk was continuously available to the monkeys, and monkeys typically spent 1 to 2 hours a day using the disk to obtain the rewards.

Figure 6B shows a picture of the hand of a monkey with the receptive field of a neuron in area 3b indicated on the tip of D2. Figure 6C shows the topographic organization of the finger region of area 3b in a monkey before training. The region highlighted in gray indicates the area where neurons responded just to touch of the tip of D2. Figure 6D shows the topographic organization of area 3B in the same monkey after about 3 months of training with the rotating disk using his index finger (D2). The cortical region that responded to touch of D2 greatly expanded (by approximately threefold) compared to before the training. In monkeys in whom training did not involve a rotating disk or time requirements, little change in the SI cortex was detected. This indicates that attention (and the associated top-down facilitation; see Figures 8 and 9, Chapter 11) is required for this kind of plasticity to occur. Overall, these results clearly demonstrate flexibility in the organization of the cortex and that additional territory can be allocated depending on need and usage. This type of plasticity associated with increased usage likely arises from synaptic strengthening in existing but otherwise relatively weak connections.

Perhaps one of the most extreme types of increased usage occurs in blind individuals who rely primarily on somatosensation and hearing to gather information about the outside world that normally is conveyed through vision. For example, reading is accomplished through tactile signals arising from the fingertips scanning raised Braille letters. It seems reasonable to hypothesize that blind individuals have expanded somatosensory cortices needed to serve the increased usage and demand on tactile (and proprioceptive) sense. This hypothesis was tested using functional magnetic resonance imaging (fMRI) to detect regions of increased blood flow (indicator of enhanced neural activity) in blind individuals as they read Braille words or sets of Braille symbols (Burton *et al.* 2002). This was done in both individuals blind from birth and those who became blind later in life. The results of these experiments were remarkable. As shown in Figure 7, little extra activity was detected in the somatosensory cortex. Instead, feeling Braille symbols led to extensive activation in the occipital lobe, where the visual cortex is located, in both congenitally blind and those who became blind later in life. It is important to recognize that in humans and other primates, the visual cortex is the most expansive of the sensory cortical regions. Therefore, it appears that tactile inputs are rerouted to the occipital lobe in blind individuals to capitalize on the vast

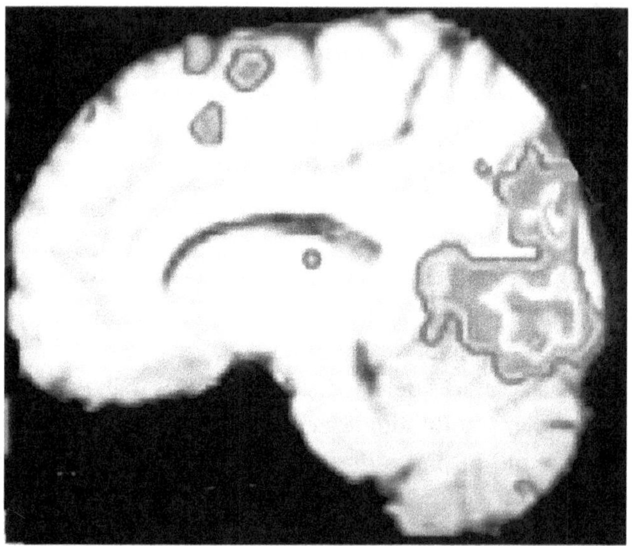

Figure 7.   Functional MRI of blind individual reading Braille text with fingertips. There was robust activation (darkened areas) in the occipital lobe—the location of visual processing in sighted individuals. Little activity was seen in the primary somatosensory cortex. The small regions of activations in the motor areas of the dorsal frontal cortex are likely a consequence of finger movements across the Braille letters. (Adapted from Burton *et al.* [2002].)

computational powers of the visual cortices. Indeed, blind individuals have greater tactile and proprioceptive acuity than sighted individuals (Norman & Bartholomew 2011). The mechanisms by which such dramatic cortical reorganization takes place in blind individuals are not yet known. It seems likely, however, that the main site of such plasticity would occur in the thalamus—a hub where the processing of most sensory modalities is concentrated—thereby (in theory) permitting cross-modality plasticity when input to one modality is eliminated.

Summary

The adult brain has the surprising capacity to reorganize in response to both increases and decreases in usage. The somatosensory cortex, because of its exquisitely detailed topographic organization, has served as an important testbed to understand the nature of such brain plasticity. In response to minor deprivations in sensory input, the somatosensory cortex reorganizes quickly. This type of reorganization appears to be due to the unmasking and synaptic strengthening of extant but weak synaptic connections arising from neighboring body regions. When the deprivation is more extensive (like that associated with a limb amputation), the reorganization may take many months. In this case, axonal branches sprout from distant sources and eventually make synapses onto neurons that have been deprived of their normal input. Oftentimes, this entirely new type of synaptic input leads to misperceptions, such as those associated with phantom limb sensations. When sensory input is enhanced, like that occurring with repeated practice or training associated with a particular task or activity, the cortical areas dedicated to processing the relevant inputs are expanded. Thus, the brain possesses some degree of flexibility to allocate resources needed to enhance performance and function based on an individual's particular circumstances.

References

Biella G & Sotgiu ML (1995). Evidence that inhibitory mechanisms mask inappropriate somatotopic connections in the spinal cord of normal rat. *Journal of Neurophysiology* **74**, 495–505.

Burton H, Snyder AZ, Conturo TE, Akbudak E, Ollinger JM & Raichle ME (2002). Adaptive changes in early and late blind: A fMRI study of Braille reading. *Journal of Neurophysiology* **87**, 589–607.

Elbert T, Pantev C, Wienbruch C, Rockstroh B & Taub E (1995). Increased cortical representation of the fingers of the left hand in string players. *Science* **270**, 305–307.

Feldman DE & Brecht M (2005). Map plasticity in somatosensory cortex. *Science* **310**, 810–815.

Florence SL, Taub HB & Kaas JH (1998). Large-scale sprouting of cortical connections after peripheral injury in adult macaque monkeys. *Science* **282**, 1117–1121.

Jenkins WM, Merzenich MM, Ochs MT, Allard T & Guíc-Robles E (1990). Functional reorganization of primary somatosensory cortex in adult owl monkeys after behaviorally controlled tactile stimulation. *Journal of Neurophysiology* **63**, 82–104.

Jain N, Florence SL, Qi HX & Kaas JH (2000). Growth of new brainstem connections in adult monkeys with massive sensory loss. *Proceedings of the National Academy of Sciences of the United States of America* **97**, 5546–5550.

Kaas JH, Florence SL & Jain N (1997). Reorganization of sensory systems of primates after Injury. *The Neuroscientist* **3**, 123–130.

Norman JF & Bartholomew AN (2011). Blindness enhances tactile acuity and haptic 3-D shape discrimination. *Attention, Perception, and Psychophysics* **73**, 2323–2331.

Nudo RJ, Wise BM, Si Fuentes F & Milliken GW (1996). Neural substrates for the effects of rehabilitative training on motor recovery after ischemic infarct. *Science* **272**, 1791–1794.

Petersen CCH (2019). Sensorimotor processing in the rodent barrel cortex. *Nature Reviews Neuroscience* **20**, 533–546.

Ramachandran VS (1993). Behavioral and magnetoencephalographic correlates of plasticity in the adult human brain. *Proceedings of the National Academy of Sciences of the United States of America* **90**, 10413–10420.

Wall PD (1977). The presence of ineffective synapses and the circumstances which unmask them. *Philosophical Transactions of the Royal Society B: Biological Sciences* **278**, 361–372.

Part 3

Motor System

Chapter 14

Motor Neurons and Motor Units

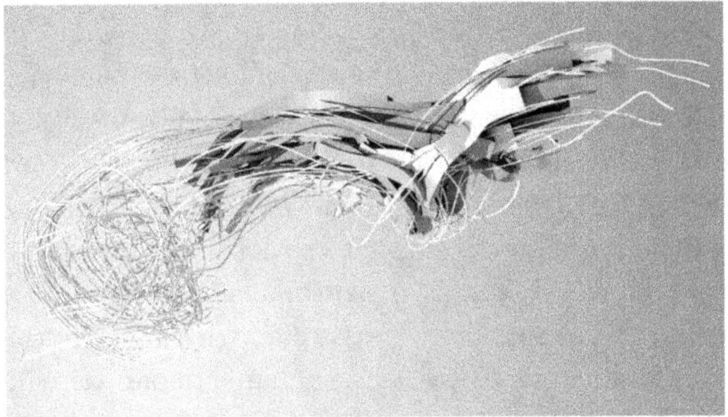

"Forms" is a collaboration between visual artists Memo Akten and Quayola, a series of studies on human motion, and its reverberations through space and time.

In previous chapters, basic ideas as to how neurons take in and process information were discussed. As mentioned in Chapter 1, information conveyed by sensory systems (and from memory) is used by the brain to make decisions about what behavior should be enacted at any moment. Virtually all forms of behavior require movement mediated by muscular activity. In the following chapters, the machinery of the nervous system that underlies the production of behavior is described. As was done for the somatosensory system, we begin this discussion in the periphery and work our way up to the primary cortex, then to higher-level cortices, and to other brain structures. However, in this case, we move opposite to the normal flow of information, beginning with the last-order neurons and progressing toward earlier stages of processing in the motor system.

Anatomy of Motor Nuclei

The last-order neurons in the central nervous system (CNS) are the **motor neurons**. *Their axons exit the CNS to target muscle fibers to provoke muscle contraction.* Motor neurons reside in the spinal cord (that control the limb and body muscles) and in the brain stem (that control the face, mouth, eye, and tongue muscles). Figure 1A indicates the lumbar region of the spinal cord containing motor neurons supplying leg muscles. Figure 1B shows the locations of motor neuron somata in the cat spinal cord supplying the left medial gastrocnemius (MG) and the right soleus muscles (Burke *et al.* 1977). *The collection of motor neurons that supply a given muscle is referred to as a* **motor nucleus**. Motor nuclei in the spinal cord form longitudinal columns that extend over several millimeters. Some of the labeled motor neurons shown in Figure 1B are **gamma motor neurons** *that innervate the small intrafusal muscle fibers of the muscle spindle* (see Figure 13, Chapter 9). Most motor neurons in a motor nucleus, however, are **alpha motor neurons** *that supply the main muscle fibers of a muscle.* For simplicity, unless otherwise noted, the term motor neuron will refer to alpha motor neurons. Furthermore, we will focus on

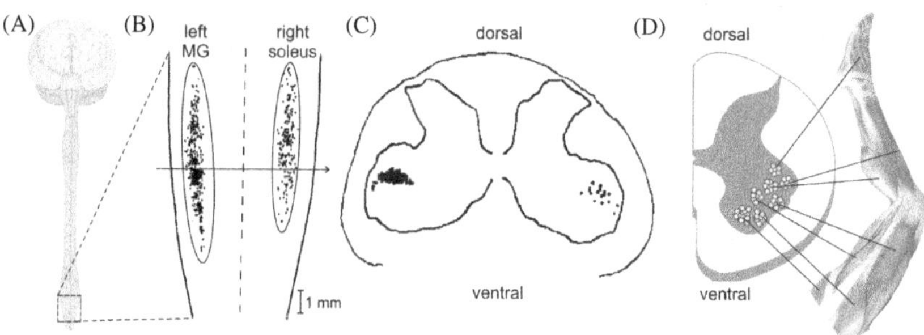

Figure 1.   Location and spatial organization of motor nuclei. (A) Spinal cord with small longitudinal segment of the lumbar region highlighted (dashed box). (B) Locations of motor neuron somas (black dots) in a longitudinal section of cat spinal cord innervating the left MG and right soleus muscles. (C) Cross-section through the spinal cord showing motor neurons of MG (on left) and soleus (on right) located in the ventral horn. (D) Schematic depicting the topographic arrangement of motor nuclei supplying different leg muscles. ([A] from BioRender.com; [B] and [C] from Burke *et al.* [1977].)

spinal motor neurons although much of what is described is also applicable to motor neurons in the brain stem.

Relative to the billions of neurons in the rest of the CNS, the typical number of motor neurons within a motor nucleus is surprisingly small, on the order of a few hundred. For example, the cat MG motor nucleus (Figure 1B) has about 250 motor neurons, whereas the soleus motor nucleus possesses about 130. There is a tendency for the motor nuclei supplying bigger muscles to possess larger numbers of motor neurons. For example, in monkeys, the biceps brachii is innervated by about 1,000 motor neurons whereas small intrinsic hand muscles are supplied by about 100 (Jenny & Inukai 1983).

When examining a cross-section of the spinal cord (Figure 1C), motor neurons are found to reside in the ventral horn. The motor nuclei supplying different muscles occupy slightly different regions of the ventral horn and are topographically organized. For example, in the lumbar spinal cord (Figure 1D), motor nuclei supplying the distal foot muscles are located dorsal-laterally. As one moves ventrally and medially across the ventral horn, motor nuclei innervating progressively more proximal muscles are encountered.

Inputs to Motor Neurons

Figure 2 (adapted from one of Ramon y Cajal's diagrams) schematically shows a column of motor neurons in the ventral horn of the spinal cord. Each motor neuron sends an axon out of the spinal cord to synapse on multiple fibers in the target muscle. Mammalian motor neurons have enormous dendritic arbors and receive on the order of 10,000 to 50,000 synaptic contacts. The sources of these synaptic inputs are diverse but can be roughly segregated into three main types. One source of synaptic input is referred to as **descending** (Figure 2). *These inputs arise from neurons in the brain, including from the cerebral cortex.* Descending inputs play an important role in voluntary movements (such as reaching for an object). *A second set of inputs are those that arise from interneurons within the spinal cord itself* and are referred to as **interneuronal** or **spinal** inputs (Figure 2). These may represent the largest source of inputs to

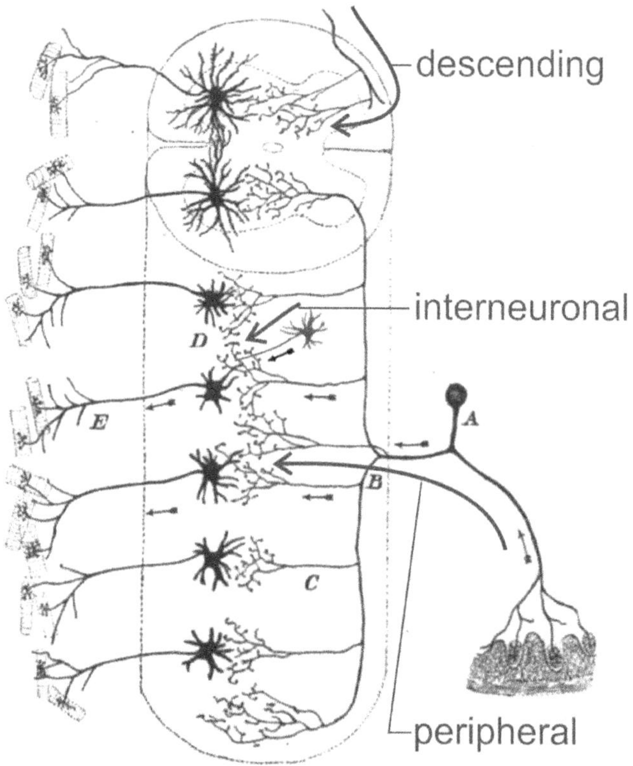

Figure 2.   Sources of input to motor neurons. Motor neurons are shown schematically as a column of neurons in the ventral horn of the spinal cord sending axons out to muscle fibers (left side of figure). Descending inputs arise from structures in the brain, spinal inputs from local interneurons in the spinal cord, and peripheral inputs from a variety of somatosensory receptor neurons. (Adapted from Cajal 1894.)

motor neurons. Such inputs are often associated with spinal circuits that carry out complex processes, for example, regulating the activities of large numbers of muscles involved in various forms of locomotion. It is important to recognize, therefore, that the spinal cord is not simply a conduit carrying information between the brain and periphery. And the third source of input, referred to as **peripheral** (Figure 2), is from *various somatosensory receptors that either directly, or through interneurons, make synaptic contacts onto motor neurons.* Peripheral inputs are often associated with various forms of reflexes.

Motor Units

A full representation of a typical motor neuron is shown in Figure 3A. The dendritic tree is massive, occupying much of the entire ventral horn and extending partially into the white matter. And while the somata of motor nuclei are clustered into columns (e.g., Figure 1), it should be kept in mind that there will be an extensive overlap of the dendrites from motor neurons supplying many different muscles. The axon exits the spinal cord through the ventral root (not shown in Figure 3A). Once the axon approaches its designated muscle (Figure 3B), it divides many times (tens to thousands

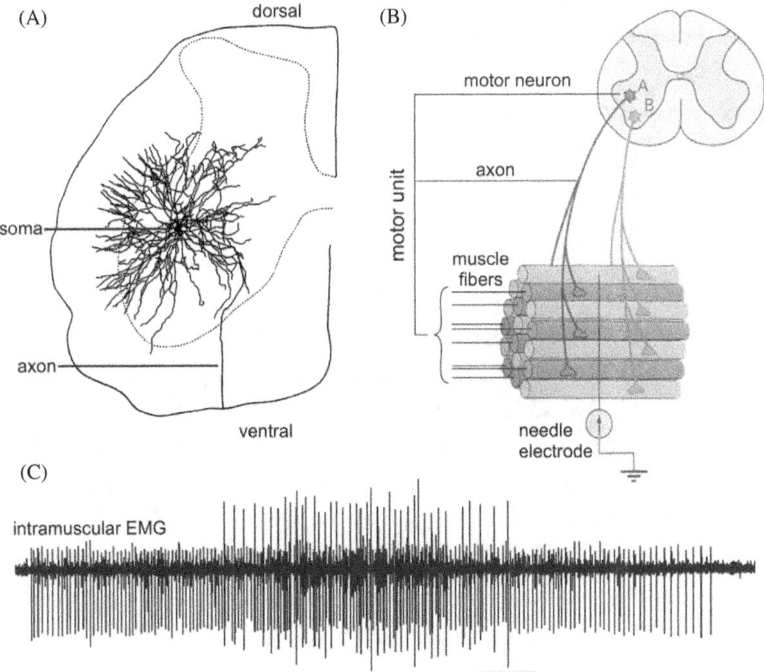

Figure 3.   (A) Expansive dendritic arbor of motor neuron in the ventral horn of spinal cord. (B) A motor unit consists of the motor neuron, axon, and all muscle fibers singularly innervated by branches of axon. Intramuscular needle electrode enables recording the spiking activity of individual motor units. (C) Intramuscular electromyographic recording of spiking activity of two motor units. ([A] from Ulfhake *et al.* [1988]; [B] from Kandel *et al.* {2012}; [C] from the author's laboratory.)

of times) with each terminal branch making a synapse onto a single muscle fiber at the neuromuscular junction. In adult muscle, each muscle fiber receives input from just one motor neuron. Recall from Chapter 6 that the neuromuscular junction is an unusually potent synapse—each action potential that arrives in the presynaptic terminal triggers an action potential in the postsynaptic muscle fiber. Therefore, each action potential set up in a motor neuron will instigate action potentials in all its axonal branches, and in turn, will cause all its innervated muscle fibers to be activated and contract together. This system, namely, *the motor neuron, its axon, and all the muscle fibers innervated by branches of the axon constitutes a functional entity*, called a **motor unit** (Figure 3B). The motor unit is the indivisible output element of the nervous system.

One interesting consequence of the configuration of motor units is that the activity of single motor neurons, otherwise secluded within the spinal cord (or brain stem), is literally broadcast and amplified through the simultaneous activation of hundreds of muscle fibers belonging to a typical motor unit. Because skeletal muscle is readily accessible, it is reasonably easy to place a thin needle electrode into the muscle (Figure 3B) and record the spiking activities of a few motor units whose muscle fibers are in the vicinity of the detection tip of the electrode. Such intramuscular electromyographic (EMG) recordings detect the electrical signals that emanate into the extracellular space from the action potentials propagated along the muscle fibers. Figure 3C shows an example intramuscular EMG signal. The spiking of just one motor unit was detected at the outset of the recording, then a second motor unit (with a larger extracellular signal) became activated before it switched off, leaving just the activity from the original motor unit. Because of these unusual features of motor units, motor neurons are the only neurons of the CNS that can be recorded in awake, healthy human subjects.

Contractile Properties of Motor Units

A great deal is known about the mechanical properties of motor units primarily through experiments in which single motor axons were microsurgically teased out from the ventral root and stimulated in anesthetized

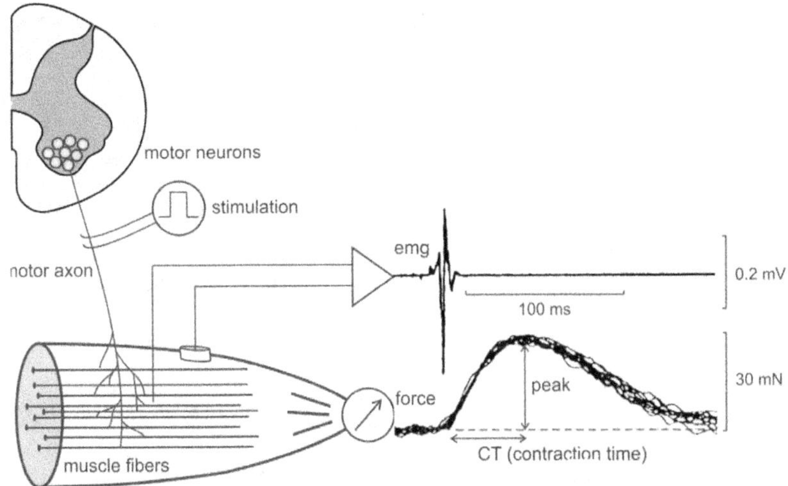

Figure 4.   Method to characterize the mechanical properties of single motor units. Single axons are stimulated, and the evoked force (twitch) and electromyographic (EMG) responses are recorded. Key measures of contractile response are peak twitch force and CT. Ten EMG and force responses from a human motor unit are shown overlaid (from Macefield *et al.* [1996].)

animals (Figure 4). It is also possible to stimulate single motor axons in human subjects using microneurographic methods (described in Chapter 9). The force response to axon stimulation is typically recorded with a transducer attached to the tendon or limb and the EMG response is detected with electrodes inserted into the muscle or placed on the skin over the muscle (Figure 4).

The force and EMG traces shown on the right side of Figure 4 were those evoked in response to a single stimuli (i.e., one action potential at a time) in a human subject (Macefield *et al.* 1996). Ten such traces are shown overlaid in Figure 4 for both force and EMG signals, demonstrating the stability of these responses. The *EMG responses to single axonal action potentials* are referred to as **motor unit action potentials**. Motor unit action potentials tend to have distinct profiles because of the unique spatial relationship between the recording electrodes and the motor unit's muscle fibers. This facilitates the ability of experimenters to distinguish one motor unit from another.

The *force response to a single action potential is called* a **twitch**. Note that the time course of the twitch is substantially longer than the motor unit action potential that triggers these contractile responses. This prolonged response is mainly due to the relatively slow time courses of calcium release and reuptake within the muscle fibers that enables cross-bridge formation and development of force by the myofibrils. The key measurements made to characterize a twitch are the peak twitch force, representing the strength of the motor unit, and the contraction time (CT), indicative of the speed of contraction.

Twitch Force

A consistent observation of experiments done in many mammalian species, including humans, is the wide range of contractile properties among motor units making up a muscle. For example, Figure 5 shows a histogram of the number of motor units observed in a single muscle that had various twitch forces (Milner-Brown *et al.* 1973). The distribution is highly

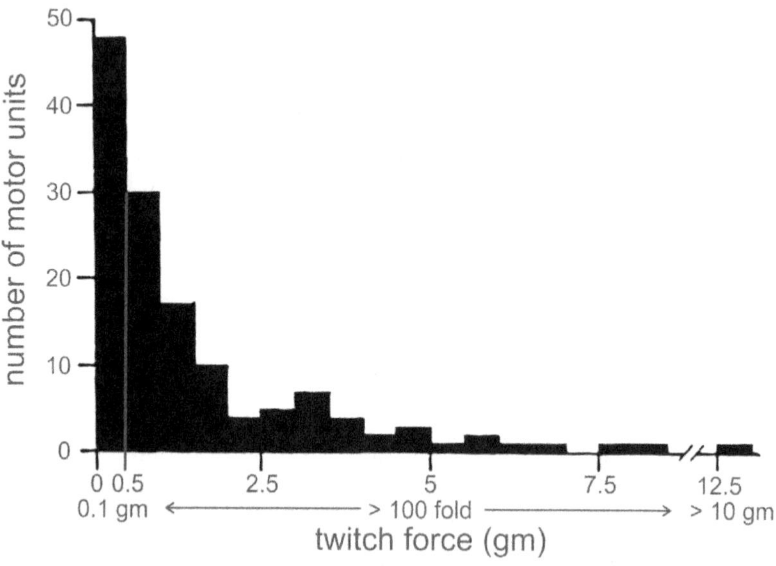

Figure 5.   Distribution of motor units from a single human muscle (first dorsal interosseus) based on twitch force. (From Milner-Brown *et al.* [1973].)

skewed—with many small-force units and few motor units that produced large forces. For example, 48 motor units had peak twitch forces less than 0.5 g (first bar on left, Figure 5) whereas only one motor unit generated greater than 12.5 g (last bar on right; *note*: 1 g force ≈ 10 mN ≈ weight of a raisin). Within the set of the 48 weakest motor units, some had forces as low as 0.1 g. As such, the force range of motor units within a muscle is large—usually greater than 100-fold. This skewed arrangement of motor unit populations based on twitch force is highly conserved across muscles and species. The utility of such an organization is discussed below.

Factors Determining the Twitch Force

A logical question to ask at this stage is what makes some motor units strong and others weak? There are many factors that could influence the force produced by a motor unit. It could be that strong motor units have larger-diameter muscle fibers than weak motor units. Also, it could be that the muscle fibers belonging to strong motor units intrinsically produce more force than that of weak units. Furthermore, strong motor units might innervate more muscle fibers than weak ones.

To answer this question, experimenters developed a clever method to be able to identify the muscle fibers in a whole muscle that belong to just one motor unit (Edstrom & Kugelberg 1968). To do this, a motor axon is first isolated (as shown in Figure 4) and stimulated to determine the force produced by the motor unit. Then, the *motor axon is stimulated continuously for long periods of time (up to 2 hours or more) to expend glycogen (a key energy source stored in muscle fibers) only from the muscle fibers belonging to that motor unit*. For this reason, this method is called the **glycogen depletion technique**. The muscle is then rapidly removed, frozen, and subsequently sliced into very thin sections. The sections are bathed in a solution containing chemicals that stain in the presence of glycogen.

Figure 6A shows a microscopic section of a rat muscle depicting muscle fibers in cross-section (Tötösy de Zepetnek *et al.* 1992). Those muscle fibers that are clear of stain were most probably those whose axons had been stimulated for a prolonged duration. Note that these motor unit fibers are intermingled with muscle fibers belonging to many other motor units. The diameter of glycogen-depleted fibers, their total number, and their

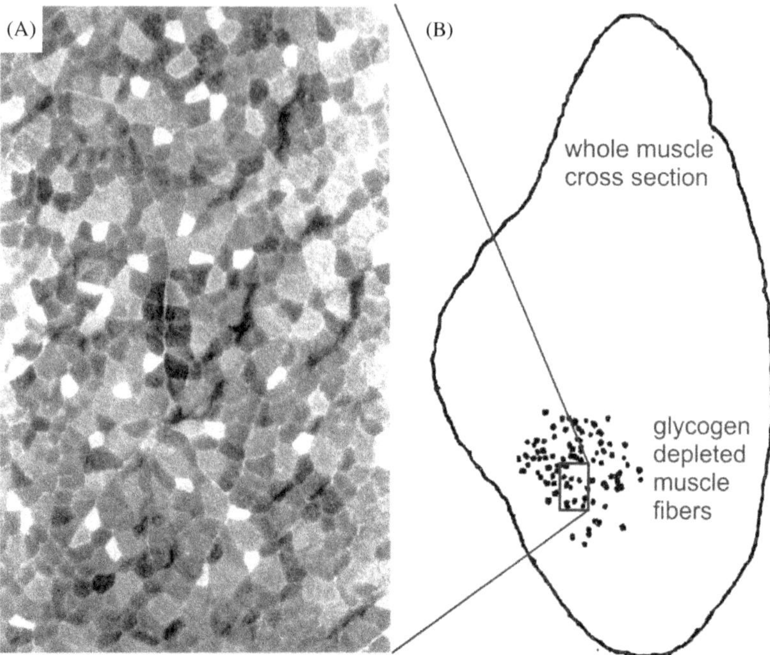

Figure 6.   Glycogen depletion to identify muscle fibers belonging to single motor unit. (A) Histological stain for glycogen applied to a small section of rat tibialis anterior after a single motor unit was stimulated for a prolonged duration. Individual muscle fibers appearing white indicate a near absence of glycogen and are those likely belonging to the motor unit that was stimulated. (B) Locations of glycogen-depleted muscle fibers in the whole muscle cross-section. (From Tötösy de Zepetnek *et al.* [1992].)

locations within the boundaries of the whole muscle (Figure 6B) can be determined. When examining the relationship between various parameters and motor unit force, *the variable that most readily accounts for the large variation in motor unit force is the number of muscle fibers innervated by branches of the motor axon.* For example, Figure 7 shows **tetanic force** (i.e., the *force produced by the temporal summation of twitches during repetitive stimulation*) plotted as a function of the number of muscle fibers identified for each tested motor unit in rat MG muscle (Kanda & Hashizume 1992). Such results indicate that greater the number of muscle fibers belonging to a motor unit, the stronger it is.

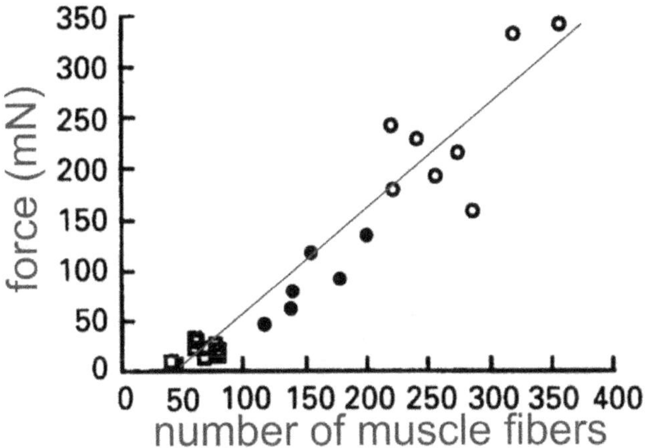

Figure 7.   Motor unit tetanic force plotted as a function of the number of identified muscle fibers (using glycogen depletion) belonging to each unit. Different symbols represent different types of motor units (see Figure 8): squares—type S, filled circles—type FR, open circles—type FF. (From Kanda and Hashizume [1992].)

Motor Unit Types

In addition to the strength of a motor unit, there are two other important contractile properties: (1) the speed of contraction and (2) the extent of fatigue during sustained activity. When characterizing these three features (strength, speed, fatiguability) for each motor unit in a population (or pool) making up a muscle, three categories (or types) of motor units often can be identified (Figure 8). One is referred to as **type S**, where the "*S*" *stands for slow—evidenced by a prolonged CT. Type S motor units also tend to be weak and highly resistant to fatigue.* Figure 8A shows an example of a type S motor unit recorded in a cat hindlimb muscle (Burke *et al.* 1973). In this case, the twitch force was about 1 g and the CT was about 60 ms. The traces immediately below the twitch show the tetanic forces produced in the motor unit when activated at 40 stimuli/s for about one-third of a second. This stimulation pattern was repeated every second for about one hour. The two tetanic responses shown below the twitch indicate the force produced for the first set of stimuli and that produced after 60 minutes of stimulation. The entire run of repeated activation is shown

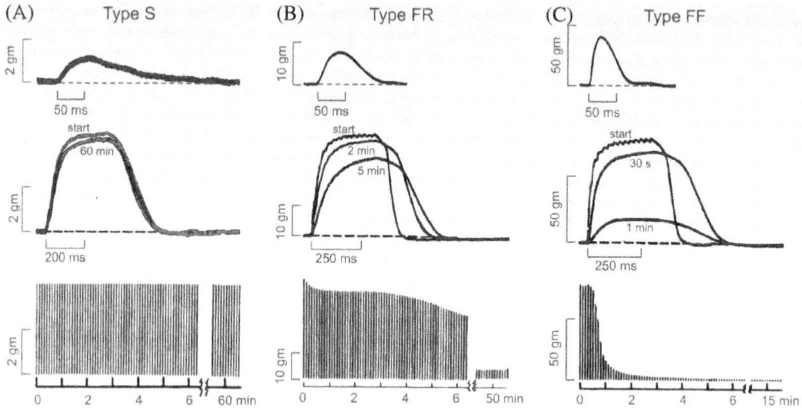

Figure 8.   Motor unit types. (A) Type S motor unit. Top trace shows relatively slow twitch response. Middle traces show tetanic force at the start and following 60 minutes of intermittent stimulation (40 stimuli/second for one-third of a second, repeated every second). Bottom trace shows repeated tetanic responses to stimulation for >60 minutes. Only every 10th response is shown. Type S units are slow, weak, and fatigue-resistant. (B) Type FR motor unit. Same arrangement as for panel A. Type FR motor units are fast (relatively brief twitch), have intermediate strength, and are relatively fatigue-resistant. (C) Type FF motor unit. Same arrangement as for panel A. Type FF motor units are fast, strong, and fatigue rapidly. (From Burke *et al.* [1973].)

in the bottom panel of Figure 8A. With this long time base, each tetanic response looks like a vertical line. This motor unit, like other type S units, exhibited almost no loss in force despite over an hour of intense activity.

Another category of motor units is called **type FR** (Figure 8B)— where the *F stands for fast contracting and the R indicates relatively resistant to fatigue. These motor units also tend to have intermediate strength.* The twitch of the FR unit shown in Figure 8B had a peak force of almost 10 g and a CT of about 45 ms. As such, it was much stronger and somewhat faster than the type S motor unit shown in Figure 8A. As shown in the middle panel of Figure 8B, the tetanic force after 2 minutes of intermittent activation (at 40 stimuli/s) was modestly reduced compared to that at the outset. After 5 minutes of stimulation, the force had dropped even more. When examining the tetanic responses over the entire course of 50 minutes of stimulation for this FR motor unit (bottom of Figure 8B), one can see that force was relatively well maintained during the first few minutes of activity but then it progressively and more steeply declined thereafter, with little force after 50 minutes of activation.

The third category of motor units is called **type FF**—*where the first F stands for fast and the second F stands for fatigable. These motor units are also the strongest.* The type FF motor unit shown in Figure 8C had a large twitch force of about 40 g and a brief CT of about 30 ms. This motor unit also exhibited substantial fatigue when repeatedly activated at 40 stimuli/s. As seen in the middle panel of Figure 8C, there was a substantial loss of force over the first minute of activity, so that by 2 minutes of activation, this unit only produced about 10% of its initial force (bottom panel, Figure 8C). A standardized way to quantify the extent of fatigue in motor units is to calculate the **fatigue index**, which is the *ratio of the force produced at 2 minutes to that at the beginning.* In the case of the type S motor unit (Figure 8A), its fatigue index was about 1.0, the fatigue index for the type FR unit (Figure 8B) was ~0.8, and the type FF motor unit (Figure 8C) had a fatigue index close to 0.1.

Factors Determining CT and Fatigability

In a nutshell, type S motor units are slow, weak, and fatigue-resistant, type FR units are fast, of intermediate strength, and are relatively resistant to fatigue, and FF units are fast, strong, and fatigue rapidly. The main mechanism underlying differences in the strength of motor units was discussed above (i.e., variation in the number of muscle fibers innervated; Figure 7). But what factors account for differences in contractile speed and fatigue resistance across motor unit types? These differences arise from distinct biochemical profiles of the muscle fibers innervated by type S, type FR, and type FF motor units.

The development of force by individual muscle fibers depends on interactions between the parallel filaments, actin and myosin. When calcium is present, heads extending from the myosin filaments latch onto binding sites on the actin filaments. The subsequent conformational change in the shape of the myosin head serves to pull on the actin filament. The myosin head then detaches and reattaches, like a rope climber's hands attaching, pulling, detaching, and then reattaching further up the rope as the climber ascends. The total force exerted by the fiber is directly related to the number of myosin heads bound to actin (i.e., cross-bridges) at any moment. Just like in a tug-of-war, the more "hands" on the rope, the stronger the pull.

This process requires energy supplied by the breakdown of ATP. The rapidity with which a portion of the myosin head (called the **myosin ATPase**) *catalyzes the breakdown of ATP to power cross-bridge cycling* is a critical determinant of how quickly force develops in muscle fibers. There are two main types of myosin ATPases that differ in the rates at which they mediate ATP hydrolysis—a fast and a slow type. As such, the muscle fibers possessing the fast myosin ATPase make up the fast motor unit types (i.e., FF and FR), whereas the muscle fibers having the slow myosin ATPase belong to type S motor units.

Related to fatigue, certain muscle fibers possess high concentrations of enzymes needed for oxidative metabolism. **Oxidative metabolism** *enables muscle fibers to use extensively available glucose and free fatty acids, carried in the blood, as fuels to power contraction for long periods of time, if oxygen is available.* Other muscle fibers rely primarily on **glycolytic metabolism**. In this case, the *glycogen stored in the muscle fibers is used as a fuel source. Such metabolism does not require oxygen.* However, glycogen stores can be rapidly depleted (and not quickly replenished), leaving such fibers drained of their energy source after short bouts of activity.

Figure 9 shows a thin section of human muscle stained with substances to identify different biochemical types of muscle fibers. Consecutive sections are stained with different chemicals to detect different types of myosin ATPase, oxidative enzymes, and glycolytic enzymes. Such staining provides a histochemical profile of the muscle fibers (Schiaffino & Reggiani 2011). One type of fiber identified with such profiling, **type I**, *has slow myosin ATPase, high concentrations of oxidative enzymes, and modest levels of glycolytic enzymes.* These muscle fibers are those innervated by **type S** motor units. Another type, called **type IIa** (the human equivalent is called type IIx), *has fast myosin ATPase, intermediate levels of both oxidative and glycolytic enzymes.* These are the muscle fibers that make up the **type FR** motor units. And lastly, **Type IIb** *muscle fibers also have fast myosin ATPase, have high levels of glycolytic enzymes, and meager amounts of oxidative enzymes.* Type IIb fibers are innervated

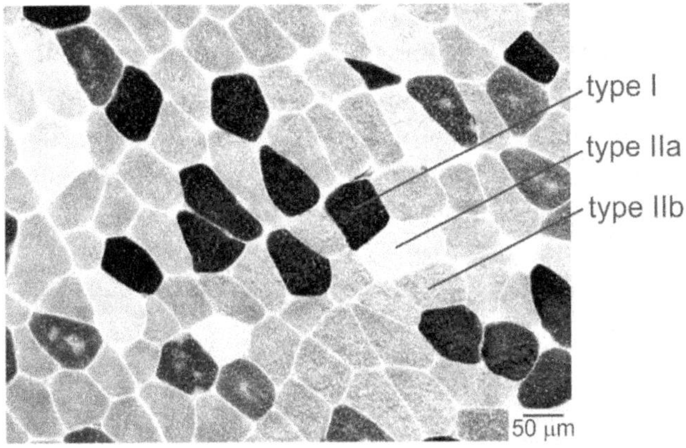

Figure 9.   Magnified view of skeletal muscle fibers in cross-section stained to reveal different fiber types (type I, IIa, and IIb). (Adapted from Neuromuscular Disease Center, https://neuromuscular.wustl.edu/.)

primarily by **type FF** motor units. It is interesting to note that the diameters of type I, IIa, and IIb muscle fibers are not markedly different from one another (Figure 9). This is consistent with the idea that the main factor underlying variation in the strengths of the different motor unit types is in the number of fibers innervated by a motor neuron and not generally because strong motor units have larger muscle fibers.

Motor Unit Populations

Different muscles may possess varying proportions of the three main types of motor units. This can endow individual muscles with distinct contractile properties. For example, the soleus muscle typically has a high proportion of type S motor units, making the soleus highly resistant to fatigue. This is fitting given its function as a postural muscle, involving long-lasting, steady, and relatively weak contractions. There can also be variation in the proportion of motor unit types for the same muscle but in different individuals. For example, some individuals may possess high proportions of type FF motor units in the quadriceps muscle whereas others may have relatively high numbers of type S motor units. Individuals with high proportions of type FF units in the quadriceps may have an advantage in activities requiring explosive muscle contractions (like jumping and sprinting), whereas those with a high prevalence of type S motor units would likely have an advantage in endurance activities (e.g., long-distance running).

Let's consider a motor unit population that has been extensively documented, namely that for the cat gastrocnemius muscle (Figure 10; adapted from Burke *et al.* [1973].). Each symbol in this 3D plot is for one motor unit. The vertical placement of the symbol indicates the strength of the motor unit produced during tetanic contraction. The left–right placement of the stems emerging from each symbol indicates the CT of the motor unit. And the location of the stem along the front–back axis indicates the

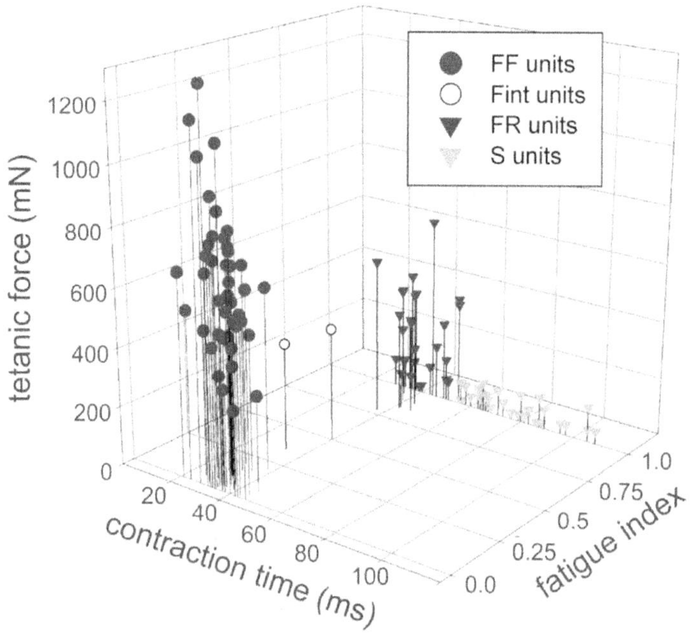

Figure 10.   Contractile properties of cat MG motor units. Type FF units are strong, have brief CTs and are very fatigable (fatigue index < 0.25). Type FR units have intermediate strength, brief CTs, and are relatively fatigue resistant (fatigue indices > 0.75). Type S units are weak, have long CTs (>50 ms), and are highly resistant to fatigue (fatigue index close to 1.0). Some motor units could not be readily classified into type S, FR, or FF, and were called type Fint (fast with intermediate fatigue, open circles). (From Bigland-Ritchie *et al.* [1998] based on data from Burke *et al.* [1973].)

fatigue index of the motor unit. Those motor units whose symbols barely sit above the "floor" of this 3D plot are the type S motor units. Note that the CTs of all these motor units sit in the long duration range (>50 ms). And all these type S motor units had fatigue index values very close to 1.0, meaning they exhibited little fatigue.

At the other extreme, type FF units (solid circles) all had relatively large tetanic forces (>200 mN), their CTs were brief (most less than 40 ms), and fatigue index values between 0 and 0.25 (meaning highly fatigable). Type FR motor units (solid triangles), on the other hand, had a range of low to intermediate strength values, brief CTs (all less than 45 ms), and fatigue index values between 0.75 and 1.0—indicating relative resistance to fatigue.

Not all motor units fall neatly into one of these three categories. For example, two motor units in this sample from the cat gastrocnemius shown in Figure 10 (open circles) had intermediate strengths, fast CTs, and moderate fatigue resistances (fatigue index values between 0.25 and 0.75). As such, the investigators termed these motor units as **type Fint** — *fast but of intermediate fatigue resistance*. Furthermore, in some muscles, there does not appear to be a clear segregation of motor unit types like that shown in Figure 10 (Bigland-Ritchie *et al.* 1998). Rather, there appears to be a continuum of motor unit properties, making it difficult to draw lines distinguishing one type of motor unit from another (Heckman & Enoka 2012).

The Selection Problem

Regardless of the specific composition of a motor unit population, a major challenge that confronts the CNS is which motor units to activate to achieve a desired level of muscle force. It should be kept in mind that (for all practical purposes) the **total muscle force** is *equivalent to the linear sum of the individual motor unit forces*. To understand the problem, consider the situation when one wants to lift and hold a coffee cup against gravity. The biceps brachii and other elbow flexor muscles rapidly and precisely develop the amount of force needed to just elevate the cup. Figure 11 is a schematic that illustrates this process. The thick outer line indicates the total muscle force produced, for example, by the biceps

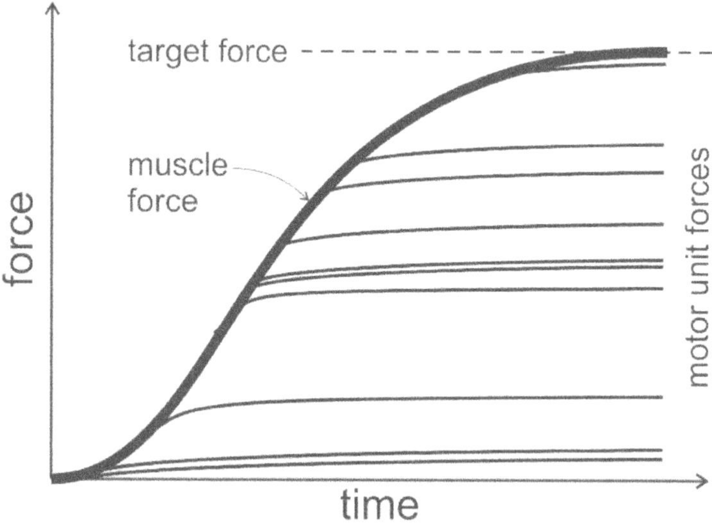

Figure 11.   Schematic depicting summation of individual motor unit forces (thin lines) to attain the desired target muscle force (thick line). In this theoretical case, motor units are selected randomly from the population of motor units making up a muscle.

during this task. The thinner lines represent the forces contributed by individual motor units in the biceps. The force of one motor unit "stacks" upon the forces of the other previously activated motor units, and the total "stack" equals the muscle force.

Now one solution to the problem (i.e., selecting the appropriate set of motor units to achieve the desired muscle force) would be for the CNS to randomly select motor units from the population until the target force is attained (like shown in Figure 11). This process is akin to a mason building a wall to a desired height by randomly grabbing and placing bricks from a pile that have widely varying thicknesses. When getting close to the desired wall height, the mason might then need to search more carefully through the pile to find just the right thicknesses of bricks to home in on the target height. Such a random selection process, however, would entail an enormous computational challenge for the CNS. As pointed out by Elwood Henneman, a Harvard neurophysiologist and trailblazer in the study of motor unit physiology (as will be discussed later), even with a population of only 100 motor units, there would be on the order of 10^{30} different combinations of motor unit forces that the CNS would need to "sort through" to find desired target muscle forces (Henneman *et al.* 1974). Instead, nature has developed an elegant solution to enable rapid, precise, and consistent selection of motor units to efficiently achieve target forces under most circumstances. So, what is that solution? We address that question in the following sections.

Fixed Sequence of Recruitment

A major clue as to how the CNS "solves" the selection problem was uncovered in the 1930s by Derek Denny-Brown, a New Zealand-born neurologist, who did his scientific training with Sir Charles Sherrington. Denny-Brown recorded motor unit action potentials using a needle electrode (like that shown in Figure 3B) while human subjects performed graded muscle contractions (Denny-Brown & Pennybacker 1938). What he observed was that the motor units recorded (each with a distinctive electrical profile, for example, see Figure 4) always seemed to be activated ("recruited") in the same sequence regardless of the type of contraction.

Figure 12 shows a modern example of such a recording made in the biceps brachii muscle of a human subject. The subject gradually increased the isometric force produced by the muscle up to the level of about 20 N and then lessened the contraction intensity back to zero force. A single needle electrode detected the discharge of five motor units during this contraction, distinguished by the shape and amplitude of their motor unit potentials. For convenience, let's call them motor unit 1 to motor unit 5 (there would have been many other motor units activated during the contraction—but only five were close enough to the electrode tip to be detected). Their times of first activation (i.e., recruitment) are shown by the numbered downward arrows above the intramuscular EMG trace. Extensive experimental work since the time of Denny-Brown has shown that regardless of the type of contraction, the speed of contraction, or even the source of the synaptic excitation (descending, spinal, or peripheral; see Figure 2), the sequence of recruitment is stable and practically immutable (Bräcklein *et al.* 2022).

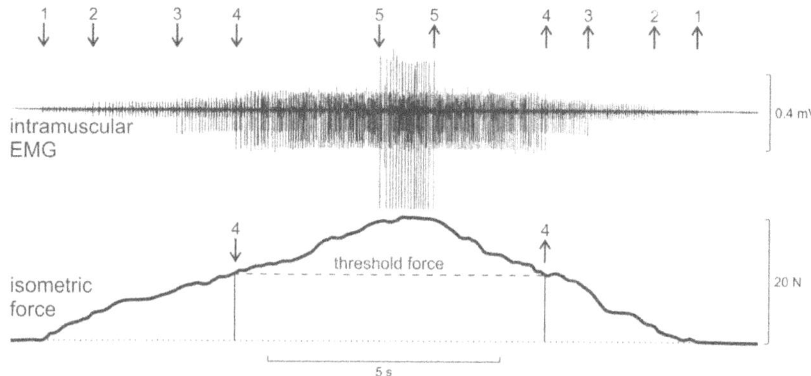

Figure 12.   Recruitment and derecruitment of human biceps brachii motor units during an isometric contraction. In this recording, the intramuscular EMG signals associated with five motor units were detected. The first motor unit recruited (1) was the last to be derecruited, whereas the last unit recruited (5) was the first to be derecruited. Threshold force (shown for motor unit 4 on the isometric force trace) represents the muscle force above which a motor unit is active. (From the author's laboratory.)

As shown on the right-hand side of Figure 12, during the decreasing force phase of the contraction, motor units turn off (i.e., are "derecruited") in the opposite sequence to that which they were recruited. Therefore, in addition to a fixed sequence of recruitment, there is a generalized rule of thumb related to recruitment and derecruitment: "first on" is "last off" (in this case, motor unit 1) and "last on" is "first off" (e.g., motor unit 5). The consistency of this inverse sequence of *derecruitment*, however, is not as robust as it is for the sequence of *recruitment*. In other words, sometimes there are swaps in the derecruitment order. Nevertheless, for the most part, the nervous system uses a consistent pattern for activating (and deactivating) motor units. But is there anything meaningful about the sequence itself?

Orderly Recruitment

To answer that question, let's look again at Figure 12. One way to think about the process of recruitment and derecruitment is that (to a first approximation) and under the constraints of an isometric contraction, a particular motor unit will start firing once a certain level of isometric force is attained (i.e., a "force threshold") and will continue to discharge if the force is above that threshold. This idea is illustrated for motor unit 4 in Figure 12. The vertical lines on the force trace indicate the isometric force at which that motor unit was recruited and derecruited. The forces associated with these two events are about the same. Consequently, whenever the force was above that threshold (dashed line, Figure 12), motor unit 4 was active; when the force dropped below that level, the activity of motor unit 4 halted. As such, early recruited motor units will have low force thresholds and later recruited units will have high thresholds.

In the early 1970s, Richard Stein and colleagues at the University of Alberta in Canada carried out a crucial set of experiments that helped answer the question as to the meaning of the fixed sequence of recruitment. They measured the threshold force at which various motor units were recruited during graded isometric contractions of a human muscle. They also estimated the twitch force produced by each of those motor units. Figure 13 shows a plot depicting the relationship between the threshold force (i.e., the muscle force at which a unit was recruited) and the motor unit twitch force. Each dot on the plot is for a different motor unit, and the data are from a single subject.

From Figure 13 it is evident that those motor units with the lowest thresholds (i.e., those recruited early in the contraction) were those that had the weakest twitches, while those with higher thresholds had progressively larger twitches. Therefore, motor units are activated in a highly organized way: *from those that are the weakest toward those that are the strongest*—referred to as **orderly recruitment**. Furthermore, this figure also illustrates the wide range of twitch forces (~100-fold) with about half the motor units having weak twitch forces within the range of 0.1 to 1 g (logarithmic vertical axis, Figure 13).

One consequence of this organization is that fine resolution of force is an in-built control feature, such that when performing delicate motor tasks involving weak muscle contractions, subtle adjustments in force can be accomplished by drawing upon a large population of weak motor units. As shown in Figure 13, more than 50% of the motor units would likely be activated during a muscle contraction that exerts less than 10% (~200 g in Figure 13) of maximal muscle force. Furthermore, the presence of a

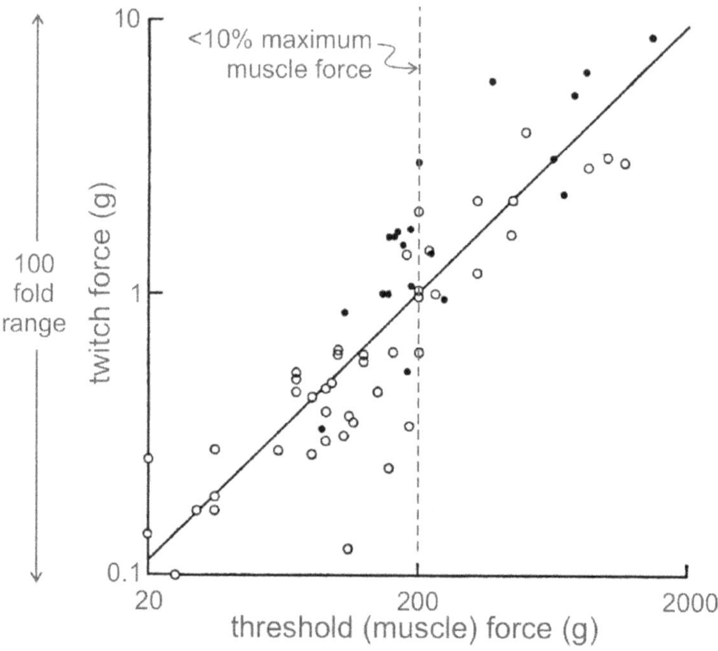

Figure 13.   Relationship between motor unit force (twitch force) and muscle force (threshold force) at which motor units were recruited. The linear relationship between these two variables indicates that motor units are recruited in order from weakest to strongest. Note the 100-fold range in twitch forces with roughly half of the motor units producing forces of 1 g or less. Also, at a muscle force of ~200 g (vertical dashed line) at least half of all units have been recruited yet this only represents about 10% of the muscle force range tested. Data were obtained from the first dorsal interosseus muscle in one human subject. The different symbols are for recordings made on different days. (Adapted from Milner-Brown *et al.* [1973].)

relatively small population of very strong motor units endows muscle with a large operational range without the added necessity of dedicating many neural elements for controlling powerful contractions.

Uniformity of Synaptic Input to Motor Neurons

Orderly recruitment implies that the CNS invariably activates motor units in a fixed sequence related to the physical strength of the motor units. But how is this trick accomplished? How would the synaptic inputs to a motor nucleus "know" which motor neuron innervates the weakest motor unit to activate it first, and which motor neuron is tied to the strongest motor unit so that it is recruited last? One possibility is that each motor neuron is contacted by a distinct set of synaptic inputs (like labeled lines) and that the neurons providing these lines of input are engaged in a fixed order. This turns out not to be the case. Indeed, it is practically the opposite. As a first approximation, all motor neurons in a motor nucleus receive practically the *same* synaptic input.

Evidence for the similarity of input across members of a motor nucleus comes both from anatomical and electrophysiological studies. For example, Figure 14 shows an anatomical reconstruction of the axon and axon terminal branches of a *single* Ia afferent arising from a muscle spindle in a cat hindlimb muscle (Brown & Fyffe 1978). To obtain this, the investigators injected a label into the axon and then allowed sufficient time for the substance to be transported to all the fine branches of the axon in the spinal cord. Subsequent histological analysis enabled the

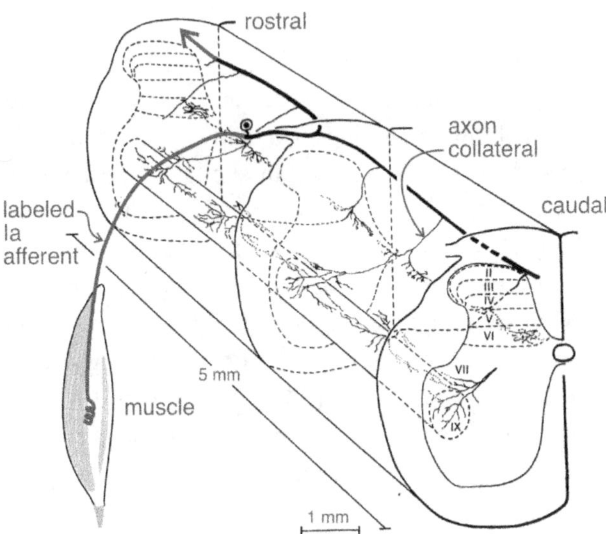

Figure 14.   Schematic reconstruction of the main axon branches and collaterals of a single Ia afferent from the triceps surae muscle group in the lumbosacral cord of the cat. (Adapted from Brown and Fyffe [1978].)

investigators to trace out the destinations of the axon terminals providing synaptic input within the 3D structure of the spinal cord.

As shown, the soma of the Ia afferent is in the dorsal root ganglion and the axon enters the spinal cord through a dorsal root. Upon entry into the dorsal column, the axon bifurcates with one branch ascending to the brainstem and the other coursing caudally down the spinal cord. Along both main branches, multiple axon collaterals are seen directed ventrolaterally to terminate in the part of the ventral horn (dashed cylinder) possessing the motor neurons supplying the muscle from which the Ia afferent originated. This diagram exemplifies the organization of most synaptic inputs to a motor nucleus: the axons of individual neurons ramify extensively to contact a large proportion of the motor neurons making up a motor nucleus. Because all the inputs supply most motor neurons, it follows that any given motor neuron receives more or less the same inputs as its companions.

Such a one-to-many organization was also demonstrated in electrophysiology studies by Mendell and Henneman (1971). In these experiments, the spiking of single Ia afferents in response to sustained muscle stretch was recorded with electrodes placed in the dorsal root. At the same time, microelectrodes were inserted into motor neurons innervating the same muscle to record changes in membrane potential (Figure 15A). In a broad survey involving recordings from multiple motor neurons, those that exhibited a clear depolarization (an excitatory postsynaptic potential [EPSP]) with short latency following afferent action potentials (Figure 15B) were identified as those receiving direct synaptic input from that Ia afferent. Overall, greater than 90% of the motor neurons recorded were supplied with synaptic input from individual Ia afferents. Less direct evidence also suggests broad connectivity for descending and spinal inputs (Jankowska 1992; Lawrence *et al.* 1985; Somjen *et al.* 1966). Collectively, such extensive projection of single inputs is consistent with the idea that most motor neurons innervating a muscle receive similar synaptic inputs.

Differences in Intrinsic Excitability Determine Recruitment Order

If all motor neurons supplying a muscle receive approximately the same synaptic input, then how is it possible that some motor neurons are

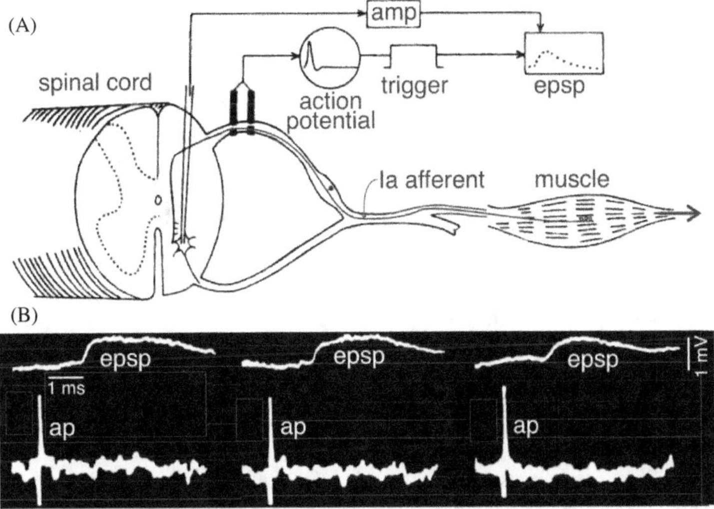

Figure 15.   (A) Method used to record the change in membrane potential in motor neurons in response to action potentials occurring in single Ia afferents. Action potentials were detected with an electrode placed on the dorsal root. The occurrence of each action potential was used to trigger a device to average the amplified (amp) excitatory postsynaptic potentials (epsp) recorded with a microelectrode inserted into a motor neuron in the cat spinal cord. (B) Examples of action potentials (ap) recorded from a Ia afferent and the associated epsps recorded in a motor neuron. The delay between detection of ap and the onset of epsp was ~1.5 ms, consistent with that expected for a monosynaptic connection. (Adapted from Mendell and Henneman [1971].)

activated (recruited) before others? It turns out that there are systematic variations in the **intrinsic excitability** of motor neurons, namely, *how readily individual neurons are depolarized in response to the same level of excitatory synaptic (or injected) current.*

To understand this idea, consider the changes in the membrane potential of a motor neuron in response to stepwise increases in the injected current shown in Figure 16. Before the current is delivered, the motor neuron's resting potential is about −60 mV. The first step of the current depolarized the membrane by about 15 mV. This was not quite sufficient to bring the neuron to the spiking threshold. An additional small step in current was then just enough to bring the motor neuron to the voltage threshold (ΔV_{Th}) and the neuron began spiking (i.e., was recruited). The *minimum* **current** *needed to just bring a neuron to the spiking threshold*

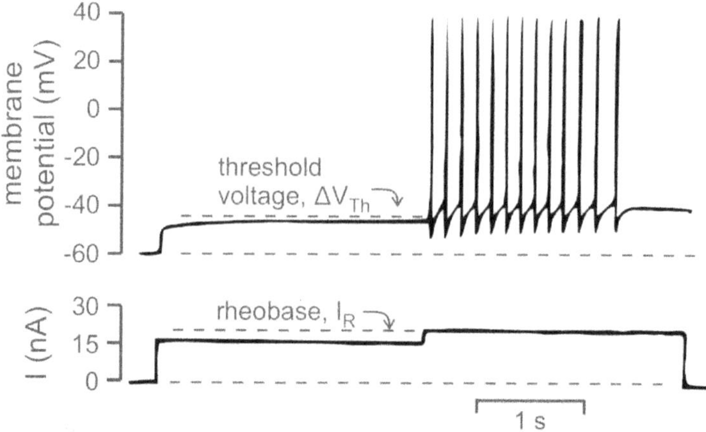

Figure 16.   Stepwise increases in current (*I*) injection and associated changes in membrane potential recorded in a motor neuron. The minimum current needed to just bring a neuron's membrane potential to the threshold for generating action potentials is called the rheobase current. (Adapted from Shepherd [1988].)

is called the **rheobase current**. Interestingly, when measured across neurons within a motor nucleus, there is a very wide range of rheobase values. This means that some neurons require much more injected (or synaptic) current to be brought to the threshold than others, that is, they are intrinsically less excitable—but why?

One possibility is that there could be large differences in the amount of membrane depolarization needed to reach ΔV_{Th}. This, however, turns out not to be the case. In general, most motor neurons have roughly the same ΔV_{Th} (~15 to 20 mV above the resting potential). For simplicity, therefore, let's assume ΔV_{Th} is a constant with a value of 15 mV. Thus, motor neurons in a motor nucleus all receive about the same synaptic input and they all have roughly the same threshold voltage, yet the amount of current needed to recruit them (rheobase current) is vastly different. What can account for this apparent incongruity?

Ohm's law helps provide the solution to this riddle. Let's write Ohm's law for the specific case representing the amount of current needed (i.e., rheobase, I_{rh}) to bring the membrane potential to the spiking threshold (i.e., ΔV_{Th}) as:

$$\Delta V_{Th} = I_{rh} \times R_i. \tag{1}$$

R_i is the so-called **input resistance** that represents the *overall resistance of a neuron to the passage of current.* It reflects a combination of both the axial and membrane resistances (see Figure 8D, Chapter 5). Keep in mind that ΔV_{Th} is a constant, around 15 mV. Therefore, the product of I_{rh} and R_i always needs to come out to the same value. As such, if R_i has 15 units of resistance, then I_{rh} must be 1 unit of current such that the product is 15. Alternatively, if R_i has only 1 unit of resistance, then I_{rh} must increase to 15 units of current in order that their product remains constant at 15. Thus, the larger the input resistance, the smaller the rheobase current, and vice versa.

An alternate way to look at this is to rearrange equation 1 to solve for the rheobase current as:

$$I_{rh} = \Delta V_{Th}/R_i. \tag{2}$$

Keeping in mind that ΔV_{Th} is a constant, then this equation indicates that the greater the input resistance (denominator on the right-hand side), the lower the rheobase current, while the lower the input resistance, the higher the rheobase. This suggests (and perhaps somewhat counterintuitively) that neurons with *high* resistances require *less* current to be brought to the threshold than neurons with lower resistances.

Equation 2 is an example of the so-called inverse function, like:

$$Y = a/X \tag{3}$$

where a is a constant. When plotted, equation 3 looks like that shown in Figure 17A.

What has been described thus far is theoretical—but is there experimental evidence to support the idea that rheobase current is indeed inversely related to input resistance? Figure 17B shows data obtained from motor neurons supplying a muscle in the cat hindlimb across several experiments (Binder 1989). The coordinate of each dot shows the measured rheobase current (on the vertical axis) and input resistance (on the horizontal axis) for single motor neurons. Drawn on this plot is a curve that provides a reasonable fit to the data. Note that it has more or less the same profile as that for the inverse function shown in Figure 17A. Those neurons that had low input resistances tended to have high rheobase

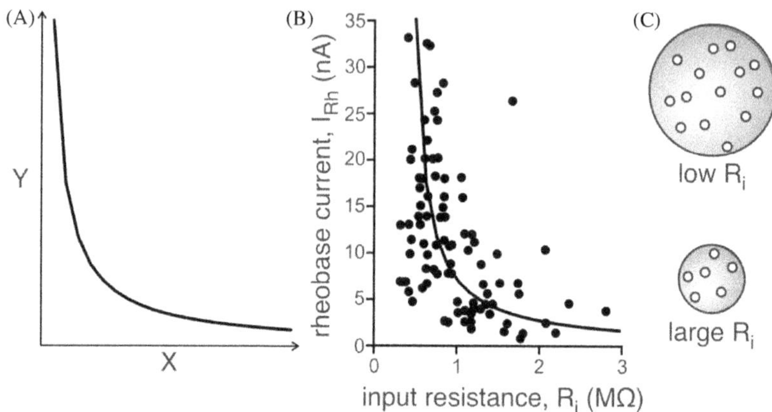

Figure 17.   (A) Plot of an inverse function of the form Y = a/X. (B) Plot of rheobase currents and input resistances measured in motor neurons supplying a hindlimb muscle of the cat. These data generally follow the form of an inverse function, as predicted by Ohm's law. (C) Schematic representation of two factors that affect input resistance (R_i): cell diameter and total number of leak channels. ([B] Adapted from Binder [1989].)

currents while those with the highest resistances had low rheobase values, just as predicted by Ohm's law.

From Figure 17B, input resistance clearly influences how readily a neuron is brought to threshold, but what general factors affect input resistance (a combination of *axial* and *membrane* resistances)? As was discussed in Chapter 5, *axial* resistance is inversely related to cross-sectional area. Therefore, large-diameter neurons should have lower resistances. In addition, the total *membrane* resistance is inversely related to the number of leak channels in the membrane. Figure 17C is a schematic showing the cross-sections through the somas of a large- and small-diameter neurons. Leak channels are indicated as holes in the membrane, and the density of the leak channels is the same for both neurons. Because of the greater surface area of the large neuron, the total number of leak channels will be higher. Recall that if we consider each leak channel to function like a resistor, then the more resistors in parallel, the lower the effective resistance. Another way to think about this is to consider the pictures of the two neurons in Figure 17C as the bottoms of two buckets of different diameters. Holes have been drilled in the bottoms. If we fill the two buckets, water will flow out more quickly from the large than the small bucket because of the greater number of pathways (channels) through which water can flow. In other words, the resistance to flow is lower in the larger bucket even though the density of holes is the same.

Henneman's Size Principle

Many of the ideas discussed above about the mechanisms underlying orderly motor unit recruitment were derived from an extensive series of experiments carried out by Elwood Henneman (Figure 18) and colleagues in the 1950 and 1960s. Figure 19A is a schematic that outlines some of the main features of those mechanisms. A set of motor neurons is depicted as containers having different diameters. Small-diameter motor neurons are shown to possess high input resistance while large motor neurons are indicated to have low input resistance. Excitatory synaptic input is shown to diverge and to supply all motor neurons with synaptic contacts, providing the same synaptic current (I_s) to all members of the motor nucleus. In addition, small motor neurons are shown to have relatively thin axons while large-diameter neurons give rise to thick axons. At the muscle, the axons give off branches to innervate muscle fibers. Small-diameter axons give rise to few terminal branches and innervate relatively few muscle fibers. Conversely, large-diameter axons ramify extensively to innervate many muscle fibers. This arrangement is not unlike upside-down trees:

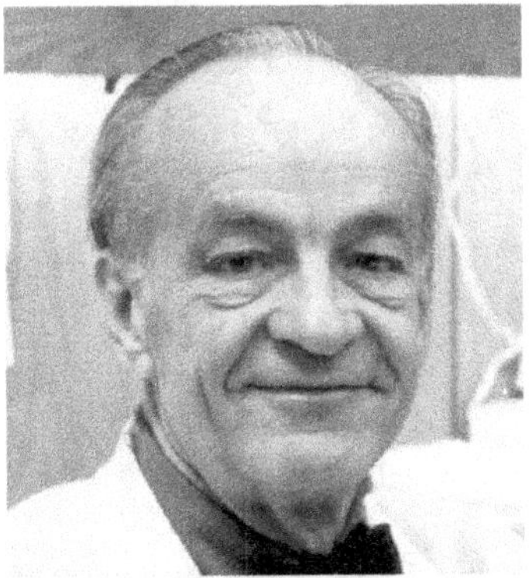

Figure 18.   Elwood Henneman.

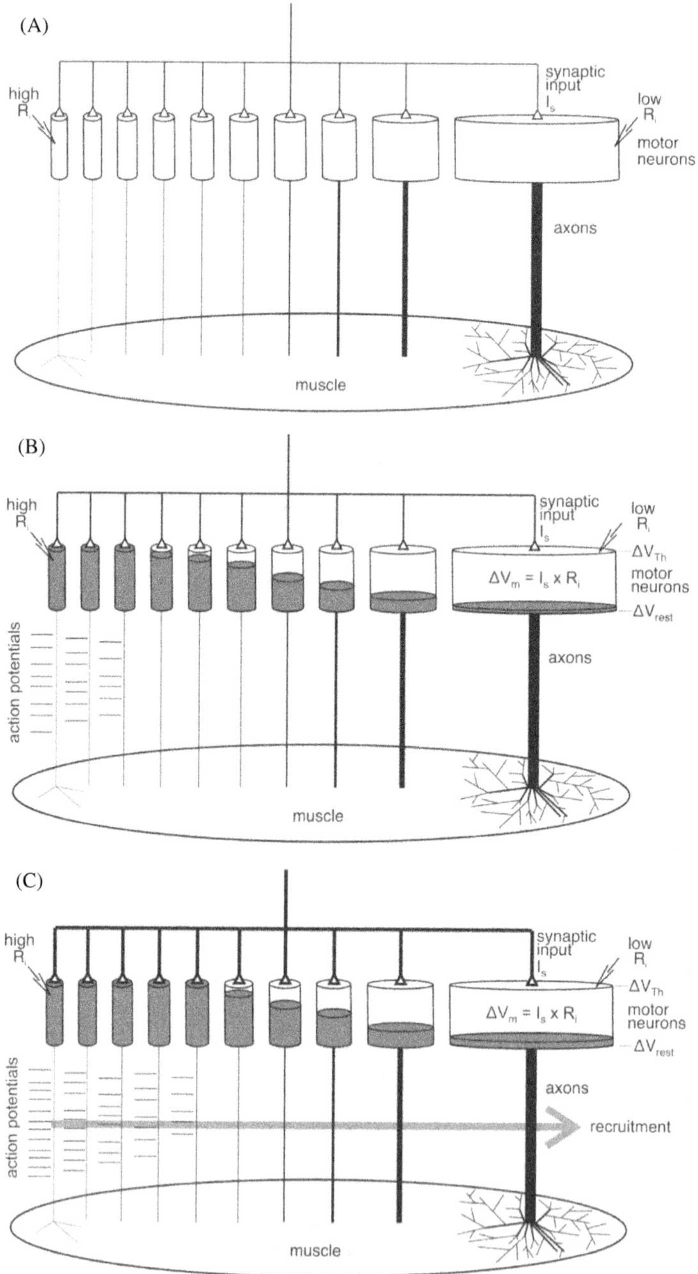
(A)
high
R_i
synaptic
input
I_s
low
R_i
motor
neurons
axons
muscle
(B)
high
R_i
synaptic
input
I_s
low
R_i
ΔV_Th
ΔV_m = I_s x R_i
motor
neurons
ΔV_rest
action potentials
axons
muscle
(C)
high
R_i
synaptic
input
I_s
low
R_i
ΔV_Th
ΔV_m = I_s x R_i
motor
neurons
ΔV_rest
action potentials
axons
recruitment
muscle

Figure 19.   (Figure on facing page) Schematic of the size principle. (A) Motor neurons (indicated as cylinders) that make up a motor nucleus possess a wide range of sizes. Small motor neurons have high input resistances (R_i) whereas large neurons have small R_i. Every motor neuron received similar synaptic current (I_s). Axons from small motor neurons are relatively thin and innervate few muscle fibers whereas large motor neurons have large axons supplying many muscle fibers. (B) Change in membrane potential (indicated by shading in cylinders) associated with weak synaptic input is sufficient to exceed the spiking threshold (ΔV_{Th}, top of cylinder) in small motor neurons (with large input resistances, R_i) but not large neurons. Neurons that have been driven above the threshold generate action potentials to cause muscle fibers to contract. (C) Change in membrane potential associated with stronger synaptic input. More motor neurons are activated leading to stronger contraction. Overall, recruitment progresses from small to large motor neurons, activating motor units from the weakest (and most fatigue-resistant) to the strongest (and most fatiguable).

skinny saplings have few branches while trees with huge trunks give rise to a multitude of branches. Also, recall that the main factor that determines motor unit strength is the number of muscle fibers innervated by branches of a motor axon (Figure 7).

From Ohm's law, the degree of membrane depolarization (ΔV_m) in any neuron will be the product of the synaptic current received (I_s) and the input resistance (R_i) of the neuron, that is, $\Delta V_m = I_s \times R_i$. At a low level of synaptic input (indicated by the slight thickening of the synaptic input line, Figure 19B), the degree of depolarization will, therefore, be largest in smaller motor neurons and least in the larger neurons. The amount of depolarization is indicated as the extent of "filling" of each container. For the case depicted in Figure 19B, depolarization has reached the threshold (the container is filled) for the first few motor neurons and they generate action potentials to cause their muscle fibers to contract. Note that all neurons have the same "height," which symbolically represents the threshold voltage, ΔV_{Th}. Slightly larger diameter neurons will be depolarized but not enough to reach ΔV_{Th} because of their lower input resistances. Despite receiving the same synaptic current (I_s) as the others, the largest motor neuron is barely depolarized above the resting level (V_{rest}) because of its exceptionally low input resistance.

If the magnitude of the synaptic input is increased further (Figure 19C), then neurons that were close to the threshold previously are now brought to the threshold and they start generating action potentials. Those that were already recruited respond to the increase in synaptic input by increasing their firing rates (which increases the force exerted by their muscle fibers; discussed later). Collectively, as synaptic input increases, motor neurons are activated in order from those that are the smallest toward those that are the largest. Furthermore, motor units associated with the smallest motor neurons are also those that produce the weakest forces while those with the biggest neurons have the strongest motor units. Consequently, motor unit recruitment (arrow, Figure 3) will progress "automatically" from those that are the weakest toward those that are the strongest.

It should also be kept in mind that those units that are the weakest are the Type S motor units. Thus, during weak muscle contractions, most of the motor units activated will be of that type. Many muscles (particularly postural muscles) may be continuously activated at low levels most of the day (e.g., neck muscles). Therefore, fatigue-resistant Type S motor units will be the main contributors to such activity, enabling long-lasting contractions with little fatigue. The set of *ideas that explain orderly recruitment of motor units based on the physical dimensions of motor neurons* is referred to as **Henneman's size principle**. The original idea, however, about smaller cells being more excitable than large ones came from the work of Katz and Thesleff (1957), as acknowledged by Henneman.

Rate Coding

Once sufficient current has been delivered to a motor neuron to recruit it, it responds to additional current by increasing its rate of discharge. Figure 20A shows the spiking of a motor neuron to a low level (trace 1) and a high level (trace 2) of injected current. The two traces have been overlaid. After an initial period of higher-frequency discharge, firing rates settle out to more or less steady values. For the low level of current injection, the time between successive spikes in the steady state was about 60 ms (~17 spikes/s) whereas for the high level of current, the time between spikes was about 15 ms (~67 spikes/s). When steady-state frequency is plotted as a function of the intensity of injected current, a linear relation often is observed (Figure 20B).

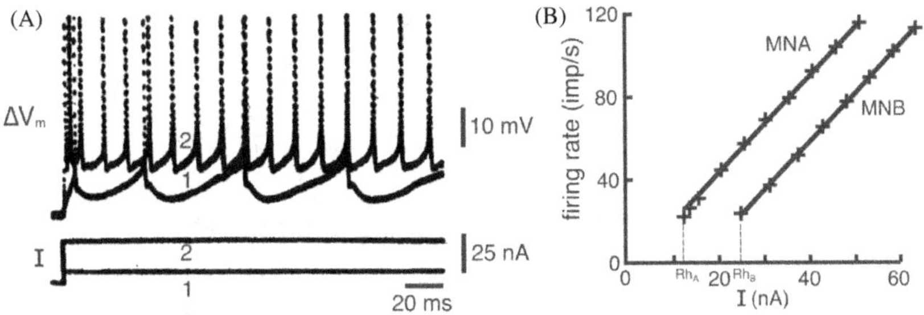

Figure 20.   Rate coding in motor neurons. (A) Spiking response of a motor neuron to two levels of current injection (1 and 2). (B) Plot of steady-state firing rate as a function of injected current (*I*) for two motor neurons (MNA and MNB) that have different rheobase (Rh) currents. ([A] From Schwindt and Crill [1984]. MNA in [B] also from Schwindt and Crill [1984]. MNB is conceptual and not from an actual experiment.)

Keep in mind, up to the rheobase current, no spikes are generated. At rheobase, this motor neuron (MNA) spiked at its lowest rate (in this case, about 20 spikes/s; Figure 20B), dictated largely by the duration of its afterhyperpolarization (see Chapter 4, Figure 3A). The maximum steady-state firing rate for MNA was about 120 impulses/s when ~50 nA of current was injected. But what would happen if higher levels of current were injected; would the firing rate continue to increase? Typically, this does not occur. Instead, with such high levels of depolarizing current, repolarization of the membrane following each spike is insufficient to draw the membrane potential low enough to remove inactivation of the voltage-gated Na^+ channels. This can cause the neuron to cease spiking altogether (see Chapter 4, Figure 3D).

The firing rate versus current relation for a second motor neuron (MNB) is also shown in Figure 20B. This neuron has a higher rheobase, so it requires more current to be activated. Its minimal spiking rate (i.e., at rheobase) is shown to be about the same as that for neuron A but it could also be somewhat higher. Regardless, if we consider the current injected (along the horizontal axis) to represent the net excitatory current delivered to a set of motor neurons, then when the higher threshold MNB is recruited (its rheobase current has been delivered), MNA's firing rate has already ascended to a higher level (about 60 spikes/s). It is as though MNA has had a "head start" with respect to the higher-threshold MNB.

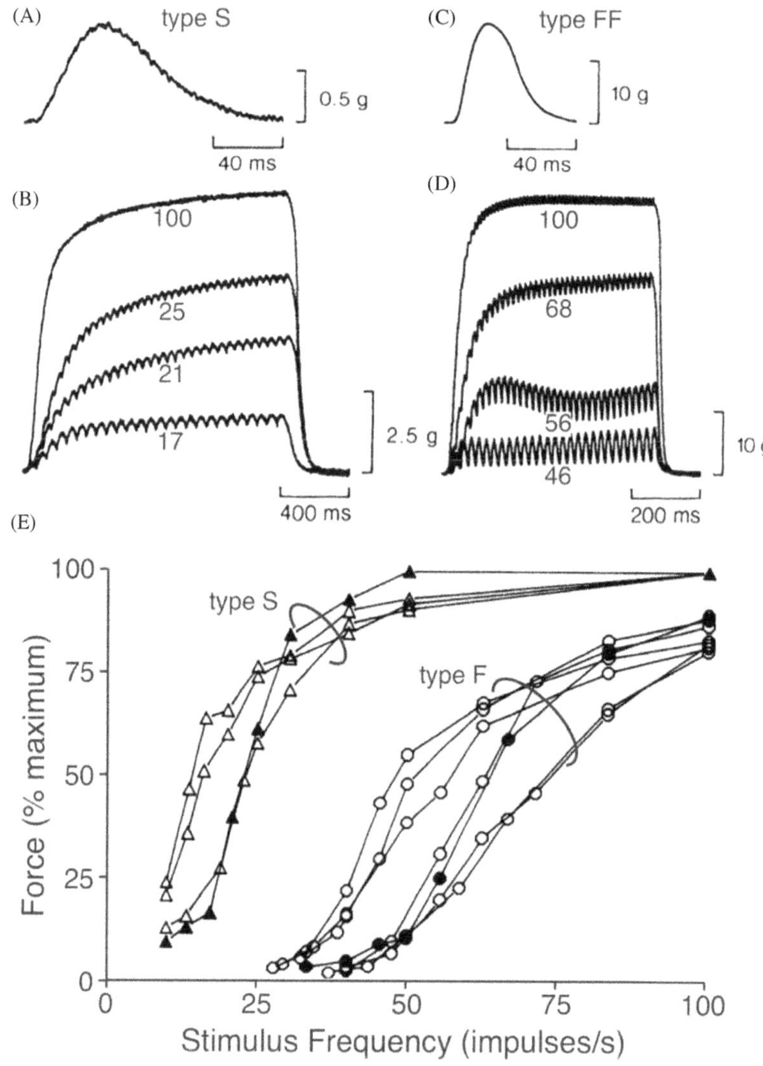

Figure 21.   Force–frequency relation for single motor units in a forelimb muscle of a cat. (A) Twitch of type S motor unit. (B) Tetanic responses of the unit shown in (A) to stimulus frequencies of 17, 21, 25, and 100 impulses/s. (C) Twitch of a type FF motor unit. (D) Tetanic responses of the unit shown in (C) to stimuli at 46, 56, 68, and 100 impulses/s. (E) Plot of steady-state force (normalized to maximum force) versus stimulus frequency for a set of type S (triangles) and type F units (circles). Units with filled symbols are those shown in panels (B) and (D). (From Botterman *et al.* [1986].)

Indeed, if the slopes of the firing rate–current relationships are similar (Kernell 1965), then the firing rates of higher-threshold neurons will tend to be less than that of the lower-threshold neurons.

Impact of Rate Coding on Modulation of Motor Unit Force

Motor neurons rarely emit single action potentials. Instead, sequences (trains) of action potentials are generated that possess varying spike rates. The contraction force of the muscle fibers supplied by a motor neuron increases markedly with increases in the rate of action potentials delivered by the motor neuron. Figure 21A shows the twitch responses of a type S motor unit. Its peak twitch force was about 1 g. Figure 21B shows the force produced by the same unit when its motor axon was stimulated to produce trains of action potentials, each lasting about 1.5 s, at frequencies from 17 to 100 impulses/s. These so-called "tetanic" responses, caused by the temporal summation of many individual twitches, lead to progressively larger forces with higher frequencies. In this case, the maximum force at 100 impulses/s was almost nine times greater than that produced by a single twitch. As such, rate coding can provide profound modulation of force produced by single motor units.

The relationship between stimulus frequency and force varies for different types of motor units. Figure 21C shows a twitch from a type FF motor unit. In this case, the peak twitch force was about 15 g and the CT was about half that of the type S motor unit in Figure 21A. For the lowest frequency of action potentials delivered to this fast motor unit (46 impulses/s), there was virtually no temporal summation because the twitch was so brief. Instead, the response was like a sequence of individual twitches (Figure 21D). Only when stimulus frequencies were above 50 impulses/s did summation occur. While not shown in the figure, such type FF motor units can continue to increase the force with increased frequencies up to about 130 to 150 impulses/s.

When steady-state force is plotted as a function of the frequency of action potentials delivered to muscle fibers, sigmoid-shaped curves are observed. Figure 21E shows a set of those curves for several type S and F motor units. The vertical axis shows force normalized to the maximum force produced by the unit. The force increases steeply at relatively low stimulus frequencies for the type S motor units. They reach near maximal forces at 50 impulses/s. Beyond that, no additional increases in force are observed. On the other hand, Type F motor units only begin to exhibit increases in force at stimulus frequencies between 30 and 50 impulses/s and have not attained maximal force at 100 impulses/s.

The sigmoid-shaped relationship between action potential frequency and motor unit force shown in Figure 21E can be considered to represent **signal transduction** in the motor system. Recall that in sensory systems, transduction involves *converting some form of external energy or signal (mechanical, chemical, light, temperature) into a biological signal,* namely a change in membrane potential in the receptor neurons (Chapter 8, Figure 1). Here, the transduction process is inverted: biological signals (i.e., action potentials delivered to muscle fibers) are transformed into

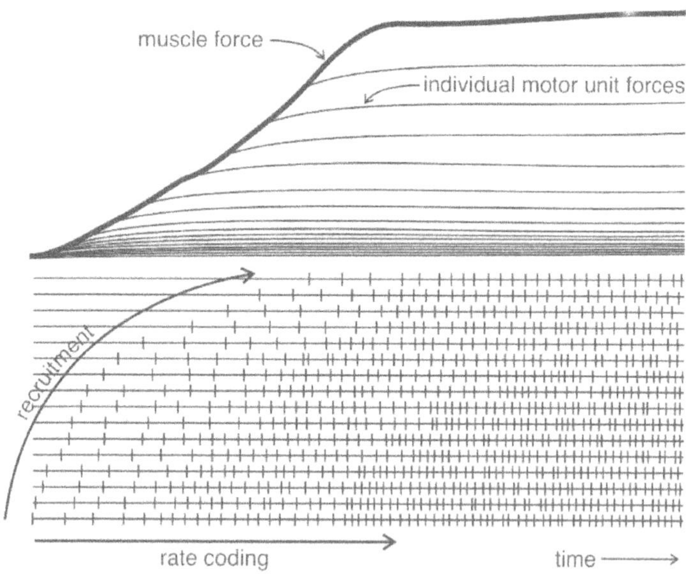

Figure 22.   Schematic representation of recruitment and rate coding among a group of motor units. Each horizontal line at the bottom represents the firing of an individual motor unit. Vertical tick marks indicate occurrences of action potentials. Recruitment and rate coding transpire together to modulate muscle force.

mechanical contractile forces that are exerted upon the outside world though the tendon and bone.

Also as occurs in sensory systems (see Chapter 8, Figure 21B), the "code" used to dictate the *intensity* of muscle contraction involves both rate coding and recruitment. These two processes play out in parallel (Figure 22). As the degree of synaptic excitation to a motor nucleus increases, progressively more motor units are recruited, increasing the total muscle force. At the same time, once the motor units are recruited, increasing the synaptic excitation causes their motor neurons to emit action potentials at higher rates (rate coding; Figure 22). This, in turn, causes their muscle fibers to produce greater amounts of force.

Summary

Motor neurons are the last-order neurons of the CNS. Virtually all forms of behavior come about by the funneling of neural activity through these neurons. Each motor neuron innervates many muscle fibers within a target muscle. The synaptic connection between the axonal branches of motor neurons and muscle fibers is potent. Consequently, every action potential emitted by a motor neuron will cause all its innervated muscle fibers to contract together as a group. Collectively, the motor neuron, its axon, and all the muscle fibers innervated by an axon represents the output element of the nervous system called a motor unit. The motor units that make up a muscle typically possess a wide array of physiological properties, varying in strength, contraction speed, and fatigue resistance.

The order in which motor units are recruited is dictated by the size principle. Namely, small motor neurons, possessing high input resistances, are more readily depolarized (due to Ohm's Law) to action potential threshold (i.e., recruited) than larger, lower-resistance neurons, in response to evenly distributed synaptic input. Furthermore, small motor neurons innervate few muscle fibers whereas large neurons innervate many muscle fibers. Consequently, the recruitment order progresses from the weakest, slowest, and most fatigue-resistant motor units to the strongest, fastest, and most fatigable. Once recruited, increased synaptic excitation causes motor neurons to increase the firing rate. Increased firing rate (rate coding) causes substantial increases in the force produced by a motor unit. It is the collective action of recruitment and rate coding that dictates the forces produced by muscles. And it is muscle forces that are the underpinnings of the remarkably diverse and exquisite movements that can be produced by humans and other animals.

References

Bräcklein M, Barsakcioglu DY, Ibáñez J, Eden J, Burdet E, Mehring C & Farina D (2022). The control and training of single motor units in isometric tasks are constrained by a common input signal. *Elife* **11**, e72871.

Bigland-Ritchie B, Fuglevand AJ & Thomas CK (1998). Contractile properties of human motor units: Is man a cat? *Neuroscientist* **4**, 240–249.

Binder MD (1989). Functional organization of the motorneuron pool. In: Patton HD, Fuchs AF, Hille B, Scher AM, Steiner R (eds.) *Textbook of Physiology: Excitable Cells and Neurophysiology*, Philadelphia: WB Saunders.

Botterman BR, Iwamoto GA & Gonyea WJ (1986). Gradation of isometric tension by different activation rates in motor units of cat flexor carpi radialis muscle. *Journal of Neurophysiology* **56**, 494–506.

Brown AG & Fyffe RE (1978). The morphology of group Ia afferent fibre collaterals in the spinal cord of the cat. *Journal of Physiology* **274**, 111–127.

Burke RE, Levine DN, Tsairis P & Zajac FE (1973). Physiological types and histochemical profiles in motor units of the cat gastrocnemius. *Journal of Physiology* **234**, 723–748.

Burke RE, Strick PL, Kanda K, Kim CC & Walmsley B (1977). Anatomy of medial gastrocnemius and soleus motor nuclei in cat spinal cord. *Journal of Neurophysiology* **40**, 667–680.

Cajal SRY (1894). The Croonian Lecture: La fine structure des centres nerveux. *Proceedings of the Royal Society of London* **55**, 444–468.

Denny-Brown D & Pennybacker JB (1938). Fibrillation and fasciculation in voluntary muscle. *Brain* **61**, 311–334.

Edstrom L & Kugelberg E (1968). Histochemical composition, distribution of fibres and fatiguability of single motor units. Anterior tibial muscle of the rat. *Journal of Neurology, Neurosurgery, and Psychiatry* **31**, 424–433.

Heckman CJ & Enoka RM (2012). Motor unit. *Comprehensive Physiology* **2**, 2629–2682.

Henneman E, Clamann HP, Gillies JD & Skinner RD (1974). Rank order of motoneurons within a pool: Law of combination. *Journal of Neurophysiology* **37**, 1338–1349.

Jankowska E (1992). Interneuronal relay in spinal pathways from proprioceptors. *Progress in Neurobiology* **38**, 335–378.

Jenny AB & Inukai J (1983). Principles of motor organization of the monkey cervical spinal cord. *Journal of Neuroscience* **3**, 567–575.

Kanda K & Hashizume K (1992). Factors causing difference in force output among motor units in the rat medial gastrocnemius muscle. *Journal of Physiology* **448**, 677–695.

Kandel ER, Schwartz JH, Jessell TM, Siegelbaum SA & Hudspeth AJ (2012). Principles of Neural Science, (5th edition). McGraw-Hill.

Katz B & Thesleff S (1957). On the factors which determine the amplitude of the "miniature end-plate potential." *Journal of Physiology* **137**, 267–278.

Kernell D (1965). The adaptation and the relation between discharge frequency and current strength of cat lumbosacral motoneurones stimulated by long-lasting injected currents. *Acta Physiologica* **65**, 65–73.

Macefield VG, Fuglevand AJ, Bigland-Ritchie B (1996). Contractile properties of single motor units in human toe extensors assessed by intraneural motor axon stimulation. *Journal of Neurophysiology* **75**, 2509–2519.

Milner-Brown HS, Stein RB & Yemm R (1973). The orderly recruitment of human motor units during voluntary isometric contractions. *Journal of Physiology* **230**, 359–370.

Schwindt PC & Crill WE. (1984). In: Davidoff RA (ed.). *Handbook of the spinal cord*, pp. 199–242, Dekker: New York.

Shepherd GM (1988). Neurobiology (2nd edition). Oxford: Oxford University Press.

Schiaffino S & Reggiani C (2011). Fiber types in mammalian skeletal muscles. *Physiological Reviews* **91**, 1447–1531.

Tötösy de Zepetnek JE, Zung HV, Erdebil S & Gordon T (1992). Innervation ratio is an important determinant of force in normal and reinnervated rat tibialis anterior muscles. *Journal of Neurophysiology* **67**, 1385–1403.

Ulfhake B, Cullheim S & Franson P (1988). Postnatal development of cat hind limb motoneurons. I: Changes in length, branching structure, and spatial distribution of dendrites of cat triceps surae motoneurons. *Journal of Comparative Neurology* **278**, 69–87.

Chapter 15

Neural Bases of Strength and Fatigue, and Nonsynaptic Excitation of Motor Neurons

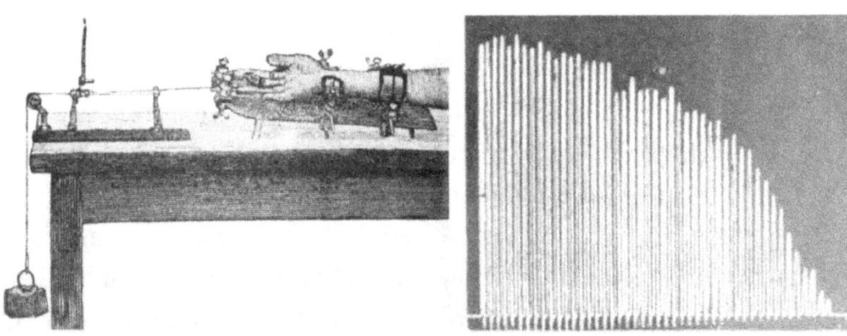

Experimental apparatus (left) for testing muscle fatigue in a human subject. Subject repeatedly lifted a load with a finger, the displacement of which (right) was recorded on a smoked drum kymograph (from Mosso [1904]).

In Chapter 14, the principles and mechanisms governing motor unit activity during normal muscle contractions were introduced. In this chapter, we consider how motor unit activity determines the maximum force that a muscle can produce (i.e., its strength) and how rapidly a muscle fatigues. In addition, this chapter describes a novel mechanism that may enable motor neurons to be driven independently of synaptic input.

Neural Basis of Muscle Strength

Clearly, the strength of a muscle is dependent on how big it is, that is, its cross-sectional area. A long-standing question in movement neuroscience, however, is whether (or to what degree) the nervous system can drive muscle to produce its maximal force capacity. For an individual to produce the maximum force from a muscle, two things must happen. One, all motor units in the muscle must be recruited, and two, every unit must be activated at firing rates commensurate with the plateau on its force–firing rate curve (Chapter 14, Figure 21E). It may be, however, that neither of these conditions are fulfilled even during maximal effort contractions. Regarding recruitment, keep in mind that large motor neurons require immense levels of synaptic current to be depolarized to threshold (Chapter 14, Figure 19). Thus, it is feasible that under normal circumstances, sufficient depolarizing current simply cannot be delivered to the motor nucleus to activate the largest motor neurons (that innervate the strongest motor units). This would imply that during maximal efforts, some fraction of the muscle may not be excited. At present, however, little direct evidence has been presented demonstrating whether recruitment is complete or not during maximum contractions in healthy humans.

There is, however, convincing evidence indicating that firing rates may not reach levels needed to produce the maximal force in individual motor units during *maximum voluntary contractions* (**MVCs**). An MVC is carried out by a *human subject exerting their absolute strongest effort (often under verbal exhortations of experimenters) against a device that measures contraction force or torque.* The typical firing rates reported for human motor units during MVCs are in the order of 15 to 30 impulses/s (Bellemare *et al.* 1983). Indeed, the firing rates of individual motor units oftentimes level off ("saturate") at quite low levels while voluntary muscle force (and excitatory synaptic drive to the motor nucleus) continues to increase (Figure 1). The mechanisms underlying this saturation are not yet understood.

Regardless, this low level of firing rate indicates that most motor units do not produce their peak capacity during MVCs. For example, the top part of Figure 2 shows five superimposed twitches and electromyographic

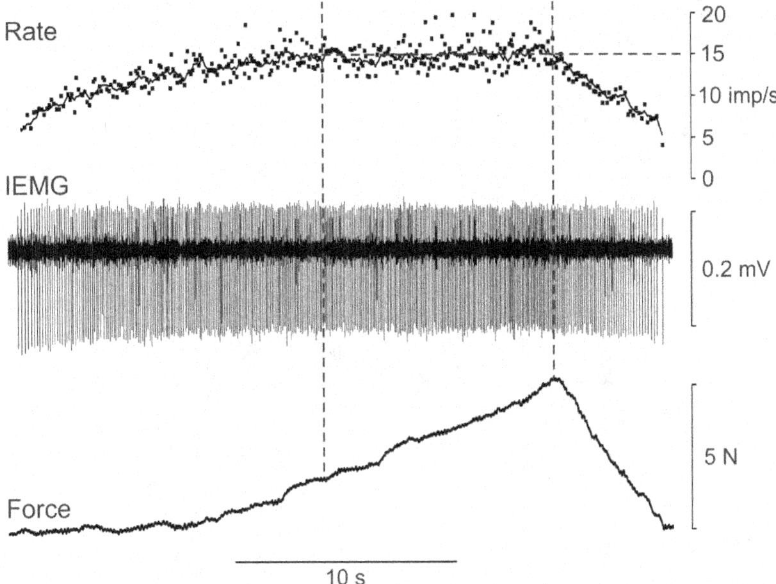

Figure 1.   Isometric force exerted by the biceps muscle in a human subject (bottom trace), intramuscular EMG (IEMG) depicting discharge of a single motor unit (middle trace), and instantaneous firing rate of the recorded unit (top trace). Vertical dashed lines indicate the period during which force was increasing yet motor unit firing rate had leveled off ("saturated") at a value of ~15 impulses/s. (From Fuglevand *et al.* [2015].)

(EMG) responses to the stimuli delivered to a single motor axon with a microelectrode placed within the median nerve of a human subject. The twitch contraction time of this motor unit was of intermediate duration (54 ms)—placing it in the middle of the range of contraction times for human motor units. The motor axon was then stimulated with trains of stimuli at progressively increasing rates from 2 to 100 impulses/s, and the evoked EMG and force responses recorded (lower part of Figure 2). This typical motor unit required 80 impulses/s to reach its peak force. This rate of action potentials is substantially higher than the rates recorded during voluntary contractions (see Figure 1). Therefore, there would seem to be a substantial reserve of force capacity that is normally not enlisted even during the strongest voluntary contractions.

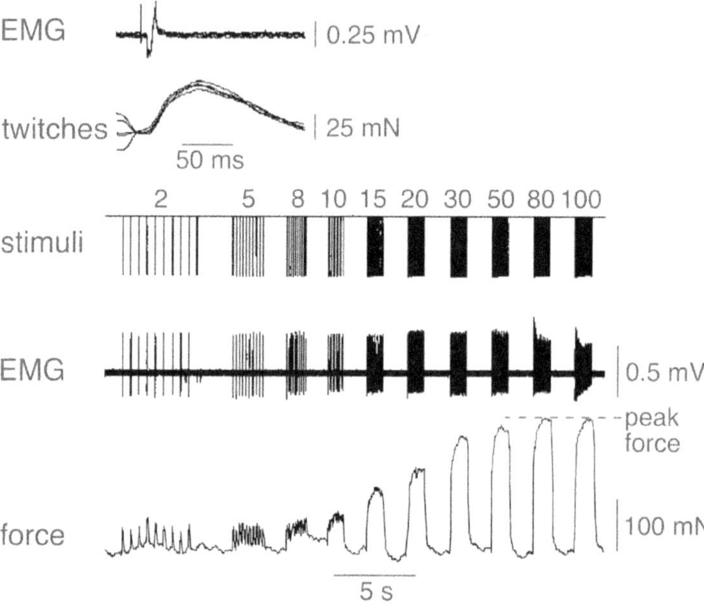

Figure 2.   Top: Five superimposed EMG responses and twitch (twitch amplitude 44 mN, contraction time 54 ms) responses to individual stimuli delivered to a single motor axon supplying a human hand muscle. Lower: Force and EMG responses to trains of stimuli from 2 to 100 impulses/s delivered to the same unit as depicted above. Peak force in this unit was attained with a stimulus rate of 80 impulses/s. (From Fuglevand *et al.* [1999].)

Neural Basis of Strength Gains with Training

Given that the firing rates of motor units during MVCs seem insufficient to produce maximum forces, is it possible to "train" the nervous system to generate higher firing rates, and thereby produce greater motor unit (and muscle) forces? There is good experimental support for this idea. For example, during the early stages of strength training (i.e., during the first few weeks), individuals significantly increase their strength but without detectable changes in the sizes of the muscles or muscle fibers of the trained muscles (Sale 1988). Also, when human subjects undergo strength training of a single limb, the strength of the contralateral, untrained limb typically increases by about 20% (Enoka 1988). Similarly, in a carefully controlled study (Yue & Cole 1992), human subjects increased MVC force by >20% following four weeks of training involving only imaginary muscle contractions.

Only recently, however, has direct evidence become available demonstrating strength-training-related increases in motor unit firing rates. In a recent study (Del Vecchio *et al.* 2019), a clever method was used to enable the firing rates of the same, identified motor units to be monitored over a four-week period of strength training. Both strength (MVC force) and motor unit firing rates increased by about the same amount over the training period. These results provided a clear demonstration that early increases in strength with training are likely caused by increases in motor unit activity.

But what mechanisms might underlie these training-related increases in motor unit activity? One possibility is that plastic changes in the motor cortex (the main site contributing descending excitation to motor neurons during voluntary contractions), triggered by repeated, vigorous cortical activity over a few weeks of training, enhanced the intensity of cortical drive to motor neurons. Alternatively (or in addition), it could be that the central nervous (CNS) "learned" to dampen some of the inhibitory synaptic input to motor neurons that often co-occurs with excitatory inputs.

And a third possibility is that the motor neurons themselves became more responsive to excitatory synaptic input with training. Such an intrinsic change might, for example, come about because of a reduction in membrane "leakiness" (Chapter 14, Figure 17C). This would increase the input resistance and enhance the magnitude of depolarization and associated firing rates of motor neurons for the same level of synaptic input. In addition, it could also be that the characteristics of the ion channels responsible for the afterhyperpolarization (which plays a key role in determining firing rate; Chapter 4, Figure 3) change with repeated intense activity accompanying strength training. Furthermore, it could be that *nonsynaptic* sources of depolarizing current (discussed later in this chapter) become more prevalent with training. While none of the proposed mechanisms for increasing motor unit firing rate have yet been clearly demonstrated, it does seem clear that muscle strength depends both on muscle and the CNS (Fuglevand 2019).

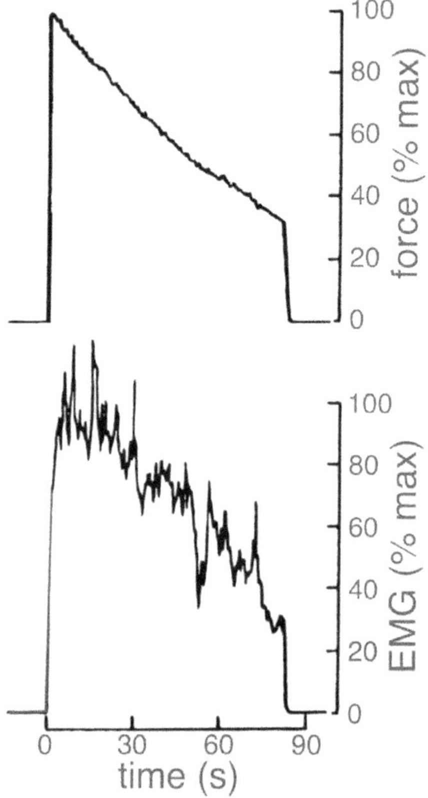

Figure 3.   Isometric force and smoothed EMG during a sustained maximum voluntary contraction of the biceps brachii muscle in a human subject. (From Bigland-Ritchie [1981].)

Fatigue

Muscle **fatigue** *is a temporary decline in the force and power capacity of skeletal muscle resulting from muscle activity.* Muscle fatigue can adversely affect the lives of workers, athletes, patients, and the elderly. Yet, the basic mechanisms underlying muscle fatigue have not been firmly established despite more than a century of systemic investigation (see frontispiece image for this chapter from Mosso [1904]). At the level of the muscle, fatigue is thought to arise mainly because of impairments in cross-bridge function between myofibrils that underlies force production by muscle fibers (Kent-Braun *et al.* 2012). These impairments are brought about by many mechanisms, including diminished release of calcium by intracellular stores that triggers cross-bridge formation, accumulation of intracellular metabolites that may interfere with the cross-bridge formation, and temporary disruption of the ionic concentration gradients across the muscle fiber membrane, reducing their excitabilities.

It also seems clear that force loss during prolonged activity is due, in part, to a failure of the nervous system to provide an adequate level of drive to muscle. Such neural fatigue (sometimes referred to as central fatigue) is manifest as an impairment in the activation of the motor neurons that drive muscle fibers. A clear demonstration of neural fatigue can be observed in the changes in EMG activity while a human subject attempts to exert maximum muscle force for a sustained period (Bigland-Ritchie 1981; Figure 3). In this case, the EMG signal was recorded with surface electrodes placed over the contracting muscle. Such signals broadly detect the collective activities of many motor units, and roughly represent the total neural input (in terms of recruitment and rate coding) driving muscle. Strikingly, the EMG signal drops precipitously (by about 50% in 60 s) and is accompanied by a similar drop in force. In this situation, much of the fatigue appears due to loss of neural drive.

Indeed, motor unit firing rates can decline markedly during sustained MVCs. For example, Figure 4 shows the spiking of a single motor unit recorded in a human muscle during a 60-s MVC (Marsden *et al.* 1983). The top trace depicts spiking during the first 2 s whereas the bottom trace shows spiking over the last 2 s of the contraction. For this motor unit, the firing rate dropped by more than 50% over the trial.

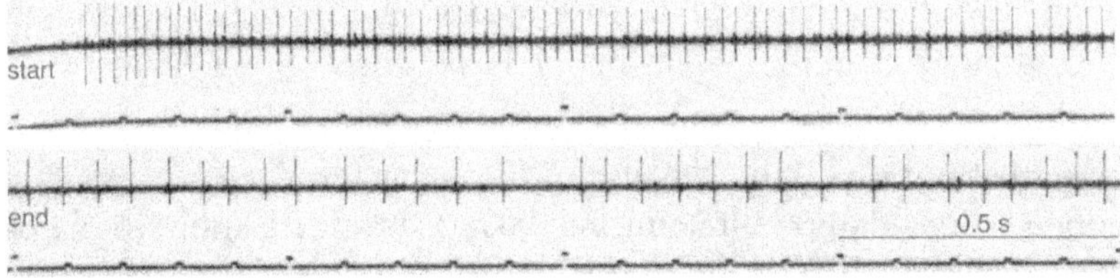

Figure 4.   Spiking activity of a single motor unit in a human hand muscle during the first 2 s (top) and final 2 s (bottom) of a 60-s sustained maximum voluntary contraction. (From Marsden *et al.* [1983].)

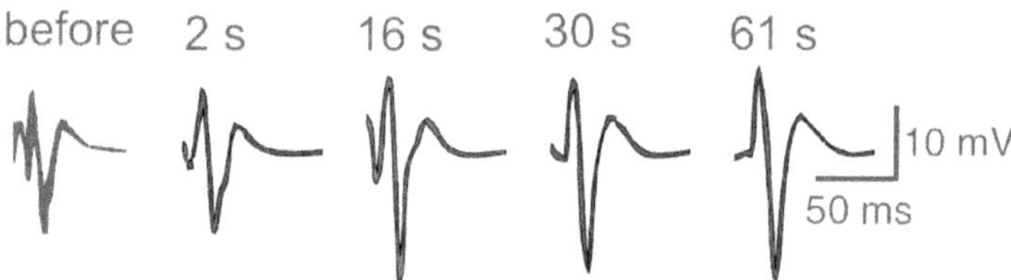

Figure 5.   EMG responses recorded in human biceps brachii to single pulse stimuli delivered to the motor cortex with TMS before and at different times during a sustained maximum voluntary contraction. (Adapted from McNeil *et al.* [2009].)

There are several factors that likely contribute to this fatigue-related decrease in the neural drive to muscle. One possibility is that the output from the higher motor centers that operate on motor neurons declines during fatiguing contractions. Perhaps surprisingly, the evidence to support this idea is not clear. For example, Figure 5 shows a set of brief EMG responses evoked in a contracting muscle of a human subject at different time points during a maximum voluntary contraction (McNeil *et al.* 2009). These responses were produced by delivering *high-intensity magnetic pulses with an electrical coil positioned above the scalp to excite the underlying cortex*, in this case, the motor cortex. This type of stimulation is relatively painless and is referred to as **transcranial magnetic stimulation** (TMS). TMS has been widely used to probe normal cortical function in human subjects and is being used diagnostically and therapeutically in association with several brain disorders (Hallett 2007). The magnitudes of the TMS-evoked muscle responses are thought to reflect the "excitability" of the motor cortex—in other words, how readily can cortical neurons be brought to threshold in response to the same stimulus. As can be seen in Figure 5, over the duration of the sustained MVC, TMS-evoked responses increased rather than decreased, implying progressively enhanced (rather than diminished) cortical excitability during fatigue.

Another possibility for the drop-off in the neural drive during fatiguing contractions could be due to increasing synaptic inhibition directed at motor neurons. One likely source of this inhibition is from nociceptors (pain receptors) that reside in skeletal muscles. Some of these nociceptors appear to be activated by increases in metabolites (like lactic acid) that accompany long-lasting contractions. Indeed, the dull, achy, burning

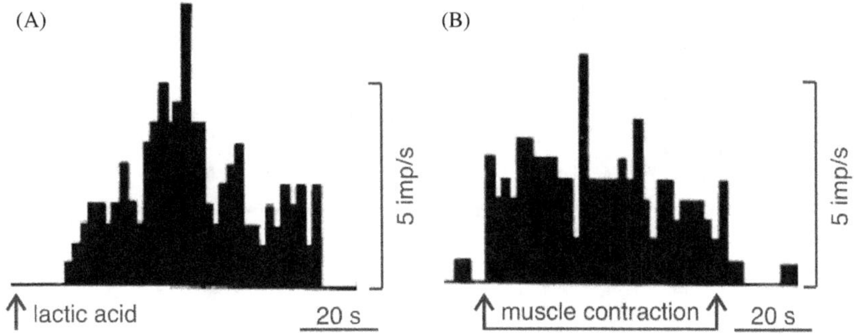

Figure 6.   Spiking activity of a group IV sensory axon arising from the cat triceps surae in response to injection of lactic acid (A) or sustained contraction. (Adapted from Rotto and Kaufman [1988].)

sensations that arise during fatiguing exercise are likely a consequence of the activation of chemosensitive receptors supplied by type IV (thin, unmyelinated) afferents in muscle. Figure 6A shows the firing rate of a type IV muscle afferent in response to injection of lactic acid into a muscle (Rotto & Kaufman 1988). This same afferent was again strongly activated during a sustained muscle contraction lasting about 60 s (Figure 6B).

But what evidence is there that such sensory receptor activity in the muscle leads to the inhibition of motor neurons? Because of technical challenges, there has not yet been direct demonstration that metabolite-sensitive afferents in muscle inhibit motor neurons. However, a clever study by Brenda Bigland-Ritchie and colleagues (1986) provided convincing circumstantial evidence of such inhibition. They measured the firing rates of motor units in human subjects performing MVCs of the quadriceps muscle. To begin, subjects exerted an MVC for 20 s (Figure 7). The average firing rates of motor units were measured over 10-s periods during this task. As shown in the lower part of Figure 7, the average firing rate was about 30 impulses/s for the first 10 s and dropped to about 24 impulses/s in the next 10-s period. To prevent blood flow from "washing away" metabolites that built up during this contraction, the investigators inflated a blood pressure cuff above the contracting muscle during and after the contraction. The subjects then rested for 3 minutes following this short 20-s contraction. After 3 minutes, subjects then performed a 10-s

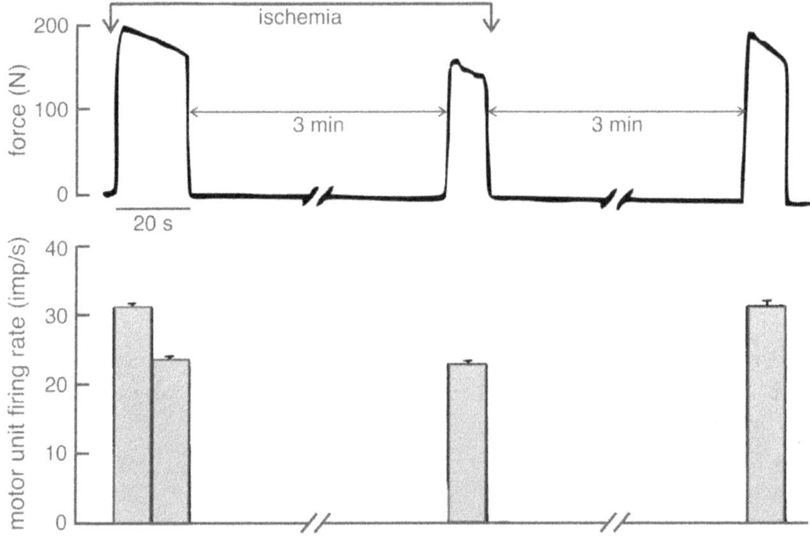

Figure 7.   (Top) Force exerted during a 20-s MVC of the human biceps brachii, and during a 10-s MVC following 3 minutes of rest. During these contractions, blood flow was occluded with a blood pressure cuff. The cuff was then released and after an additional 3 minutes of rest, a second 10-s MVC was performed. (Bottom) Average firing rates over 10-s periods in biceps motor units recorded during the MVCs indicated in the top trace. (Adapted from Bigland-Ritchie *et al.* [1986].)

MVC. At this time point, the firing rates of the motor units and MVC force remained depressed. Only once the cuff was removed and metabolites cleared from the muscle did firing rates and MVC force return to their original levels. These results suggested that motor neurons were likely inhibited by sensory feedback from metabolite-sensitive receptors in the muscle that are activated during sustained contractions.

A third possible source of reduced activity in motor neurons during sustained contractions is the motor neurons themselves. As discussed previously in the context of sensory receptors (see Chapter 8, Figure 4), the firing rates of neurons can progressively diminish in the presence of a constant stimulus—a phenomenon referred to as spike-frequency adaptation. As demonstrated by Daniel Kernell and colleagues in Amsterdam, motor neurons also exhibit spike-frequency adaptation. Figure 8 shows the firing rate of a cat motor neuron over a 4-minute period during which a

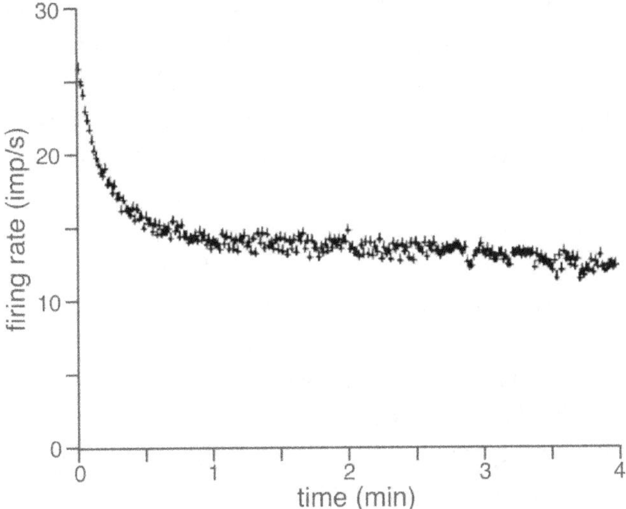

Figure 8.   Spike-frequency adaptation in motor neurons. Firing rate of motor neuron supplying cat gastrocnemius during 4 minutes of constant current injection into the soma. (Adapted from Kernell and Monster [1982].)

constant level of depolarizing current was injected into the neuron (Kernell & Monster 1982). Despite the stable current injection, the firing rate of the motor neuron dropped steeply (~50% in 1 minute), not unlike what occurs during natural voluntary contractions in humans (e.g., Figure 4).

Collectively, therefore, it appears that inhibitory feedback from muscle metaboreceptors (and perhaps from other neurons as well) and spike-frequency adaptation (intrinsic to motor neurons themselves) both contribute to the reduction in the firing rates of motor units (decreasing the forces produced) during fatiguing contractions. The degree to which impaired drive from the cerebral cortex to the motor neurons occurs during fatigue remains an open question.

Nonsynaptic Excitation of Motor Neurons

The conventional view of synaptic integration in motor neurons (and other neurons as well) is that the firing rate output is roughly proportional to the net depolarizing current delivered to the spike-initiating zone by a variety of synaptic inputs. However, investigators in the 1980s observed changes in membrane potential that could not be readily accounted for by external inputs (synaptic or microelectrode-injected). Indeed, they identified a new, nonsynaptic source of excitation in motor neurons (Schwindt & Crill 1980). This source was intrinsic to the neuron itself and involved the activation of voltage-gated channels. These channels were not at the spike-initiating zone but out on the dendrites and soma of the neuron. The depolarizing ionic currents passing through these channels were exceptionally long-lasting. *Such nonsynaptic currents were referred to as persistent (i.e., long-lasting) inward (i.e., depolarizing) currents, or* **PICs**. *PICs, in turn, could lead to a sustained and marked depolarization of the membrane referred* to as a **plateau potential**.

Two conditions typically must be met to activate the channels underlying PICs: (1) the membrane must be substantially depolarized (through the action of external inputs) and (2) the channels must be enabled through an intracellular biochemical cascade (Hounsgaard & Kiehn 1985). This cascade is triggered by the binding of substances referred to as neuromodulators to metabotropic receptors on the neuron membrane. **Neuromodulators** *(such as serotonin and noradrenaline) are neurochemicals that tend to be widely broadcast within the CNS and thereby influence relatively large regions of the brain or spinal cord.* Because they act on metabotropic receptors, neuromodulators also tend to have long-lasting effects. Neuromodulators, therefore, are unlike the pinpoint, selective, and rapid effects of neurotransmitters released at presynaptic terminals and acting at ionotropic (directly gated) receptors.

Figure 9A shows the firing rate response of a motor neuron to a constant level of depolarizing current injected through a microelectrode. In this case, the motor neuron was within a thin slice of the spinal cord that was kept alive in a dish immersed in a control physiological solution. As expected, the neuron spiked continuously during the stimulation and exhibited a moderate degree of spike-frequency adaptation. As soon as the stimulation was halted, the neuron ceased to fire. On the other hand, when the neuromodulator serotonin was added to the solution, a very different response was recorded (Figure 9B). During the stimulation, the firing rate accelerated during the period of constant current injection (+0.5 nA). Most remarkably, when stimulation was halted, the neuron continued

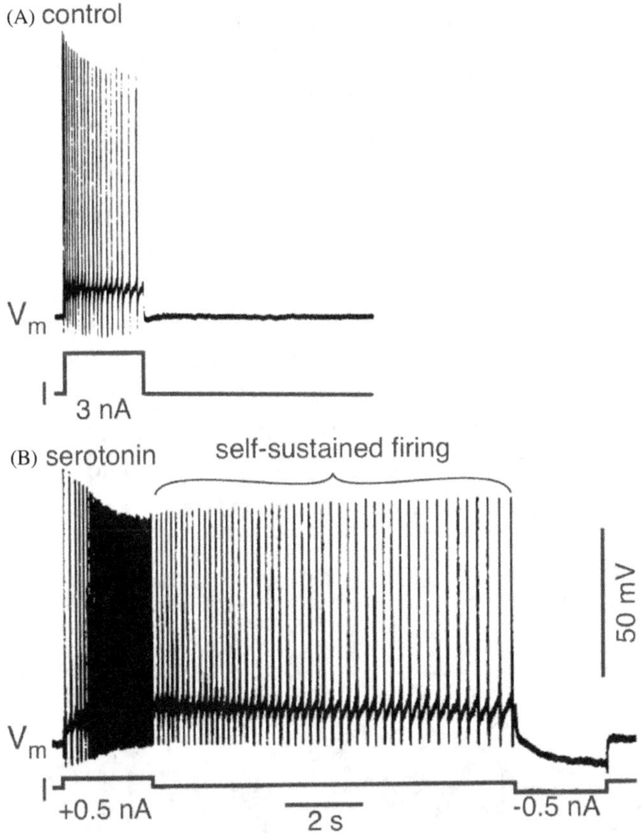

Figure 9.   (A) Firing response of the spinal motor neuron to constant current stimulation in a control solution. (B) Response of the motor neuron when the neuromodulator serotonin was added to the bathing medium. Weak depolarizing current (+0.5 nA) activated the neuron and caused spike-frequency acceleration during the constant pulse. When stimulation was halted, the neuron continued to fire (self-sustained firing) due to activation of PICs. To terminate firing, a hyperpolarizing current pulse (−0.5 nA) injected into the neuron was needed. (Adapted from Hounsgaard and Kiehn [1989].)

to fire. This meant that the neuron, without any external source of input, was generating action potentials on its own. Such activity in the absence of input is sometimes referred to as "self-sustained firing." Indeed, to halt this self-sustained firing, the experimenters needed to inject a hyperpolarizing current (−0.5 nA; Figure 9B).

Subsequent work showed that the channels primarily responsible for PICs in motor neurons are the so-called **L (for long-lasting)-type Ca²⁺ channels**. *These calcium channels have a relatively high voltage threshold for activation and exhibit little inactivation.* L-type Ca²⁺ channels and PICs have now been shown to be involved in a variety of functions throughout the CNS. They are also found in other tissues; for example, they play an important role in excitation–contraction coupling in skeletal, cardiac, and smooth muscles.

Theoretical notions as to how neurons process synaptic inputs to generate spiking outputs are, in some respects, upended by the discovery of PICs. In the conventional view (Figure 10A), the firing rate output of a neuron is roughly proportional to the sum of the depolarizing currents delivered to the spike-initiating zone from active excitatory synapses. On the other hand (Figure 10B), when neuromodulators are present, and the

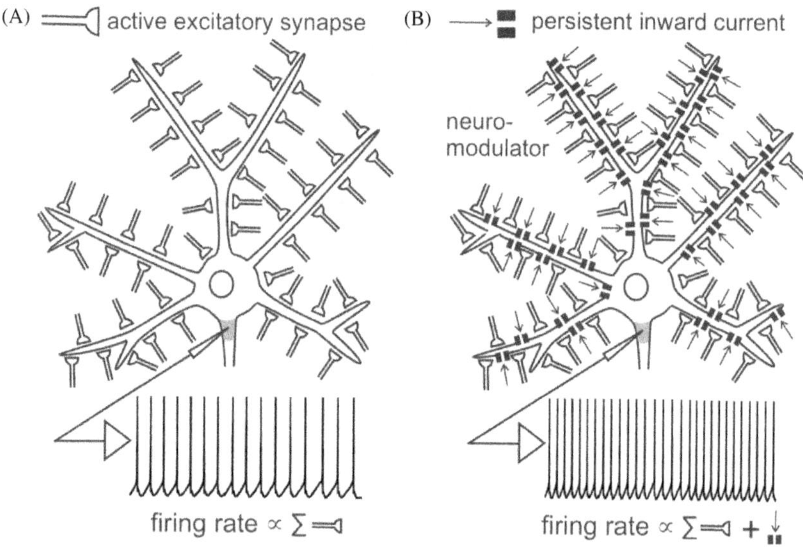

Figure 10.   (A) In the conventional view of synaptic integration, the firing rate output of a neuron is roughly proportional to the sum of the excitatory synaptic inputs. (B) When neuromodulators are available, PICs in the dendrites can be activated. In such cases, the firing rate output of a neuron will be related to the sum of depolarizing currents delivered to the spike initiation zone by excitatory synaptic inputs and that conveyed by channels mediating PICs.

membrane potential is depolarized enough to activate L-type Ca^{2+} channels, the firing rate of a neuron will be theoretically proportional to the sum of the inputs from active synapses *and* the depolarizing inputs arising from PICs (see "equation," bottom Figure 10B). Indeed, one can remove all synaptic input from this equation and still have sufficient PIC input to drive spiking.

The physiological function of PICs in motor neurons remains a matter of debate. On one hand, it has been suggested that the added depolarization provided by PICs is necessary for the normal operation of motor neurons (Binder *et al.* 2020). This reasoning is based on speculation that under typical circumstances, synaptic inputs alone may not be able to drive motor neuron discharge at anything but minimal firing rates. Furthermore, the self-sustained (autonomous) firing mediated by PICs may enable continuous activity in motor neurons during long-lasting contractions (such as in postural muscles) without the need for the continuous bombardment of motor neurons with synaptic input.

On the other hand, it may be that the PICs are engaged only under periods of high arousal. The neuromodulators most associated with enabling PICs are noradrenaline and serotonin. Both these substances are broadly released throughout the nervous system from brainstem nuclei during stressful or arousing events (Foote *et al.* 1980; Takase *et al.* 2004). It could be that the PICs activated under such situations provide an added boost of depolarization leading to augmented firing rates, increased motor unit force, and enhanced muscle strength. Indeed, there are numerous anecdotal accounts of extreme strength under highly stressful conditions; for example, an individual lifting a car to rescue a person pinned underneath following an accident (Wise 2011). The degree to which PICs are involved in day-to-day activities versus only during "emergencies," however, is yet to be determined.

Summary

The maximum force capacity of a muscle can only be achieved when all the motor units making up the muscle are recruited, and each motor unit fires at a rate corresponding to the plateau on its force–frequency curve. Under normal circumstances, however, it appears that most humans are not capable of driving motor units to such high firing rates. Consequently, there could be a substantial reserve of muscle force that typically remains untapped. With strength training, early (and substantial) increases in muscle force appear to be due to neural adaptations that enable motor neurons to be driven to higher rates to capitalize on some of this force reserve. Fatigue of muscle during sustained activity also appears to be partially due to neural factors. Indeed, the firing rates of motor units drop off quite quickly (by ~50% in 60 s) during maximal effort contractions, contributing to the diminution of muscle force. Possible candidates for the loss in neural activity during fatigue include inhibitory feedback from metabolite-sensitive sensory receptors in muscle and spike-frequency adaptation—an intrinsic property of motor neurons themselves. And finally, it appears that motor neurons (and other neurons) possess the ability for self-excitation through the activation of PICs. Such activation requires both the presence of neuromodulators and initial depolarization by synaptic inputs. Once activated, PICs provide an additional long-lasting source of depolarization that can sustain motor neuron activity even when synaptic input is removed. The added boost of depolarization associated with PICs during stressful situations might also serve to augment firing rates to provide a temporary enhancement of muscle strength.

References

Bellemare F, Woods JJ, Johansson R & Bigland-Ritchie B (1983). Motor-unit discharge rates in maximal voluntary contractions of three human muscles. *Journal of Neurophysiology* **50**, 1380–1392.

Bigland-Ritchie BR, Dawson NJ, Johansson RS & Lippold OC (1986). Reflex origin for the slowing of motoneurone firing rates in fatigue of human voluntary contractions. *Journal of Physiology* **379**, 451–459.

Binder MD, Powers RK & Heckman CJ (2020). Nonlinear input-output functions of motoneurons. *Physiology* **35**, 31–39.

Del Vecchio A, Casolo A, Negro F, Scorcelletti M, Bazzucchi I, Enoka R, Felici F & Farina D (2019). The increase in muscle force after 4 weeks of strength training is mediated by adaptations in motor unit recruitment and rate coding. *Journal of Physiology* **597**, 1873–1887.

Enoka RM (1988). Muscle strength and its development. *Sports Medicine* **6**, 146–168.

Foote SL, Aston-Jones G & Bloom FE (1980). Impulse activity of locus coeruleus neurons in awake rats and monkeys is a function of sensory stimulation and arousal. *Proceedings of the National Academy of Sciences* **77**, 3033–3037.

Fuglevand AJ (2019). The brain can make you stronger. *Journal of Physiology* **597**, 1779–1780.

Fuglevand AJ, Lester RA & Johns RK (2015). Distinguishing intrinsic from extrinsic factors underlying firing rate saturation in human motor units. *Journal of Neurophysiology* **113**, 1310–1322.

Fuglevand AJ, Macefield VG & Bigland-Ritchie B (1999). Force-frequency and fatigue properties of motor units in muscles that control digits of the human hand. *Journal of Neurophysiology* **81**, 1718–1729.

Hallett M (2007). Transcranial magnetic stimulation: A primer. *Neuron* **55**, 187–199.

Hounsgaard J & Kiehn O (1985). Ca^{2+}-dependent bistability by serotonin in spinal motoneurones. *Experimental Brain Research* **57**, 422–425.

Hounsgaard J & Kiehn O (1989). Serotonin-induced bistability of turtle motoneurones caused by a nifedipine-sensitive calcium plateau potential. *Journal of Physiology* **414**, 265–282.

Kent-Braun JA, Fitts RH & Christie A (2012). Skeletal muscle fatigue. *Comprehensive Physiology* **2**, 997–1044.

Kernell D & Monster AW (1982). Time course and properties of late adaptation in spinal motoneurones of the cat. *Experimental Brain Research* **46**, 191–196.

McNeil CJ, Martin PG, Gandevia SC & Taylor JL (2009). The response to paired motor cortical stimuli is abolished at a spinal level during human muscle fatigue. *Journal of Physiology* **587**, 5601–5612.

Mosso A (1904). Fatigue. GP Putnam's Sons.

Rotto DM & Kaufman MP (1988). Effect of metabolic products of muscular contraction on discharge of group III and IV afferents. *Journal of Applied Physiology* **64**, 2306–2313.

Sale DG (1988). Neural adaptation to resistance training. *Medicine and Science in Sports and Exercise* **20**, S135–S145.

Schwindt PC & Crill WE (1980). Properties of a persistent inward current in normal and TEA-injected motoneurons. *Journal of Neurophysiology* **43**, 1700–1724.

Takase LF, Nogueira MI, Baratta M, Bland ST, Watkins LR, Maier SF, Fornal CA & Jacobs BL (2004). Inescapable shock activates serotonergic neurons in all raphe nuclei of rat. *Behavioural Brain Research* **153**, 233–239.

Wise J (2011). *Extreme Fear: The Science of Your Mind in Danger*. St. Martin's Griffin, New York.

Yue G & Cole KJ (1992). Strength increases from the motor program: comparison of training with maximal voluntary and imagined muscle contractions. *Journal of Neurophysiology* **67**, 1114–1123.

Chapter 16

Reflexes

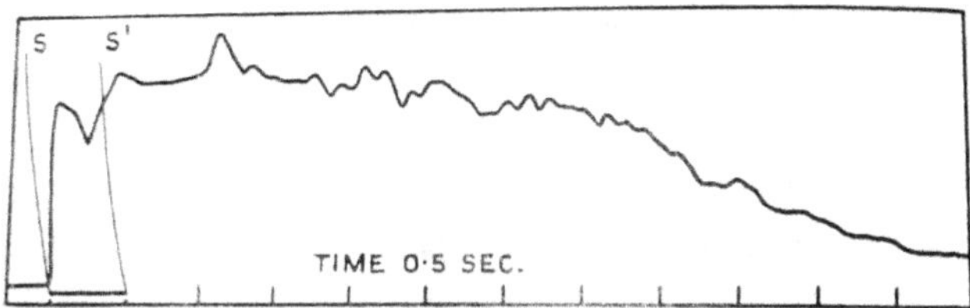

Flexion reflex in the hindlimb muscles of a spinalized dog. Electrical stimulation was applied to the skin of the hind paw for a period of 0.5 s. Flexion contraction force began soon after onset of stimulation (at S) and was maintained for several seconds after stimulation ceased (at S'). (Sherrington 1906.)

In Chapters 14 and 15, mechanisms that underlie the activation of motor neurons and the production of muscle force were outlined. The following chapters describe how various spinal cord and brain structures engage motor neurons across multiple motor nuclei to produce a variety of movements. This topic is discussed in the context of three broad categories of movements: reflexes, rhythmical motor behaviors, and voluntary actions (Table 1).

Reflexes (the main topic of this chapter) are considered the simplest forms of motor behavior. They consist of relatively automatic, fast, stereotyped responses to external stimuli. The neural circuitry that produces most reflexes resides in the "low levels" of the central nervous system (CNS), namely, in the spinal cord or the brain stem. A few examples of the many types of reflexes include sneezing, pupil constriction, and tendon tap (stretch) responses. As highlighted by these examples, it is not readily possible to "will" a reflex to occur. For example, one typically

Table 1.   Three main categories of movement.

Movement Type	Characteristics
Reflexes	- Simplest forms of movement - Stereotyped, "automatic," and fast response - Controlled by "low-level" circuitry in the spinal cord or brain stem - Triggered by specific external stimuli - Can't be willed into action - Can be modulated
Rhythmical behaviors	- Repetitive, cyclical movements (e.g., walking, chewing, breathing) - Involves low-level circuitry called "central pattern generators" - Activated and modulated by higher CNS centers
Voluntary movements	- Most complex movements - Willed, consciously activated movements - Involves the highest level of the CNS - Can involve learning, improvement with practice

cannot produce a sneeze upon command. And while reflexes may seem to be an all-or-nothing phenomenon, in many cases, reflexes can be modulated (made weaker or stronger) or suppressed altogether by input from other parts of the CNS.

At the other extreme, are **voluntary movements** (Table 1). These are movements that are consciously willed into action. A wide range of behaviors can be categorized as voluntary, such as reaching for a cup, playing a musical instrument, typing, hitting a tennis ball, buttoning a shirt, and speaking. Voluntary movements can be quite complex and can improve with practice. Indeed, the cerebral cortex (the highest level of the CNS) is needed to produce voluntary movements.

In terms of complexity and type of control, **rhythmical motor behaviors** are situated between reflexes and voluntary movements (Table 1). Virtually all animal species exhibit rhythmical movements of one type or other, including most forms of locomotion (crawling, walking, running, swimming, flying), chewing, scratching, and breathing. Such behaviors are like reflexes in that the main circuits producing them (called central pattern generators) are found within the low levels of the CNS. On the other hand, instigation and modulation of rhythmical behaviors oftentimes derives from commands issued from higher levels (e.g., cerebral cortex in mammals).

It should also be noted that there are some types of motor behaviors that do not fit neatly into one of these three categories. For example, there are many so-called **innate** behaviors that tend to be *specific to individual species*. Examples of these *include courtship displays, social vocalizations, defensive or escape responses, maternal and mating behaviors, and emotional facial expressions*. Many of these innate behaviors in vertebrates appear to be controlled by distinct regions within the periaqueductal gray matter of the brainstem (discussed briefly in Chapter 11, Figure 3; Silva & McNaughton 2019). In addition, maintenance of posture and balance has both reflexive and voluntary aspects to it, and therefore, does not accord readily with either category. Nevertheless, the three main categories of movement (Table 1) do encompass a wide span of motor behaviors that are the main focus of the following chapters.

It is important to recognize that virtually all movements, from the simplest reflex to the most complex voluntary movement, involve the coordination of multiple muscles. Furthermore, such coordination not only involves the excitation of some muscles but inhibition of others. For example, during running, it is crucial that the leg extensor muscles, used to propel the body forward by thrusting against the ground, be briskly silenced as the toes leave the ground so as to not counteract the leg flexor muscles that lift the leg during the early part of the swing phase of the gait cycle. Linking together the contractions and relaxations of several muscles to produce a particular movement is the essence of motor coordination.

Involvement of Somatosensory Receptors in Reflexes

Many of the somatosensory receptors (muscle spindles, Golgi tendon organs, tactile receptors, nociceptors, etc.) discussed in Chapter 9 are involved in triggering different types of reflexes. Before describing the circuitry associated with some example reflexes, it is useful to briefly recall the destinations of somatosensory receptor axons. As shown in Figure 1, tactile and proprioceptive afferents enter the spinal cord through the dorsal roots, whereupon they ascend all the way to the dorsal column nuclei in the brain stem. Second-order neurons in the dorsal column nuclei then project to the thalamus, and the recipient thalamic neurons send tactile and proprioceptive information to the primary somatosensory cortex. In addition, upon entering the spinal cord, sensory afferents give off

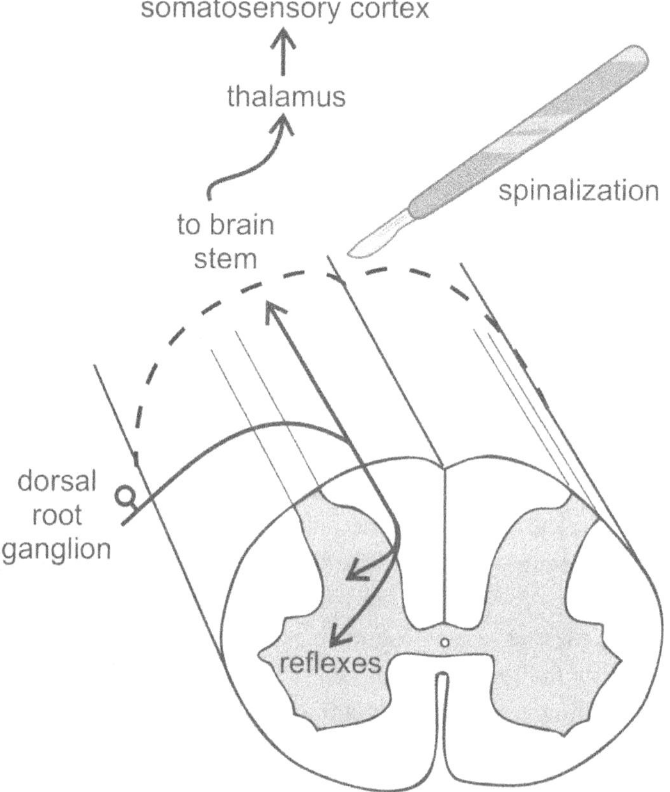

Figure 1.   Destination of somatosensory afferents. Somatosensory afferents (such as those from tactile and proprioceptive receptors) enter the spinal cord through the dorsal roots and ascend in the dorsal column to the brainstem. Secord-order neurons in the brainstem convey somatosensory information to the thalamus, and third-order neurons in the thalamus project to the somatosensory cortex. In addition, upon entry into the spinal cord (or brainstem) axon collaterals project into the gray matter of the spinal cord. These projections are the source of many reflexes. The study of reflexes often employed spinalized or decerebrate animal preparations.

collaterals that project into the gray matter of the spinal cord. It is the activity on these spinal collaterals of sensory afferents that can instigate reflexes.

Charles Sherrington studied reflexes as a tractable type of behavior from which general principles about neural circuits could be revealed. One significant challenge to such studies is that anesthetics must be given to the experimental animal to prevent pain associated with surgical access to the parts of the nervous system under investigation. Anesthetics, however, largely depress the excitability of the nervous system. Therefore, the very behaviors one might wish to study are suppressed by anesthetics. Sherrington and others developed experimental preparations that partially mitigated that problem. One such approach is referred to as a **decerebrate preparation**, *in which the cerebrum is first removed under anesthesia, leaving only the brainstem intact.* Because the animal no longer possesses a cerebral cortex, all conscious awareness is extinguished. Therefore, the animal cannot "feel" pain and anesthesia can be discontinued. Furthermore, the vital functions carried out by the brainstem remain intact, thereby keeping the animal alive.

A similar approach is referred to as **spinalization** (Figure 1) *in which the spinal cord is transected and experiments are carried out in parts of the nervous system below the lesion.* As Sherrington noted, both types of preparations lead to robust, stable, and maybe even exaggerated responses (see frontispiece for this chapter). This is partly due to the elimination of the descending influences that normally moderate reflexes. It was under spinal and decerebrate experimental conditions that Sherrington worked out the circuitry underlying several reflexes. Some of these are described in the following sections.

Stretch Reflex

Probably the most widely investigated reflex is the **stretch reflex** (also called the myotatic reflex or tendon tap reflex). The stimulus that triggers the reflex is an external perturbation that causes a muscle to be abruptly lengthened. For example, as shown in Figure 2, an unexpected knock to the forearm will cause the elbow to extend and thereby will lengthen the biceps muscle (agonist). Such lengthening potently activates Ia afferents emerging from muscle spindles in the agonist muscle. That activity, in addition to ascending in the dorsal column (not shown in Figure 2), is directed to and excites motor neurons in the spinal cord. The motor neurons that receive that excitation are primarily those that innervate the same muscle from which the Ia afferents originate. The consequent activation of those motor neurons will cause the stretched muscle to contract,

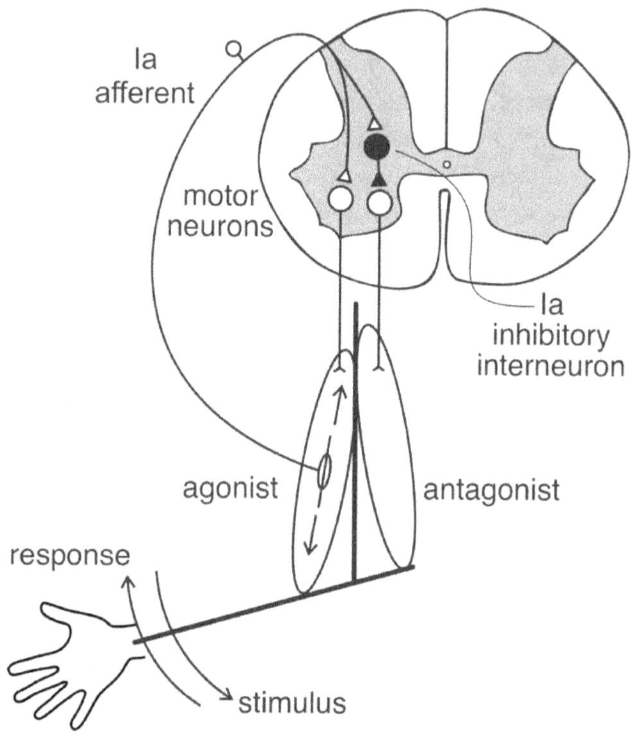

Figure 2.   Stretch reflex. Abrupt displacement of a joint (stimulus) causes lengthening of the agonist muscle. Such lengthening leads to activity on muscle spindle Ia afferents that make excitatory synaptic connections onto motor neurons supplying the stretched muscle. This leads to a reflex contraction to restore the limb (response) to its original configuration. Branches of the Ia afferents also excite inhibitory interneurons to suppress activity in the antagonistic muscles.

restoring the limb to its original configuration before the perturbation. Furthermore, activity on the Ia afferents also excites inhibitory interneurons (Figure 2) that, in turn, suppresses ongoing activity in antagonist (triceps) muscles, which otherwise would impede the restoring actions of the agonist. Such *reflex suppression of antagonistic muscles when agonist muscles are induced to contract* is sometimes referred to as **reciprocal inhibition**. Thus, even the simplest of motor behavior involves coordination across more than one muscle (excitation of agonist and inhibition of antagonist).

Beyond its role to rapidly respond to external perturbations that displace parts of the body, the stretch reflex is thought to play other important roles. For example, maintaining an upright human body represents a substantial control problem for the nervous system given the precarious nature of bipedal standing. The external force of gravity acts to pull the body downward. The stretch reflex, however, continuously operates across multiple muscles in the legs, trunk, and neck to prevent such falling. As shown in Figure 3, a small sway forward of the body from its stable position will lead to lengthening of the muscles in the back of the leg. Such lengthening triggers a stretch reflex to cause the stretched muscles to contract and pull the body back into a more stable configuration. Likewise, a backward sway will cause muscles in the front of the leg to lengthen, triggering a stretch reflex in them to pull the body forward toward a more stable configuration. This kind of activity operates

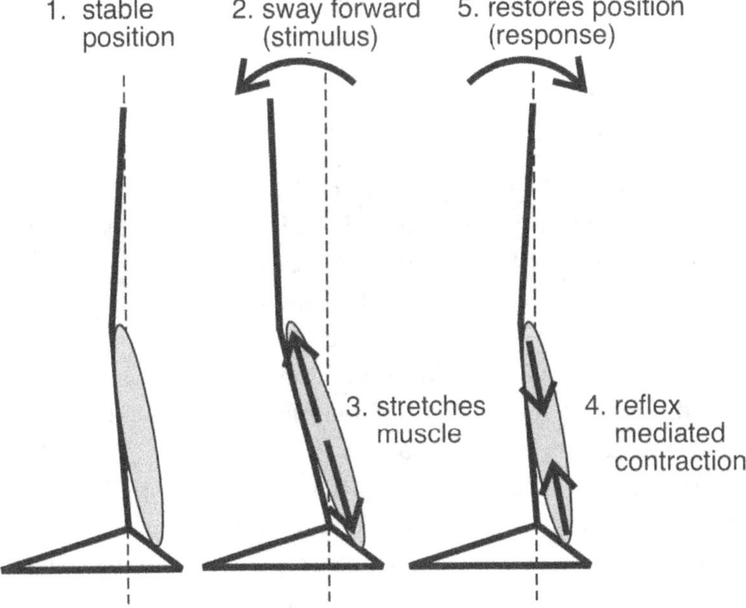

Figure 3.   Stretch reflex to help maintain upright posture. Sway forward (2) from a stable position (1) will cause lengthening of the muscles (3) in the back of the leg. This lengthening triggers a stretch reflex contraction (4) of those muscles to pull the body back into a stable position (5).

continually in the background involving only the lowest levels of the CNS, but serving an important and complex function.

It is also the stretch reflex that is frequently evaluated by physicians during clinical evaluations using a little hammer. The physician strikes a tendon with the hammer causing a rapid (albeit small) muscle stretch. Because Ia afferents are highly sensitive to the *rate* of the muscle stretch (see Chapter 9, Figure 15), the tendon tap elicits an intense, brief barrage of activity on Ia afferents, triggering a stretch reflex. The physician observes the response, oftentimes by palpating the target muscle. But what is the diagnostic value of such a maneuver? The tendon tap is a simple and efficient way to ascertain the likelihood of an array of neurological disorders. If the response is weak or absent, this can indicate a dysfunction in the peripheral nerves (referred to as neuropathies) that may occur with, for example, diabetes, kidney dysfunction, vitamin deficiencies, or alcoholism. If the response is exaggerated, this may indicate damage to brain centers or corticospinal pathways that normally act to modulate reflexes.

Flexor Reflex

Another important reflex that we all experience is the **flexor reflex**. This behavior is triggered by activity on Aδ afferents from nociceptors. Aδ axons are the faster of the two types of nociceptor axons and are thought to underlie first pain (see Chapter 9). As shown in Figure 4, activity on these receptors is instigated by an acute, painful stimulus, like stepping on a tack. The Aδ activity is communicated to an array of neurons in the dorsal horn of the spinal cord. One set of dorsal horn neurons gives rise to the spinothalamic pathway (not shown in Figure 4) that ultimately underlies the conscious perception of pain.

Another set activates a series of excitatory interneurons that culminate with the excitation of motor neurons on the same side of the spinal cord and that supply the flexor muscles over the entire limb (Figure 4). Coactivity of the limb flexor muscles generally pulls a limb inward toward the body. Thus, this reflex will quickly withdraw the limb away from the offending stimulus. As with the stretch reflex, another branch of Aδ axons will activate a different set of interneurons, leading to the reciprocal

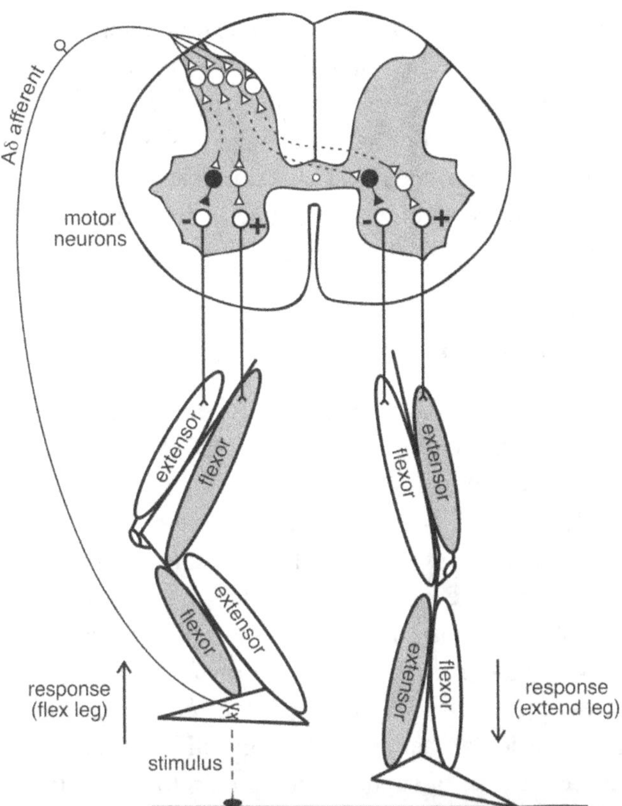

Figure 4.   Flexor (left side of figure) and crossed extensor reflexes (right side). An abrupt painful stimulus (e.g., stepping on a tack) activates the Aδ nociceptive afferents in the skin of the foot. That activity, upon entry into the spinal cord, excites arrays of interneurons in the dorsal horn. One set culminates in excitation (+) of the motor neurons, provoking contraction (dark shading) in the flexor muscles across the entire limb. This causes the limb to quickly retract away from the noxious stimulus. Another set of interneurons simultaneously leads to inhibition (−) of the extensor muscles on the same side of the body to prevent them from impeding the action of the flexor muscles. In addition, activation of further sets of interneurons project to the opposite side of the spinal cord to induce contraction in extensor muscles (shaded muscles) and suppression of activity in flexor muscles. This causes that limb to push outward, providing a stable base of support and helping to push the body away from the painful stimulus.

inhibition of the motor neurons supplying extensor muscles on the same side of the spinal cord. This inhibition serves to reduce activity in the antagonistic (in this case, extensor) muscles that otherwise would impede the desired withdrawal action of flexor muscles. Collectively, this low-level neural circuitry mediates a quick, coordinated response to a painful stimulus, such as immediately withdrawing the hand upon touching a hot burner on a stove.

Crossed Extensor Reflex

In some situations, the flexor reflex is coupled to another reflex, referred to as the **crossed-extensor reflex**. Nociceptive Aδ activity on one side of the body triggers responses in the opposite limb. Thus, the same signals triggering a flexor reflex engage the crossed-extensor reflex through sets of interneurons that "cross over" to the opposite side of the spinal cord (Figure 4). As the name of the reflex implies, one set of interneurons excites the motor neurons supplying the extensor muscles in the unaffected limb, while another set inhibits the motor neurons innervating the flexor muscles. This leads to rapid limb extension (pushing the limb away from the body). Such an action in the leg will push the leg downward, providing a secure base of support and helping to propel the body away from the noxious stimulus.

Other Reflexes

The neural bases of the stretch, flexor, and crossed-extensor reflexes are just some of the reflexes that Sherrington brought to light in the early part of the 20th century. It is important to recognize, however, that some reflexes identified and studied in decerebrate or spinalized preparations would seem to serve little function in intact animals. For example, the so-called "**inverse myotatic reflex**" *resembles that of a stretch (myotatic) reflex except that excitation and inhibition of target motor neurons are inverted.* In this case, the triggering stimulus is muscle force leading to the excitation of Ib afferents arising from the Golgi tendon organs. Through sets of interneurons in the spinal cord, the Ib input is transformed into inhibition of the contracting muscle (the agonist) and excitation of the antagonist muscle. As such, this reflex (sometimes called the "clasped-knife" reflex) would seem largely counterproductive by shutting down a muscle that is contracting and exciting its antagonist. Probably, this reflex has little practical use and is only "revealed" when normal descending influences have been artificially removed (Rymer *et al.* 1979). Indeed, this reflex may only become evident in humans after an injury to the corticospinal pathways.

Similarly, the **Babinski reflex** can be *elicited in healthy infants by stroking the skin on the sole of the foot. This causes a reflex hyperextension of the large toe and splaying of the other toes.* With development of the CNS, however, this reflex disappears. It emerges in adults only when there is damage to the corticospinal pathways that normally prevent this reflex. As such, like the tendon tap reflex, the Babinski reflex is often tested in neurological patients to evaluate the integrity of the corticospinal system. It should be said that Sherrington was somewhat circumspect about attributing functional significance to many reflexes. In his 1906 monograph, he stated that a simple reflex *"is probably a purely abstract conception because all parts of the nervous system are connected together and no part of it is probably ever capable of reaction without affecting or being affected by various other parts."*

Primary Role of Somatosensory Receptors

Sherrington was awarded the Nobel Prize in Physiology (1932), largely for his work on reflexes—in particular, for his demonstrations of the active (and substantial) role that inhibition plays in the CNS. Sherrington's incisive thinking, clarity of experiments, and broad ideas had a profound influence on motor control scientists throughout the 20th century and beyond. With the development of extracellular and intracellular microelectrodes, a large body of meticulous work was initiated (and continues today) to identify the actual neural elements involved in the production of reflexes. As done by Sherrington, much of this work was carried out in "reduced" (e.g., decerebrate, spinalized, or "in vitro"—involving the removal of part of the nervous system and keeping the tissue alive in a dish) experimental preparations.

This intense focus on reflexes in the second half of the 20th century may have led to a nearsighted view of the role of somatosensory receptors. For example, some current textbooks imply that the main function of the muscle spindle is to mediate the stretch reflex. Yet, the most prominent function of many somatosensory receptors, such as proprioceptors and tactile receptors, may be in enabling and shaping *voluntary* movements. This idea was vividly demonstrated by Sherrington in the late 19th century. Sherrington, with his student Fredrick Mott, cut the dorsal roots on one side of the spinal cord in monkeys. Following recovery from the surgery, Sherrington and Mott carefully observed the types of deficits incurred by the removal of somatosensory input to the CNS. The outcome was dramatic: *"From the time of the performance of the [dorsal root] section onwards, the movements of the hand and foot are abolished; the movements of grasping, which is so useful to the monkey, never occurs at all in our experience"* (Mott & Sherrington 1895). If the limb with intact sensation was restrained, monkeys still would not use the deafferented limb to reach for food despite the animal being hungry following a period of food deprivation. Even if a piece of fruit was placed in the hand, the monkeys would not lift the hand to the mouth. Such considerable and persistent loss of voluntary function of the limb occurred even though the descending motor pathways remained fully intact. Indeed, Mott and Sherrington demonstrated that electrical stimulation of the motor cortex evoked movements as readily in the deafferented limbs as in intact limbs.

These striking findings highlight the essential role that somatosensory signals play in voluntary motor behaviors. As will be discussed in a later chapter, prominent sources of input to the motor cortex are from somatosensory cortex and somatosensory thalamus. The motor cortex, therefore, depends on somatosensory signals to formulate and shape the commands that underlie voluntary movements. While visual input to the motor cortex is also important, complex voluntary movements can be performed in the absence of vision (e.g., highly skilled musicians often perform with their eyes closed). One the other hand, as demonstrated by the experiments of Mott and Sherrington (and by the rare cases of humans who lose somatosensory input due to disease, as described in Chapter 9), even simple movements cannot be produced in the absence of somatosensation. The importance of somatosensory afferents, therefore, is greatly undervalued by solely emphasizing their role in reflexes or in feedback corrections.

Reflex Interference with Voluntary or Rhythmical Movements

Every movement, regardless of type, causes profound activation of somatosensory afferents. Under canonical representations of reflex circuitry (like Figures 2 and 4), such activity on various sensory afferents should obligatorily trigger reflexes. But that does not happen. For example, consider what occurs when rapidly extending the elbow to reach out to grab a low-flying fast ball. Descending commands are conveyed to the triceps motor neurons (arrow 1, Figure 5A) to cause the triceps muscle to contract (arrow 2, Figure 5B), thereby extending the elbow and driving the hand

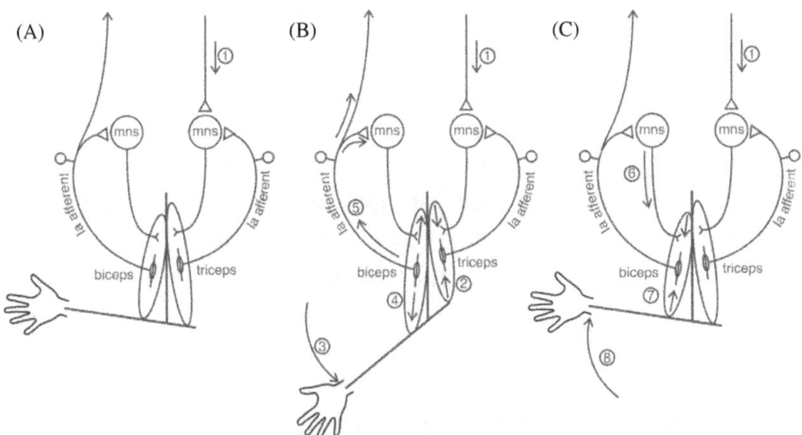

Figure 5.   Interference of reflexes in the elaboration of voluntary movement. (A) Descending command (arrow 1) to activate the motor neurons (mns) supplying the elbow extensor muscles such as the triceps. (B) Contraction of the triceps (arrow 2) causes the elbow to extend (arrow 3) and lengthening of the biceps (arrow 4) on the opposite side of the joint. Lengthening of the biceps will instigate activity on the biceps muscle spindle Ia afferents (arrow 5). Such activity will be conveyed along the ascending pathways to the brain and to the biceps motor neurons in the spinal cord. (C) Ia activity will excite the motor neurons supplying the biceps muscle (arrow 6), causing it to contract (arrow 7), leading to elbow flexion and countermanding the desired action of elbow extension.

downward (arrow 3, Figure 5B). The extension of the elbow will cause the biceps muscle to be lengthened (arrow 4, Figure 5B), provoking a barrage of activity to be set up on the Ia afferents emerging from the biceps muscle spindles (arrow 5, Figure 5B). Such activity is delivered along the ascending pathways to the brain and to the motor neurons supplying the biceps muscle (Figure 5B). If nothing else were to happen, excitation of the biceps motor neurons (arrow 6, Figure 5C), within tens of milliseconds of the onset of the stretch, would cause the biceps to contract (arrow 7, Figure 5C) and flex the elbow (arrow 8, Figure 5C), preventing the elbow extension needed to catch the ball.

Convergence onto Common Interneurons

Fortunately, mechanisms are available to override reflexes that otherwise would interfere with voluntary or rhythmical behaviors (McComas 2016). One mechanism entails **convergence onto common interneurons**, namely that *interneurons identified in conventional representations of reflexes are not the "private property" of a reflex pathway. Instead, such interneurons receive converging synaptic input from many sources. Thus, a reflex will be instigated only if the collective synaptic input is sufficient to activate the interneurons.* This concept was thoroughly brought to light through the work of Anders Lundberg and Elzbieta Jankowska of Sweden.

A typical type of experiment they carried out involved recording changes in the membrane potential of motor neurons in response to stimulation of peripheral afferents (site 1, Figure 6A), descending pathways (site 2, Figure 6A), and near-simultaneous stimulation of both. As shown in the schematic in Figure 6B, when stimulating either site 1 or site 2, no membrane potential response was recorded in the motor neuron. However, when both sites were activated near the same time, a robust depolarization occurred. Based on this type of observation, the investigators inferred that the sensory afferent and descending pathways converged upon a set of common excitatory interneurons (Figure 6C). (*Note*: The word "common" in this context refers to a "shared" neuron, not an "ordinary" one.) Activation of either pathway by itself was insufficient to excite the interneurons. However, when the excitatory inputs from these two

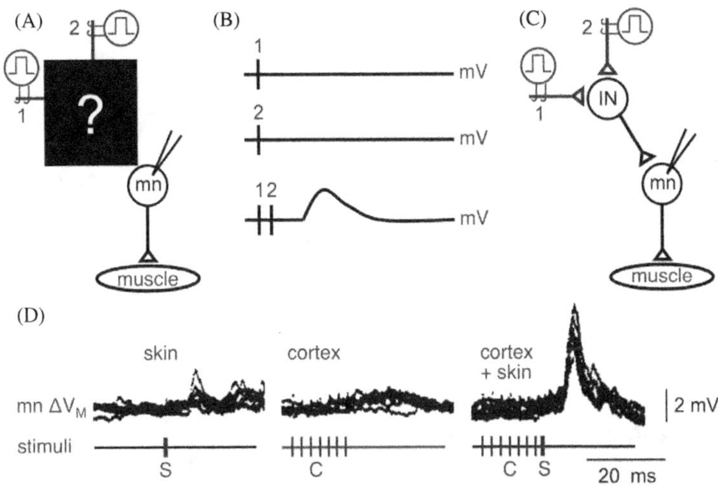

Figure 6. Convergence onto common excitatory interneurons. (A) Membrane potential responses are recorded in a motor neuron (mn) to stimulation of peripheral afferents (site 1) and/or stimulation of a descending pathway (site 2). (B) Schematic indicates that neither stimulation of site 1 nor site 2 by themselves yield a response in the motor neuron. However, when activated together, depolarization of the motor neuron occurs. Vertical tick marks indicate the time when the stimulus was delivered. (C) Convergence of excitation from the two pathways onto common excitatory interneurons (IN) could account for the type of responses depicted in (B). (D) Actual recordings of membrane potential changes in a motor neuron supplying a hindlimb flexor muscle in the cat to stimulation of the sural nerve, supplying the skin (S) of the hind paw (left), or of the motor cortex (C; middle). When the two pathways were activated at about the same time, robust depolarization of the motor neuron occurred (from Lundberg *et al.* [1962]).

pathways coincided, it was sufficient to bring the interneurons to the threshold and to deliver synaptic excitation to the motor neurons.

Figure 6D shows the type of actual recordings made in these types of experiments (from Lundberg *et al.* 1962). The left side shows four or five overlaid traces of membrane potential recorded in a motor neuron when a nerve supplying the skin (S) of the cat paw was stimulated. Similarly, the middle traces show the membrane potential recordings when the cortex (C) was stimulated with a train of seven pulses. Neither of these stimulations led to a consistent change in membrane potential. However, when the two pathways were coactivated (cortex slightly earlier because of the

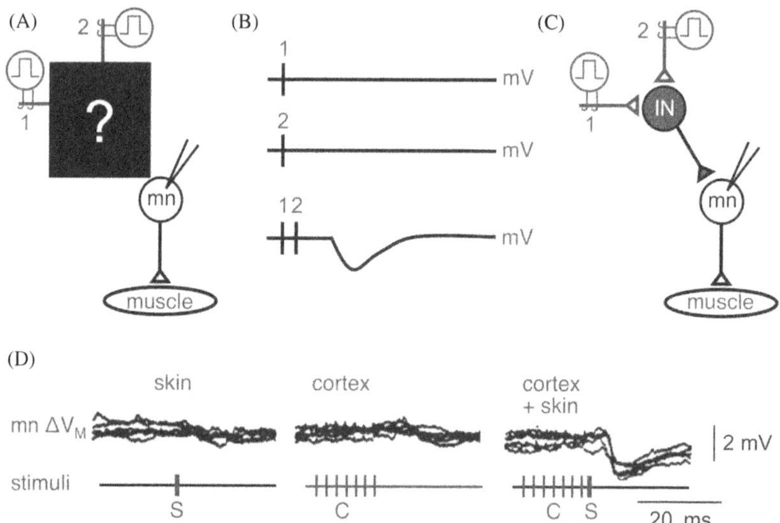

Figure 7.   Convergence onto common inhibitory interneurons. (A) Membrane potential responses are recorded in a motor neuron (mn) to the stimulation of peripheral afferents (site 1) and/or stimulation of a descending pathway (site 2). (B) Schematic indicates that neither stimulation of site 1 nor site 2 by themselves yield a response in the motor neuron. However, when activated together, hyperpolarization of the motor neuron occurs. (C) Convergence of excitation from the two pathways onto common inhibitory interneurons (IN) could account for the type of responses depicted in (B). (D) Actual recordings of membrane potential changes in a motor neuron supplying a hindlimb extensor muscle in the cat to stimulation of the sural nerve, supplying the skin (S) of the hind paw (left), or of the motor cortex (C; middle). When the two pathways were activated at about the same time, robust hyperpolarization of the motor neuron occurred (from Lundberg *et al.* [1962]).

longer distance from cortex to lumbar spinal cord), reliable depolarization of the motor neuron occurred.

Likewise, Lundberg *et al.* (1962) recorded from motor neurons supplying a different muscle to stimulation of the same sensory nerve or cortex (Figure 7A). When stimulated on their own, no responses were evoked (Figure 7B). However, when the two pathways were activated at nearly the same time, hyperpolarization was recorded in the motor neuron (Figures 7B, D). This result implied that, in this case, the two pathways acted upon a set of common inhibitory interneurons (Figure 7C), and that the convergence of those inputs activated interneurons to hyperpolarize the motor neurons.

Based on these types of experiments, Jankowska & Lundberg (1981) discovered that virtually all spinal interneurons studied received converging inputs from wide arrays of sensory and descending inputs. For example, classically defined Ia inhibitory interneurons receive excitatory inputs not only from Ia afferents of muscle spindles (as emphasized in classical representations, e.g., Figure 2) but also from sensory afferents arising in the skin and joints (Figure 8A). Furthermore, these interneurons also receive inhibitory input from Ia inhibitory interneurons of the antagonistic muscle. In addition, several descending pathways project to Ia inhibitory interneurons.

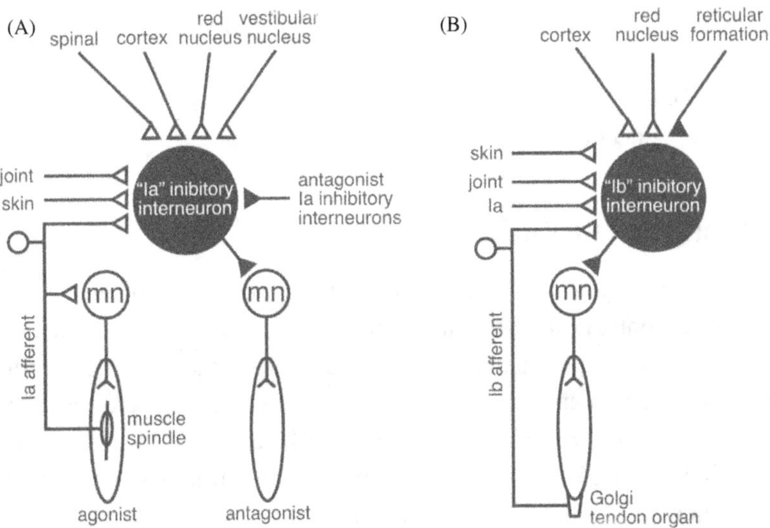

Figure 8.   Converging inputs to the interneurons of reflex pathways. (A) Ia inhibitory interneurons of the stretch reflex not only receive excitation from muscle spindle Ia afferents but also from sensory afferents arising in the skin and joints. The Ia inhibitory interneurons also receive inhibitory input from Ia inhibitory interneurons of the antagonist muscle. In addition, Ia inhibitory interneurons are also sites of convergence from descending projections originating in the rostral regions of the spinal cord (spinal also called propriospinal), cortex, and brainstem centers including the red and vestibular nuclei. (B) The Ib inhibitory interneurons of the inverse myotatic reflex receive input from the Golgi tendon organ Ib afferents, Ia afferents from muscle spindles, and sensory afferents from skin and joints. They also receive descending inputs from the cortex, red nucleus, and reticular formation. ([A] adapted from Baldissera *et al.* [1981]; [B] adapted from Jankowska and Lundberg [1981].)

In a similar vein, Ib inhibitory interneurons (Figure 8B) are a nexus of inputs from an array of sensory afferents (muscle spindle Ia, skin, and joint), and descending pathways. In some respects, the labels "Ia" or "Ib" inhibitory interneurons are misnomers as those interneurons could have equivalently been designated "red nucleus" or "joint afferent" inhibitory interneurons. The original labels have been maintained as handy designators of specific interneurons. Functionally, it is important to recognize that activation of interneurons that give rise to reflexes likely depends on cooperation across sets of inputs. Thus, activity on one type of sensory afferent alone may be insufficient to trigger a reflex. Furthermore, inhibition directed at the reflex pathway interneurons can effectively veto a reflex from occurring. In addition, excitatory inputs from other than the "named" source can likely activate the designated interneuron. For example, descending inputs (e.g., cortex, red nucleus) theoretically could activate the Ia inhibitory interneurons (Figure 8A) when inhibition to an antagonist muscle is needed to perform a movement.

Presynaptic Inhibition

One aspect of reflex modulation that cannot be accomplished through convergence onto common interneurons is that associated with the Ia afferent input onto motor neurons. This is because there are no interneurons imposed between the sensory afferent and the motor neurons (Figure 8A). Yet, as mentioned above (Figure 5), reflexes are not triggered when performing a rapid voluntary movement that stretches muscles and strongly activate Ia afferents. How can this be?

The "solution" to this problem is the existence of *inhibitory synaptic inputs that do not target dendrites or somas but that synapse onto the presynaptic terminals of sensory afferents*—in other words, synapses onto synapses. This type of synaptic interaction is referred to as **presynaptic inhibition**. Presynaptic inhibition was identified by Karl Frank and Michelangelo Fuortes in 1957. As shown in Figure 9A, they were carrying out experiments not unlike those described above (Figures 6, 7) by Lundberg and colleagues. In this case, they were recording changes in membrane potential in motor neurons supplying a lower leg muscle. When stimulating Ia afferents arising from that muscle (site 1, Figure 9A),

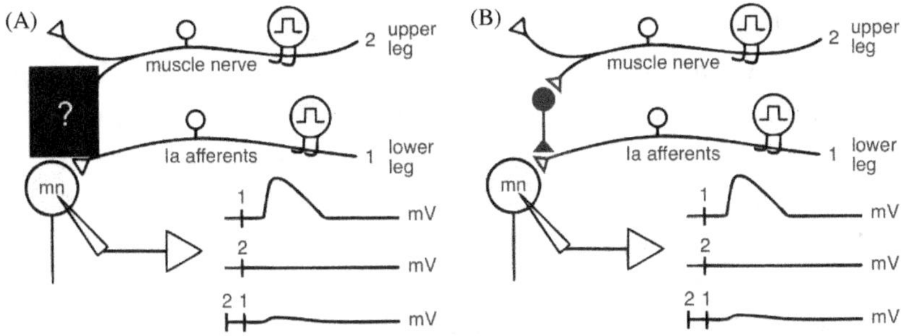

Figure 9. Presynaptic inhibition. (A) Experimental arrangement used by Frank and Fuortes (1957) in the discovery of presynaptic inhibition. Membrane potential responses are recorded in a motor neuron (mn) supplying a lower leg muscle to stimulation of Ia afferents arising from the lower leg muscle (site 1) and/or stimulation of a whole nerve emerging from an upper limb muscle (site 2). Schematic membrane potential response (1) shows strong depolarization in the motor neuron to the stimulation of the Ia afferents (as expected). Stimulation of the upper leg muscle nerve had no effect on the lower leg motor neuron (response 2). However, when both sites 1 and 2 were activated at about the same time, the direct excitation caused by activation of the Ia afferents was greatly reduced (response 2-1). (B) Excitation of interneurons by stimulation of the upper limb muscle nerve that inhibited the presynaptic terminal (i.e., presynaptic inhibition) of the Ia afferents arising from the lower leg muscle could account for the type of responses depicted in (A).

they recorded the expected depolarization associated with the direct, monosynaptic connection to the motor neuron (response 1, Figure 9A). Perhaps in preparation for examining connections to other motor neurons, Frank and Fuortes set up a second stimulating electrode to activate the nerve emerging from a different muscle in the upper leg (site 2, Figure 9A). Also (as perhaps anticipated), when stimulating this nerve in the upper leg, no response was detected in the motor neuron supplying the lower leg muscle (response 2, Figure 9A). Inexplicably, however, when stimulating the upper leg nerve and the Ia afferents emerging from the lower leg muscle at about the same time, the direct excitation from the Ia afferents was greatly suppressed (response 2-1, Figure 9A).

Puzzled by this outcome, Frank and Fuortes did a number of other tests to ensure that stimulating site 2 by itself had no influence on the lower limb motor neuron. For example, as discussed previously (Chapter 6, Figure 10), inhibitory synapses often operate by increasing the permeability of the membrane to Cl^- ions. Because the equilibrium potential of Cl^-

can reside close to the resting potential (~–60 mV), increasing Cl⁻ permeability by activating inhibitory synapses may not result in an overt change in membrane potential in a resting neuron. Therefore, Frank and Fuortes injected steady current into the motor neuron to depolarize it away from the equilibrium potential for Cl⁻. When then stimulating site 2, they again observed no change in the membrane potential, confirming that it had no direct effect on the motor neuron.

Such results led Frank and Fuortes to tentatively propose a radical idea: that stimulation of site 2 caused inhibition of the presynaptic terminals of the Ia afferents. This presumably occurred through the action of a previously unidentified class of inhibitory interneurons (Figure 9B). They referred to this type of synaptic interaction as presynaptic inhibition. Later work by Nobel Prize winner John Eccles and colleagues fully validated this idea (e.g., Eccles *et al.* 1961). Subsequent studies showed that virtually all somatosensory afferents were subject to presynaptic inhibition. Furthermore, presynaptic inhibition is not only in the spinal cord but is found in many structures throughout the CNS, such as the brainstem, cerebellum, hippocampus, amygdala, and retina (Kullmann *et al.* 2005). Also, it was later demonstrated that the interneurons that mediate presynaptic inhibition are GABAergic, and work by driving the membrane potential of sensory afferent presynaptic terminals toward the equilibrium potential of Cl⁻. Action potentials entering the presynaptic terminal of the sensory afferent are thus attenuated, reducing activation of voltage-gated Ca^{2+} channels in the terminal, and lessening the likelihood of neurotransmitter release by the sensory afferent.

Sources of Input to Interneurons Mediating Presynaptic Inhibition

A fundamental question that has yet to be fully resolved is: what are the sources of input that drive the inhibitory neurons that mediate presynaptic inhibition? Early work from Eccles and colleagues indicated that virtually all somatosensory afferents can induce presynaptic inhibition in other sensory afferents (Schmidt 1971). Importantly, early investigations by Eccles's and Lundberg's groups also showed substantial presynaptic inhibition of somatosensory afferents in the spinal cord caused by stimulation of somatosensory and motor cortices (Andersen *et al.* 1964; Carpenter *et al.* 1963), and the brainstem (Carpenter *et al.* 1962). More recently, Moreno-Lopez and colleagues (2021), clearly demonstrated direct projections from somatosensory and motor cortices to genetically identified interneurons that mediate presynaptic inhibition in the spinal cord of sensory afferents. Furthermore, they showed that these descending inputs are distinct from those that produce movements. In addition, robust presynaptic inhibition of somatosensory afferents has been shown to arise from the central pattern-generating circuits (Gosgnach *et al.* 2000) to mitigate interference of reflexes during rhythmical motor behaviors, such as those associated with locomotion.

All investigations indicated in the above discussion used anesthetized or decerebrate animal preparations. Therefore, knowledge of the natural circumstances under which presynaptic inhibition is actually deployed is limited. An important advance in this regard, however, is from the work by Seki *et al.* (2003). They stimulated peripheral sensory afferents in awake monkeys while resting and during voluntary movements. Presynaptic inhibition greatly attenuated the responses in spinal neurons receiving the sensory input only during voluntary movements. This finding indicated that presynaptic inhibition was engaged in parallel with the descending voluntary commands to minimize interference of voluntary behaviors by reflexes.

Voluntary Movements Unimpeded by Reflexes

To illustrate some of the ideas discussed above, let's reconsider the example depicted in Figure 5 of a voluntary movement (extending the elbow) impeded by the stretch reflex. Let's now add to that schematic, simplified representations of convergence onto common interneurons and presynaptic inhibition (Figure 10). As outlined before, descending commands originating in the cortex (arrow 1) excite the triceps motor neurons to cause the triceps muscle to contract (arrow 2). The shortening of the triceps will extend the elbow (arrow 3) and will cause the biceps to be stretched (arrow 4). Lengthening of the biceps will instigate activity on the Ia afferents emerging from muscle spindles in the biceps (arrow 5).

Now to prevent the stretch reflex from impeding the voluntary movement, two things could happen. First, inhibitory interneurons classically

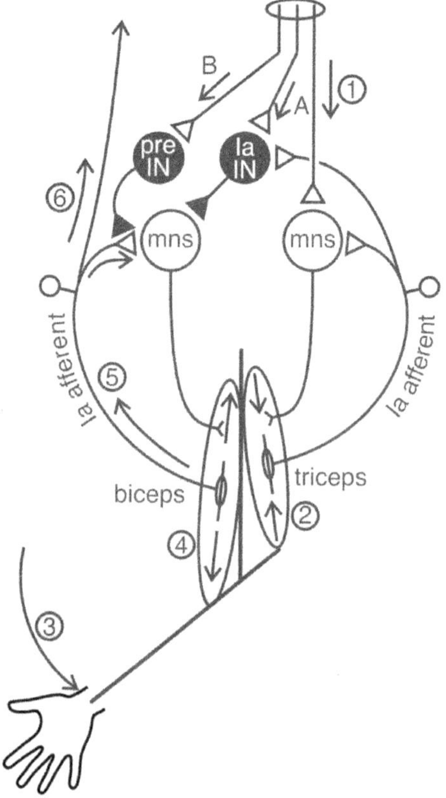

Figure 10.   Mechanisms to prevent stretch reflex in biceps during voluntary extension of the elbow. Descending command (arrow 1) to activate motor neurons (mns) supplying the triceps muscle. Contraction of the triceps (arrow 2) causes the elbow to extend (arrow 3) and lengthening of the biceps (arrow 4). Lengthening of the biceps will instigate activity in Ia afferents arising from the biceps (arrow 5). Commands (arrow A) descending in parallel with those that activate triceps motor neurons (arrow 1) may excite Ia inhibitory interneurons (Ia IN) to prevent activation of the biceps muscle. Likewise, parallel descending commands (path B) may activate interneurons that presynaptically (pre IN) inhibit Ia afferent from exciting the biceps motor neurons.

defined as "belonging" to Ia afferents from the triceps muscle (Ia IN, Figure 10), could be enlisted to directly inhibit the motor neurons supplying the biceps muscle. Such enlistment would not likely arise from the Ia afferent of the triceps muscle because the triceps is shortening, not lengthening. However, it seems feasible that descending pathways converge onto and excite those "common" interneurons (path A, Figure 10) in parallel with those exciting triceps motor neurons (path 1, Figure 10). Indeed, Jankowska *et al.* (1976) have clearly demonstrated such convergence of corticospinal inputs onto Ia inhibitory interneurons.

Second, it seems likely that descending inputs (path B, Figure 10) are activated in parallel with those that drive the triceps motor neurons but that target interneurons mediating presynaptic inhibition (pre IN, Figure 10; Moreno-Lopez *et al.* 2021). Such presynaptic inhibition would limit the transmission of the Ia activity onto the biceps motor neurons, keeping the biceps muscle relatively quiescent during volitional elbow extension. A further important aspect of this organization is that the crucial sensory signals associated with voluntary movement are not blocked but are still conveyed to the brain (arrow 6, Figure 10).

The importance of such modulation of reflexes has recently been strikingly demonstrated for voluntary reaching and during locomotion. Using genetic methods to selectively delete the inhibitory interneurons that cause presynaptic inhibition (pre IN, Figure 10), Fink *et al.* (2014) showed pronounced oscillations of the forelimb while the genetically modified animals reached for morsels of food. The oscillations were due to the alternating stretch reflexes between the flexors and the extensors that were not overridden by presynaptic inhibition. Just as shown in Figure 5, extending the limb triggered stretch reflexes in the flexor muscles, causing the limb to flex. The flexion action then caused the extensor muscles to be lengthened, sparking a stretch reflex in them, and so on.

Similarly, Koch *et al.* (2017) genetically deleted interneurons mediating presynaptic inhibition driven by central pattern generators that produce rhythmical behaviors, such as locomotion. While walking, these animals exhibited extraordinarily excessive motion of their hindlimbs. This was particularly evident during the swing phase, when the hind paw was lifted well above the walking surface, presumably because unimpeded stretch reflexes of flexor muscles caused exaggerated flexion of the hindlimb.

Such findings also provide insight into certain dysfunctions following damage to descending motor pathways, such as occurs with cerebral palsy, stroke, spinal cord injury, or traumatic brain injury. Individuals with these kinds of injuries oftentimes develop *uncontrolled and sometimes long-lasting muscle contractions*, referred to as **spasticity**. It is thought that the damage to the descending pathways that act to suppress reflexes (like that shown in Figure 10) may be partially responsible for spasticity. For example, stretch reflexes below the level of the lesion may become stronger and longer lasting in these individuals. The gentle stroking of the skin of the thigh in an individual with spinal cord injury may provoke a powerful extension of the leg. Such spastic contractions can lead to several complications. In individuals with sustained spastic contractions (referred to as hypertonia), the joints and bones may become deformed. Furthermore, spastic contractions can impede the ability of the individual to perform basic activities of daily living such as dressing, feeding, and bathing. In addition, spastic contractions can be painful.

One clinical approach to treating spasticity is to cut the dorsal roots (referred to as dorsal rhizotomy) that are the sources of sensory afferent input triggering reflexes (Oakes & Rocque 2015). Another less destructive method involves continuous infusion of a GABA (the inhibitory neurotransmitter) agonist directly into the space surrounding the spinal cord below the level of the lesion using a small, implanted pump. The GABA agonist dampens the excitability of spinal reflex circuits and markedly reduces the extent of spasticity in patients with damage to descending pathways (Penn *et al.* 1989).

Summary

Reflexes are the simplest type of motor behavior. They are typically triggered by some form of external stimulus. The external stimulus is detected by peripheral sensory receptors leading to activity on primary sensory afferents. In the somatosensory system, such activity can excite local circuits in the spinal cord or the brainstem to provoke a rapid response to an unexpected perturbation or painful stimulus. Yet, all willed movements, such as reaching for a cup or walking down the street, also excite many of the same somatosensory receptors and sensory afferents that cause reflexes. In these instances, however, reflexes would interfere with the desired action.

To prevent reflexes from occurring during self-produced movements, two systems are in place to abrogate reflexes. One involves interneurons through which signals must pass to instigate reflexes. These interneurons receive input not only from reflex-designated sensory afferents but also from a rich array of descending, interneuronal, and peripheral sources. Thus, these common interneurons serve as decision hubs, either enabling or disabling reflexes from occurring. Furthermore, because these interneurons are shared, they can be activated by inputs other than from reflex-designated sensory inputs. For example, descending input may access these common interneurons to strategically deliver inhibition or excitation to motor neurons needed to accomplish a desired voluntary movement. The other system involves presynaptic inhibition whereby sensory signals are suppressed by inhibitory interneurons that act at the terminal branches of primary afferents in the spinal cord (or the brain stem). This greatly reduces the delivery of sensory signals to local reflex circuitry while preserving the delivery of sensory information to higher centers. Both systems of reflex suppression appear to be driven, in part, by inputs that descend in parallel with commands to produce voluntary movements or with commands emanating from central pattern generators to produce rhythmical movements.

References

Andersen P, Eccles JC & Sears TA (1964). Cortically evoked depolarization of primary afferent fibers in the spinal cord. *Journal of Neurophysiology* **27**, 63–77.

Baldissera F, Hultborn H & Illert M (1981). Integration in spinal neuronal systems. Republished in: Comprehensive Physiology (2011), pp. 509–595.

Carpenter D, Engberg I & Lundberg A (1962). Presynaptic inhibition in the lumbar cord evoked from the brain stem. *Experientia* **18**, 450–451.

Carpenter D, Lundberg A & Norrsell U (1963). Primary afferent depolarization evoked from the sensorimotor cortex. *Acta Physiologica Scandinavica* **59**, 126–142.

Eccles JC, Eccles RM & Magni F (1961). Central inhibitory action attributable to presynaptic depolarization produced by muscle afferent volleys. *Journal of Physiology* **159**, 147–166.

Fink AJP, Croce KR, Huang ZJ, Abbott LF, Jessell TM & Azim E (2014). Presynaptic inhibition of spinal sensory feedback ensures smooth movement. *Nature* **509**, 43–48.

Frank K & Fuortes MGF (1957). Presynaptic and postsynaptic inhibition of mono-synaptic reflexes. *Federation Proceedings* **16**, 39–40.

Gosgnach S, Quevedo J, Fedirchuk B & McCrea DA (2000). Depression of group Ia monosynaptic EPSPs in cat hindlimb motoneurones during fictive locomotion. *Journal of Physiology* **526**, 639–652.

Jankowska E & Lundberg A (1981). Interneurones in the spinal cord. *Trends in Neurosciences* **4**, 230–233.

Jankowska E, Padel Y & Tanaka R (1976). Disynaptic inhibition of spinal motoneurones from the motor cortex in the monkey. *Journal of Physiology* **258**, 467–487.

Koch SC, Barrio MGD, Dalet A, Gatto G, Günther T, Zhang J, Seidler B, Saur D, Schüle R & Goulding M (2017). RORβ spinal interneurons gate sensory transmission during locomotion to secure a fluid walking gait. *Neuron* **96**, 1419–1431.e5.

McComas AJ (2016). Hypothesis: Hughlings Jackson and presynaptic inhibition: Is there a big picture? *Journal of Neurophysiology* **116**, 41–50.

Moreno-Lopez Y, Bichara C, Delbecq G, Isope P & Cordero-Erausquin M (2021). The corticospinal tract primarily modulates sensory inputs in the mouse lumbar cord. *Elife* **10**, e65304.

Mott FW & Sherrington CS (1895). Experiments upon the influence of sensory nerves upon movement and nutrition of the limbs. Preliminary communication. *Proceedings of the Royal Society of London* **57**, 481–488.

Kullmann DM, Ruiz A, Rusakov DM, Scott R, Semyanov A & Walker MC (2005). Presynaptic, extrasynaptic and axonal GABAA receptors in the CNS: Where and why? *Progress in Biophysics and Molecular Biology* **87**, 33–46.

Lundberg A, Norrsell U & Voorhoeve P (1962). Effects from the pyramidal tract on spinal reflex arcs. *Acta Physiologica Scandinavica* **56**, 201–219.

Oakes WJ & Rocque BG (2015). Dorsal rhizotomy for spasticity. Nerves and Nerve Injuries. Academic Press. http://dx.doi.org/10.1016/B978-0-12-802653-3.00074-9.

Penn RD, Savoy SM, Corcos D, Latash M, Gottlieb G, Parke B & Kroin JS (1989). Intrathecal baclofen for severe spinal spasticity. *New England Journal of Medicine* **320**, 1517–1521.

Rymer WZ, Houk JC & Crago PE (1979). Mechanisms of the clasp-knife reflex studied in an animal model. *Experimental Brain Research* **37**, 93–113.

Seki K, Perlmutter SI & Fetz EE (2003). Sensory input to primate spinal cord is presynaptically inhibited during voluntary movement. *Nature Neuroscience* **6**, 1309–1316.

Sherrington CS (1906). The integrative action of the nervous system. New Haven: Yale University Press.

Schmidt RF (1971). Presynaptic inhibition in the vertebrate central nervous system. *Ergebnisse Der Physiologie Rev Physiology* **63**, 20–101.

Silva C & McNaughton N (2019). Are periaqueductal gray and dorsal raphe the foundation of appetitive and aversive control? A comprehensive review. *Progress in Neurobiology* **177**, 33–72.

Chapter 17

Rhythmical Movements

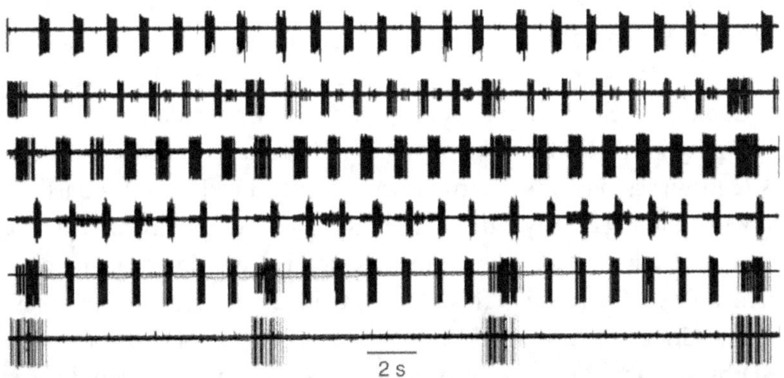

Recording from some of the several nerves emerging the stomatogastric ganglion that controls the rhythmic process of grinding food in the lobster stomach. (Adapted from Marder and Bucher [2007].)

As mentioned in Chapter 16, virtually all creatures use rhythmical, repetitive movements to propel them through their environments. This can involve undulations of the body wall for swimming, flapping of wings for flying, wiggling for crawling, and a vast array of cyclic leg motions for walking and running. In addition, rhythmical motions serve a variety of other purposes, such as scratching, mastication (see frontispiece above), and breathing. In this chapter, we will focus mostly on the neural control of mammalian terrestrial locomotion. Nevertheless, many of the principles identified underlying control of this type of behavior are similar to those governing other forms of rhythmical movements.

The study of the neural basis of mammalian locomotion has an interesting history (Stuart & Hultborn 2008). Sherrington proposed that repetitive stepping associated with locomotion was likely the outcome of different types of reflexes being linked together in sequence. For example, he stated in 1910 that: *"In stepping, a pair of antagonistic reflexes E [extensor] and F [flexor] alternate . . . the flexion phase of the step exhibits the same principles of coordination of the limb musculature as were shown for the flexion reflex. Similarly, the muscles employed in the extension phase of the step are those employed in the crossed extension-reflex."* Furthermore, he points out that *"alternation of the two intermittent proprioceptive stimulations arise in the limb itself,"* asserting that the reflexes are triggered by activity arising in proprioceptive afferents caused by movements of the limbs.

Around the same time, Thomas Graham Brown, who was working in Sherrington's lab, carried out a set of experiments to test these ideas of his boss. Contrary to Sherrington's concept, Graham Brown demonstrated stepping activity in the lower limbs of spinalized animals even when the dorsal roots (carrying axons of somatosensory receptors) had been lesioned. This remarkable finding clearly indicated that the source of the rhythmical behavior was not from the *"limb itself"* (as asserted by Sherrington), and did not involve reflexes, because reflexes require input from peripheral sensory receptors. Graham Brown modestly and succinctly summarized these results (1911) by stating: *"the act of progression [i.e., locomotion] may be essentially a central and not a peripheral phenomenon."* In other words, the circuits that control the activities of muscles associated with a rhythmical motor act (like walking) reside within the central nervous system (CNS) and do not require a sensory input to be produced. Surprisingly, and for reasons that are not entirely clear, these findings were not embraced by Sherrington. Likely because of Sherrington's prominence in the field, his (rather than Graham Brown's) ideas were broadly accepted by the scientific community and Graham Brown's findings were largely ignored for half a century.

Midbrain Locomotor Region

Advances in understanding the control of locomotion languished until the 1960s, when a landmark discovery by a group of USSR investigators working in Moscow thoroughly reinvigorated the study of the neural bases of rhythmical motor behaviors. These researchers (Mark Shik, Fyodor

Severin, Grigori Orlovsky) identified a small region (~1 mm diameter) in the dorsal midbrain, which when activated with nonrhythmic, continuous electrical stimulation, evoked full-blown, sustained walking movements in a decerebrate cat. As stated by the authors (Shik *et al.* 1966): "The cat, which before stimulation was immobile, suddenly 'came to life', stood up on its legs and began to move, setting in motion or accelerating the treadmill belt." Figure 1A shows the location of this region, which was called the **midbrain locomotor region** (**MLR**). It was later shown that the

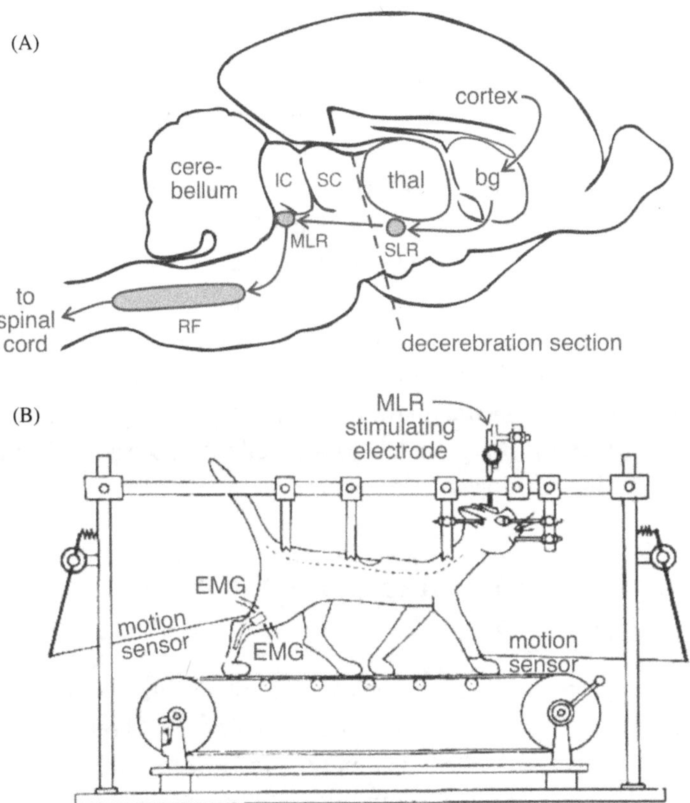

Figure 1.   Locomotion induced in the decerebrate cat. (A) Sagittal section of the cat brain showing key relays in the commands to engage locomotion. Dashed line indicates the location of the lesion for decerebration. SLR—subthalamic locomotor region, MLR—midbrain locomotor region, RF—reticular formation. (B) Setup for studying characteristics of evoked locomotion in the decerebrate cat caused by stimulation of the MLR. ([A] adapted from Whelan [1997]; [B] adapted from Severin *et al.* [1967].)

output of the MLR fed through the reticular formation (RF, Figure 1A), the dense interconnected region in the core of the pons and medulla, which in turn projected to the spinal cord.

To carefully evaluate the qualities of the evoked locomotion, these investigators developed a sophisticated experimental setup (Figure 1B), in which a decerebrate cat was held by a frame over a free-to-move treadmill belt. Actions evoked with MLR stimulation were detected with movement sensors placed on the limbs and electromyography (EMG) electrodes inserted into muscles. The signals measured during MLR-evoked locomotion in decerebrate cats were, for all practical purposes, no different than those recorded in intact cats walking on the treadmill.

When the intensity of the MLR stimulation was increased, the decerebrate cat increased walking speed, and if stimulation intensity increased further, the gait pattern switched from walking to trotting to galloping. Likewise, when the treadmill motor was engaged and the speed of the belt progressively increased, the decerebrate cat with *constant* low-level MRL stimulation appropriately altered gaits from walking to trotting to galloping. Because a decerebrate cat would have no awareness of changing treadmill belt speeds, this latter finding implied that sensory feedback of the limbs being moved more briskly by the belt as the treadmill speed increased, must have played a key role in adapting the gait pattern to the pace of the treadmill. But is such sensory feedback necessary for the production of the locomotion?

Decerebrate Cat Locomotion without Sensory Feedback

Sten Grillner, a Swedish investigator who trained in the laboratory of Anders Lundberg (see Chapter 16), visited the Moscow group to learn the methods to evoke controlled locomotion in decerebrate cats. Back in Sweden, and in the experiments reminiscent of Graham Brown's, Grillner evaluated the ability of MRL stimulation to produce locomotion in decerebrate cats when the dorsal roots of those animals had been severed. Figure 2A shows EMG recordings from four sample muscles during MLR-evoked locomotion in a cat with dorsal roots intact (Grillner &

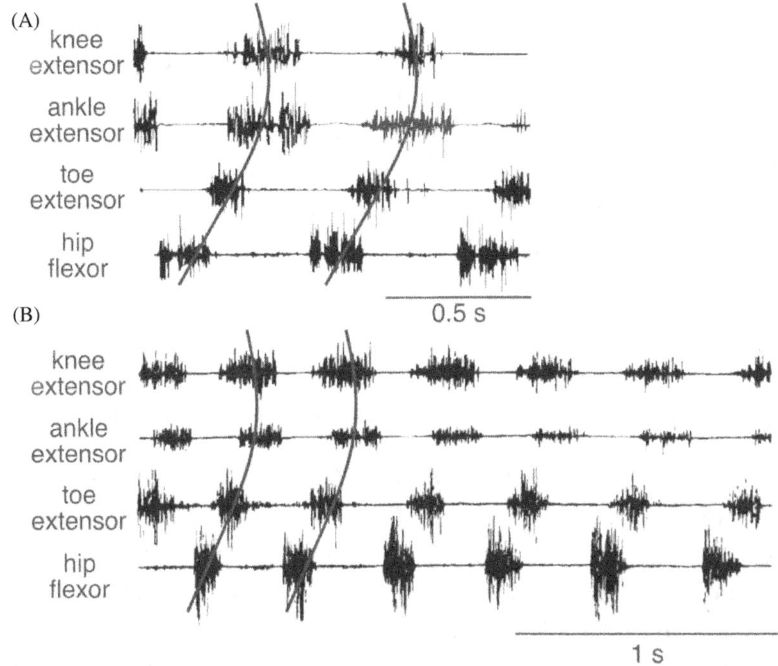

Figure 2.   MLR-evoked locomotion in decerebrate cat (A) with and (B) without dorsal roots intact. EMG signals from four representative hindlimb muscles. Patterns of EMG activity were largely the same for the two situations (the time scale is different for the two panels). Curved lines superimposed on EMG signals for two consecutive walking strides provided is an aid to visualize the temporal pattern across muscles. (Adapted from Grillner and Zangger [1984].)

Zangger 1984). The curved lines superimposed on the EMG signals provide a visual guide to the temporal patterning of those muscles during two consecutive walking strides.

Figure 2B shows the EMG signals in the same muscles and cat in response to MLR stimulation but following bilateral sectioning of the lumbar (hindlimb) dorsal roots. The movements and pattern of muscle coordination seen in the cat following removal of sensory input (Figure 2B) was nearly the same as for the cat with intact dorsal roots. Therefore, the complex motor patterns produced during locomotion do *not* require sensory input (a conclusion similar to that made by Graham

Brown in 1911). However, as pointed out by Grillner and Zangger (1984), following several well-coordinated steps in the cat with dorsal roots severed (e.g., Figure 2B): "the pattern of activity may become more variable and may breakdown altogether." This result implied that while signals from somatosensory afferents are not necessary to produce the basic pattern of locomotion, sensory feedback is important for maintaining and adjusting the pattern to small step-by-step alterations in limb placements and subtle variations in the pathway upon which an animal locomotes.

Locomotor Activity Is Produced in the Spinal Cord

Another fundamental question addressed by Grillner and colleagues had to do with the location within the CNS where the locomotor pattern is generated. It seemed feasible that the MLR, for example, could be the region that coordinates muscle activities associated with locomotion. Previous qualitative findings from the 19th century and Graham Brown's experiments in the early 20th century suggested, however, that the circuitry producing locomotion might reside within the spinal cord itself. To test this idea rigorously, Grillner and colleagues surgically lesioned the spinal cords of kittens at a thoracic level, leaving the hindlimbs paralyzed (Forssberg *et al.* 1980). Presumably, kittens were used because of the high degree of plasticity in the nervous system in the early stages of development. Following recovery from the surgery, the kittens were "trained" to walk on a treadmill. This involved daily sessions during which the experimenters displaced the hindlimbs on the moving treadmill to approximate the action of walking. The nonparalyzed forelimbs of the kitten stood on a platform, while the hindquarters of the animal were supported by the experimenters holding the tail (Figure 3A). After only a few days of such training, the kittens began to produce rhythmical hindlimb movements on their own. Eventually, the patterns of movements and muscle activities were similar to that of intact cats walking on a treadmill (Figures 3B, C). This remarkable result clearly demonstrated that the circuitry for controlling complex locomotor activity resides in the spinal cord.

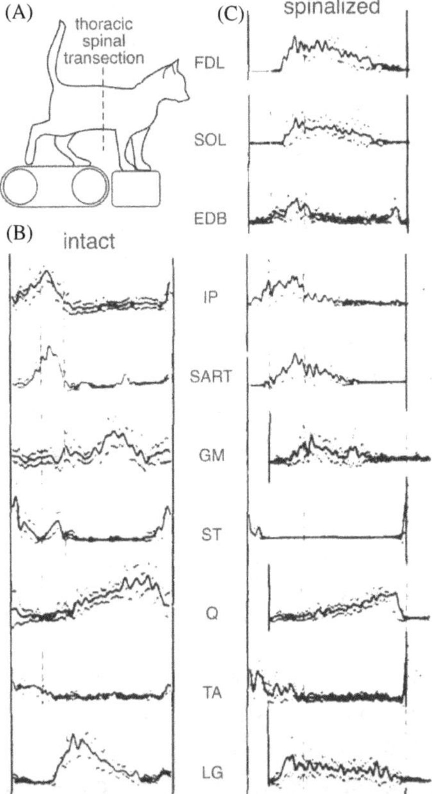

Figure 3.   Walking in spinalized animal. (A) Setup showing a spinalized kitten (transection in thoracic spinal cord) with forelimbs standing on a platform and hindlimbs walking on a treadmill. Experimenters held the tail to stabilize the hindquarters above the treadmill. (B) Rectified, filtered, and averaged EMG signals (dashed lines indicate ±1 standard deviation) in intact kitten walking on the treadmill. (C) EMG signals recorded in the spinalized kitten after a few weeks of treadmill training. FDL—flexor digitorum longus, SOL—soleus, EDB—extensor digitorum brevis, IP—iliopsoas, SART—sartorius, GM—gluteus medius, ST—semitendinosus, Q—quadriceps, TA—tibialis anterior, LG—lateral gastrocnemius. (Adapted from Forssberg *et al.* [1980].)

Central Pattern Generators and Instigation of Rhythmical Movements

Such findings led to the fundamental concept of **central pattern generators** (CPGs) as *low-level central circuits that produce the* *complex spatiotemporal patterns of muscle activity associated with rhythmic behaviors without requiring sensory input.* Keep in mind that for many forms of locomotion, up to 100 muscles or more might be involved. The orchestration of such complex activity is thereby relegated to noncortical structures requiring little conscious involvement. However, because the decision to engage in locomotion is essentially a volitional act, the cerebral cortex is involved in instigating locomotion. As shown in Figure 1A, such commands probably issue from the motor cortex to activate regions of the basal ganglia (bg), which in turn operate on a region in the diencephalon, referred to as the subthalamic locomotor region (SLR). The SLR is most likely housed within a slender nucleus called the zona incerta (Milner & Mogenson 1988). Output from the SLR activates the MLR, which then drives projections from the reticular formation (RF) to excite spinally located CPGs to produce locomotion.

Figure 4 depicts a simplified representation of the key elements likely involved in activating CPGs for mammalian locomotion. A small region of the cerebral cortex (highlighted in gray in Figure 4) sends out the volitional command to initiate locomotion. The actual cortical site responsible for instigating locomotion has not been definitively identified, although some indirect evidence (Wang *et al.* 2009) points to the supplementary motor area (discussed in Chapter 18). The cortical command is then relayed through the basal ganglia, SLR, MLR, and RF before being sent to the spinal cord to activate CPGs. While one could consider the sequential activation of brain structures (i.e., those above the horizontal dashed line in Figure 4) as serving as a "switch" for engaging the CPG, perhaps a more apt analogy would be that of a controller knob on a variable speed fan. As such, the activity in this pathway not only "turns on" locomotion, but also dictates the speed of locomotion.

The intensity of the command received then determines the rapidity by which activity in the spinal CPGs cycles. In each cycle, similar time-distributed patterns of output are delivered to large numbers of motor nuclei (MN, Figure 4), driving the activities of many muscles needed for the basic production of locomotion. Feedback from peripheral sensory receptors (Figure 4) continuously update and adjust the activity in the CPG to maintain successful locomotion in the face of modest changes

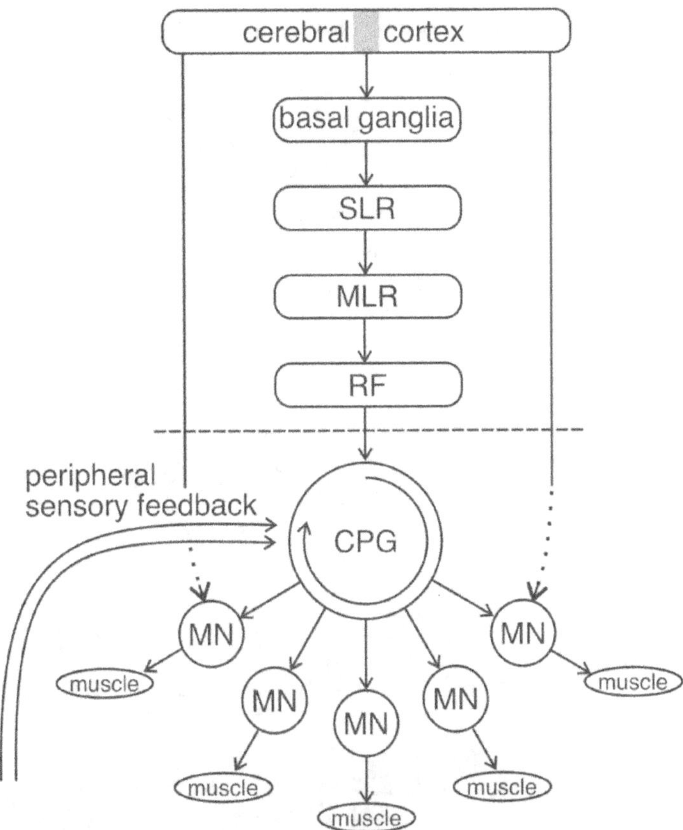

Figure 4.   A CPG is an ensemble of interneurons situated at a low level in the CNS that produces the repeating, spatiotemporal patterns of muscle activity associated with rhythmic movements. Higher brain centers (above the dashed horizontal line), originating from a small region of the cortex (gray area), send commands to initiate activity in the CPG but do not fundamentally dictate the pattern. Separate corticospinal projects (dashed arrows) can converge with output from CPG onto motor nuclei (MN) to adjust locomotor patterns to the specific needs of the individual. Feedback from peripheral sensory receptors helps correct errors and keep the overall pattern on target. SLR—subthalamic locomotor region, MLR—midbrain locomotor region, RF—reticular formation.

in the stepping environment and slight errors in the production of the movements. For more overt challenges and obstacles in the locomotor environment, separate descending commands originating in other areas of the cerebral cortex (dotted arrows, Figure 4) can converge with CPG commands on motor nuclei to smoothly adjust gait to turn a corner or step over an object (Drew 1991).

An extraordinary demonstration of the pathway shown in Figure 4 was provided by the Russian group, which originally identified the MLR and the SLR. In these experiments (Sirota & Shik 1973), only the SLR was lesioned, and stimulating electrodes were placed below that level into the MLR (Figure 5A). Following recovery from surgery, these otherwise fully intact (not decerebrated) cats looked perfectly normal. They were attentive

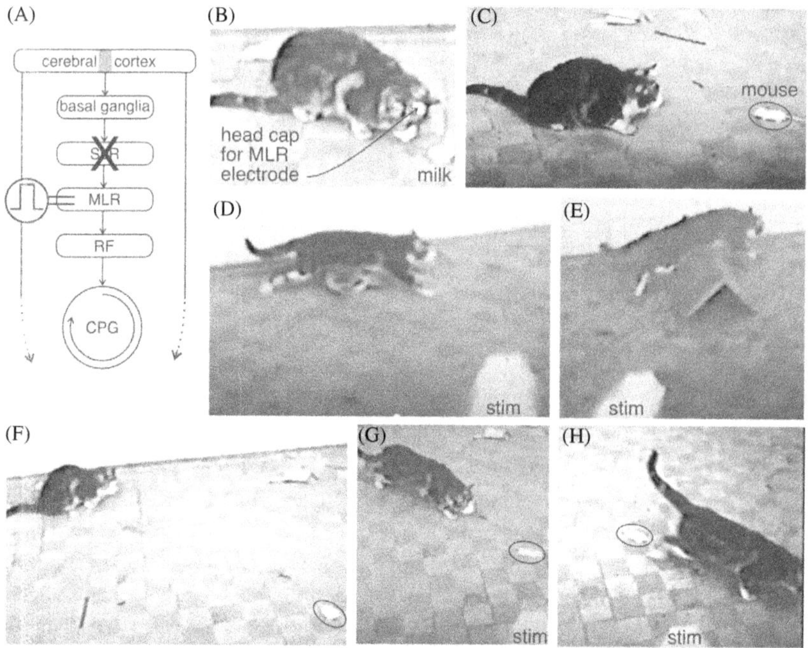

Figure 5.   MLR-evoked locomotion in cat. (A) Cats had small lesions of the SLR and stimulating electrodes placed in the MLR. (B)–(H) Movie frames depicting the cat with the SLR lesion and its responses to MLR stimulation (stim). (B) With the stimulator turned off, the cat was unable to walk forward to drink milk. (C) With the stimulator off, the cat was unable to pursue a mouse placed in the room. (D) When the stimulator was turned on (small light displayed at bottom of the movie frame), the cat immediately began walking or running throughout the room, and could (E) readily jump over obstacles and make turns to avoid walls. (F)–(G) Movie frames from a single sequence. (F) The cat was unable to stalk the mouse (oval) when the stimulator was off. (G) The cat immediately approached the mouse when the stimulator was turned on, but (H) could not halt locomotion to attack the mouse under the continued stimulation of the MLR. (Film courtesy of the late Mikhail Sirota.)

to what was going on in their surroundings and maintained typical sitting postures of cats. However, they could not locomote despite that they were not "paralyzed" in the conventional sense. Even when enticed with a cup of milk placed a small distance away from them (Figure 5B) or with the release of a mouse inside of the room where they were sitting (Figure 5C), the cats did not locomote. As seen in Figure 5A, a lesion of the SLR would prevent volitional commands from the cortex to be conveyed downstream to the MLR, RF, and to the spinal CPG. However, when the MLR was stimulated, the cats immediately stood up and started to walk (Figure 5D) or run (with higher stimulus intensities) about the large room they were housed in. They made the perfectly normal turns needed to avoid running into walls and readily jumped over obstacles (Figure 5E) placed in the room. This retained maneuverability was due to the actions of unaffected parallel corticospinal pathways (dotted lines in Figure 5A). The cats continued to locomote as long as the MLR stimulation was maintained.

Indeed, it appeared as though the cats could not cease to locomote with sustained MLR stimulation, even if they desired to do so. This was strikingly demonstrated as shown in the movie frames of Figures 5F, G, and H. With the stimulator turned off, the cat was attentive to a mouse placed in the room but did not move toward it (Figure 5F). When the stimulator was turned on (Figure 5G), the cat stalked the mouse . . . but could not halt its locomotion (Figure 5H), thereby, bypassing it and leaving the mouse to live another day. The cat continued to ambulate ceaselessly under the drive to its locomotor CPG by the MLR stimulation. Apparently, the KGB (security agency of the Soviet Union) encouraged these experiments (personal communication with the late Mikhail Sirota, also see Feldman [2015]). Perhaps the KGB was looking to create a spy "robo-cat," instrumented with microphones and cameras, to be adopted into the White House. Regardless, these phenomenal experiments provide one of the most important and graphic demonstrations of the crucial sites involved in the instigation of locomotion.

Clinical Implications of CPGs

As shown in Figure 4, a spinal cord injury (e.g., at the level of the dashed horizontal line Figure 4) will permanently impair or eliminate the ability of the brain pathway (cortex → basal ganglia → SLR → MLR → RF) to activate the central pattern generating circuity in the spinal cord. In such circumstances, it seems reasonable to consider whether an alternate means might be provided to "turn on" the CPG and reinstate basic locomotor function. Indeed, as shown by the experiments on kittens with complete lesions of the thoracic spinal cord, after a period of training, the otherwise paralyzed hindlimbs generated locomotion (Figure 3). This was not because of some regrowth of axons across the lesion. Therefore, what was the origin of signals activating the CPG? The most likely source was from the peripheral sensory receptors, which have access to the CPG (Figure 4). Presumably, the repetitive and persistent moving of the hindlimbs on the treadmill contributed to the synaptic plasticity of those connections onto the neural circuitry making up the CPG. Furthermore, as discussed in Chapter 13, when a region of the CNS is deprived of much of its normal input (in this case the CPG in the spinal cord), several mechanisms can be unleashed, such as enhanced synaptic efficacy (Manabe *et al.* 1989) and axonal sprouting (Murray & Goldberger 1974) of peripheral afferents, which can lead to the reactivation of those circuits.

A pressing clinical question was whether the recovery of locomotion shown to occur in kittens with spinal cord lesions could also occur in adults. This was shown to be the case by Serge Rossignol and colleagues in Montreal using an experimental setup similar to that used for the kitten experiments (Figure 6A). Using implanted EMG electrodes and video capture of reflective markers placed over the joints to track limb movements, features of hindlimb locomotion were recorded in adult cats. The forelimbs stood on a platform and the hindlimbs were placed over a treadmill. Figure 6B shows the pattern of EMG activities recorded from a variety of left (L) and right (R) hindlimb muscles in the intact cat. Following these recordings, a complete surgical lesion was made in the thoracic region of the spinal cord. These cats were then trained a few times a week to walk on the treadmill with the experimenters moving the hindlimbs to mimic walking. After about 3 weeks of such training, these cats began to exhibit reasonably normal locomotor patterns on the treadmill with robust muscle activities and expansive movements (Barbeau & Rossignol 1987). Figure 6C shows EMG signals in an adult cat 32 days following a complete spinal cord transection and training to walk on the treadmill. While there are some subtle differences in the EMG patterns,

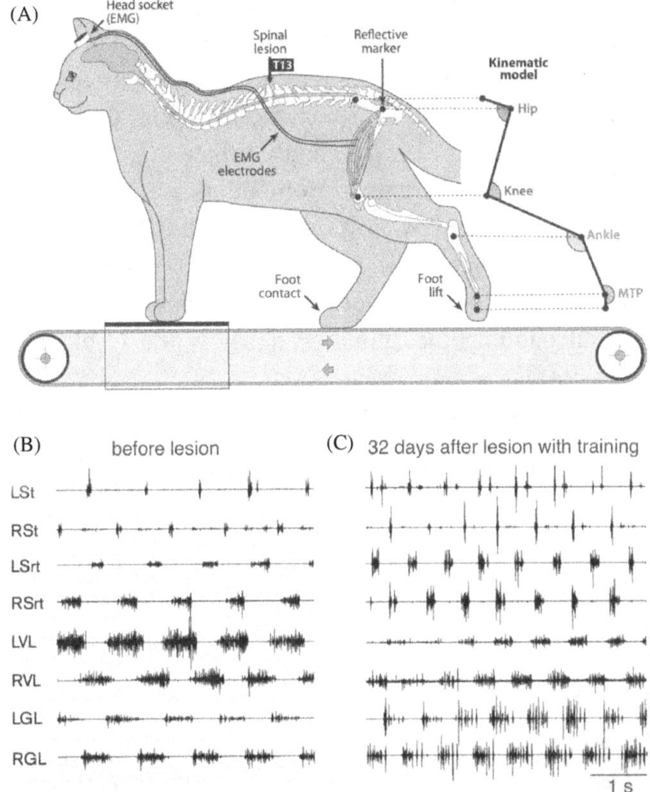

Figure 6. (A) Experimental setup showing an adult cat with a thoracic spinal cord lesion. The forelimbs stand on a platform and the paralyzed hindlimbs are positioned over a treadmill. The leads of EMG electrodes from several hindlimb muscles are led to a socket on the head for connecting to amplifiers. Small reflective markers are placed over bony landmarks to record limb movements (kinematics) with video. (B) EMG activity recorded in left (L) and right (R) hindlimb muscles in the intact cat. (C) EMG recordings from the same cat 32 days after the spinal cord lesion and with treadmill training showing robust locomotor activity. St—semitendinosus, Srt—sartorius, VL—vastus lateralis, GL—lateral gastrocnemius. ([A] Adapted from Rossignol and Frigon [2011]; [B] and [C] Adapted from Rossignol [2000].)

the overall movements were quite similar to those recorded when the cat was intact. This finding opened the doors to the possibility of reactivation of CPG activity and restoration of walking in humans with spinal cord injury.

It should be said that training an animal (or person) with a spinal cord lesion to walk on a treadmill requires substantial time and effort by the trainers. Perhaps there might be a more immediate way to activate CPG circuitry below the level of a spinal cord lesion. Early work from Lundberg's (Jankowska *et al.* 1967) and Grillner's (Forssberg & Grillner 1973) labs suggested that various neuromodulators (like noradrenaline or serotonin) might serve as activating signals of the CPG in the spinal cord. To systematically address this possibility, Rossignol and colleagues directly injected an agonist of noradrenaline (clonidine) into the fluid-filled space surrounding the spinal cord below the level of the lesion (Chau *et al.* 1998).

Figure 7A shows the EMG patterns and stick figures representing the configuration of the hindlimb from successive video frames during one

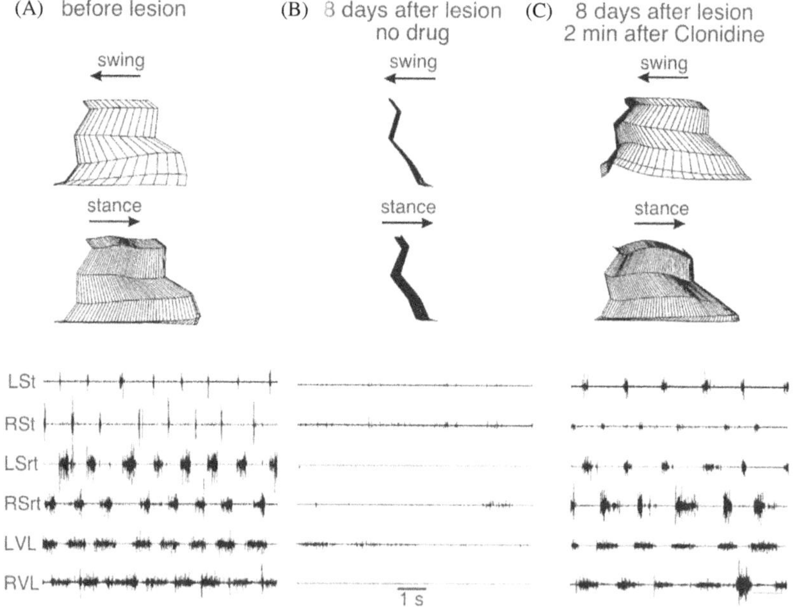

Figure 7.   Limb movements (top) and EMG activity (bottom) in (A) adult cat before complete thoracic spinal cord lesion, (B) eight days following lesion, and (C) eight days following lesion and 2 minutes following injection of noradrenaline agonist clonidine into the space surrounding the spinal cord below the level of the lesion. Muscle abbreviations defined in legend of Figure 7. (Adapted from Chau *et al.* [1998].)

walking stride of an intact cat on a treadmill (like that in Figure 6A). The top set of stick figures depicts the forward movement of the leg during the swing phase of walking, and the next set indicates the backward movement of the leg during the stance phase with the paw on the treadmill. This animal was then subjected to a complete transection of the thoracic spinal cord. Figure 7B shows that when this animal was placed on the treadmill eight days after the surgery, there was virtually no muscle activity, and the legs were simply dragged backward by the treadmill. On the same day and after the recordings of Figure 7B were made, the investigators injected clonidine into the spinal cord. Almost immediately, fully coordinated and vigorous locomotion was produced in the cat (Figure 7C) that moments before had exhibited complete paralysis of the hindlimbs.

Translation to Humans with Spinal Cord Injuries

The possibility to translate the astounding results of Chau *et al.* (1998; Figure 7) carried out in cats to human patients was taken up by several groups of investigators. Disappointingly, and for reasons that remain unclear, injection of clonidine into the spinal cord below the level of complete lesions in human paraplegics did not induce locomotion (Dietz *et al.* 1995). Consequently, much effort was directed toward reanimating locomotion in paraplegics with treadmill training. In one study, despite four-and-a-half months of daily training on a treadmill, none of the individuals with complete spinal cord injuries could produce stepping movements (Wirz *et al.* 2001). This disheartening finding was partially offset by improvements in walking capabilities with training in individuals with incomplete spinal cord injuries. Nevertheless, the absence of locomotion following clonidine injection or with treadmill training in patients with complete spinal cord injuries raised questions about the existence of locomotor CPGs in the human spinal cord.

Recently, treadmill training was combined with electrical stimulation of the spinal cord (Angeli *et al.* 2018) in patients with motor complete spinal cord injuries. Electrodes, surgically implanted below the level of the lesion of the spinal cord, were used to excite the CPGs presumed to exist in the lumbar spinal cord. The patients then underwent up to a year and a half of treadmill training combined with stimulation delivered to the spinal cord. Impressively, two of the four individuals regained the ability to walk slowly overground using a walker for support. Although not definitive, this finding strongly suggests the presence of spinal CPGs in humans.

Neural Circuitry of CPGs

Up to this point, CPGs have been discussed as though they were black boxes. But what is inside the box? How might groups of neurons be interconnected to give rise to reliable, repeating patterns of muscle activation needed to produce rhythmical motor behaviors? This question was first given serious consideration by Graham Brown (1914). Graham Brown recognized that many forms of rhythmical motion involve alternating activations of antagonistic muscle groups, such as knee flexors and extensors operating at different phases of the gait cycle. Accordingly, Graham Brown hypothesized that there might exist a minimum of two competing subcircuits (which he called "**half centers**"), *one that tends to activate one group of muscles and another that activates the other. When one half center is active (say that exciting knee flexors), it inhibits the other half center of the antagonistic group (i.e., the knee extensors), and vice versa.*

Figure 8A shows the basic architecture of Graham Brown's half-center model for controlling cyclical activation of antagonistic muscle groups. The CPG (oval) contains the two half centers. The half centers consist of excitatory (E) and inhibitory (I) interneurons. Each set of E neurons projects to motor nuclei (MN) controlling the activation of a muscle or muscle group. In addition, each E neuron group excites inhibitory (I) neurons that suppress the activity of E neurons of the opposite half center. Both half centers receive more or less equivalent tonic (nonpatterned) excitation from brainstem centers (Figure 8A). As such, when the command to locomote first descends from the brainstem, both sets of E neurons are driven toward the threshold for generating action potentials.

Let's assume that the E neurons supplying muscle$_1$ in Figure 8A (E_1) reach the threshold just ahead of those supplying muscle$_2$ (E_2). At that moment, E_1 will excite the motor neurons supplying muscle$_1$. At the same time, E_1 will also excite its I neurons (I_1) to inhibit and prevent spiking in E_2. Therefore, muscle$_1$ will be activated and muscle$_2$ will be silent. In this

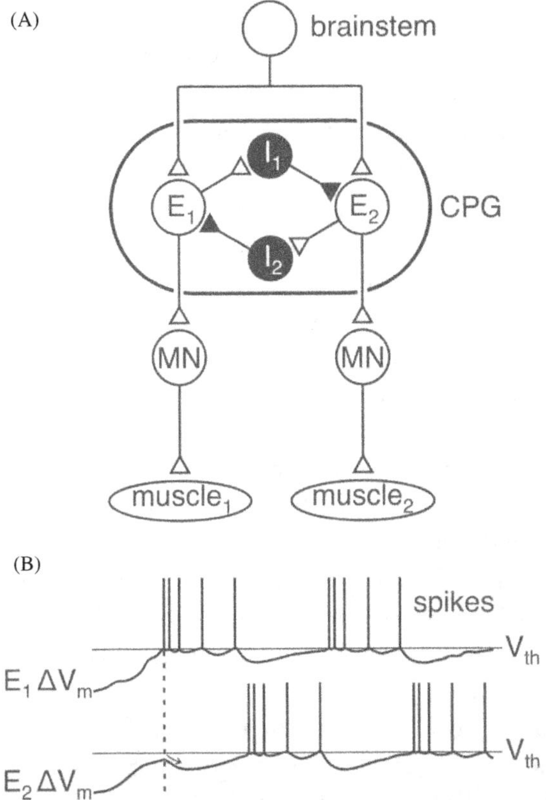

Figure 8.   (A) Half-center circuit for generating alternating activity to a pair of antagonistic muscles. Excitatory (E) neurons provide the drive to motor nuclei controlling individual muscles. Output from E neurons also excite inhibitory (I) neurons that suppress activity in the E neurons of the opposing half center. Both sets of E neurons receive steady excitation from the brainstem. Such a circuit provides a simplified framework for how CPGs might work. (B) Schematic representation of membrane potential (ΔV_m) recorded from two E neurons, one driving muscle$_1$ (E_1) and the other driving muscle$_2$ (E_2). Activating command from brainstem drives membrane potential for both E neurons toward spike threshold (V_{th}). If E_1 reaches threshold first (vertical dashed line), its activity will excite I_1 to drive ΔV_m of E_2 away from the threshold (downward curved arrow) and prevent E_2 from spiking. During sustained excitation from the brainstem, spiking of E_1 diminishes due to spike frequency adaptation. This lessens the inhibition of E_2. Ultimately, E_1 may cease to discharge, lifting inhibition from E_2, whereupon E_2 will become active and suppress activity in E_1. The process of alternating activities of E_1 and E_2 (and of muscle$_1$ and muscle$_2$) will persist with ongoing excitation from the brainstem.

scenario, the first E neuron to reach the threshold would persistently dominate, and all subsequent activity would be exclusively directed toward its muscle—a "winner-take-all" situation. So how might activity be switched from one side to the other under the equivalent and continuous excitatory input to both half centers from the brainstem?

To resolve this conundrum, Graham Brown speculated that each half center might undergo some form of "fatigue," whereby, despite continued excitation, the spiking output of E neurons progressively diminish and may cease altogether. Indeed, this prescient idea was later identified as that associated with spike-frequency adaptation. Recall from Chapter 8 (Figure 4) and Chapter 15 (Figure 8) that many types of neurons undergo such reductions in spike frequency during sustained excitation. To conceptualize this process, consider simultaneous intracellular recordings from an E_1 and an E_2 neuron (Figure 8B). At the onset of excitation from the brainstem, both neurons depolarize toward the spiking threshold (horizontal lines, Figure 8B). For whatever reason, let's assume E_1 reaches the spike threshold first. Spiking in E_1 will excite I_1 (Figure 8A) to deliver inhibition to E_2, pushing its membrane potential away from the threshold (curved arrow, Figure 8B). E_1 generates spikes for a period of time driving its motor neurons to excite its muscle. However, during the sustained excitation from the brainstem, E_1 undergoes spike-frequency adaptation, leading to lower spiking rates and less inhibition of E_2. Eventually, E_1 ceases to fire, whereupon E_2 is immediately relieved of inhibition, and it starts to spike, causing its muscle to be activated and E_1 to be temporarily suppressed (Figure 8B). This process then continues indefinitely in the presence of the descending excitation, with activity switching from one half center to the other, reciprocally activating the two antagonistic muscles.

Some of the basic ideas outlined by Graham Brown for the production of such rhythmical muscle activation were confirmed in later studies involving intracellular and extracellular recordings of neurons within CPGs (McCrea & Rybak 2008). Clearly, however, locomotion (and other forms of rhythmical behaviors) does not involve simple alternating activation between antagonistic muscle groups. Therefore, the cellular architecture of CPGs is much more complex than that represented by the half-center model, enabling subtle timing and activation differences across large numbers of muscles during each cycle of a rhythmic pattern (Arber 2012; Goulding 2009; Kiehn 2016; Marder & Bucher 2007). Nevertheless, the half-center model provides a good starting point to understand how interconnected sets of neurons can underlie the production of various types of stereotyped behavior, such as that associated with locomotion.

Summary

Many forms of motor behavior involve repetitive activation of large numbers of muscles. The detailed patterns of muscle activation associated with these behaviors are generated by low-level circuits, referred to as CPGs. Typically, descending commands from higher brain centers are needed to engage CPGs to drive rhythmical movements. While sensory feedback from peripheral sensory receptors is not needed by CPGs to produce the basic forms of rhythmical movements, such feedback is important for keeping the patterned activity operating properly in the face of unpredictable variations in the environment and in movement production. Furthermore, independent commands from the cerebral cortex can be combined with ongoing patterns generated by CPGs to fluently adjust rhythmical movements to the needs of the animal, such as avoiding obstacles and making turns. Lastly, our deepening understanding of the nervous system's organization for controlling rhythmical movements is crucial for developing clinical strategies to restore such movements in paralyzed individuals.

References

Angeli CA, Boakye M, Morton RA, Vogt J, Benton K, Chen Y, Ferreira CK & Harkema SJ (2018). Recovery of over-ground walking after chronic motor complete spinal cord injury. *New England Journal of Medicine* **379**, 1244–1250.

Arber S (2012). Motor circuits in action: specification, connectivity, and function. *Neuron* **74**, 975–989.

Barbeau H & Rossignol S (1987). Recovery of locomotion after chronic spinalization in the adult cat. *Brain Research* **412**, 84–95.

Brown TG (1911). The intrinsic factors in the act of progression in the mammal. *Proceedings of the Royal Society B* **84**, 308–319.

Brown TG (1914). On the nature of the fundamental activity of the nervous centres; together with an analysis of the conditioning of rhythmic activity in progression, and a theory of the evolution of function in the nervous system. *The Journal of Physiology* **48**, 18–46.

Chau C, Barbeau H & Rossignol S (1998). Effects of intrathecal alpha1- and alpha2-noradrenergic agonists and norepinephrine on locomotion in chronic spinal cats. *Journal of Neurophysiology* **79**, 2941–2963.

Dietz V, Colombo G, Jensen L & Baumgartner L (1995). Locomotor capacity of spinal cord in paraplegic patients. *Annals of Neurology* **37**, 574–582.

Drew T (1991). Visuomotor coordination in locomotion. *Current Opinion in Neurobiology* **1**, 652–657.

Feldman AG (2015). Running away from KGB informers to neuroscience. In: Referent Control of Action and Perception, Challenging Conventional Theories in Behavioral Neuroscience. New York: Springer, pp. 1–11.

Forssberg H & Grillner S (1973). The locomotion of the acute spinal cat injected with clonidine i.v. *Brain Research* **50**, 184–186.

Forssberg H, Grillner S & Halbertsma J (1980). The locomotion of the low spinal cat. I. Coordination within a hindlimb. *Acta Physiologica* **108**, 269–281.

Goulding M (2009). Circuits controlling vertebrate locomotion: Moving in a new direction. *Nature Publishing Group* **10**, 1–12.

Grillner S & Zangger P (1984). The effect of dorsal root transection on the efferent motor pattern in the cat's hindlimb during locomotion. *Acta Physiologica Scandinavica* **120**, 393–405.

Jankowska E, Jukes MGM, Lund S & Lundberg A (1967). The effect of DOPA on the spinal cord 5. Reciprocal organization of pathways transmitting excitatory action to alpha motoneurones of flexors and extensors. *Acta Physiologica Scandinavica* **70**, 369–388.

Kiehn O (2016). Decoding the organization of spinal circuits that control locomotion. *Nature Reviews Neuroscience* **17**, 224–238.

Manabe T, Kaneko S & Kuno M (1989). Disuse-induced enhancement of Ia synaptic transmission in spinal motoneurons of the rat. *Journal of Neurophysiology* **9**, 2455–2461.

Marder E & Bucher D (2007). Understanding circuit dynamics using the stomatogastric nervous system of lobsters and crabs. *Annual Review of Physiology* **69**, 291–316.

McCrea DA & Rybak IA (2008). Organization of mammalian locomotor rhythm and pattern generation. *Brain Research Reviews* **57**, 134–146.

Milner KL & Mogenson GJ (1988). Electrical and chemical activation of the mesencephalic and subthalamic locomotor regions in freely moving rats. *Brain Research* **452**, 273–285.

Murray M & Goldberger ME (1974). Restitution of function and collateral sprouting in the cat spinal cord: The partially hemisected animal. *Journal of Comparative Neurology* **158**, 19–36.

Rossignol S (2000). Locomotion and its recovery after spinal injury. *Current Opinion in Neurobiology* **10**, 708–716.

Rossignol S & Frigon A (2011). Recovery of locomotion after spinal cord injury: Some facts and mechanisms. *Annual Review of Neuroscience* **34**, 413–440.

Severin FV, Orlovsky GN & Shik ML (1967). Work of the muscle receptors during controlled locomotion. *Biophysics* **12**, 575–586.

Sherrington CS (1910). Flexion-reflex of the limb, crossed extension-reflex, and reflex stepping and standing. *Journal of Physiology* **40**, 28–121.

Shik ML, Severin FV & Orlovsky GN (1966). The control of locomotion by means of electrical stimulation of the brain stem. *Biofizika* **11**, 659–666.

Sirota MG & Shik ML (1973). Lokomotsiia koshki pri stimuliatsii srednego mozga [Locomotion of the cat on stimulation of the mesencephalon]. *Fiziol Zh SSSR Im I M Sechenova.* **59**, 1314–1321.

Stuart DG & Hultborn H (2008). Thomas Graham Brown (1882–1965), Anders Lundberg (1920–), and the neural control of stepping. *Brain Research Reviews* **59**, 74–95.

Wang J, Wai Y, Weng Y, Ng K, Huang Y-Z, Ying L, Liu H & Wang C (2009). Functional MRI in the assessment of cortical activation during gait-related imaginary tasks. *Journal of Neural Transmission* **116**, 1087–1092.

Whelan PJ (1997). Control of locomotion in the decerebrate cat. *Progress in Neurobiology* **49**, 481–515.

Wirz M, Colombo G & Dietz V (2001). Long term effects of locomotor training in spinal humans. *Journal of Neurology, Neurosurgery, and Psychiatry* **71**, 93.

Chapter 18

Voluntary Movement and Motor Cortex

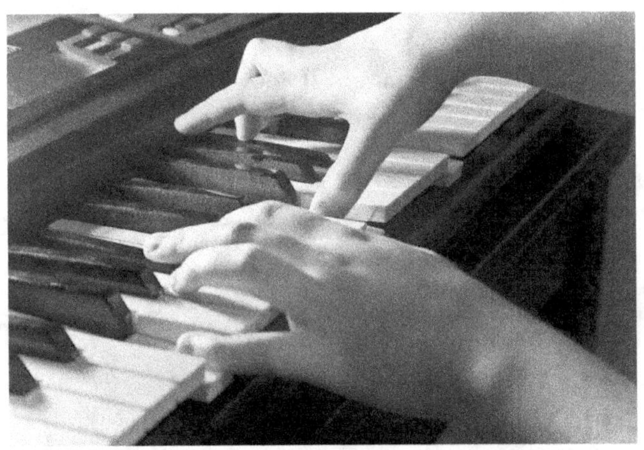

Simply defined, voluntary movements are consciously willed behaviors that involve the cerebral cortex. Probably no aspect of movement neurophysiology has undergone more of an evolution in our understanding than that associated with voluntary movements. One reason for this evolution is the remarkable advances in methods that enable the recording of hundreds of neurons simultaneously in animals performing complex tasks and the manipulation of specific types of neurons through genetic targeting. Yet, in some respects, our concept of how the brain controls voluntary behaviors has gone from a civilized place of relatively straightforward ideas to a wilderness of new, intricate findings that are sometimes difficult to fathom. Perhaps it is only reasonable that control over such awe-inspiring behaviors produced by the concert pianist, prima donna ballerina, professional basketball player, or opera singer (or even the mundane actions of making a coffee, buttoning a shirt, or reciting a poem) would require highly complex coordination among millions of different types of neurons. Nevertheless, some basic discoveries over the past 100 years have provided insight into the framework underpinning the control of voluntary movements. It is these discoveries that are the main (but not exclusive) focus of this chapter.

Sources of Descending Input Driving Voluntary Movements

It is helpful for understanding the control of voluntary movements to consider the topographic organization of motor nuclei in the spinal cord. Figure 1 is a schematic depicting a cross-section through the cervical

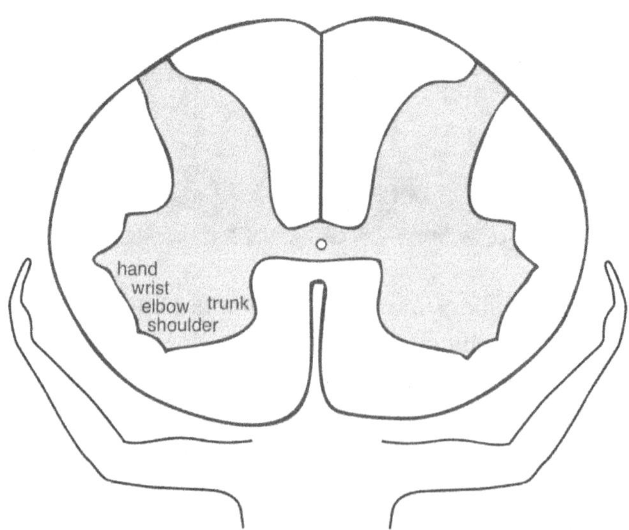

Figure 1.   Topographic arrangement of motor nuclei in the cervical spinal cord. Hand muscle motor nuclei are located most laterally in the ventral horn, whereas trunk muscle nuclei are medial.

spinal cord. Shown in the gray matter of the ventral horn are approximate indications of motor nuclei locations that project to muscles in various parts of the upper limb and trunk. The motor nuclei controlling hand muscles tend to be situated most dorsolateral in the ventral horn. Then, moving ventromedial, motor nuclei are encountered that project to more proximal muscles of the limb. The most medial portion of the ventral horn possesses motor nuclei controlling trunk/axial muscles. The cartoon of the person "holding up" the spinal cord provides an easy-to-remember image of the approximate topographic arrangement of the motor nuclei. (A similar type of topographic organization for the lumbar spinal cord and leg muscles was shown in Chapter 14, Figure 1D.)

The origins of descending pathways that provide input to motor neurons (either directly or through intervening spinal interneurons) underlying voluntary movements arise from two main regions in the brain. One encompasses a variety of cortical areas on either side of the central sulcus (Figure 2). These include Brodmann's areas 6 (premotor area), 4 (primary motor cortex), and the somatosensory cortices (Brodmann's areas 3a, 3b, 1, 2, 5). The other source of descending projections to the spinal cord is the brainstem, mainly from the reticular formation and the vestibular nuclei (Figure 2).

As with the somatosensory system, in which there are two main ascending pathways conveying sensory information to the brain (see Chapter 11), there are two principal descending pathways involved in the control of movement. One, referred to as the **medial pathway** (Figure 3A), *arises from brainstem nuclei, descends primarily in the ventral column of the spinal cord, and largely terminates in the medial aspects of the intermediate and ventral gray matter of the spinal cord.* Two main brainstem regions represent the origins of this pathway: the **vestibular nuclei** (*which integrate information about head motion from the sensory apparatus in the inner ear*) and the **reticular formation** (*the dense interconnected core of the pons and medulla*). Because the medial part of the spinal cord provides excitation to proximal and axial muscles, the medial pathway provides commands needed to maintain upright posture and balance. It is also likely to be involved in integrating body movements and stabilization during whole limb movements, such as might occur during actions like throwing. Furthermore, as discussed in the previous chapter, the reticular

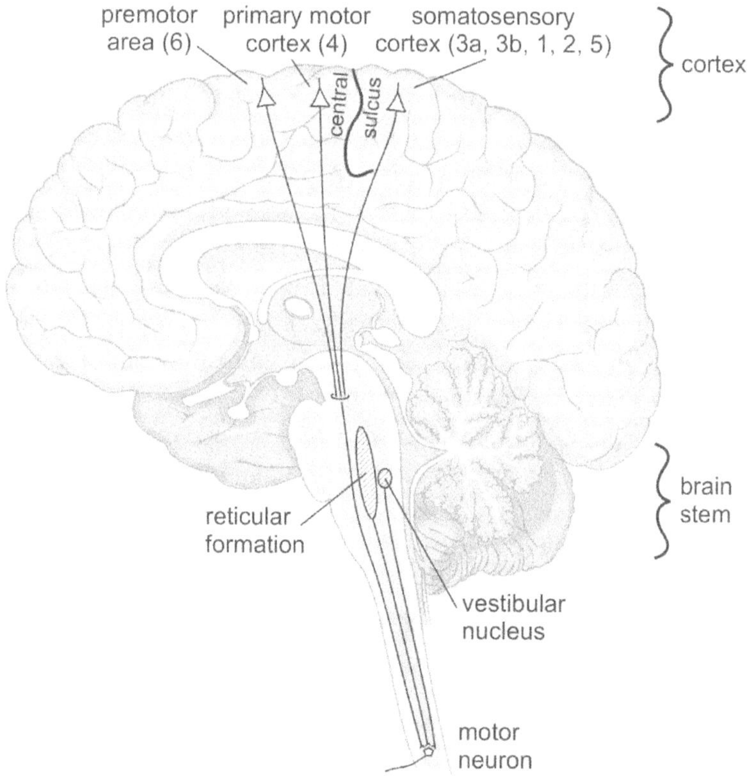

Figure 2.   Two main sources of descending inputs from the brain to motor neurons include those from the cerebral cortex and those from the brain stem. The image only shows the medial portions of the cortex that provide descending inputs. (made using BioRender.com)

formation is the last-order station for activating central pattern generators for locomotion, which likely reside in the medial gray matter of the spinal cord. Thus, the medial pathway is also important for instigating locomotion. Both the vestibular nuclei (Akbarian *et al.* 1994) and the reticular formation (Fregosi *et al.* 2017) receive input from the cerebral cortex (see Figure 3A). Such *cortical inputs to the brainstem* (sometimes referred to as **corticobulbar** projections) may enable some degree of volitional control over the actions of the medial pathway.

The other pathway is referred to as the **lateral pathway** (Figure 3B). *It originates from layer 5 neurons in several regions, including in the*

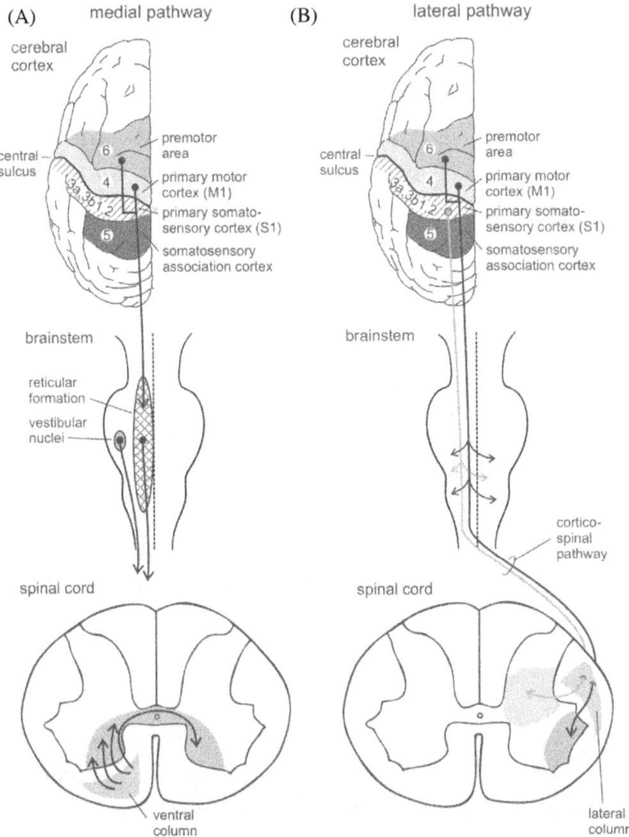

Figure 3.   Descending motor pathways. (A) The medial pathway originates in the vestibular nuclei and reticular formation of the brainstem. Axons descend mainly in the ventral column of the spinal cord to target motor nuclei and interneurons bilaterally in the medial part of the ventral horn and intermediate zone of the spinal cord. This region of the spinal cord controls muscles involved in posture and balance and in instigating locomotion. The brainstem nuclei that give rise to the medial pathway receive input from motor areas of the cerebral cortex. (B) The lateral pathway originates in the primary motor, premotor, primary somatosensory, and area 5 cortical regions. Corticospinal axons descend through the brainstem and cross over to the opposite side at the base of the medulla oblongata. Axon collaterals targeting brainstem structures are given off by some corticospinal axons. In the spinal cord, corticospinal axons are carried in the lateral column. Corticospinal axons from the motor cortex primarily target motor nuclei in the lateral part of the ventral horn that control muscles of the limbs and distal extremities. Corticospinal axons from the somatosensory cortex target interneurons in the dorsal horn and intermediate zone to modulate local circuits and promote presynaptic inhibition to suppress reflexes from interfering with voluntary movement.

primary motor cortex (M1, Brodmann's area 4) just rostral to the central sulcus and the premotor area (Brodmann's area 6), rostral to M1. In addition (perhaps surprisingly), axons from the primary somatosensory cortex (Brodmann's areas 3a, 3b, 1, 2) and the somatosensory association cortex (Brodmann's area 5) also project to the spinal cord and are involved in voluntary movement control. Axons from these cortical regions are bundled together within prominent longitudinal protuberances on the ventral side of the medulla oblongata called the pyramids. As such, *this mass of axons* (~1 million in humans, Lemon 2008) *is sometimes called the* **pyramidal tract** or equivalently the **corticospinal pathway**. Most of these axons (~90%, Lemon 2008) *cross over from one side of the brain to the opposite side of the spinal cord at the base of the medulla oblongata,* at a site called the **pyramidal decussation**. The remaining 10% descend ipsilaterally to the spinal cord. Such ipsilateral projections influence movements on the same side of the body. They may also play an important role in facilitating recovery from unilateral damage to the motor cortex, as occurs with stroke. In addition, corticospinal axons give off collaterals to brainstem structures bilaterally (Figure 3B, middle) (Keizer & Kuypers 1989).

The lateral pathway descends in the lateral column of the spinal cord (Figure 3B). The axons of this pathway terminate in two main regions: in the lateral part of the ventral horn (where motor nuclei controlling muscles of the limb/hand/foot are located) and in the more intermediate and dorsal regions of the spinal cord. The projections to the lateral part of the ventral horn primarily originate from the primary motor cortex (M1). Indeed, in higher primates (including humans), many of these axons make direct excitatory synapses onto motor neurons. Such direct connections from the motor cortex to motor neurons do not exist in low primates or other mammals. It is thought that direct connections facilitate independent and flexible control over individual muscles. These direct connections are particularly prominent for motor nuclei of hand muscles (Buys *et al.* 1986), enabling humans (and some other high primates) to perform exquisitely complex and discrete movements of the fingers.

The other set of corticospinal projections largely terminate in the intermediate region and dorsal horn of the spinal cord (Figure 3B). These arise, in large part, from the somatosensory cortex (Coulter & Jones 1977).

This region of the spinal cord contains interneurons that are part of spinal reflex circuits and those that mediate presynaptic inhibition. Therefore, as discussed in Chapter 16, it seems likely that an important function of the corticospinal projections from the *somatosensory* cortex is to suppress reflexes that otherwise would tend to interfere with the elaboration of voluntary movements (Lemon 2008; Moreno-Lopez *et al.* 2021).

The different roles of the medial and lateral pathways were strikingly demonstrated in a set of lesion experiments carried out by Donald Lawrence and Henricus Kuypers in the 1960s. Monkeys with lesions to the medial pathway showed severe postural deficits, inability to sit upright, impaired proximal limb movements, and disability in locomotion (Lawrence & Kuypers 1968a). However, when these animals were supported in a seated position, they could skillfully remove morsels of food from small holes using independent movements of their fingers. In contrast, following surgery that lesioned the lateral (corticospinal) pathway in monkeys, "there was an immediate ability to sit with the head up and to stand, walk, run and climb ... Yet during this early post-operative phase they were apparently unable to use their extremities, especially their hands, independently of total body movements. Thus, although they could not pick up food with their hands, they could use them in clinging to the cages and in climbing" (Lawrence & Kuypers 1968b).

It should be mentioned that there is another descending pathway, the **rubrospinal pathway**, that has features of both the medial and lateral pathways. Like the medial pathway, *it arises in the brainstem—in a nucleus of the midbrain called the red nucleus ("rubro" means red). Like the lateral pathway, it descends together with corticospinal axons in the lateral column and tends to target the more lateral aspects of the ventral horn*. Interestingly, however, the rubrospinal pathway seems to be relatively sparse in humans (Nathan & Smith 1982; Yang *et al.* 2011). It may be that the expansion of the motor cortex and the corticospinal pathways in humans has largely supplanted the role of the rubrospinal tract.

Topography of the Primary Motor Cortex

The main contributor to the lateral pathway is from axons arising in the primary motor cortex (M1). Early work using electrical stimulation of the brain demonstrated that the strip of cortex just rostral to the central sulcus (i.e., Brodmann's area 4) can evoke different types of movements. Movements could also be produced by stimulating in the more rostral premotor area (Brodmann's area 6), but substantially larger stimulus intensities were needed. Leyton & Sherrington (1917) carried out an extensive investigation of the types of movements produced using threshold stimulation (minimal current needed to just elicit a movement) in M1 of various types of apes. Figure 4A shows a summary of the movements evoked at different sites along M1 in the anesthetized gorilla. In general, moving laterally and ventrally from the midline across the convexity of M1, stimulation produced movements of the leg, arm, hand, and face/mouth/tongue. Movements were mostly produced in body parts contralateral to the stimulation site. *Eye movements were produced by stimulating sites quite rostral to the primary motor cortex, in a region called the* **frontal eye fields** (labeled "EYE" in Figure 4A). In this case, both eyes moved in a coordinated manner, typically directed toward the opposite side of stimulation.

As mentioned in Chapter 12, Sherrington's trainee, Wilder Penfield adopted similar procedures for identifying sites in the cortex that provoke epileptic seizures in human patients. When stimulating just rostral to the central sulcus, a variety of movements in the patients were documented. Based on work performed on hundreds of patients, Penfield and Rasmussen (1952) summarized the organization of the motor cortex as a

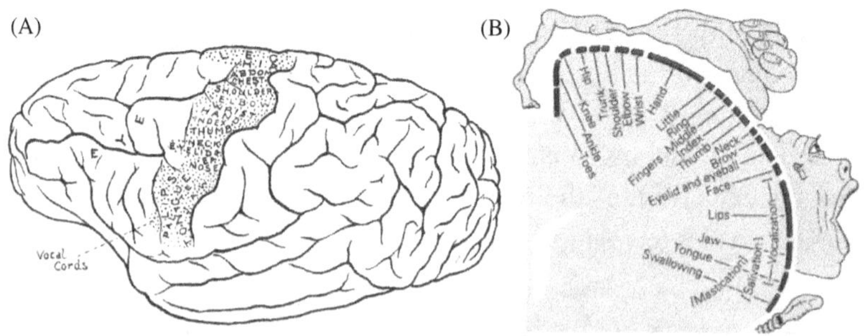

Figure 4.   Topographic representation of movements evoked by electrical stimulation of the primary motor cortex. (A) in the gorilla and (B) in man. ([A] adapted from Leyton and Sherrington [1917], [B] adapted from Penfield and Rasmussen [1952].)

homunculus, not unlike that done for the somatosensory cortex. This iconic image (Figure 4B) sets forth a clear representation of the motor cortex as one in which separate regions are dedicated to controlling different parts of the body.

Based on such an organization, it seemed reasonable to assume that if one wished to move the index finger, for example, then its associated region of M1 would need to be activated. This, in turn, would engage motor nuclei in the spinal cord innervating index finger muscles to move that finger. Likewise, to move the thumb, its dedicated region of M1 would need to be engaged. To move the finger and the thumb together, say as occurs during the precision grip, then both index and thumb M1 regions would need to be enlisted in unison. In some respects, therefore, M1 was considered like a keyboard, wherein complex movements could be created by the particular sequence and combinations of "keys" played. Accordingly, a pervasive idea in clinical neuroscience is that M1 neurons are "upper motor neurons"—keys to be struck that actuate designated movements.

Evidence Challenging Somatotopy of M1

Despite its appealing simplicity, many concepts about M1 function derived from considerations of the motor homunculus (Figure 4B) are unlikely to be correct. Indeed, evidence of something unusual in the spatial organization of M1 can be found in the works of both Sherrington and Penfield. Leyton and Sherrington (1917) reported that the responses to stimulation of M1 in anesthetized animals were highly labile. For example, they "observed that a cortex point which ordinarily evoked as its primary response flexion of the elbow would evoke, when stimulated next and soon after a distant point giving adduction of thumb". Such functional instability is not readily accounted for in a homuncular representation of M1.

More tellingly are findings presented in the original publication of Penfield and Boldrey (1937) describing the results of cerebral cortex stimulation in human patients. For example, a map depicting the sites of stimulation that evoked movements of the fingers did not have segregated regions for each finger. Instead, all the fingers and thumb sites were fully

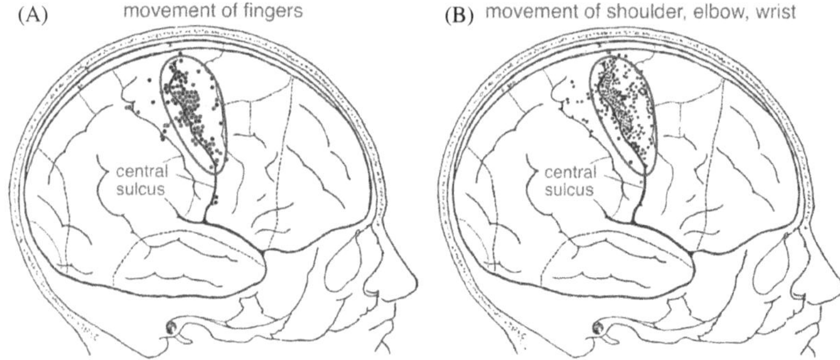

Figure 5.   (A) Sites evoking movements of the fingers and (B) movements of the shoulder, elbow, or wrist in response to electrical stimulation in patients undergoing surgery for intractable epilepsy. The oval enclosing most response sites is placed over the same brain region in A and B. (A from Figure 12 and B from Figure 14 in Penfield and Boldrey [1937].)

intermingled across a wide expanse of M1, extending from the "shoulder" to the "face" regions on the homunculus (Figure 5A). Furthermore, more sites were indicated that caused movements of all fingers together than of individual digits. Moreover, the figure in Penfield and Boldrey (1937) depicting the region of M1 from which finger movements could be evoked (Figure 5A) almost perfectly overlaps the region from which movements of the shoulder, elbow, and wrist were elicited (Figure 5B). Penfield and Boldrey made only one small comment about this overlap, namely: "from practically the same general cortical area as that from which we have already reported finger movements, there appear those of the hand, arm and shoulder." Inexplicably, however, no mention was made of this striking incompatibility with the concept of the motor homunculus in the widely cited book summarizing Penfield's studies (Penfield & Rasmussen 1952).

Since the publication of that book, the concept of a clearly delineated motor homunculus has made its way into neurology and neuroscience textbooks. Nevertheless, a scattering of neuroanatomical (Shinoda *et al.* 1981), electrophysiological (Andersen *et al.* 1975; Schieber & Hibbard 1993), and imaging (Remy *et al.* 1994; Sanes *et al.* 1995) studies presented results incompatible with partition of the motor cortex into distinct subregions.

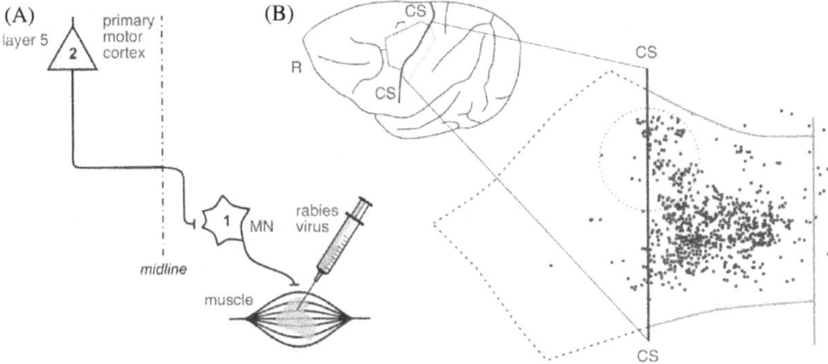

Figure 6.   Rabies-virus labeled identification of motor cortical neurons projecting to hand muscle motor nucleus in the monkey. (A) Injection of rabies virus into target hand muscle. Virus first infects motor neurons (1) making synaptic contact onto injected muscle. The virus then infects layer 5 cortical neurons (2) that make synaptic contact with infected motor neurons. (B) The top panel shows a lateral view of the monkey brain (CS—central sulcus, R—rostral). The dashed section is the region highlighted in the "flattened" portion of the cortex shown to the right. Dots indicate layer 5 neurons infected with the virus, and therefore, are corticospinal neurons that made direct contact with motor neurons supplying the injected muscle. Portion to the right of the vertical line is along the bank of the central sulcus. (Adapted from Rathelot and Strick [2006].)

The strongest evidence against a strictly homuncular view of the motor cortex has come from the laboratory of Peter Strick involving trans-synaptic labeling of neurons using rabies virus (Rathelot & Strick 2006). As shown in Figure 6A, the virus was injected into a target muscle (in this case, a diminutive muscle controlling movements of the thumb in a monkey). The virus replicates and crosses the neuromuscular junction to infect the motor axons innervating the muscle. The virus is then transported in a retrograde (backward) fashion up the axon to infect the soma and dendrites of the motor neurons within the motor nucleus. The virus then infects the axons, making synapses onto the motor neurons. The virus then again retrogradely travels up the axons to infect the somas of the last order neurons (such as layer 5 neurons in M1), contacting the motor neurons that control the targeted muscle. Each stage of infection takes a certain period of time. Accordingly, the animals were sacrificed after a time period associated with two stages of infection. Infected cells were then identified by examining thin sections of the brain under the microscope.

What Rathelot and Strick (2003) found was astonishing: infected cortical neurons in layer 5 of M1 were found distributed over a wide expanse of M1 (Figure 6B). Instead of a tightly clustered band of neurons within a narrow region of M1 (as predicted by the motor homunculus), the cortical neurons controlling an individual muscle were practically spread over the entirety of the "arm/hand" region of the M1. Similar experiments involving other muscles revealed equivalent arrangements with extensive intermingling of the locations of cortical neurons supplying various muscles of the upper limb. Thus, M1 seems less organized as a homunculus than as a pointillistic painting with intermingled dots (neurons) of various colors (target muscles). The general regions controlling the face/head, arm/hand, and leg/foot, however, are more-or-less separated. Nevertheless, the sharply delineated and distinct areas representing even minute body parts in the primary somatosensory cortex (e.g., see Chapter 12, Figure 8) are not a feature of the primary motor cortex.

And lastly in this regard, there is an additional feature of M1 organization that should be considered. Namely, the extent to which corticospinal axons diverge to contact multiple motor nuclei. Shinoda *et al.* (1981) addressed this issue by performing an exceptionally difficult experiment involving the injection of a labeling substance into single corticospinal axons in monkeys. Reconstruction and identification of the terminations of those axons in the spinal cord was possible in only a few cases. Nevertheless, what they found was clear: single axons arising from the motor cortex projected to multiple motor nuclei. For example, Figure 7 shows terminations of a single corticospinal axon onto motor neurons in at least four different motor nuclei of the cervical spinal cord. Therefore, instead of single corticospinal neurons controlling particular muscles, this finding suggested that such neurons would tend to enlist the activities of multiple muscles together. Indeed, electrophysiological studies have shown that individual neurons in the motor cortex frequently facilitate more than one muscle (Fetz & Cheney 1980), including proximal and distal muscles together (McKiernan *et al.* 1998). In some cases, corticospinal axons directly facilitate certain sets of muscles while simultaneously (through inhibitory spinal interneurons) suppress other muscles (Cheney *et al.* 1985). Motor nuclei that control intrinsic finger muscles acting on individual digits, however, seem to have relatively independent inputs (Buys *et al.* 1986). Presumably, such segregated input enables high

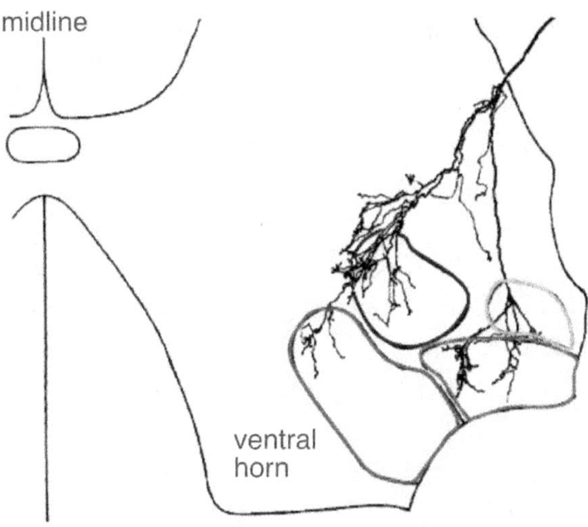

Figure 7.   Reconstruction of terminations of single corticospinal axon in the spinal cord of a monkey. Oval areas indicate different motor nuclei supplying separate muscles. (Adapted from Shinoda *et al.* [1981].)

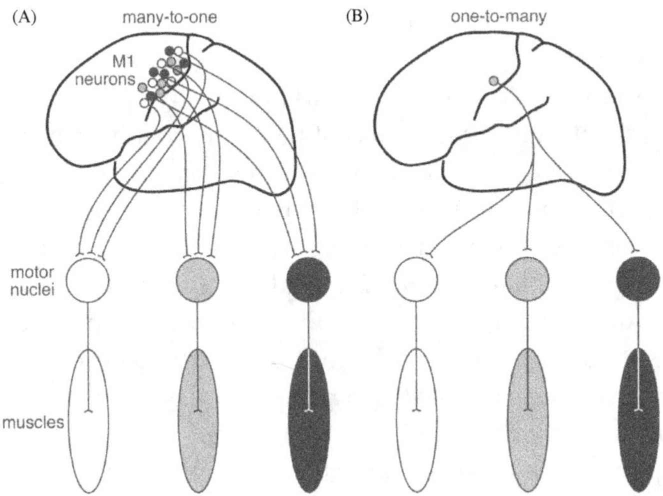

Figure 8.   Output arrangement of motor cortex. (A) Corticospinal neurons that project to a particular motor nucleus are broadly distributed across the arm/hand region of primary motor cortex and intermingle with corticospinal neurons projecting to other motor nuclei. Such an arrangement can be considered as "many (locations)-to-one." (B) Individual corticospinal neurons may diverge to contact multiple motor nuclei, thereby possessing a "one-to-many" configuration.

primates (including humans) to exert fine-grained control over individual fingers.

Figure 8 is a schematic that summarizes the complex output organization of the primary motor cortex. First, other than broad regions supplying the leg, arm, and head, there is little topographic organization within M1. Individual corticospinal neurons supplying a particular motor nucleus can be distributed over a wide expanse of M1 and are intermingled with neurons supplying other muscles (Figure 8A). This can be considered a kind of "many (locations)-to-one" organization, with corticospinal neurons from many different sites in M1 converging upon a single motor nucleus.

At the same time, there also exists a "one-to-many" arrangement (Figure 8B), such that single corticospinal neurons can project to multiple motor nuclei. It may be that the specific patterns of connectivity across motor nuclei might partially underlie the assemblage of muscles into synergistic groups needed to generate elemental movements that are the building blocks of the behavioral repertoire of an animal (Hockensmith *et al.* 2005; Schieber 1990). For example, when reaching for an object, many muscles are co-activated, controlling the shoulder, elbow, wrist, and fingers. Such co-activity even occurs for simple finger movements. As a case in point, Wood Jones (1941) originally observed that when extending the thumb by the actions of the extensor pollicis brevis (EPB) muscle, there is robust, synchronized activation of the extensor carpi ulnaris (ECU) (Figure 9). But why would a wrist extensor muscle be activated when extending the thumb? This is because EPB not only extends the thumb but also tilts the hand toward the thumb side (radial deviation of the hand). To prevent that unwanted action, the ECU is concurrently engaged because it tends to tilt the hand in the opposite direction (ulnar deviation), thereby counteracting the radial deviation torque produced by EPB. Collectively, therefore, there may exist certain corticospinal neurons that simultaneously enlist the activities of multiple muscles needed for a voluntary action based on their synaptic connections across multiple motor nuclei. The degree to which such "hard-wired" coordination of muscles is implemented in voluntary movements, however, is not presently known.

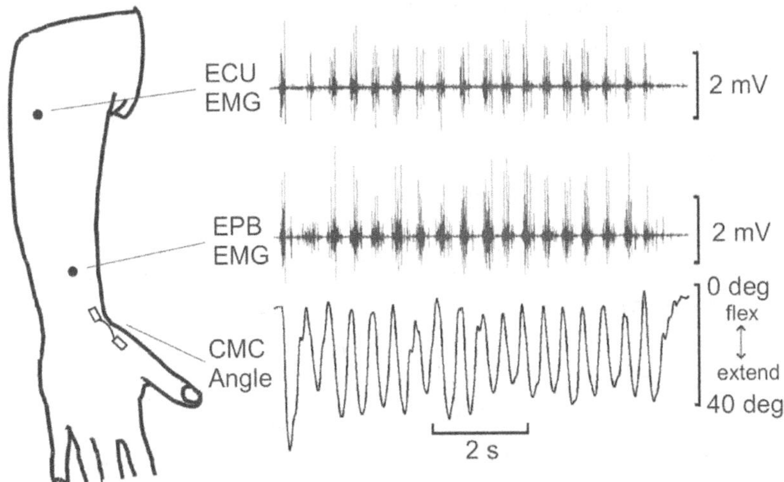

Figure 9.   Electromyographic (EMG) activity recorded from extensor pollicis brevis (EPB) and from extensor carpi ulnaris (ECU) during repeated extension-flexion movements of the carpometacarpal (CMC) joint of the thumb. EMG signals were recorded with intramuscular electrodes inserted into the sites indicated on the drawing of the arm. Joint angle was detected with a transducer taped in place over the CMC joint of the thumb. Each burst of EPB activity was accompanied by activity in ECU. (from the author's laboratory.)

Representation of Muscle Activity by Individual Corticospinal Neurons

Regardless of the spatial configuration of neurons in the motor cortex, what does the spiking activity of individual neurons in M1 correspond to in terms of movement? Edward Evarts at the National Institutes of Health in the United States was one of the first investigators to address this question systematically. To do so, he helped pioneer a new method to enable the recording of activity from individual neurons in awake, behaving animals. This method involved surgically *removing a small piece of the skull* while the animal was anesthetized and then surrounding the opening (a **craniotomy**) with a protective chamber that could be hermetically sealed. Following recovery from surgery, the chamber could be opened, and thin microelectrodes inserted directly into the brain to record activities from a few neurons near the tip of the electrode while the animal performed various types of previously trained motor tasks. Because the brain does not possess pain receptors, this type of recording caused the animal no discomfort. Furthermore, after each experimental session, the chamber could be sealed to protect the craniotomy from infection. In this way, a single animal could be tested repeatedly without discomfort for long periods of time.

One prescient issue addressed by Evarts had to do with whether M1 neural activity is directly associated with muscle activity or may be related to more abstract features of a motor behavior such as movement direction. This question is difficult to address because movement direction is almost always directly related to which muscles are activated. So how could one distinguish muscles from movements in association with recorded M1 activity? Evarts developed a clever protocol to differentiate between these two possibilities (Evarts 1968). A monkey was trained to move a lever by flexing the wrist from an extended wrist position. Using a pulley system, loads of different weights could be added to alter the wrist torque (and associated flexor muscle activity) required to move the lever (Figure 10A). In a separate configuration, the load could be added on the opposite side of the lever such that the load itself would pull the wrist from the extended to the target flexed position (Figure 10B). In this case, flexor muscle activity was not required to perform the task—instead, wrist extensor muscle activity was needed (in an eccentric or lengthening contraction) to control the rotation of the wrist from the starting extended position to the target flexed position. In both cases, the movement direction (wrist flexion) was the same, but the muscles activated were different.

Evarts then recorded the firing of neurons in the primary motor cortex while the monkey performed both types of the task. It is of crucial importance to point out that Evarts did not just record from any type of neuron in the motor cortex. He specifically targeted M1 neurons that send axons to the pyramidal tract, that is, corticospinal neurons originating in layer 5 of the cortex. How did Evarts "know" that he was recording from layer 5 neurons and not from neurons in other layers? He first tested each recorded neuron by stimulating the corticospinal pathway with an electrode placed in the pyramid of the medulla oblongata. A single high-intensity stimulation pulse triggered a single action potential in most of

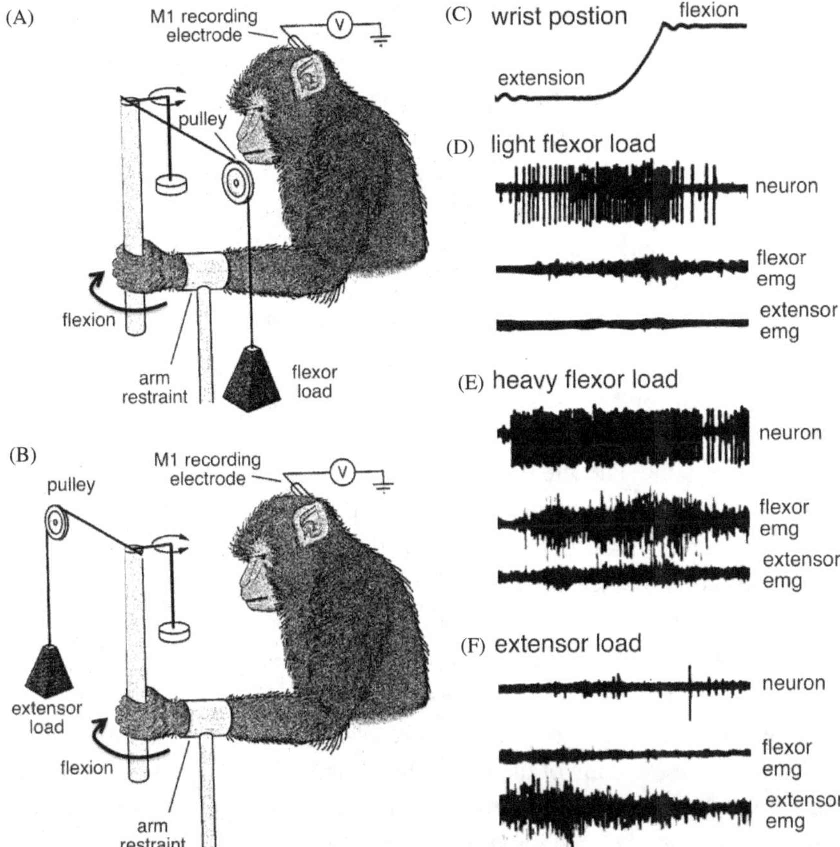

Figure 10.   Experiment to distinguish the role of corticospinal neurons in the encoding of muscle activity or limb movements. (A) A monkey was trained to flex its wrist with varying flexor loads while spiking activities of identified corticospinal neurons were recorded. (B) Modification of task involving a load opposing extension (but promoting flexion) of the wrist. In this case, the monkey needed to activate wrist extensor muscles in lengthening contractions to control wrist flexion. (C) Example angular displacement of the wrist that occurred during the tasks. The bottom position of the trace occurred when the wrist was fully extended, while the top position occurred with the wrist fully flexed. (D) Corticospinal neuron activity during wrist flexion with light flexion load. Also shown are EMG signals from wrist flexors and extensors. (E) Same as for (D) but with heavier flexion load, showing increased corticospinal neuron and flexor EMG activities. (F) Under extensor load (but for the same movement), little activity in the same neuron shown in panels (D) and (E), with minimal flexor muscle EMG but substantial activity in extensor muscle. ([A] adapted from Kandel *et al.* [2012], [C–F] from Evarts [1966].)

the corticospinal axons. Those action potentials, instigated midway along the axons, not only traveled to the spinal cord but also *traveled "backwards"* (**antidromically**) along the axon up to the soma. If the cortical neuron recorded in M1 responded with an action potential linked to the stimulation of the pyramid, then Evarts reasonably concluded that the neuron was a corticospinal neuron in layer 5.

Figure 10C shows an example wrist flexion movement performed by the monkey during these tasks. The movement was more or less the same under the different conditions. Figure 10D shows the activity of an identified pyramidal tract M1 neuron recorded during the wrist flexion task with a light load. The spiking of this neuron accelerated just prior to wrist flexion and slightly led the EMG activity of the wrist flexor muscle responsible for the movement. The same neuron is shown in Figure 10E for the same task but with a heavier load. In this case, spiking was much more intense and was paralleled by greater EMG activity in the wrist flexor muscle needed to move the heavier load. However, when the load was placed on the opposite side of the wrist such that the load itself pulled the wrist to the target flexed position (Figure 10B), little activity was recorded in the M1 neuron (Figure 10F). In this situation, negligible EMG activity was detected in the wrist flexor, but strong activity was seen in the wrist extensor while it controlled the lowering of the load. Therefore, even though the movement and movement directions were the same (wrist flexion), the neuron seemed to be active only when the wrist flexor muscles were involved.

Most of the pyramidal tract neurons recorded by Evarts that were active during wrist flexion responded in this way. Therefore, Evarts concluded that the firing rates of pyramidal tract (layer 5 corticospinal) neurons in M1 code for the intensity of muscle contraction (and associated muscle force) needed to perform various tasks. While this may seem an expected finding, as will be discussed next, there are M1 neurons that seem to do the opposite, code for movements and not necessarily muscle activity.

M1 Neurons Coding Movement Direction

When you ponder reaching for an object, like a coffee cup, your conscious awareness is of the direction you need to move your hand to reach the cup, not which muscles need to be activated nor how the joints of the arm must rotate to accomplish the task. Likewise, when you move a cursor from one location to another on a computer screen using a mouse, your mental attention is on the trajectory of the cursor on a vertically oriented monitor and not necessarily on the horizontal motions of your hand holding the mouse. Could activity in primary motor cortex be partially responsible for the abstract cognitive process of representing desired movements (even of objects that are not part of our body, like a computer cursor) rather than of the muscle activities needed to make the movements?

As mentioned in the context of Evarts' work above, it is difficult to dissociate muscle activities from the movements they produce. However, some clever experimental protocols (like Evarts') have been used to separate movements from the muscles involved while recording the activity of neurons in the motor cortex. For example, Shen and Alexander (1997) trained monkeys to move a cursor from a center position on a computer screen to one of four targets using a long joystick. In the standard joystick configuration, moving the cursor to a target on the right side of the screen required moving the joystick to the right (Figure 11A). Such rightward movements of the arm involved activity of the brachialis muscle with little participation of the deltoid (right side, Figure 11A). Likewise, to move the cursor upward to a target at the top of the screen required a forward movement of the joystick.

In a separate configuration, monkeys performed the task with the joystick rotated 90 degrees. In this case, to move the cursor on the screen to the right required that the monkey pull back on the joystick (Figure 11B). This different arm movement was accomplished with strong activity in the deltoid and minimal activity in the brachialis (Figure 11B, right). Such a rotated configuration is similar to that required to control movements of a cursor on a computer screen when the mouse is rotated 90 degrees from the way it is typically held. The monkeys learned both configurations of the task such that their ability to hit the targets was similar for both.

Figure 12 shows the activity of a typical neuron recorded in M1 during both these configurations. Figure 12A shows the movements of the hand for several repeat trials when the target was on the right side of the screen under the standard joystick configuration. Across the different target directions (not shown), this particular situation elicited the greatest

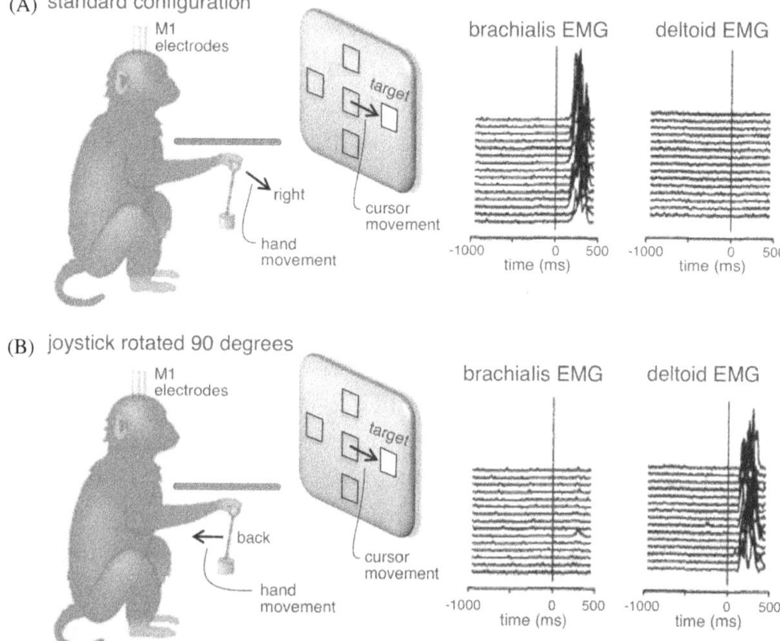

Figure 11.   Experiment evaluating encoding of movement direction in motor cortical neurons. (A) Monkey was trained to move the cursor from the center of a computer screen to illuminated targets using a long joystick. During the task, motor cortical and muscle activities were recorded. Traces in the right panel show several trials of EMG activity recorded from the brachialis and deltoid during the rightward movements of the hand toward the target on the right of the screen. Time 0 indicates the display of the target. (B) In a separate version of the task, the monkey moved the joystick to capture targets displayed on screen with the cursor, but in this case, the joystick was rotated 90 degrees from the standard configuration. As such, to move the cursor to the right required that the monkey pull back on the joystick. Such a motion of the hand involved a different pattern of muscle activation (right panel) compared to that for the standard configuration. (Adapted from Shen and Alexander [1997].)

activity in the neuron (Figure 12A, right). The vertical dashed line indicates when the target was displayed, which was soon followed by strong spiking in this neuron. Figure 12B shows the movements of the hand in the rotated joystick configuration. Under this 90-degree rotated condition, to hit the target at the top of the screen with the cursor required

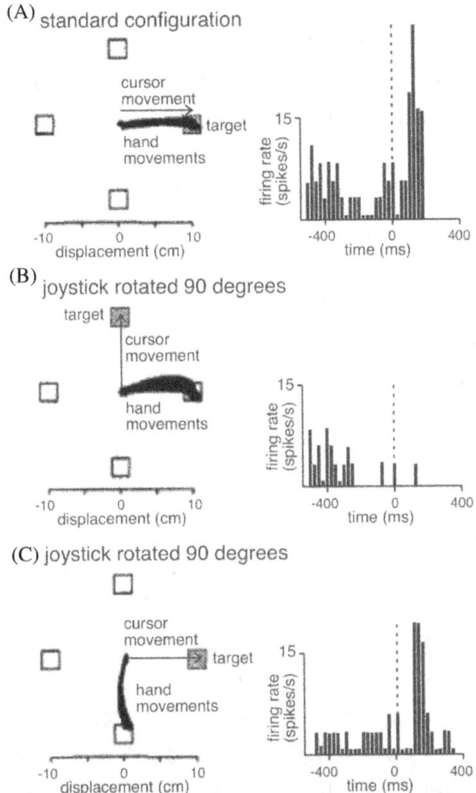

Figure 12. Motor cortical activity associated with movement of cursor on computer screen and not hand movements or muscle activity. (A) Left—repeated trials showing hand trajectories superimposed on a layout of the computer screen associated with movements of the cursor to the right target using the standard joystick configuration. Right—peristimulus time histogram (PSTH—see Figure 13 for description) for one motor cortical neuron that showed robust activation during this task. Time 0 indicates the time of target display. (B) Same as for (A) except with the joystick rotated. In this case, the target was at the top of the screen, requiring the same hand movements as for that shown in (A). However, in this case, there was little activity of the neuron (PSTH on the right). (C) situation for which the target was on the right side of the screen involving rightward movements of the cursor. Because of the rotated joystick, such movements of the cursor required backward movements of the hand on the joystick. Despite the different movements of the hand as compared to (A), activity in the neuron was again robust. (Adapted from Shen and Alexander [1997].)

rightward movements of the hand. As such, the movements of the hand in this situation were practically identical to that as shown in Figure 12A for the standard configuration. Yet, there was little activity in this M1 neuron under this circumstance (Figure 12B, right). Importantly, in the joystick-rotated configuration, and in trials for which the target was on the right side of the screen (Figure 12C), neural activity was again robust even though hand movements were entirely different from that shown in Figure 12A.

Therefore, it appears as though this neuron was representing rightward movements of the *cursor* independently of how those cursor movements were enacted. Over half of the M1 neurons recorded by Shen and Alexander (1997) exhibited this property, namely, of seeming to encode movement direction of the task-relevant effector (in this case, the cursor) and not which muscles or limb movements were involved. A similar finding using a different ingenious method to dissociate movements from the muscles involved was reported by Kakei *et al.* (1999). It is important to point out that in neither the Alexander and Shen (1997) nor the Kakei *et al.* (1999) studies were the M1 neurons identified (as Evarts had done) in terms of the cortical layers in which they were situated. Therefore, it seems likely that many of the ~30% of neurons recorded in M1 that responded to the muscles activated and not effector movements (Kakei *et al.* 1999) could have been layer 5 corticospinal neurons.

Confronting Complexity in the Organization of the Motor Cortex

As highlighted by the findings described above, the motor cortex is not a homogenous entity involved only in sending commands to drive muscles. Indeed, it is important to keep in mind just how complex the motor cortex is (or other cortical regions for that matter). There are millions of neurons in the primate motor cortex. Each of these neurons receives on the order of ten thousand synaptic contacts from other neurons, and each neuron in turn may send synaptic contacts to hundreds of other neurons.

To illustrate this complexity (but still in a highly simplified way), we can borrow the architecture of connections among artificial neurons used in

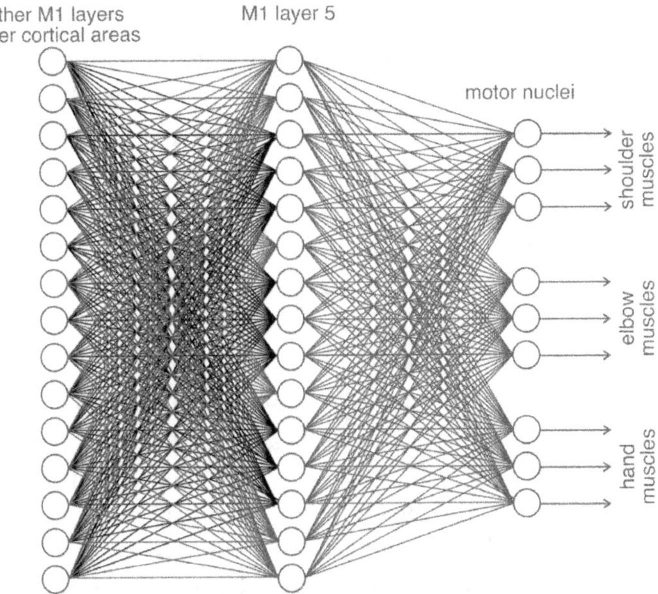

Figure 13.   Representation of the motor cortex like an artificial neural network. The left layer shows many neurons (spheres) in other cortical regions and within the motor cortex connecting to many neurons in the output layer (layer 5) of the primary motor cortex (M1). The output of layer 5 is too many spinal interneurons (not shown) and motor nuclei, which in turn project to muscles of the shoulder, elbow, and wrist/hand.

artificial neural networks (Figure 13). Each line represents a synaptic connection from a neuron at a "higher" level (on the left) to a neuron at a "lower" level (on the right). This in itself is simplified because many real *neurons also connect to other neurons at the same level with axon collaterals* (called **recurrent connections**). Because there is little question that the main output entity of the motor cortex comprises layer 5 corticospinal neurons, it has been represented as a distinct layer in the network of Figure 13. In keeping with the organization of corticospinal neurons indicated in Figure 8, output neurons from many different locations in M1 are shown to converge upon single motor nuclei ("many-to-one") and an individual layer 5 neuron in M1 is shown to project to many motor nuclei ("one-to-many").

The motor nuclei shown are for those controlling different joints of the shoulder, elbow, and hand. The spheres representing each motor nucleus would contain a few hundred motor neurons innervating a particular muscle. As described in Chapter 14, the motor neurons within a sphere (a motor nucleus) would receive similar synaptic inputs and are activated largely based on the dictates of the Size Principle.

The inputs to M1 layer 5 neurons arise from other layers in M1 and from other cortical regions (discussed in Chapter 19). It is important to point out that the strength of each input (synapse) from one neuron to any of the others it contacts can vary markedly.

In artificial intelligence applications, this type of architecture proves extremely powerful in performing highly complex tasks. This is accomplished by having the network attempt to perform a desired task and then compare what was produced by the network to what was intended. The error is then used to adjust the synaptic strengths. This process of trial, error, and synaptic adjustments is performed repeatedly until the network, through the plastic changes in synaptic strengths, learns to perform the task. This process not only enables the network to perform the tasks on which it was trained, but to perform a wide range of similar tasks with good accuracy for which it has no previous experience.

The parallels between artificial and real neural networks were explicitly built-in when the original artificial neural networks were designed (e.g., Hopfield & Tank 1986). Thus, the general organization of the network shown in Figure 13 is probably not an unreasonable starting representation of the motor cortex. Indeed, such an architecture was used to predict, with good fidelity, that patterns of activities of ~30 arm muscles during a wide range of complex movements (Hasse *et al.* 2022). In some respects, that artificial network functioned like a motor cortex. Namely, given the intention to move the hand along some path or to some location, the network computed, moment-by-moment the associated activities of the muscles needed to accomplish the task.

It should be said that data scientists and machine-learning experts put little emphasis on the behavior of individual artificial neurons. Instead, the power of artificial intelligence derives from the collective action of widespread, large-scale, plastic interconnections among many simple units. Individual elements in an artificial neural network can display a wide range of responses that, by themselves, are difficult to reconcile in the context of the desired or produced action. Similarly, individual neurons from a recorded population of neurons in the motor cortex may exhibit diverse firing-rate behaviors that have no straightforward relation to the movement (Sussillo *et al.* 2015). Yet, exquisitely controlled voluntary movements emerge from the broadly distributed and interconnected activities of thousands of motor cortical neurons. Thus, it seems important to focus attention in neurophysiological studies on the performance of neural populations.

Neural Population Analyses

One of the earliest attempts to consider neural populations as a whole, rather than cataloguing firing activities of individual neurons, was that carried out by Donald Humphrey and colleagues at the NIH in the United States (Humphrey *et al.* 1970). They used multiple electrodes to record activities from several M1 neurons simultaneously in monkeys performing a simple task. Individual neurons showed a wide range of firing patterns that were oftentimes not reliably related to any particular movement variable (e.g., muscle activity, movement direction). However, when their firing rates were combined in simple mathematical ways, prediction of a variety of movement parameters could be made with good accuracy from the same set of neurons. This suggests that information about many aspects of a movement is broadly represented in the activities of large numbers of motor cortical neurons.

Another group that significantly advanced the idea of neural population coding was led by Apostolos Georgopoulos at Johns Hopkins University. They recorded hundreds of neurons in the motor cortex while monkeys made repeated arm reaches from a center start position to one of eight radially displaced targets (Figure 14A). During a single reach to *one* of the targets, a typical M1 neuron showed increased activity ~150 ms after the target was illuminated (Figure 14B). This activity was then sustained for another ~150 ms prior to movement onset and then dissipated soon after. When the spike times of the neuron were registered with respect to movement onset (indicated as time = 0 ms) for repeated reaches to a specific target, it was evident that the neuron exhibited similar responses for each trial (Figure 14C, bottom).

The type of plot in Figure 14C (bottom) *displaying spike times for repeated trials of the same behavior or sensory input, aligned to a*

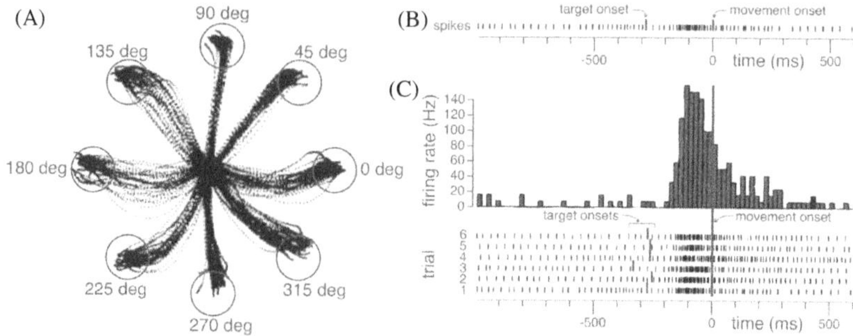

Figure 14.   (A) Hand trajectories of monkey reaching from center position to 8 radially displaced targets in the horizontal plane. (B) Example of spiking (tick marks) of one motor cortical neuron during a reach to one of the targets. Time 0 is used to indicate the onset of movement. (C) Peri-stimulus time histogram (PSTH) showing firing rates averaged over 20 ms bins for six trials (bottom) of reaches to the same target. For this PSTH, the average number of spikes/bins that occurred before the stimulus was presented (i.e., the baseline) was subtracted from the average number of spikes/bins in all bins to obtain the response (firing rate) above baseline. (Adapted from Georgopoulos *et al.* [1982].)

particular event, and then "stacked" above one another is referred to as a **raster plot**. The averaged response across trials can be obtained by counting up the total number of spikes across trials occurring in successive time bins (e.g., 20 ms bins in Figure 14C) and dividing by the number of trials. This average count can then be divided by the duration of the bin to get the firing rate. The *resulting histogram* (Figure 14C, top) *is called a* **peri-stimulus time histogram (PSTH)**, so called because it *shows the response of the neuron around the time (both before and after, i.e., "peri") that the stimulus was presented, or behavior instigated.*

Figure 15A shows rasters for a single neuron obtained across eight movement directions. For this neuron, one can discern that spiking activity was generally stronger (i.e., the density of spikes was greater) when the monkey made movements toward the left (i.e., 180 degrees) while weaker for movements to the right (0 degrees). Georgopoulos and colleagues calculated the average firing rate over a time window from target onset to the end of the movement and then plotted those values for each movement direction (Figure 15B). Those data were then fitted with a sinusoidal curve. The movement direction associated with *peak* firing rate based on this curve was called the preferred direction (PD) of movement (dashed

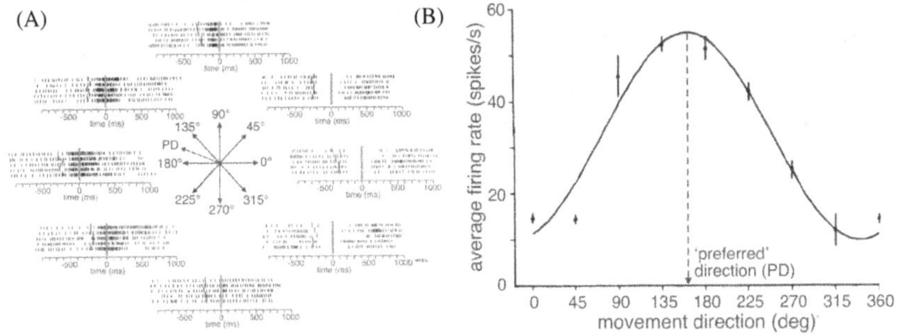

Figure 15.   (A) Rasters indicating firing of a single motor cortical neuron during repeated reaches to targets in eight different directions. Time 0 indicates the onset of reach. Longer tick marks around −300 ms indicate times of target display. (B) Plot of the firing rates of the neuron shown in (A) averaged over the time from target onset to movement end for each movement direction. Short vertical lines are standard errors of the mean. Data are fit with a sinusoidal curve. The movement direction associated with peak firing rate (estimated from the curve) was designated as the neuron's preferred direction (PD). (Adapted from Georgopoulos *et al.* [1982].)

line, Figure 15B) for that neuron. For this M1 neuron, the PD was at about 170 degrees. A dashed arrow showing the PD is also indicated in Figure 15A. When this process was repeated for the ~600 motor cortical neurons recorded in monkeys during the center-out reach task (Figure 14A), about 40% exhibited responses like that shown in Figure 15, with each of these neurons having distinct PDs (Georgopoulos *et al.* 1982).

Because of the broad "tuning" of individual neurons (i.e., neurons are active over a wide range of movement directions, just not at the PD), many neurons (probably tens of thousands) will be active during a movement in a given direction. Georgopoulos and colleagues reasoned that the collective action of the entire array of active neurons must somehow prescribe the impending movements of the limb. To understand how this might come about, these investigators proposed that each neuron "votes" for the upcoming movement to be in *its* PD only. The strength of a neuron's vote is directly related to the firing rate of the neuron. The votes of all active neurons are tallied up to determine the overall direction that the movement will follow.

To formalize this idea both mathematically and graphically, the activity of each neuron was represented as a vector (keeping in mind that a vector has both magnitude and direction). These vectors always pointed in the PD for each neuron. For example, Figure 16A shows the PDs for three pretend neurons (n1, n2, n3). Then, the length of each vector is scaled based on how close the PD of the neuron is to the impending movement

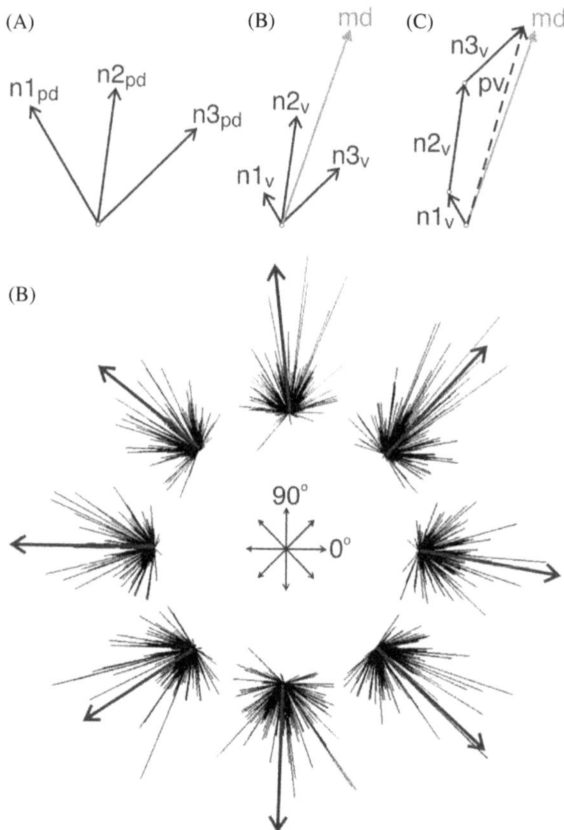

Figure 16.   Population vector analysis. (A) Arrows represent preferred directions (pd) for three theoretical neurons, n1, n2, n3. (B) Dark arrows indicate individual neuron vectors (v) that point in each neuron's preferred direction. The length of the vector represents the firing rate of a neuron associated with a particular movement direction (md). The closer the movement direction is to a neuron's preferred direction, the longer the length of the neuron vector. (C) The population vector (pv) is the vector sum of all individual neuron vectors. The population vector (based on neural activity) points in a direction similar to the actual movement. (D) Individual vectors (thin lines) for 241 neurons recorded in monkeys during reaches in eight directions. The arrows indicate the population vectors computed based on the individual neuron vectors. Those population vectors closely align with the eight movement directions (center). ([D] adapted from Georgopoulos [1988].)

direction (*md*, Figure 16B). For example, the PD of neuron 2 is quite close to that of the movement direction, so its length has only been modestly reduced (Figure 16B) compared to its nominal length (Figure 16A). On the other hand, the length of neuron 1's vector has been greatly reduced because its PD is far from (nearly 90 degrees away) the movement direction.

The tallying of the votes is then conceptualized as performing vector summation among all the active neurons. Graphically, vector summation is performed by successively placing the tail of one vector to the tip of the preceding one (Figure 16C). The sum is the vector (called the population vector, *pv*) that points from the base of the first neural vector to the tip of the last (dashed line, Figure 16C). In this simple schematic (Figure 16C), the population vector points close to the direction of the intended movement direction.

When Georgopoulos and colleagues used this approach on the few hundred motor cortical neurons from which they could identify PDs, the results were striking. The calculated population vector (shown as solid arrows in Figure 16D) closely pointed in the direction of the eight different movements that monkeys made. The starbursts of lines at the bases of the population vectors indicate the individual vectors for each of the 241 M1 neurons from which the population vectors were determined. Keep in mind that while the orientation of each neural vector remains the same for all movements, the lengths (firing rates) of those vectors can change markedly based on the angular distance between the PD and movement direction. On the whole, this work demonstrated how the combined actions of populations of cortical neurons can precisely represent the desired actions to be performed.

The population vectors shown for the eight movement directions in Figure 16D were computed based on neural activity averaged over entire movement trials. There is no reason, however, as to why population vectors cannot be computed on much finer time scales. When this was done in successive 20-ms time windows during a reach in a particular direction, an array of population vectors was produced (Figure 17A). Following the display of a target at 45 degrees, population vectors started to emerge about 100 ms later. For this reach, the orientations of the vectors were more or less the same and in the direction of the target throughout the reach. The changes in lengths of the population vectors are thought to represent changes in the speed of movement along the direction indicated

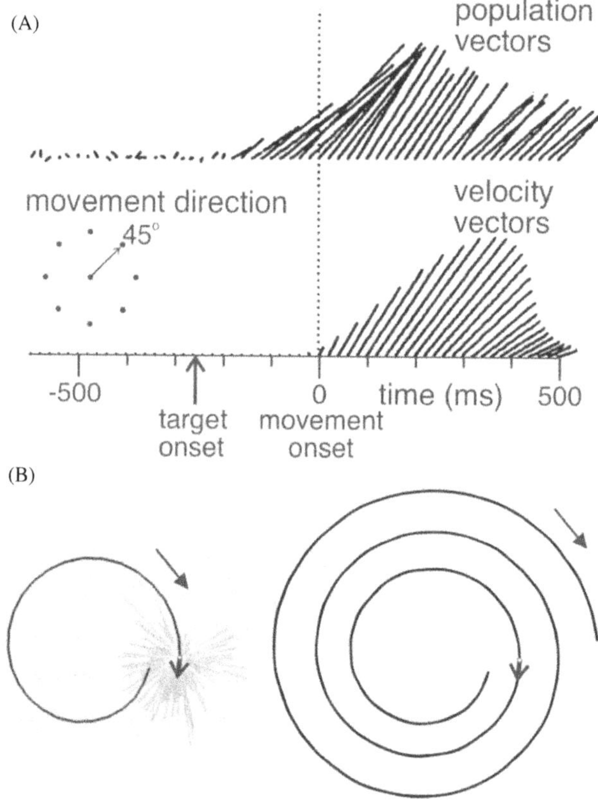

Figure 17.   Temporal evolution of population vectors. (A) Population vectors computed every 20 ms (top) from the activities of motor cortical neurons for a movement to a target at 45 degrees (inset). The base of each vector indicates the time point at which the vector was calculated. The different lengths of the vectors are related to variations in the intensity of neural activity at different times. The bottom set of vectors indicate the velocity of the hand at different time points. Note that the neural population vectors point roughly in the same direction as the movement and lead movement by about 200 ms. (B) Left—set of population vectors (shown as small dark line segments) computed in brief time windows and placed tail to head based on motor cortical recordings made while a monkey traced an inside-out spiral (direction indicated by large arrow) with his finger. At the moment shown, the last population vector in the sequence up to that point is shown as a small arrow. The starburst of light lines indicates the individual neuron vectors at that time point. Right— entire population vector trajectory. ([A] adapted from Georgopoulos [1988], [B] adapted from Schwartz [2007] [left] and Moran and Schwartz [1999] [right].)

by the vector. Indeed, with a lag of about 150–200 ms, the movements of the hand (indicated by the velocity vectors in Figure 17A, bottom) roughly parallel that of the neural population vectors. For example, peak hand velocity occurred midway along the duration of the reach, which was preceded 150–200 ms earlier by the peak lengths of the population vectors. The exact nature of these relatively long delays (at least in neural terms) is not completely understood, but likely relates to processing times needed to engage downstream brainstem and spinal circuits and delays associated with relatively long conduction distances from brain to muscle.

When reaching for an object, the hand typically follows a straight-line trajectory to the object. As such, the velocity and population vectors shown in Figure 17A maintained roughly the same orientations through-out the reach. However, many movements possess complex trajectories, such as those made during drawing. Andrew Schwartz (who trained with Georgopoulos and is now at the University of Pittsburgh) and his students taught monkeys to trace out complex figures displayed on a touch screen with their fingers. They applied population vector analysis to the activities of >300 motor cortex neurons recorded while monkeys made the tracing movements. At brief time intervals, population vectors were computed with the tail of each vector aligned to the tip of the previous one to gener-ate a population vector trajectory. Figure 17B (left side) shows a popula-tion vector (small arrow) computed based on the summation of many individual neural vectors (starburst) at one point in time while a monkey made a center-out spiral tracing. The right side of Figure 17B shows the complete spiral, drawn entirely from computations derived from the activities of neural populations. Its fidelity to the actual movements made by the monkey's finger was remarkable.

Brain–Machine Interfaces

One way to consider the results of the neural population analysis shown in Figure 17 is that it *predicts* what the monkey will do ~150 ms before the monkey does it. In some respects, this idea was the basis of the devel-opment of **brain–machine interfaces (BMIs)**. In a BMI, *activity recorded from many neurons with arrays of implanted microelectrodes are* *processed with an algorithm (like population vector analysis) that predicts intended behavior. Such predictions are then used to control, in real time, a device like a computer or robotic arm (Figure 18A). The development and utility of BMIs were first demonstrated in rats and monkeys in*

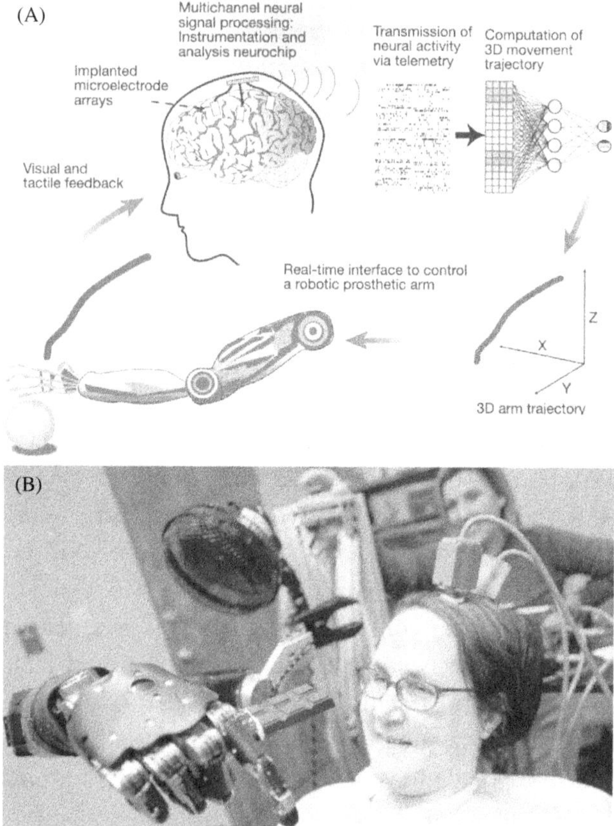

Figure 18.   Brain–machine interfaces (BMIs). (A) schematic depicting stages of a BMI to enable a paralyzed individual to control a robotic arm. The activities of populations of neurons recorded from the cerebral cortex with implanted microelectrodes are deciphered in real time using algorithms to extract the movement intention of the subject (e.g., 3D arm trajectory). The identified trajectory is then used to control the motion of a robotic arm. Visual feedback and artificial somatosensory (including tactile) feedback help shape appropriate cortical commands. (B) Image of paralyzed subject controlling robotic arm to feed herself based on neural activity recorded from her brain. The blocks on the skull hold electronics for processing signals detected with microelectrode arrays in the brain. ([A] adapted from Nicolelis [2001], [B] credit University of Pittsburgh Medical Center.)

the early 2000s by a number of investigators (e.g., Chapin *et al.* 1999; Taylor *et al.* 2002; Velliste *et al.* 2008; Wessberg *et al.* 2000). In 2012–2013, John Donoghue and colleagues at Brown University (Hochberg *et al.* 2012) and Andrew Schwartz and colleagues (Collinger *et al.* 2013) implanted BMIs in the motor cortex of human patients paralyzed from the neck down (Figure 18B). Targets placed in various locations were first presented to the patients while they imagined using their arms to reach the targets, and the activities of many neurons were recorded simultaneously. The firing rates of the recorded neurons were used to predict the direction the patient desired to reach and grasping actions in real time. Over a period of a few months, during which the algorithms were refined, the performance of the patients controlling the robotic arms improved steadily and allowed them to perform basic activities important for daily living, vividly illustrated by one subject feeding herself a bar of chocolate based entirely on brain control of the robotic arm (Figure 18B).

Summary

There are two main pathways by which commands from the brain are conveyed to the spinal machinery that engages muscles to produce motor behaviors: (1) the medial pathway, which originates from nuclei in the brainstem and acts on spinal circuits and motor neurons in the medial aspects of the spinal gray matter involved in posture, balance, and locomotion, and (2) the lateral or corticospinal pathway, which descends from layer 5 neurons in the cerebral cortex to target neurons mainly in the lateral regions of the ventral spinal cord that control movements of the limbs, hands, and fingers. The main source of axons in the corticospinal pathway is from the primary motor cortex (M1). Surprisingly, there is little clear-cut topographic organization within the main subdivisions (leg, arm/hand, head) of M1. Indeed, cortical neurons projecting to individual spinal motor nuclei are distributed across a wide expanse of M1 and are intermingled with neurons projecting to other motor nuclei. In addition, the axons of individual corticospinal neurons may diverge to contact multiple motor nuclei.

The spiking activity of layer 5 (corticospinal) neurons seems to encode the intensity of muscle activation. However, the activities of neurons in other layers of M1 can represent quite complex and abstract features of desired movements, such as the trajectory of an effector (like that of a cursor on a computer screen) independently of the muscles involved. Insight as to how such a vast and widely interconnected system as the motor cortex control movements has been gained by considering the collective action of a large population of neurons. Such approaches not only deepen our knowledge about this still mysterious entity but can also be leveraged to identify movement intentions and drive devices to aid paralyzed individuals.

References

Akbarian S, Grüsser O & Guldin WO (1994). Corticofugal connections between the cerebral cortex and brainstem vestibular nuclei in the macaque monkey. *The Journal of Comparative Neurology* **339**, 421–437.

Andersen P, Hagan PJ, Phillips CG & Powell TP (1975). Mapping by micro-stimulation of overlapping projections from area 4 to motor units of the baboon's hand. *Proceedings of the Royal Society B: Biological Sciences* **188**, 31–36.

Buys EJ, Lemon RN, Mantel GW & Muir RB (1986). Selective facilitation of different hand muscles by single corticospinal neurones in the conscious monkey. *The Journal of Physiology* **381**, 529–549.

Chapin JK, Moxon KA, Markowitz RS & Nicolelis MAL (1999). Real-time control of a robot arm using simultaneously recorded neurons in the motor cortex. *Nature Reviews Neuroscience* **2**, 664–670.

Cheney PD, Fetz EE & Palmer SS (1985). Patterns of facilitation and suppression of antagonist forelimb muscles from motor cortex sites in the awake monkey. *Journal of Neurophysiology* **53**, 805–820.

Collinger JL, Wodlinger B, Downey JE, Wang W, Tyler-Kabara EC, Weber DJ, McMorland AJC, Velliste M, Boninger ML & Schwartz AB (2013). High-performance neuroprosthetic control by an individual with tetraplegia. *Lancet* **381**, 557–564.

Coulter JD & Jones EG (1977). Differential distribution of corticospinal projections from individual cytoarchitectonic fields in the monkey. *Brain Research* **129**, 335–340.

Evarts EV (1968). Relation of pyramidal tract activity to force exerted during voluntary movement. *Journal of Neurophysiology* **31**, 14–27.

Fetz EE & Cheney PD (1980). Postspike facilitation of forelimb muscle activity by primate corticomotoneuronal cells. *Journal of Neurophysiology* **44**, 751–772.

Fregosi M, Contestabile A, Hamadjida A & Rouiller EM (2017). Corticobulbar projections from distinct motor cortical areas to the reticular formation in macaque monkeys. *European Journal of Neuroscience* **45**, 1379–1395.

Georgopoulos AP (1988). Neural integration of movement: Role of motor cortex in reaching. *The FASEB Journal* **2**, 2849–2857.

Georgopoulos AP, Kalaska JF, Caminiti R & Massey JT (1982). On the relations between the direction of two-dimensional arm movements and cell discharge in primate motor cortex. *Journal of Neuroscience* **2**, 1527–1537.

Hasse BA, Sheets DEG, Holly NL, Gothard KM & Fuglevand AJ (2022). Restoration of complex movement in the paralyzed upper limb. *Journal of Neural Engineering* **19**, 046002.

Hochberg LR, Bacher D, Jarosiewicz B, Masse NY, Simeral JD, Vogel J, Haddadin S, Liu J, Cash SS, van der Smagt P & Donoghue JP (2012). Reach and grasp by people with tetraplegia using a neurally controlled robotic arm. *Nature* **485**, 372–375.

Hockensmith GB, Lowell SY & Fuglevand AJ (2005). Common input across motor nuclei mediating precision grip in humans. *Journal of Neuroscience* **25**, 4560–4564.

Hopfield JJ & Tank DW (1986). Computing with neural circuits: A model. *Science* **233**, 625–633.

Humphrey DR, Schmidt EM & Thompson WD (1970). Predicting measures of motor performance from multiple cortical spike trains. *Science* **170**, 758–762.

Kakei S, Hoffman DS & Strick PL (1999). Muscle and movement representations in the primary motor cortex. *Science* **285**, 2136–2139.

Kandel ER, Schwartz JH, Jessell TM, Siegelbaum SA & Hudspeth AJ (2012). Principles of Neural Science (5th Edition). McGraw-Hill.

Keizer K & Kuypers HGJM (1989). Distribution of corticospinal neurons with collaterals to the lower brain stem reticular formation in monkey (*Macaca fascicularis*). *Experimental Brain Research* **74**, 311–318.

Lawrence DG & Kuypers HGJM (1968a). The functional organization of the motor system in the monkey: II. The effects of lesions of the descending brain-stem pathways. *Brain* **91**, 15–36.

Lawrence DG & Kuypers HGJM (1968b). The functional organization of the motor system in the monkey: I. The effects of bilateral pyramidal lesions. *Brain* **91**, 1–14.

Lemon RN (2008). Descending pathways in motor control. *Annual Review of Neuroscience* **31**, 195–218.

Leyton ASF & Sherrington CS (1917). Observations on the excitable cortex of the chimpanzee, orang-utan, and gorilla. *Quarterly Journal of Experimental Physiology* **11**, 135–222.

McKiernan BJ, Marcario JK, Karrer JH & Cheney PD (1998). Corticomotoneuronal postspike effects in shoulder, elbow, wrist, digit, and intrinsic hand muscles during a reach and prehension task. *Journal of Neurophysiology* **80**, 1961–1980.

Moran DW & Schwartz AB (1999). Motor cortical activity during drawing movements: Population representation during spiral tracing. *Journal of Neurophysiology* **82**, 2693–2704.

Moreno-Lopez Y, Bichara C, Delbecq G, Isope P & Cordero-Erausquin M (2021). The corticospinal tract primarily modulates sensory inputs in the mouse lumbar cord. *Elife* **10**, e65304.

Nathan PW & Smith MC (1982). The rubrospinal and central tegmental tracts in man. *Brain* **105**, 223–269.

Nicolelis MA (2001). Actions from thoughts. *Nature* **409**, 403–407.

Nicolelis MAL & Lebedev MA (2009). Principles of Neural Ensemble Physiology Underlying the Operation of Brain–Machine Interfaces. Nature Publishing Group, pp. 1–11.

Penfield W & Boldrey E (1937). Somatic motor and sensory representation in the cerebral cortex of man as studied by electrical stimulation. *Brain* **60**, 389–443.

Penfield W & Rasmussen T (1952). The Cerebral Cortex of Man. New York: Macmillan.

Rathelot J-A & Strick PL (2006). Muscle representation in the macaque motor cortex: An anatomical perspective. *Proceedings of the National Academy of Sciences of the United States of America* **103**, 8257–8262.

Remy P, Zilbovicius M, Leroy-Willig A, Syrota A & Samson Y (1994). Movement- and task-related activations of motor cortical areas: A positron emission tomographic study. *Annals of Neurology* **36**, 19–26.

Sanes JN, Donoghue JP, Thangaraj V, Edelman RR & Warach S (1995). Shared neural substrates controlling hand movements in human motor cortex. *Science* **268**, 1775–1777.

Schieber MH (1990). How might the motor cortex individuate movements? *Trends Neuroscience* **13**, 440–445.

Schieber MH & Hibbard LS (1993). How somatotopic is the motor cortex hand area? *Science* **261**, 489–492.

Schwartz AB (2007). Useful signals from motor cortex. *The Journal of Physiology* **579**, 581–601.

Shen L & Alexander GE (1997). Neural correlates of a spatial sensory-to-motor transformation in primary motor cortex. *Journal of Neurophysiology* **77**, 1171–1194.

Shinoda Y, Yokota J-I & Futami T (1981). Divergent projection of individual corticospinal axons to motoneurons of multiple muscles in the monkey. *Neuroscience Letters* **23**, 7–12.

Sussillo D, Churchland MM, Kaufman MT & Shenoy KV (2015). A neural network that finds a naturalistic solution for the production of muscle activity. *Nature Neuroscience* **18**, 1025–1033.

Taylor DM, Tillery SIH & Schwartz AB (2002). Direct cortical control of 3D neuroprosthetic devices. *Science* **296**, 1829–1832.

Velliste M, Perel S, Spalding MC, Whitford AS & Schwartz AB (2008). Cortical control of a prosthetic arm for self-feeding. *Nature* **453**, 1098–1101.

Wessberg J, Stambaugh CR, Kralik JD, Beck PD, Laubach M, Chapin JK, Kim J, Biggs SJ, Srinivasan MA & Nicolelis MA (2000). Real-time prediction of hand trajectory by ensembles of cortical neurons in primates. *Nature* **408**, 361–365.

Wood Jones F (1941). The Principles of Anatomy as Seen in the Hand. Baltimore, MD: Williams & Wilkins.

Yang H-S, Kwon HG, Hong JH, Hong CP & Jang SH (2011). The rubrospinal tract in the human brain: Diffusion tensor imaging study. *Neuroscience Letters* **504**, 45–48.

Chapter 19

Inputs to Motor Cortex

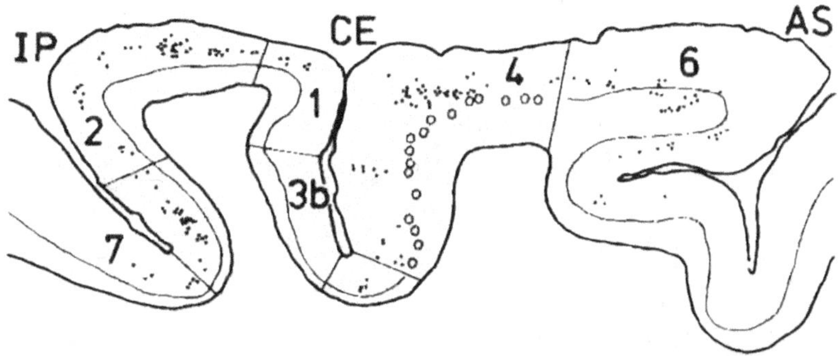

Cortical inputs to primary motor cortex. Sagittal section (80 μm thick) passing through frontal and parietal lobes on either side of the central sulcus (CE) of a monkey. Retrograde label was injected into a small area of primary motor cortex (M1, Brodmann's area 4) about 1 mm lateral to this section. Labeled neurons that project into that area of M1 are shown as dots. Circles indicate corticospinal neurons in layer 5 of M1 that had axon collaterals in the injected region of M1. Shown from left to right (caudal to rostral) are Brodmann's areas 7, 5 (not labeled), 2, 1, 3b, 3a (not labeled), 4, and 6. IP—intraparietal sulcus, AS—arcuate sulcus. (Adapted from Ghosh et al. [1987].)

In Chapter 18, the organization and operations of the primary motor cortex were outlined. Yet the primary motor cortex is not a self-contained entity that generates myriad voluntary behaviors on its own. Instead, the primary motor cortex (M1) receives convergent inputs from a wide array of sources that underlie the formation of motor commands that issue from M1. In this chapter, some of the main inputs to M1 will be described.

Somatosensory Afferent Input to M1

At first glance, it may seem surprising that many neurons in M1 possess somatosensory receptive fields similar to those in primary somatosensory cortex. Figure 1 shows example somatosensory receptive fields of neurons recorded in a monkey along two electrode tracks in M1

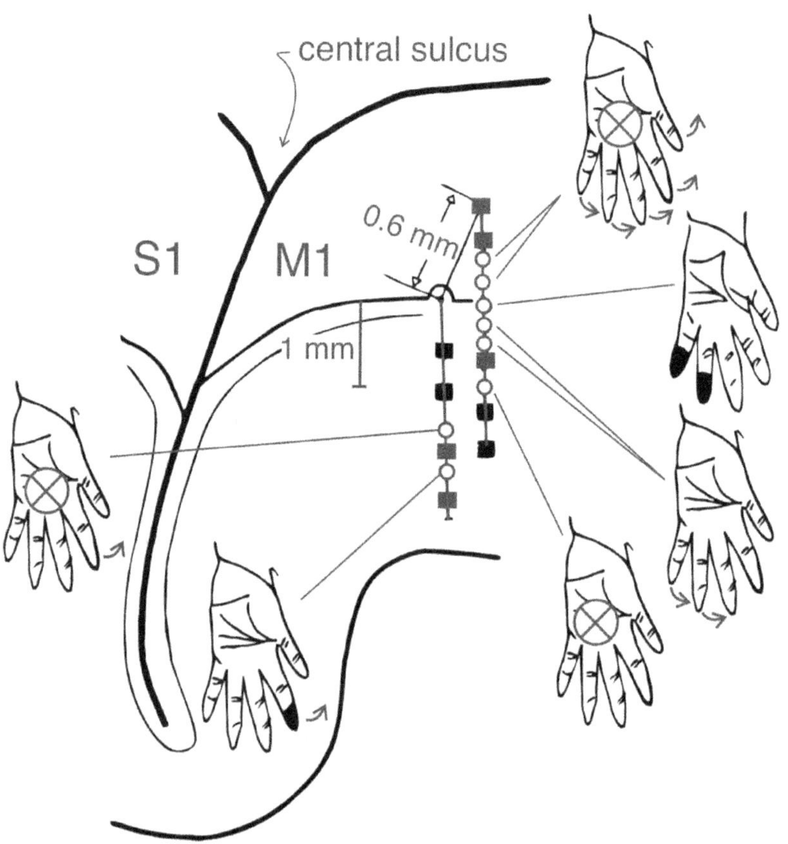

Figure 1.   Somatosensory receptive fields in primary motor cortex (M1). Electrode tracts (vertical lines) through M1. Open circles indicate recording sites at which movements (curved arrows), tactile input (black areas), or pressure (circle with X) applied to the contralateral hand elicited spiking responses in M1 neurons. Black squares indicate sites at which receptive fields were not identified. Electrical stimulation along these pathways evoked finger movements. S1—primary somatosensory cortex. (Adapted from Rosén and Asanuma [1972].)

(Rosén & Asanuma 1972). The sites indicated with open circles show locations where sensory receptive fields were identified. Along the leftmost track, the most superficial of such sites responded to deep pressure (represented by a circle with an X through it) applied to the hand. The other site on this track responded to tactile stimuli (brushing of the skin) applied to the tip of the index finger (blackened area) and to passive extension of the index finger (curved arrow). Along the other track, six sites responded to somatosensory stimuli, including two sites that responded to deep pressure and extension of all fingers, one that responded to tactile stimuli of distal segments of the ring and little fingers, two that responded to extension of the ring and little fingers, and one that responded to just deep pressure applied to the hand. The sites that responded to the extension of the fingers likely were activated by sensory receptors stretched by the stimulus, such as muscle spindles in finger flexor muscles. Deep pressure stimuli likely activated receptors in finger flexor muscles whose tendons pass through the palm of the hand. It is important to note that electrical stimulation along these two pathways mostly caused flexion or extension of the fingers. Therefore, the sensory inputs to this region of M1 were coherent with the actions that would be caused by output from this region.

Of 257 neurons tested by Roger Lemon and Robert Porter (1976) in the hand/arm region of M1 in monkeys, 210 had clear somatosensory receptive fields arising from the contralateral arm. Most of these responded to movements in one direction only of the shoulder, elbow, wrist, or fingers, or palpation of muscles—all likely arising from activation of proprioceptors. Only 10% of the neurons responded to tactile stimulation (light touch), and generally these had small receptive fields (like shown in Figure 1). Collectively, such findings indicate that M1 receives rich somatosensory input providing detailed information about the configuration and movements of body parts needed by M1 to organize commands associated with voluntary motor behaviors.

In general, there could be two sources of such somatosensory input to M1: from the somatosensory cortex or more directly from somatosensory afferents via the dorsal column pathway and thalamus (see Figure 1, Chapter 11). This issue has long been debated. There is no doubt that M1 receives rich input from the thalamus but much of that is from the cerebellum and basal ganglia (Kievit & Kuypers 1977; Strick 1976) (as will be discussed in the next two chapters).

In addition, there is good evidence of significant input to M1 directly from the somatosensory thalamus. This evidence involved recording from thalamic neurons that were shown to receive short latency excitatory inputs from somatosensory afferents (tactile and proprioceptive) (Horne & Tracey 1979; Lemon & van der Burg 1979). It was also shown that these same neurons were excited antidromically (backwards traveling action potentials) by stimulation in M1, indicating that their axons projected into M1. Furthermore, it was found that these same neurons could *not* be driven antidromically by stimulating in primary somatosensory cortex (S1). Therefore, it seems likely that two separate populations of neurons in the thalamus transmit information from tactile and proprioceptive afferents to M1: one indirectly through S1 and another directly to M1 (Figure 2). More recent findings using sophisticated anatomical and electrophysiological methods have confirmed the existence of such direct inputs to the motor cortex from the sensory thalamus (Hooks *et al.* 2013).

Cortical Inputs to M1

The primary motor cortex also receives a rich array of inputs from other cortical regions. The frontispiece at the beginning of this chapter shows one ultrathin slice of cortex indicating neurons within that slice that project to primary motor cortex (Brodmann's area 4). Those neurons reside in Brodmann's areas 7, 5, primary somatosensory cortex, and Brodmann's area 6. Figure 3 depicts schematically the main *cortical* connections into M1. As mentioned above, one source of input to M1 is from the primary somatosensory cortex (Ghosh et al. 1987; Jones et al. 1978). Such input provides additional and more highly processed somatosensory information than that supplied more directly from the thalamus (Figure 2). Interestingly, little of the input from S1 derives from the tactile region Brodmann's area 3b. This does not mean, however, that M1 receives little cortically processed tactile information because Brodmann's area 1, like area 3b, also processes tactile signals and has extensive inputs to M1.

The most extensive inputs to M1 arise from *Brodmann's area 6* (Ghosh et al. 1987), *just rostral to M1 and called the* **premotor cortex**.

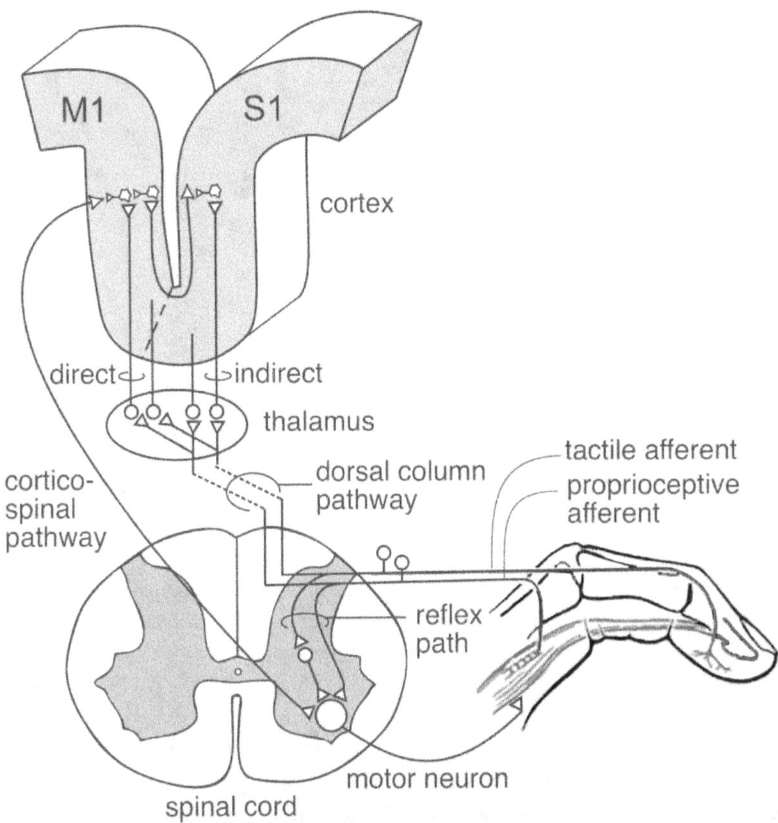

Figure 2.   Schematic showing somatosensory input to motor cortex. Tactile and proprioceptive (e.g., muscle spindle) afferents project into the spinal cord and ascend to the dorsal column nuclei (not shown) along the dorsal column pathway. Projections from dorsal column nuclei cross over to contact two sets of neurons in the thalamus. One set ascends to various subregions of the primary somatosensory cortex (S1), and the other directly to primary motor cortex (M1). Projections from S1 indirectly relay sensory information to M1. Corticospinal output from layer 5 pyramidal cells in M1 can excite motor neurons that activate muscles operating on the body part from which sensory input arises. Motor neurons also receive input more directly from spinal collaterals of somatosensory afferents that underlie reflexes. (Adapted from Asanuma [1981] and Kandel *et al.* [2012].)

The premotor cortex has two main subdivisions, *a more dorsal medial region called the* **supplemental motor area (SMA)** and a *more lateral region referred to as the* **lateral premotor cortex (LPMC)** (Figure 3). Both of these regions are generally considered to be involved in organizing

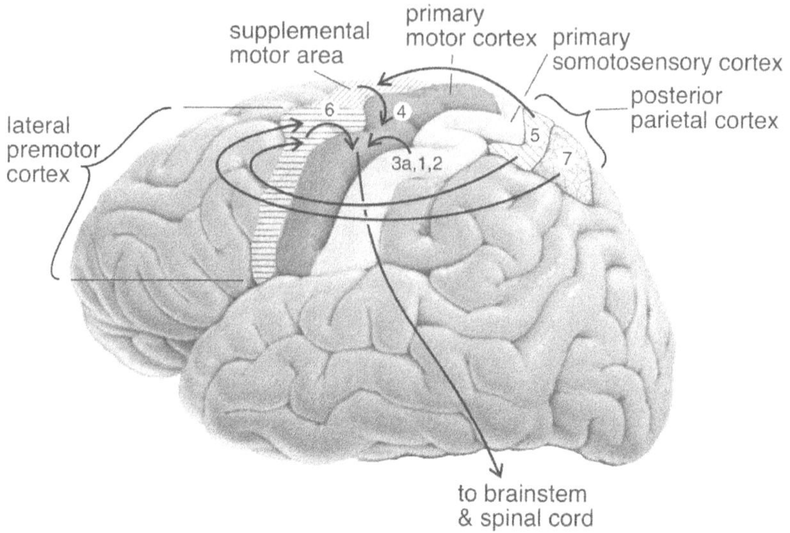

Figure 3.   Cortical inputs to primary motor cortex (Brodmann's area 4) arise from primary somatosensory cortex and premotor cortex (area 6). The premotor cortex has two subdivisions, a more dorsal medial region called the supplementary motor area (SMA), and the more lateral ventral region called the lateral premotor cortex (LPMC). The SMA helps organize plans for internally generated voluntary movements, whereas the LPMC is involved in planning externally guided movements. Proprioceptive information about limb orientation and target location are forwarded to the premotor cortex from areas 5 and 7, respectively, in the posterior parietal cortex. Output signals from the primary motor cortex act on interneurons and motor neurons in the brainstem and spinal cord to produce movements.

the plans for impending voluntary movements. Such plans might include information about which muscles to activate and when to activate them in order to achieve a desired movement goal. In a simplistic way, one can think of the premotor areas as the architects of voluntary movements whose plans are conveyed to the construction company M1 to execute the plans by commanding the motor-neuron laborers to do the needed physical work.

The SMA and LPMC are thought to be involved in planning two different types of voluntary behaviors. The SMA generally is considered to plan for **internally generated movements**. *These are movements that don't involve an overt physical target*. For example, if one randomly waves their hand around in space, that is an internally generated movement. Likewise, if one plays out a memorized piece of music on a keyboard without looking at the keys, that too would be considered internally generated. The impetus for such movements arises entirely within the brain. On the other hand, the LPMC is thought to be involved in the planning of **externally guided movements**, *movements guided to (or by) an external signal or object.* For example, hitting a tennis ball or reaching for a coffee cup would both be externally guided movements.

In order to formulate a movement plan, critical information needs to be provided to the premotor areas. Let's take, for example, reaching for a coffee cup (Figure 4A). Two main items of information are needed. One is the location of the cup (i.e., x, y, z_{cup}) relative to the body. Such information is typically derived from the visual system. In addition, one needs to know the orientation of the limb and the associated position of the hand (x, y, z_{hand}) identified through high-level processing of proprioceptive information. Given that knowledge, the brain (and in this case, the LPMC) can prepare a reach plan involving particular muscles activated at various intensities to drive the hand to the cup. If the cup is in the same location but the arm is configured differently (Figure 4B), then a different reach

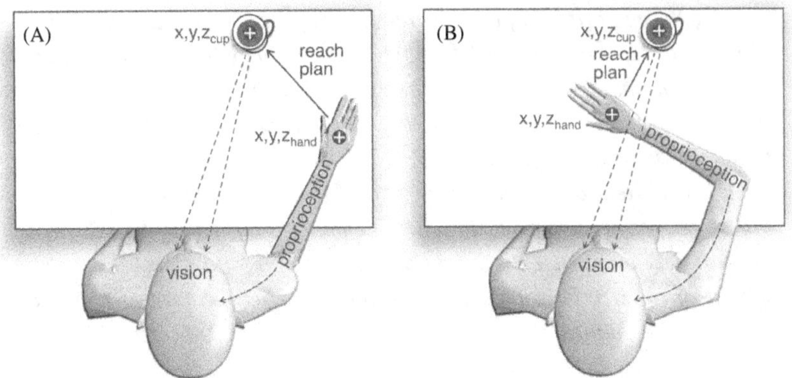

Figure 4.   Information needed by the premotor cortical region to formulate reach plans to an object. (A) Location of the target (x, y, z_{cup}) is identified using the visual system and the location of the hand (x, y, z_{hand}) from the proprioceptive system. If hand position changes but the object remains in the same location (B), then a new plan is formulated based on new proprioceptive information.

plan is devised based on new proprioceptive information arising from the limb.

But from where does such visual and proprioceptive information get relayed to the premotor cortex? There are two regions in the dorsal, posterior parietal cortex (Figure 3) that provide rich inputs to area 6 (Petrides & Pandya 1984) and are likely important sources of this information. One is **Brodmann's area 7**, *a high-order association cortex that is part of the dorsal stream of visual processing*. The **dorsal stream** is *mostly dedicated to extracting spatial information from visual signals*, for example, identifying the relative locations of objects in a visual field. This is in contrast to the **ventral stream** of visual processing that *seems more dedicated to extracting the identity of objects in the visual field* (Mishkin et al. 1983). As such, these two streams are sometimes referred to as the "where" and "what" pathways of the visual system.

As part of the "where" pathway, Area 7 seems to encode only the locations of objects that are within reaching distance and of interest to grasp. This fascinating function of area 7 was documented by Mountcastle and colleagues (1975) while recording neural activity from this region in awake behaving monkeys. The following quote from their paper exemplifies the type of neural responses recorded in area 7:

> *The discharge of [area 7] cells increase abruptly when the animal [visually] fixates certain objects. The object must, to be effective, be of interest to the animal, such as food. The effect of such an object is maximal if it is located within arm's reach, and the associated discharge on fixation decreases with object distance . . . Such a cell may, for example, be completely silent as the animal explores his environment visually fixating in sequence experimenter, instruments, books, etc., to be followed immediately by intense discharge on fixation of a food object presented within arm's length. That discharge increases as the target is moved closer to the animal.*

Presumably, projections from area 7 into the LPMC (Figure 3) provide spatial information about target objects as one ingredient needed by LPMC to devise a reach plan (Figure 4). The other ingredient has to do with information about the configuration of the limb that will be used to reach the target. As discussed in Chapter 12, Brodmann's area 5 seems a good candidate for this function. It integrates information from the various primary somatosensory cortices that could be used to generate a coded representation of the overall limb orientation (Lacquaniti et al. 1995), which is then relayed to the LPMC (Figure 3) and SMA. Based on converging information about object location (from area 7) and arm/hand orientation (from area 5), the premotor cortex could put together a movement plan. That plan is then forwarded to M1, which enacts the plan through commands sent to interneurons and motor neurons in the brainstem and spinal cord (Figure 3).

Supplementary Motor Area

Some of the original evidence pinpointing the supplementary motor area (SMA) as an area involved in planning internally generated movements came from early experiments that set the foundation for brain imaging (Roland et al. 1980). In these experiments, brain activity was detected as increased blood flow using a large array of radioactivity detectors surrounding the skull. A short-acting radioactive substance was injected into the bloodstream in healthy human subjects. Then, when certain regions of the brain required more blood supply to support neural activity associated with a given task, the detectors positioned over those regions registered the increased blood flow as enhanced radioactivity.

The subjects were asked to perform a few tasks. In one, subjects repetitively squeezed and released a spring placed between their thumb and index finger (Figure 5A). Increased blood flow was detected on either side of the central sulcus (Figure 5B)—in M1, as anticipated for such a voluntary task, and in S1 as a consequence of tactile and proprioceptive signals arising during the task. In a second task, subjects were first trained to learn a 16-step sequence of taps of different fingers to the thumb (Figure 5C). Then, while performing this memorized sequence, increased blood flow (as an index of increased neural activity) was observed not only in M1 and S1, but also in the dorsal, medial region of Brodmann's area 6 (Figure 5D), the SMA. Because the playout of a remembered sequence represents a prototypical *internally* generated behavior, SMA

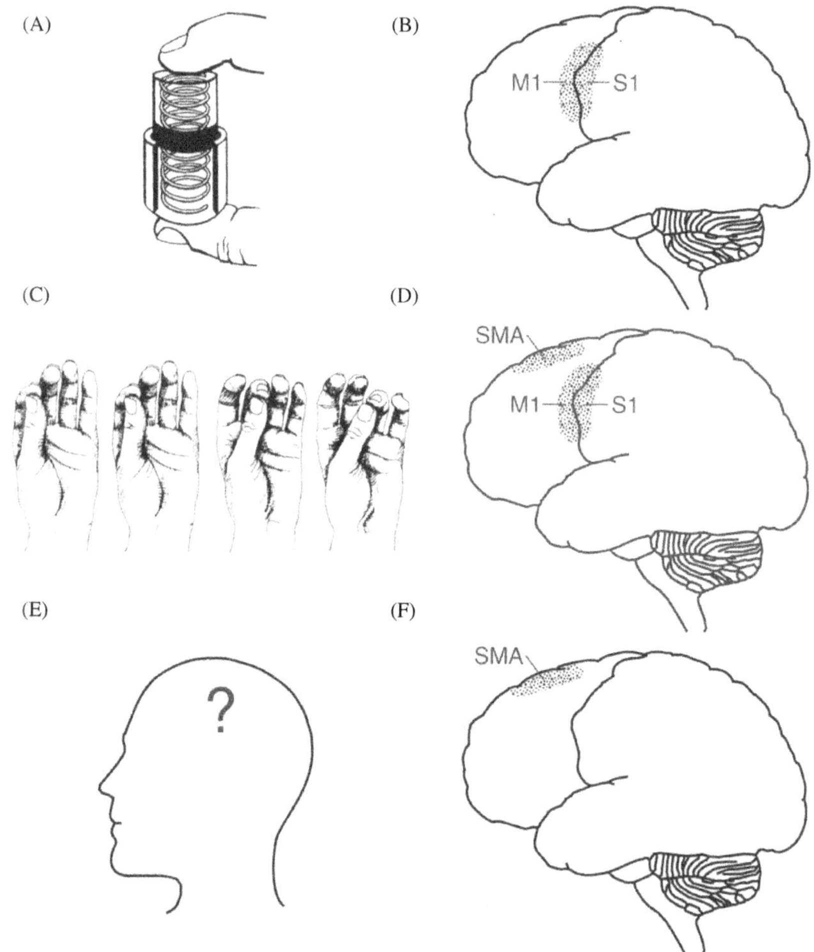

Figure 5.   Involvement of supplementary motor area (SMA) in planning internally generated movements. (A) During a simple task involving squeezing a spring between the fingers, primary motor (M1) and somatosensory (S1) cortex were activated (B). When subjects performed a 16-step finger tapping sequence from memory (C—only four of the taps are shown), the SMA, as well as M1 and S1, was active. When subjects were asked to mentally rehearse the tapping sequence without doing any movements (E), only the SMA was active. (Adapted from Roland *et al.* [1980].)

was thus implicated in the production of such behaviors. Finally, and one of the most critical aspects of these experiments, the investigators then had the subjects mentally rehearse the memorized sequence without actually moving the fingers (Figure 5E). In this case, the only region of the brain that was significantly activated was the SMA (Figure 5F). These results provided strong evidence that the SMA was involved in the planning—but not necessarily the execution—of internally generated movements.

Lateral Premotor Cortex

The other cortical region implicated in the planning of voluntary movements is also part of Brodmann's area 6, the LPMC (Figure 3). This region, however, seems more involved in planning movements associated with *externally* guided behaviors, like reaching for an object. The electrophysiological evidence supporting such a role came mostly from studies involving monkeys trained to wait for a go cue before reaching to a displayed target, as shown in Figure 6 (Weinrich & Wise 1982). Monkeys were trained to reach to one of three or four targets as they became illuminated. The monkeys were also trained to keep their hand on the target until instructed to reach to the next target. As such, even though the next target was illuminated, the monkey had to wait varying periods of a few seconds until a "go-cue" (a small LED in front of the target) was turned on.

Figure 6A shows the spiking activity of a single neuron recorded in the dorsal region of the LPMC during multiple trials for which the hand was on the third target from the right and the upcoming target was immediately to the left of that one. The raster of spikes (one row for each trial) was aligned to the time at which the target to the left was illuminated (arrow). Even though the order of targets and wait times varied randomly during the experiment, the raster has been sorted in order of increasing wait times (~1.5, 2, and 3 s). The large black dots in the raster indicate times of go-cue onset. As is evident in Figure 6A, the neuron started firing immediately when the target was illuminated and maintained its activity throughout the wait period. Once the go-cue was displayed, the monkey initiated its reach to the target, and the activity of the neuron dissipated.

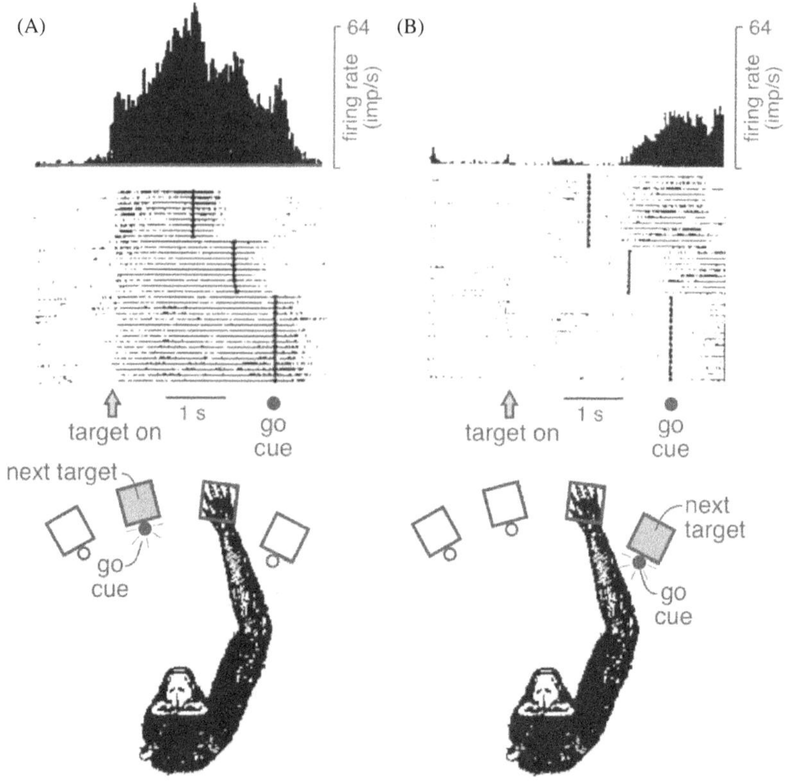

Figure 6.   Activity of neuron recorded in the dorsal region of the lateral premotor cortex (LPMC) during reaches to targets. The monkey was trained to hold hand position when the next target was displayed until a go cue was illuminated, immediately after which the monkey reached to the target. (A) When the upcoming target was to the left of the hand, robust activity commenced with target display (shaded square) and was maintained for a period of seconds until the go cue was activated. Rasters show spike times of the neuron, aligned to target onset, for repeated trials involving three different wait periods. (B) Same neuron as in A but for a target to the right of the current hand position. In this case, little activity occurred during the wait period. (Adapted from Weinrich and Wise [1982], Wise [1985].)

The activity of the same neuron is shown in Figure 6B, but for reaches to the right. In this case, there is little activity upon display of the target. After the monkey had reached the rightmost target, however, neural activity can be seen to increase as if in preparation for upcoming movements (all of which would have been to the left). Therefore, it appears that this particular neuron was involved in the planning of leftward movements to targets. Of course, thousands of neurons would be involved in preparation for upcoming movements to visual targets, many of which are likely "tuned" to different movement directions.

Concurrent Activities in SMA, LPMC, and M1

Further evidence of the distinction between SMA and LPMC was provided in experiments involving monkeys trained to carry out sequential reaching movements to targets under two conditions (Figure 7) (Mushiake *et al.* 1991). In one, monkeys reached to and touched targets that were illuminated in a random sequence (Figure 7A). In this case, planning of each movement was based on information about external, visual targets. In the other, the same monkeys were trained to carry out a memorized, learned sequence of reaches to three targets (Figure 7B). The trigger to perform the learned sequence was activation of a go-cue light. This type of behavior required the use of internally generated movement plans. Although the sequence of reaches to illuminated targets was pseudo-randomized (Figure 7A), imbedded in the sequence were the same set of reaches as for the remembered sequence (Figure 7B). Thus, neural activity could be directly compared for these two conditions because the movements were the same with only the planning contingencies different (e.g., external vs. internally generated cues).

Neural activity was recorded from M1, SMA, and LPMC for both conditions. Figure 7C shows example neurons recorded from each of the three areas during the visually cued (top row) and internally cued (bottom row) conditions. The activity of the M1 neuron (left column, Figure 7C) was very similar for both conditions, with three distinct bursts, one for each target. The LPMC neuron (middle column, Figure 7C) was strongly activated only during the visually guided movements but not during the internally cued movements. Conversely, the SMA neuron (right column, Figure 7C) was little activated during the visually guided reaches while more robustly engaged during the internally cued movements. Such findings reinforce the idea that LPMC is involved in planning externally

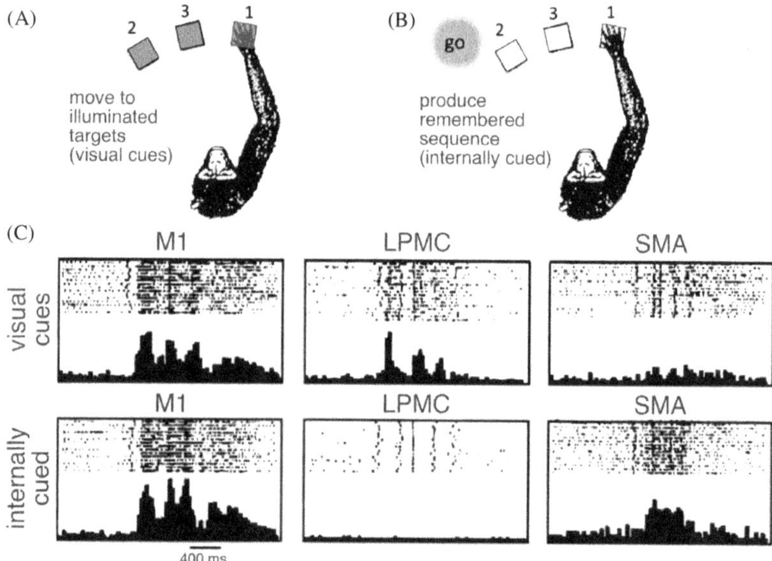

Figure 7.   Activities recorded from neurons in monkey primary motor cortex (M1), lateral premotor cortex (LPMC), and supplemental motor area (SMA) during two types of reaching: (A) successive reaches to illuminated targets (1, 2, 3) presented in a pseudorandom order and (B) playout of a memorized sequence of reaches to non-illuminated targets (1, 2, 3) triggered by the display of a go cue. (C) The top row shows neural activity recorded from the three brain areas during the externally guided (visually cued) reaches. Three bursts of activity (one for each reach) are seen in M1 and LPMC but with little activity in the SMA neuron. The bottom row shows the activity of the same neurons but for internally cued reaches to the same locations associated with the memorized sequence. Again, three bursts of activity are seen in M1 but with little activity in the LPMC neuron, while strong activity arises in SMA. (Adapted from Mushiake *et al.* [1991].)

guided movements, SMA in planning internally generated movements, and M1 in executing the plans forwarded to it from these premotor areas.

Distinct Planning for Reaching and Grasping

When performing a typical reaching behavior, there are two separate functions carried out. One is to propel the hand to the target object—a kind of transportation function. The other has to do with configuring the hand and fingers to interact effectively with the object to be grasped or touched, namely, a manipulation function. As discussed above, planning the transportation aspect of reaching depends on the location of the hand and the location of the target (Figure 4). Such planning involves Brodmann's area 5 to identify hand position based on proprioceptive signals and Brodmann's area 7 to register the location of the target with respect to the body based on visual information.

For successful grasping and manipulation, planning areas also need to know the current configuration of the hand and fingers, derived from proprioceptive information. It seems likely that a different subregion of area 5 is responsible for encoding the spatial dispositions of the hand and fingers. Likewise, the plan for manipulating an object depends critically on the *physical geometry and characteristics of the target object*. Evidence suggests that such data is extracted from visual information *in a region of the posterior parietal cortex that separates area 5 from area 7, namely in the intraparietal sulcus*. Figure 8 shows recordings from a neuron recorded in this region, specifically in a region called the **anterior intraparietal (AIP) area**, in a monkey viewing different objects (Figures 8A–F). The objects were placed in the same position in front of the animal, and in some trials, monkeys reached and grabbed the objects. In the trials shown, the monkey was trained just to stare at ("fixate") the object but not reach for it. In this case, the neuron's activity was strong as soon as it fixated on the plate (Figure 8A), moderately active when fixating on the ring (Figure 8B) or small cube (Figure 8C), and little active for the other objects. In trials when the monkey was allowed to grab the objects, these general patterns of activity were maintained throughout the reach. Other neurons had preferences for other reachable objects. Therefore, neurons in this region (AIP) appear to represent the spatial configuration and orientation of objects that might be grasped.

One of the main destinations of projections from AIP is the *ventral region of LPMC,* **PM$_V$** (Luppino et al. 1999). *Neurons in this region appear to be involved in setting up the appropriate plan to be used to grasp objects of various shapes and dimensions.* Figure 9 shows an example recording of a neuron recorded in monkey PM$_V$ (Murata et al. 1997). The monkey sat in front of a box containing a turntable divided into sectors, with each sector holding a different-shaped object. The objects were presented to the monkey in random order by rotation of the turntable. The

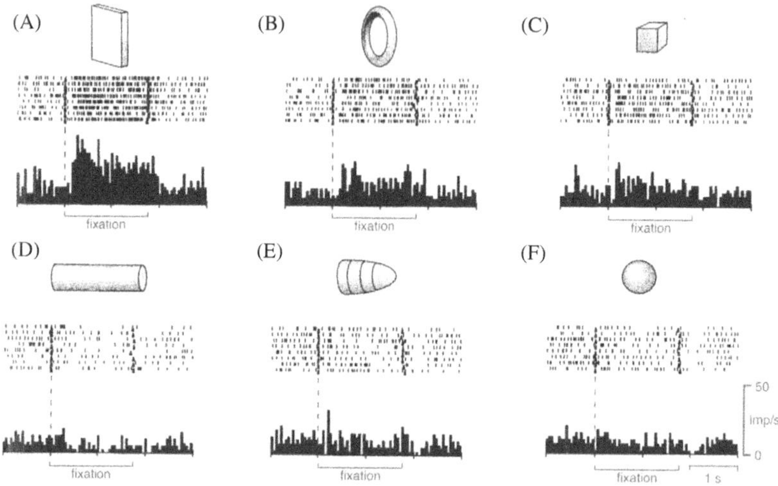

Figure 8.   Responses of a neuron recorded in the monkey anterior interparietal (AIP) region of the posterior parietal cortex in response to the presentation of various graspable objects (A–F) at the same location in front of the monkey. In this case, the monkey was trained only to visually fixate on the object presented for a period of ~2 s. For this AIP neuron, presentation of the plate (A) provoked strong activity while presentation of other objects (e.g., in D, E, F) was associated with little change in activity. (Adapted from Murata et al. [2000].)

presented object was then illuminated (small vertical arrows in Figure 9) to make it visible to the monkey. Monkeys were trained to wait for about 1.5 seconds after seeing the object before a go-cue (filled circles, Figure 9) instructed the animal to reach and grab the object.

Little activity was seen in this neuron for most of the objects. However, upon visual illumination of the ring, the neuron was strongly activated (Figure 9), which was maintained until just after the go-cue was displayed. Some modest activity also occurred upon presentation of the sphere. Different neurons in PMv showed selective activity during the wait period for different objects. Such preparatory activity is not unlike what was shown for the LPMC neuron in Figure 6 in advance of reaching to targets in different locations. In that case, the neuron was recorded in the *dorsal region of the LPMC, namely the* **PMd**. For the PMv neuron depicted in Figure 9, the locations of the objects were all the same but were of different shapes. In general, therefore, PMd appears to be involved

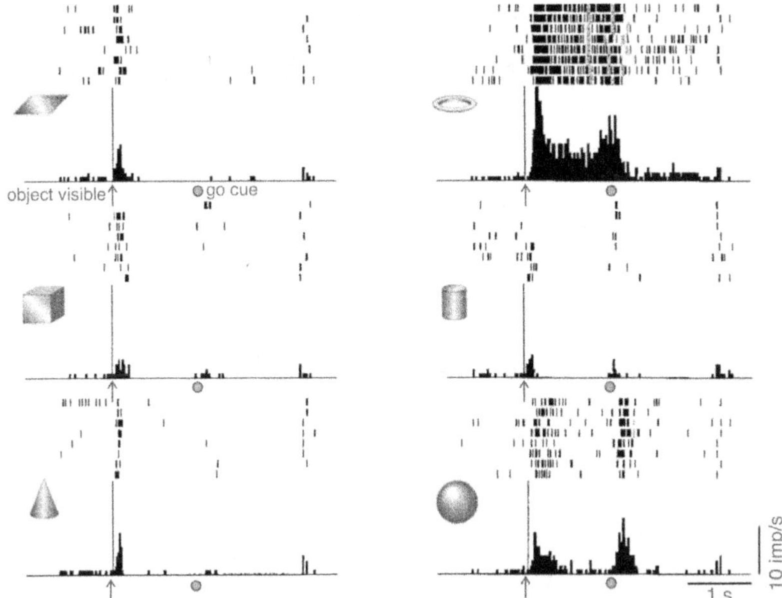

Figure 9.   Recording of neuron in the ventral region of the monkey lateral premotor cortex (PMv) during repeated presentation and grasping of various shaped objects. Objects were located on a turntable placed in front of the monkey and were presented in random order by rotating the table. Upon illumination of the object (arrows), the monkey was trained to wait for a period of 1.5 seconds before a go cue (filled circle) instructed the animal to reach to grab the object. For this neuron, the visual presentation of the ring led to substantial activity during the wait period that subsided soon after the go cue. (Adapted from Murata et al. [1997].)

in planning of reaching (i.e., transporting the hand to a given location), whereas PMv seems to plan how to move the fingers and hand to interact with objects in the environment.

Mirror Neurons

Some neurons recorded in PMv responded in a fascinating way. They not only were *active prior to a monkey grasping a particular object but were also active when the monkey observed another monkey or human grasping the same object.* Figure 10 depicts the activity of such a **mirror neuron** (Rizzolatti et al. 1996). In Figure 10A, the monkey repeatedly watched a

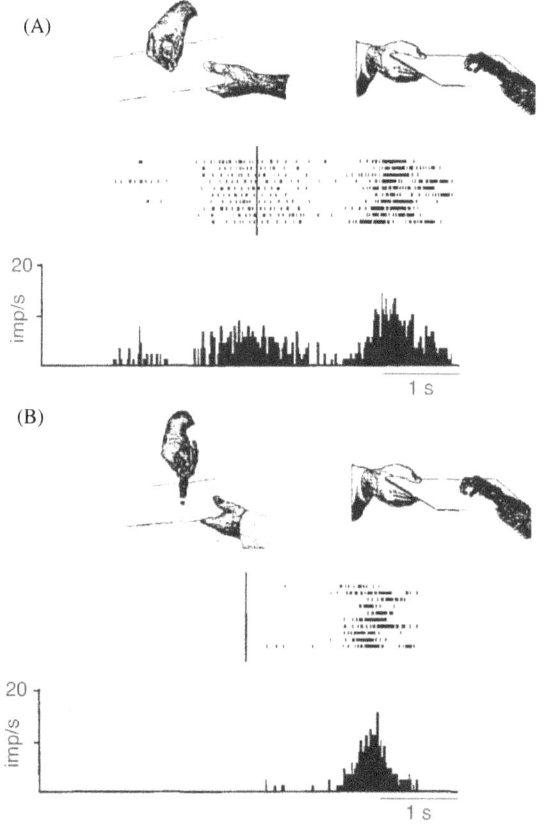

Figure 10.   Activity of mirror neuron recorded in the ventral region of the monkey lateral premotor cortex (PMv). (A) Response of the neuron over several trials during which the monkey first observed a human grasping a food morsel and then grasped a morsel offered by the human. (B) Same neuron as in A, but in this case, the human grasped the morsel with a pair of pliers before offering a morsel to the monkey to grasp. This neuron's activity during observation "mirrored" that associated with performing the same action. (Adapted from Rizzolatti et al. [1996].)

human experimenter pick up a morsel of food with his hand, immediately followed by the monkey also picking up a food morsel offered to him from the experimenter. The neuron was robustly activated both by observing the action of others ("monkey see") and performing the action himself ("monkey do"). Such mirroring of activity during watching and preparing to do an action only occurred if the watched action was similar to the specific action that engaged the neuron prior to an actual movement. For example, Figure 10B shows the responses of the same neuron when the experimenter picked up the morsel with a pair of pliers. In this case, there was very little activity in the neuron during the observation phase, but strong activity occurred when the monkey picked up the morsel with his fingers.

Since the discovery of mirror neurons in the PMv, there has been considerable debate as to the meaning of mirror neuron activity. For example, it might simply represent a kind of inadvertent mental rehearsal associated with planning to perform a movement, triggered by the observation of someone else doing it. It has also been suggested that such mirror neuron activity might underlie the learning of new motor behaviors based on observation of others, like when a coach demonstrates the correct way to carry out some athletic skill. At the other extreme, mirror neurons have been suggested to play a key role in social cognition (Keysers & Gazzola 2006). In this regard, it is thought that the ability of an individual to understand the intentions, actions, or emotions of others partly derives from the activity of mirror neurons that "simulate," in the observer's mind, the neural activity that would occur if the observer were to be involved in the same action. For example, when we observe someone weeping, activation of mirror neurons associated with that behavior might impart in us a feeling of sadness even though we are not weeping or may not even know the reason why the other person is crying. While these ideas are appealing, the function of such mimicking activity by mirror neurons is not yet fully understood.

Neural Population Dynamics

In this chapter, the activities of *single* neurons have been used to illustrate the types of inputs conveyed to the primary motor cortex. Yet, a deeper understanding of how neural activity associated with movement planning actually leads to a particular pattern of descending motor commands requires consideration of representative populations of the tens of thousands of neurons simultaneously actually involved. A new conceptual framework, known as **neural population dynamics**, has been used to gain important insight into how the collective actions of many neurons during the planning stages of movement give rise to the complex motor commands that drive muscles during voluntary behaviors (Shenoy et al. 2013).

The concept of neural population dynamics derives from the field of **dynamical systems**, *used in mathematics and physics to describe systems whose properties change over time*, like the weather, the flight of a rocket, the growth of bacteria, and even the membrane potential of a neuron. In some cases, like that of a swinging pendulum, the time-varying trajectory of the system is predictable given knowledge of the initial conditions (the position of the pendulum upon its release).

Insight into the behavior of a dynamical system is gained by graphical depiction of key variables that characterize the system. For a pendulum (Figure 11A), the horizontal axis might indicate how far to the right or to the left of the straight down position the pendulum is at any moment (Figure 11B). The vertical axis might represent the velocity of the pendulum (with rightward velocities indicated as positive and leftward as negative, Figure 11B). In this case, the plot will have a circular-shaped trajectory: when the pendulum is at its far-left position (just before

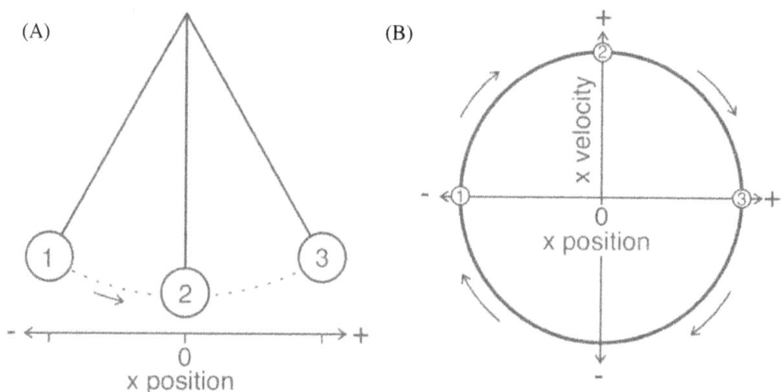

Figure 11.   (A) Pendulum as a dynamical system. Points 1, 2, and 3 indicate when the pendulum is at the leftmost, middle, and rightmost locations of the pendulum trajectory. B) Plot of x—position and velocity of an ideal pendulum. Points on the circle (1, 2, 3) indicate the position and velocity of the pendulum at the particular moments in time indicated in A.

initiating its movement to the right), its velocity is zero (position 1, Figure 11). Then, as it starts to move to the right, the velocity increases, reaching a maximum (and highest point on the vertical axis) as it passes through the zero (straight down position) on the horizontal axis (position 2, Figure 11). Then the velocity progressively slows down until it again reaches zero at the far-right position (position 3, Figure 11), and so on. Any point on this trajectory indicates the state (position, velocity) of the pendulum at that moment and is predictive of forthcoming states.

In neural population dynamics, the key variables representing the brain system of interest are the firing rates of individual neurons, like position and velocity for a pendulum. The collective spiking activity across a population can be plotted where each axis on the graph represents the firing rate of an individual neuron. For example, Figure 12A shows the spiking activity of three make-believe neurons. For each successive brief time period (shaded regions), the spiking rates of each neuron can be determined and plotted as points in 3D space (one dimension for each neuron, n1, n2, n3, Figure 12B). For example, for the first time period (no shading, Figure 12A), neuron 1 (n1) generated zero spikes, neuron 2 four spikes, and neuron 3 zero spikes. The activities of these neurons at this time are then represented as the white dot in the 3D firing-rate space (sometimes called the **neural state space**) (Figure 12B). During the next time period (pale gray, Figure 12A), neuron 1 emitted 3 spikes, neuron 2 reduced its output to 2 spikes, and neuron 3 again produced no spikes. This "state" of our population of three neurons at that moment is indicated as the light gray dot in Figure 12B. This process is continued throughout the segments of the behavioral period of interest (different shades of gray). "Connecting the dots" across each successive state produces a path through the neural state space called a **neural trajectory** (Figure 12B).

One appealing aspect of this type of representation is that it provides a clear visual depiction of how the activities of multiple neurons evolve over time during the elaboration of some behavior or mental process. Yet to provide a reasonable representation of a neural population requires recording the activities of a few hundred neurons simultaneously—something now possible using electrodes possessing hundreds of detection sites (Jun et al. 2017). While a computer has no inherent difficulty dealing with a neural state space consisting of hundreds of orthogonal dimensions, it is

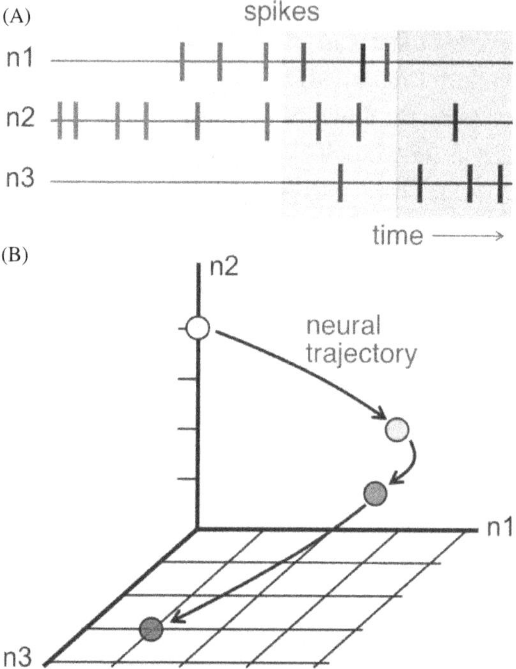

Figure 12.   Population neural dynamics. (A) Spiking behavior over time of three make-believe neurons (n1, n2, n3). (B) Such population neural activity shown in (A) can be represented in neural state space with each dimension of the space indicating the firing rate of one neuron. A point in this 3D space indicates the composite activities of the three neurons over a small epoch of time (shaded regions in A). The progression of neural states through this space is referred to as a neural trajectory. (Adapted from Vyas *et al.* [2020].)

exceptionally difficult for humans to visually imagine more than three. Fortunately, data scientists have "tricks" that *maintain the richness of large-scale multidimensional data while simplifying the representation to a few visual dimensions.* This approach is referred to as **dimensionality reduction**. In part, this approach capitalizes on common (or correlated) behaviors among some neurons (or other entities in a dynamical system). In other words, if one recorded 100 neurons during some behavior, not all of those neurons would fire in ways completely independent of all other neurons. Indeed, different neurons oftentimes show strong correlations in their activities with other neurons.

Figure 13 shows a simplified depiction of this idea. The simultaneous spiking activities of two neurons (n1, n2) are illustrated in Figure 13A. To represent the neural dynamics of this population of two neurons requires a two-dimensional state space (Figure 13B). The firing rates of the two neurons at different epochs of time (1, 2, 3, and 4, Figure 13A) are shown

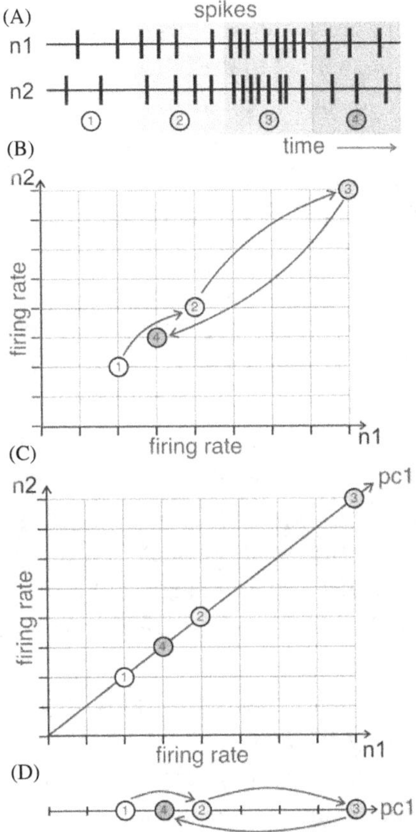

Figure 13.   Dimensionality reduction. (A) Spiking of two pretend neurons. (B) Neural state space for firing rates of the two neurons (n1, n2) shown in A. Numbered circles correspond to time periods shown as shaded regions in A. (C) Because the activity of neuron 1 correlates with that of neuron 2, all neural states are confined to a line in the 2-D state space. This axis that encompasses most of the activities of neurons 1 and 2 is called a principal component (pc). (D) Therefore, the co-activities of neurons 1 and 2 can be captured as points located along this single pc axis.

as points in this space (Figure 13B). Note that these points do not visit most of the possible locations in this plane but rather seem constrained to reside along a single line. Indeed, as shown in Figure 13A, the firing rates of the two neurons appear to go up and down together, as if the activity of one neuron was harnessed to the activity of the other. There are a number of physiological reasons as to why this might be. For example, the two neurons may receive similar synaptic inputs (like motor neurons in the spinal cord) and therefore are driven in tandem. Also, one neuron might provide potent excitatory input to the other—thereby the second neuron's spiking response mimics that of the first.

Regardless, two separate dimensions are not required to represent the activities of our two neurons. Instead, we can characterize their firing along a single tilted axis that passes through most of the data points (Figure 13C). A *method used to identify such axes that can account for much of the data along fewer axes than the original dimensions* is called **principal components analysis**, with each new axis called a principal component (pc, Figure 13C). Therefore, we can envision the activities of our two neurons as moving together along a single pc axis (Figure 13D). Thus, in this simple example, we have lessened the number of dimensions of our neural state space from two to one. In reality, we might have 10, 50, or 100 neurons that could be readily represented along such an axis. For neurons whose activities do not follow along such a path, or for more complex neural activity, we would need additional pc dimensions. Furthermore, it should be recognized that while a set of principal components might effectively represent activity among a group of neurons for one behavior or mental process, a different set might be needed for other situations.

Because the concept of dimensionality reduction is very helpful for understanding neural population dynamics, let's revisit the example shown in Figure 12 involving three neurons. Figure 14A again shows that neural trajectory. It can be seen, however, that the population activity does not appear to visit all possible regions of the 3D space, like a fly would buzzing around inside a room. Instead, the population activity seems largely confined to a single plane. As mentioned before, such constraints on activity can arise due to the nature of the connectivity to and between the neurons. Because a plane can be defined using just two orthogonal axes (in this case, pc1 and pc2), we can nicely illustrate the simultaneous activities of our 3-neuron population using two dimensions (Figure 14B).

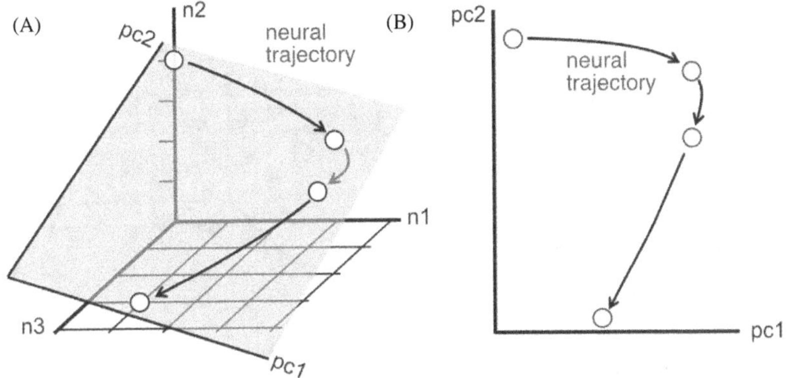

Figure 14.   (A) Activities of three neurons shown in the 3D state space of Figure 12 reside within a plane. (B) Therefore, this population activity can be represented in a 2D space with two principal components (pc) as orthogonal axes.

Neural Population Dynamics During Movement Planning

We now return to the issue raised at the outset of the previous section, namely, how might neural activity distributed over a population of neurons involved in planning a movement in premotor areas lead to a particular pattern of descending motor commands? Krishna Shenoy at Stanford University, Mark Churchland at Columbia University, and their colleagues proposed that such neural activity before movement (which they refer to as "preparatory" activity) positions the neural population at a particular site in neural state space. This preparatory state then seeds and dictates the impending neural dynamics associated with movement execution (Churchland et al. 2006; Lara et al. 2018). In a coarse way, preparatory activity is like positioning a pendulum to some location prior to letting it go. The position of the pendulum at release dictates the movement dynamics that follow.

For example, consider a large population of premotor cortex neurons whose activities can be represented by three principal components. Figure 15A shows activity in the neural state space associated with planning and making movements to a target on the right. Prior to the target display, the neurons discharge somewhat randomly at relatively low intensities, referred to as baseline activity. However, once a right target has

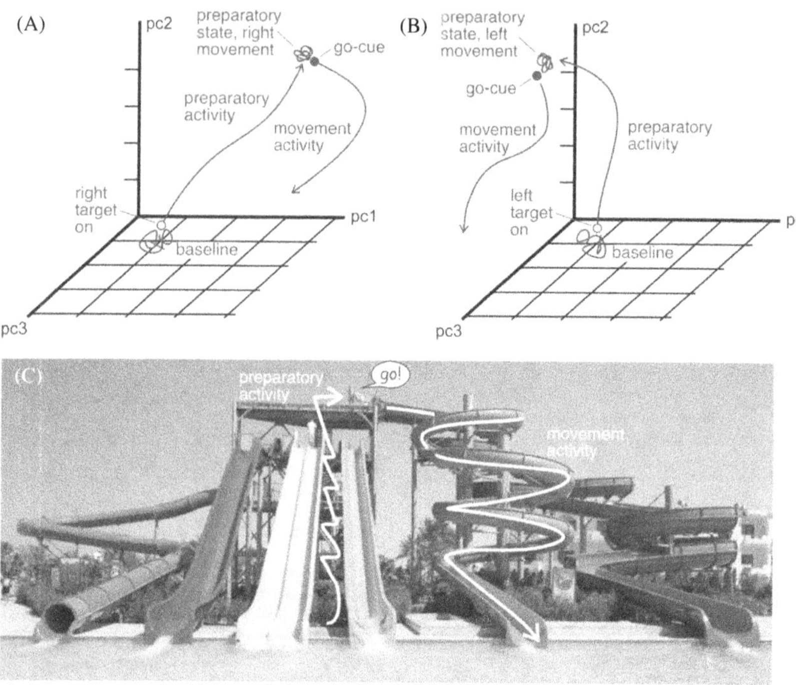

Figure 15.   Conceptual representation of preparatory and movement execution activities in neural state space. (A) Firing rates of a large population of neurons can be reduced to three principal components (pc). Before a target is presented, baseline neural activity is weak and desultory. Upon display of a target on the right side, preparatory activity drives the population to a particular preparatory state for movements to the right. This preparatory state seeds the impending movement-related activity for the rightward movement when the go cue is given. (B) When the target is presented on the left, preparatory activity ascends to a different preparatory state that seeds leftward movement activity when a go cue is given. (C) An analogy for preparatory and movement-related neural activities is the behavior of a person at a water slide park. Preparatory activity involves climbing stairs/ladders to the landing of the desired slide (i.e., the preparatory state). Upon receiving the go cue from the attendant, subsequent movement activity and exit site is dictated by the physical structure of the slide.

been displayed, preparatory activity arises, driving the neural population to a new state. Neural activity will then hover at this preparatory state for rightward movements (like a pendulum pulled to a particular position) until a go-cue is given (the pendulum is released). Immediately following, a particular pattern of neural activity ensues (the swinging of the pendulum). This is registered as a trajectory through neural state space (movement activity, Figure 15A), which impels primary motor cortex to emit signals driving muscles to perform the desired rightward movement. In the case of movements to a target on the left (Figure 15B), preparatory activity pushes the neural population to a different state that seeds neural activity associated with movement to the left. It should be pointed out that if there were no requirement to wait for a go-cue, movement activity would immediately follow once preparatory activity attained the desired preparatory state.

Perhaps a simple way to envision such preparatory and movement activities is to imagine a person at a waterslide park (Figure 15C). Preparatory activity would involve climbing stairs and ladders to the landing in front of the entrance to a desired slide. The person may be required to "hover" at this preparatory state before the attendant gives the "go" signal. The ensuing movement activity is then dictated by the physical characteristics and linkages among the structural components of that specific slide. These mechanical linkages are analogous to the robust synaptic connections that have been built up among large populations of neurons. Different slides will propel the individual to different locations in the pool. As such, preparatory activity situates the individual at a particular start point needed to seed a forthcoming dynamical ride on a desired slide.

A real example of the preparatory activity of a neural population is shown in Figure 16 (Elsayed et al. 2016). In this case, monkeys were trained to reach to one of eight targets from a center position displayed on a touch screen (Figure 16A). As is typical for these experiments, monkeys were required to wait for up to 1 second after the target was displayed before a go-cue instructed the monkey to reach to the target. Figure 16B shows the normalized firing rates of 127 neurons (recorded mainly in PMd) represented in neural state space with just two dimensions (PC1 and PC2) during the wait period prior to reaching to the different targets. Such preparatory activity propelled the neural population from baseline (dots, Figure 16B) to one of eight distinct preparatory states (arrowheads, Figure 16B) that were maintained until the go-cue was presented. Following the go-cue (not shown in Figure 16B), a unique neural trajectory emerged from each state associated with movement execution to each

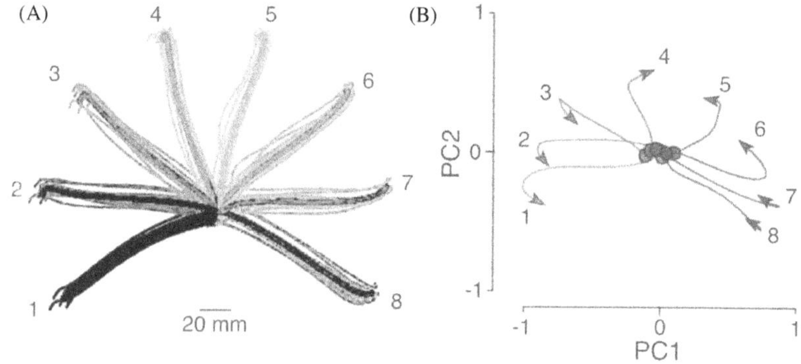

Figure 16.   (A) Trajectories of the hand of a monkey reaching from a central position to eight different targets displayed on a touch screen. After one of the eight targets was displayed, the monkey was trained to wait for about 1 s before a go cue instructed the monkey to make the reach. (B) Neural state space for 127 neurons, recorded mainly in the dorsal lateral premotor cortex, reduced to two principal components (PCs). Trajectories show preparatory activity during the wait period before reaching each target. Arrowheads show preparatory states that were maintained until the go cue. (Adapted from Elsayed et al. [2016].)

of the targets. A remarkable aspect of these neural data is that the locations of the preparatory states (keeping in mind that these are abstract representations of the activities of 127 different neurons) largely mimic the spatial arrangements of the targets in physical space. For example, target 4 is physically situated between targets 3 and 5. Likewise, preparatory state 4 is located in neural state space between those for targets 3 and 5. This indicates that population neural activity during preparation for movement to target 4 is more similar to that for targets 3 and 5 than to target 8, which seems logical but would be difficult to convey using conventional analyses of neural data.

Summary

The primary motor cortex heavily depends on sensory input and preparatory information from other parts of the brain to generate movement commands. To summarize such inputs as discussed in this chapter, let's

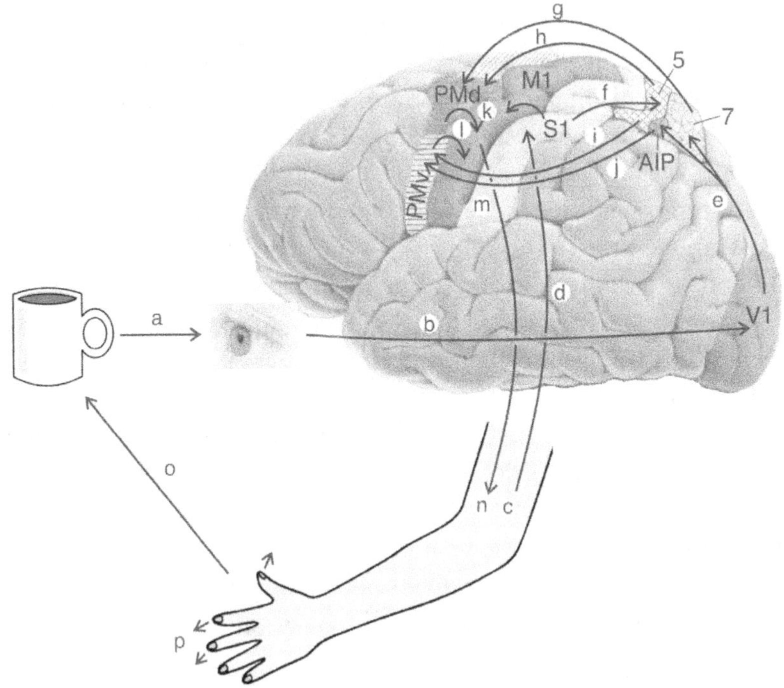

Figure 17.   Sequence of neural events involved in planning and execution of a movement to reach and grab an object. See text for details.

consider the sequence of events that might occur during reaching to an object (Figure 17). The image of the object is registered on the retinas (a). That information is conveyed (b) through the visual thalamus to the primary visual cortex, V1. At the same time, proprioceptors in the arm and hand register their orientations (c) and convey that information (d) through a different region of the thalamus to the primary somatosensory cortex, S1. Visual information about the location of the cup and its physical dimensions are processed along the dorsal visual stream (e). In Brodmann's area 7, the location of the object with respect to the body is likely encoded, whereas the spatial configuration of the object to be grasped is represented in the AIP cortex. Similarly, information from the various subdivisions of S1 converge in Brodmann's area 5 (f) to holistically represent the position of the hand and configuration of the fingers.

Signals from areas 7 (g) and 5 (h), representing critical information about target and hand locations (see Figure 4), respectively, are then passed onto the planning region for arm movements, the dorsal premotor cortex (PMd). Likewise, information about finger configurations and object attributes is forwarded from area 5 (i) and AIP (j) to the planning region for grasping actions, the ventral premotor cortex (PMv). The plans for moving the arm (k) and fingers (l) are then relayed to the primary motor cortex (M1), perhaps by seeding particular preparatory states that dictate the neural dynamics underlying the complex patterns of descending commands (m). Those commands operate on interneurons and motor neurons in the brainstem and spinal cord to engage muscles in the arm and hand (n). Finally, that muscular activity transports the hand (o) to the vicinity of the desired object and arranges the digits of the hand (p) appropriately for grasping the object. Importantly, it needs to be noted that if no overt external target were the goal of the movement, then the SMA (not labeled in Figure 17) would provide the planning information conveyed to M1 to execute such internally generated movements.

References

Asanuma H (1981). Functional role of sensory inputs to the motor cortex. *Progress in Neurobiology* **16**, 241–262.

Churchland MM, Yu BM, Ryu SI, Santhanam G & Shenoy KV (2006). Neural variability in premotor cortex provides a signature of motor preparation. *Journal of Neuroscience* **26**, 3697–3712.

Elsayed GF, Lara AH, Kaufman MT, Churchland MM & Cunningham JP (2016). Reorganization between preparatory and movement population responses in motor cortex. *Nature Communications* **78**, 1–15.

Ghosh S, Brinkman C & Porter R (1987). A quantitative study of the distribution of neurons projecting to the precentral motor cortex in the monkey (*M. fascicularis*). *The Journal of Comparative Neurology* **259**, 424–444.

Hooks BM, Mao T, Gutnisky DA, Yamawaki N, Svoboda K & Shepherd GMG (2013). Organization of cortical and thalamic input to pyramidal neurons in mouse motor cortex. *Journal of Neuroscience* **33**, 748–760.

Horne MK & Tracey DJ (1979). The afferents and projections of the ventroposterolateral thalamus in the monkey. *Experimental Brain Research* **36**, 129–141.

Jones EG, Coulter JD & Hendry SHC (1978). Intracortical connectivity of architectonic fields in the somatic sensory, motor and parietal cortex of monkeys. *The Journal of Comparative Neurology* **181**, 291–347.

Jones EG, Wise SP & Coulter JD (1979). Differential thalamic relationships of sensory-motor and parietal cortical fields in monkeys. *The Journal of Comparative Neurology* **183**, 833–881.

Jun JJ et al. (2017). Fully integrated silicon probes for high-density recording of neural activity. *Nature* **551**, 232–236.

Kandel ER, Schwartz JH, Jessell TM, Siegelbaum SA & Hudspeth AJ (2012). Principles of Neural Science (5th edition). McGraw-Hill.

Keysers C & Gazzola V (2006). Towards a unifying neural theory of social cognition. *Progress in Brain Research* **156**, 379–401.

Kievit J & Kuypers HGJM (1977). Organization of the thalamo-cortical connexions to the frontal lobe in the rhesus monkey. *Experimental Brain Research* **29**, 299–322.

Lacquaniti F, Guigon E, Bianchi L, Ferraina S & Caminiti R (1995). Representing spatial information for limb movement: Role of area 5 in the monkey. *Cerebral Cortex* **5**, 391–409.

Lara AH, Elsayed GF, Zimnik AJ, Cunningham JP & Churchland MM (2018). Conservation of preparatory neural events in monkey motor cortex regardless of how movement is initiated. *eLife* **7**, 555.

Lemon RN & Porter R (1976). Afferent input to movement-related precentral neurones in conscious monkeys. *Journal of the Royal Society of London, Series B* **194**, 313–339.

Lemon RN & van der Burg J (1979). Short-latency peripheral inputs to thalamic neurones projecting to the motor cortex in the monkey. *Experimental Brain Research* **36**, 445–462.

Luppino G, Murata A, Govoni P & Matelli M (1999). Largely segregated parieto-frontal connections linking rostral intraparietal cortex (areas AIP and VIP) and the ventral premotor cortex (areas F5 and F4). *Experimental Brain Research* **128**, 181–187.

Mishkin M, Ungerleider LG & Macko KA (1983). Object vision and spatial vision: Two cortical pathways. *Trends Neuroscience* **6**, 414–417.

Mountcastle VB, Lynch JC, Georgopoulos A, Sakata H & Acuna C (1975). Posterior parietal association cortex of the monkey: Command functions for operations within extrapersonal space. *Journal of Neurophysiology* **38**, 871–908.

Murata A, Fadiga L, Fogassi L, Gallese V, Raos V & Rizzolatti G (1997). Object representation in the ventral premotor cortex (Area F5) of the monkey. *Journal of Neurophysiology* **78**, 2226–2230.

Murata A, Gallese V, Luppino G, Kaseda M & Sakata H (2000). Selectivity for the shape, size, and orientation of objects for grasping in neurons of monkey parietal area AIP. *Journal of Neurophysiology* **83**, 2580–2601.

Mushiake H, Inase M & Tanji J (1991). Neuronal activity in the primate premotor, supplementary, and precentral motor cortex during visually guided and internally determined sequential movements. *Journal of Neurophysiology* **66**, 705–718.

Petrides M & Pandya DN (1984). Projections to the frontal cortex from the posterior parietal region in the rhesus monkey. *The Journal of Comparative Neurology* **228**, 105–116.

Rizzolatti G, Fadiga L, Gallese V & Fogassi L (1996). Premotor cortex and the recognition of motor actions. *Brain Research: Cognitive Brain Research* **3**, 131–141.

Roland PE, Larsen B, Lassen NA & Skinhoj E (1980). Supplementary motor area and other cortical areas in organization of voluntary movements in man. *Journal of Neurophysiology* **43**, 118–136.

Rosén I & Asanuma H (1972). Peripheral afferent inputs to the forelimb area of the monkey motor cortex: Input-output relations. *Experimental Brain Research* **14**, 257–273.

Shenoy KV, Sahani M & Churchland MM (2013). Cortical control of arm movements: A dynamical systems perspective. *Annual Review of Neuroscience* **36**, 337–359.

Strick PL (1976). Anatomical analysis of ventrolateral thalamic input to primate motor cortex. *Journal of Neurophysiology* **39**, 1020–1031.

Vyas S, Golub MD, Sussillo D & Shenoy KV (2020). Computation through neural population dynamics. *Annual Review of Neuroscience* **43**, 249–275.

Weinrich M & Wise S (1982). The premotor cortex of the monkey. *Journal of Neuroscience* **2**, 1329–1345.

Wise SP (1985). The primate premotor cortex: Past, present, and preparatory. *Annual Review of Neuroscience* **8**, 1–19.

Chapter 20

Cerebellum

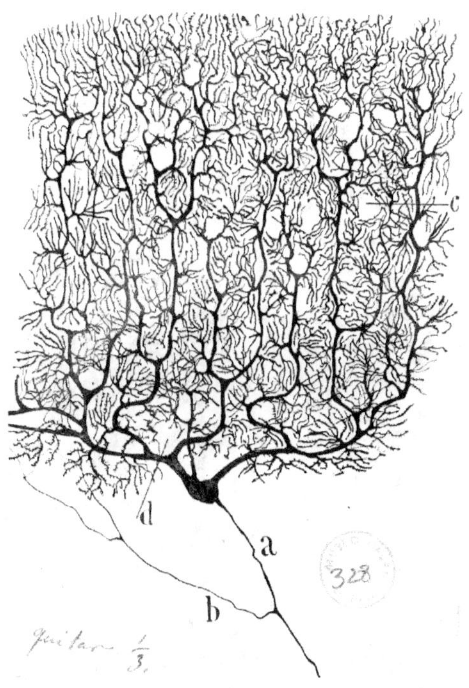

Purkinje cell of the human cerebellum drawn by Santiago Ramon y Cajal, 1899.

The cerebellum is a somewhat mysterious structure that participates in the control of movement. It receives input from several somatosensory and motor regions of the central nervous system (CNS) and projects back to many of those regions. However, unlike the motor cortex or various brainstem nuclei, the cerebellum does not send projections directly to the spinal cord to drive movement on its own. Instead, as will be discussed in this chapter, the cerebellum plays a supportive role in movement control.

Anatomy of the Cerebellum

The cerebellum sits in a depression in the base of the occipital bone of the skull. It is attached to the rest of the brain at the pons by *enormous white matter tracts* called **peduncles**. The volume of the cerebellum is about 10% of the entire brain (Filipek *et al.* 1994), hence its name (cerebellum means "little brain"). Despite its relatively small volume, the cerebellum possesses *more than half of all the neurons in the entire human brain* (Herculano-Houzel 2009). The combination of a highly folded outer covering of gray matter (the cerebellar cortex, Figure 1A), which greatly

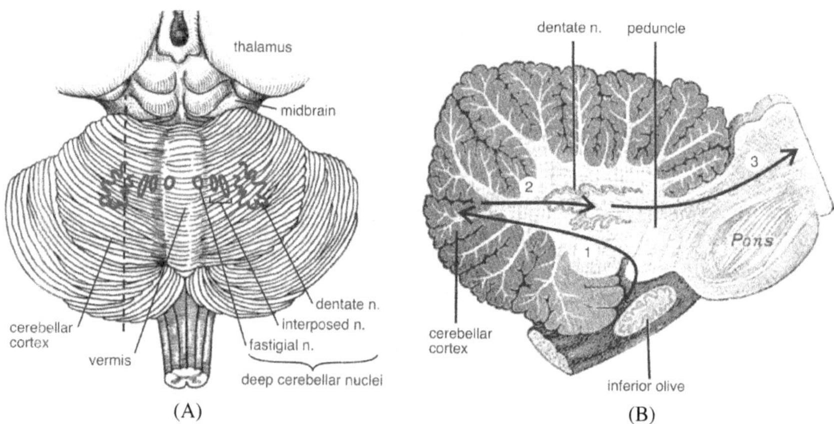

Figure 1.   Anatomy of the cerebellum. (A) Dorsal view showing folded cerebellar cortex and deep cerebellar nuclei. (B) Sagittal view (approximately at the level of the dashed line in (A) depicting the basic processing pathway through the cerebellum. Inputs (1) arrive from many regions of the CNS and project directly to the cerebellar cortex. Outputs from the cerebellar cortex (2) are conveyed to the deep cerebellar nuclei (in this case, the dentate). Output from the deep cerebellar nuclei communicates with brainstem nuclei or with regions of the cerebral cortex (via the thalamus) involved in motor control. (Adapted from plate Gray707, commons.wikimedia.org/wiki/Category:Gray's_Anatomy_plates.)

expands its surface area, and a high density of neural packing underlies the impressive neuron count in the cerebellum.

The cerebellar cortex has different subdivisions (called lobules), including a *prominent ridge along the midline* called the **vermis** (Latin for worm) (Figure 1A). Tucked under the inferior aspect of the cerebellum is a *small appendage of the cerebellar cortex* (not visible in Figure 1) called the **flocculus** (meaning tuft of wool). Deep in the interior of the cerebellum are three sets of nuclei on either side of the cerebellum (Figure 1A). If one likens the cerebellum to an orange hanging on a branch (the brainstem), with its outer peel the cerebellar cortex, then these nuclei would correspond to seeds in the interior. The nucleus nearest the midline is called the **fastigial nucleus** (meaning roof—this nucleus is situated near the "roof" of the fourth ventricle). The *largest and the most lateral of these nuclei* is the **dentate nucleus** (Figure 1A). Its convoluted perimeter brings to mind the impression teeth would leave from biting into an object, hence its name. *Interposed between the dentate and fastigial nuclei is a pair of small nuclei called the* **interposed nuclei** (Figure 1A). As discussed below, each of these nuclei processes different kinds of information. Collectively, *these nuclei of the cerebellum* are called the **deep cerebellar nuclei.**

Flow of Information through the Cerebellum

As a first step toward understanding the operations of the cerebellum, it is useful to consider the general flow of information through the cerebellum (Figure 1B). Inputs from many locations within the CNS enter the cerebellum via the peduncles and project directly to the cerebellar cortex (arrow 1, Figure 1B). Processing occurs in the cerebellar cortex, and its output projects to one of the deep cerebellar nuclei (DCN) (arrow 2, Figure 1B). The DCN then send output signals to several targets in the brain (arrow 3, Figure 1B). This general pattern holds throughout most of the cerebellum. Also shown in Figure 1B is a *prominent structure in the rostral portion of the medulla oblongata,* called the **inferior olive**. It *provides a distinct and important set of inputs to the cerebellar cortex* that will be discussed below.

Functional Subdivisions

The cerebellar cortex can be segregated into four main regions that have different functions (Figure 2): the **vermis** situated on the midline, the **intermediate zone** immediately lateral to the vermis, the large **lateral zone** occupying the most lateral region of the cerebellar cortex, and the **flocculus**, the small, hidden tailpiece. Each region receives input from distinct parts of the CNS that underlie their differing functions (Figure 2).

The flocculus receives input directly from the vestibular nerve of the vestibular apparatus in the inner ear that detects head motion (Nagao *et al.* 1997). It also receives processed vestibular information from nuclei in the brainstem. Thus, the *flocculus is designated* as the **vestibulocerebellum** (Figure 2).

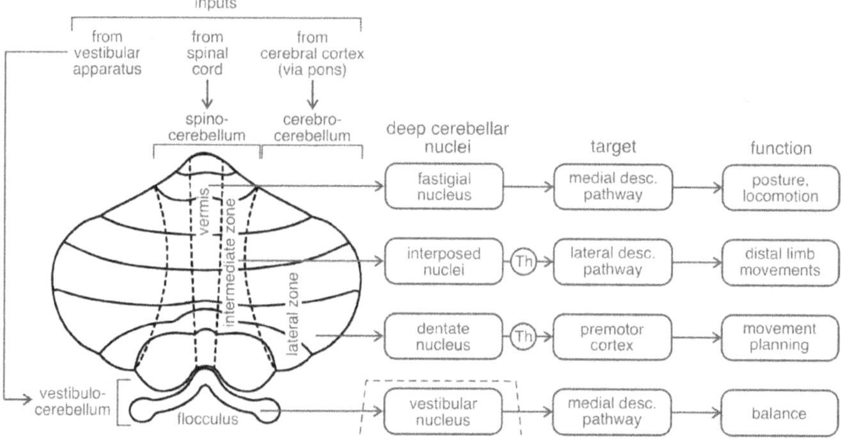

Figure 2.   Input/output organization of cerebellar cortex. Vestibulocerebellum (flocculus) receives input from the vestibular apparatus and projects to the vestibular nucleus to influence the medial descending pathway. Sensory inputs from the leg and torso traveling in the spinal cord project to the vermal portion of the cerebellar cortex. The output of the vermis, via the fastigial nucleus, is to brainstem centers that are part of the medial descending pathway. Sensory inputs from the arms, traveling in the spinal cord, project (via the dorsal column nuclei) to the intermediate zone of the cerebellar cortex. The intermediate zone sends outputs to the interposed nuclei, which project, via the thalamus, to the origins of the lateral pathway, mainly the motor cortex. The lateral zone receives inputs from sensorimotor areas of the cerebral cortex (via nuclei in the pons). Lateral zone output acts on the dentate nucleus, which projects, via the thalamus, to premotor cortical areas. Based on these patterns of connectivity, the likely supportive functions of each region of the cerebellar cortex are shown on the right. (Adapted from Purves *et al.* [2001].)

The vermis and the intermediate zone receive much of their input from ascending pathways arising in the spinal cord (Figure 2). Collectively, these regions of the cerebellar cortex are referred to as the **spinocerebellum**. The inputs to the spinocerebellum largely carry proprioceptive and tactile information (Oscarsson 1965). That information arising from the legs/hindlimbs is delivered by *neurons with cell bodies in the medial part of the lumbar gray matter of the spinal cord,* called **Clark's column**. Those neurons receive strong synaptic connections from collaterals of primary sensory axons running in the dorsal column pathway (see Chapter 11). The axons of those neurons in Clark's column ascend in the **spinocerebellar tract** directly to the cerebellar cortex. They largely project to the vermal portion of the spinocerebellum. Similarly, proprioceptive and tactile information from the arms/forelimbs are delivered to the cerebellum from second-order neurons with cell bodies in the dorsal column nuclei of the medulla oblongata. That pathway is called the **cuneocerebellar tract** (named for the cuneate nucleus—one of the dorsal column nuclei that receives sensory input from the arm and hand). It mostly projects to the intermediate zone of the spinocerebellum. The spinocerebellum is topographically organized.

In humans and other primates, the *largest functional subdivision of the cerebellar cortex is in the lateral zone and is called the* **cerebrocerebellum** *based on its inputs from the cerebral cortex* (Figure 2). The main regions of the cerebral cortex providing that input are those associated with sensorimotor function on either side of the central sulcus, namely: primary motor cortex, primary somatosensory cortex, premotor cortex, posterior parietal cortex (areas 5 and 7), and the frontal eye fields (rostral to the premotor cortex). Those inputs, however, do not project directly to the cerebellar, but are relayed through a set of nuclei in the pons of the brainstem. The density of inputs from those cortical regions is greatest for those areas closest to the central sulcus (i.e., primary motor and somatosensory cortices) and progressively diminishes for regions farther away (Wiesendanger *et al.* 1979). It should also be noted that there are significant cortical inputs to the cerebellar cortex (via the pons) from non-sensorimotor areas, such as from the prefrontal cortex (Kelly & Strick 2003).

According to the flow-of-information diagram in Figure 1B, output from different regions of the cerebellar cortex should be routed to one of the DCN. This is true in all cases except for the phylogenetically oldest part of the cerebellum, the vestibulocerebellum. Outputs from the vestibulocerebellum instead leave the cerebellum altogether to contact neurons in the vestibular nuclei (Figure 2) that are part of the medial descending pathway (see Chapter 18). As such, the vestibulocerebellum contributes to the control of balance and keeping the body upright in the face of gravitational or other physical perturbations.

Outputs from the vermal portion of the spinocerebellum project primarily to the most medial of the DCN, the fastigial nucleus (Figure 2). Outputs from the fastigial nucleus project into the origins of the medial descending pathway, and thereby provide a supportive role in the control of posture and locomotion. The intermediate zone of the spinocerebellum sends its output to the interposed nuclei of the DCN (Figure 2). Those nuclei then mainly project, via the thalamus, to the origin of the lateral descending pathway, the motor cortex. Consequently, the intermediate zone/interposed nuclei play a role in governing voluntary movements of the extremities (e.g., arms/hands). And last, the laterally situated cerebrocerebellum sends its output to the most lateral of the DCN, the dentate nucleus (Figure 2). Outputs from the dentate must also pass through nuclei in the thalamus to mainly target the premotor cortex. It is thought, therefore, that this part of the cerebellum is involved in planning and initiation of voluntary movements.

Much of what is known about the function of the cerebellum (as depicted in Figure 2) has been based on two main sources of information. One, is from meticulous anatomical studies delineating the connectivity between different components of the cerebellum and the connection of those components to other parts of the CNS. And two, that inferred from behavioral changes associated with damage to different regions of the cerebellum caused by disease or injury in human patients, or from lesions or temporary inactivation of parts of the cerebellum in experimental animals, as described in the following sections.

Vestibulocerebellum Damage

A rare patient with selective damage to the *flocculus* (part of the vestibulocerebellum) due to a stroke presented with dizziness, unsteadiness, vertigo, nausea, and nystagmus (Park *et al.* 2013). **Nystagmus** is *uncontrollable, repeated, rapid eye movements*. The symptoms of dizziness and unsteadiness seem consistent with the interconnections of the flocculus with the vestibular apparatus and nuclei. Nystagmus also makes sense given the importance of coordinating head movements (signaled by the vestibular system) with countervailing eye movements (controlled by the superior colliculus in the midbrain) to ensure visual images remain relatively fixed on the retina. Damage to the flocculus, therefore, interferes with this coordinated reflex (called the **vestibulo-ocular reflex**), leading to the uncontrolled eye movements. It should be noted that a few days after the stroke, these symptoms largely resolved, and the patient had no symptoms on follow-up evaluation.

Spinocerebellum—Vermis Damage

One of the most notorious causes of damage to the *vermis* is alcoholism. The vermis degenerates in alcoholics and is associated with a number of disturbances in motor function (Sullivan *et al.* 2000). These include excessive postural sway, problems with balance, and *dyscoordination* (**ataxia**) of gait that typically presents with a widened base of support, short, irregular steps, slow speed, and veering off to the side. These symptoms are consistent with interconnections of the vermis (and fastigial nucleus) to the medial descending pathway (involved in control of posture and gait). The reduced size of the vermis associated with alcoholism seems mostly related to degeneration of Purkinje cells (PCs) (discussed below) in the cerebellar cortex (Phillips *et al.* 1987). The reason why the vermis is particularly susceptible to excessive alcohol consumption is not really understood at this time.

Spinocerebellum—Intermediate Zone Inactivation/Damage

Selective damage in humans to the *intermediate zone* or interposed nuclei is rare. Consequently, understanding the types of motor disorders associated with dysfunction of these parts of the cerebellum has come primarily through lesion or temporary inactivation in experimental animals. For example, individual DCN can be selectively silenced for a few hours by targeted injection of the drug **muscimol**, *an agonist of the inhibitory neurotransmitter GABA.* When such inactivation or lesions are directed at the interposed nuclei, few deficits are seen when the animal makes simple movements, like those involving a single joint (Thatch *et al.* 1992). However, dysfunction is evident when multiple joints are involved, such as that which occurs during reaching.

For example, in experiments involving inactivation of individual DCN in cats trained to reach to a target, severe ataxia in the forelimb was observed when the interposed nuclei were inactivated (Martin *et al.* 2000; Milak *et al.* 1997). Little impairment, however, was detected during reaching when either fastigial or dentate nuclei were targeted with muscimol injection. Figure 3 shows the type of disordered (ataxic) movements that occurred with the inactivation of the interposed nuclei (Milak *et al.* 1997). For these experiments, the cat was trained to reach to and pull a lever when a go-cue (tone) was played (Figure 3A). The experimenters tracked the displacements of the shoulder, elbow, and wrist during the reaches to the lever. Before inactivation, movements were highly stereotyped across trials, with the wrist making a more-or-less straight trajectory to the target

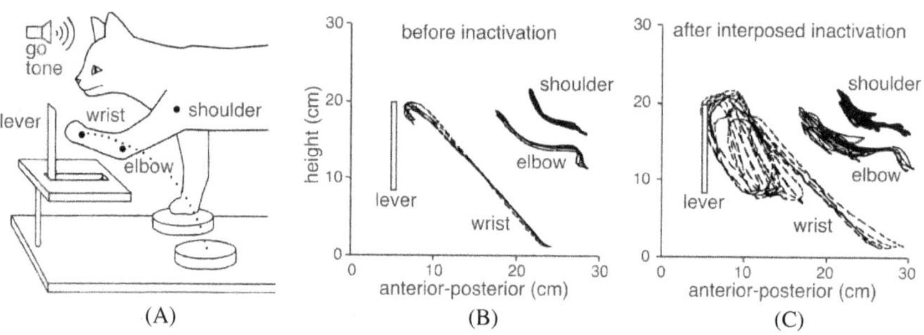

Figure 3.   Impaired reaching with inactivation of the interposed nuclei. (A) Movements of the shoulder, elbow, and wrist were recorded while cats reached to pull a lever. (B) Displacement of wrist, elbow, and shoulder during normal reaching in cats. Several trials superimposed. Wrist trajectory is practically straight. (C) After inactivation of the interposed nuclei, trajectories of forelimb joints exhibited wide variations, with clear oscillations of the wrist as it approached the lever. (Adapted from Milak *et al.* [1997].)

(Figure 3B). After inactivation of the interposed nuclei (Figure 3C), movements across all joints were highly variable from trial to trial, and the path of the wrist became quite complex, oftentimes exhibiting multiple loops or oscillations near the endpoint.

Indeed, such ataxia during reaching is one of the cardinal signs used by neurologists for an initial diagnosis of cerebellar disease or damage affecting the intermediate zone/interposed nuclei. A standard evaluation is the finger-to-nose test, in which the patient repeatedly moves their index finger from their nose to various target locations indicated by the neurologist (Figure 4A). In healthy individuals, the trajectory of the fingertip to the target during the reach is relatively straight. However, in individuals with certain cerebellar disorders, the path of the finger from nose to target (or from target to nose) is more meandering.

More quantitative evaluation of such ataxias in human patients has revealed important insights about the putative function of the intermediate zone and interposed nuclei. For example, Bastian *et al.* (1996) measured wrist trajectories and angular displacements of the shoulder and elbow in healthy subjects and in cerebellar patients while they reached to touch a target (small ball suspended from a string) with their fingertip (Figure 4B). In healthy subjects (Figure 4C), the path of the wrist was relatively straight and highly consistent across trials. In the cerebellar patient (Figure 4D), the wrist trajectory was variable across trials and typically took a curvilinear, complex path during the reach. Also, the fingertip end points (small open circles in Figure 4D) were often not on the target. These results are similar to those of the cat with inactivated interposed nuclei (Figure 3C). Because of the more widespread nature of the damage in the human patients, the deficits cannot be solely attributed to impaired function of the intermediate zone/interposed nuclei, but the similarity with the animal experimental results is suggestive.

An important aspect of the study by Bastian and colleagues is that they also examined the coordination *across* joints of the arm during the reaching task. In healthy subjects, rotations occurred simultaneously at both the shoulder and elbow joints (Figure 4E). With such coordination (one joint flexing while the other is extending), the resulting trajectory of the hand is straight. In the cerebellar patient shown in Figure 4F, one can see that this coordination is disrupted: namely, first the shoulder rotates

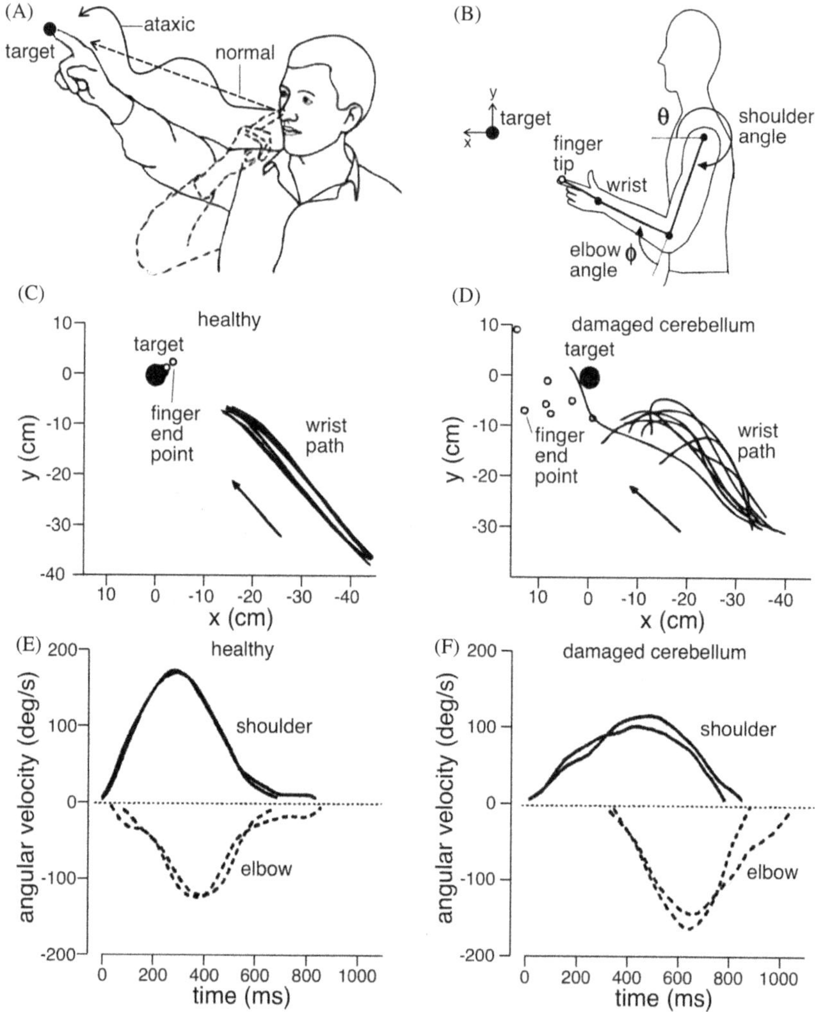

Figure 4.   (A) Ataxia (disordered) movement associated with cerebellar damage revealed in the finger-to-nose test. (B) Set up to measure arm movements in healthy subjects and cerebellar patients. Subjects reached for a target ball suspended from a string while arm kinematics were recorded. (C) In healthy subjects, wrist path is relatively straight, and the fingertip at the end of the reach is near the target (small open circles). (D) In cerebellar patients, wrist path tends to be curved, and finger end points are inaccurate. (E) In healthy subjects during reaching, shoulder and elbow joints rotate simultaneously. (F) In cerebellar patients, coordination between shoulder and elbow is disrupted. (Adapted from Bastian *et al.* [1996].)

and then the elbow. The consequence of such sequential (rather than simultaneous) rotations is the production of complex, curved trajectories of the hand.

Based on these kinds of observations of ataxia during multi-joint arm movements, two (non-mutually exclusive) ideas have been proposed as to the function of the intermediate zone/interposed nuclei. One is that they serve to enlist concurrent actions of multiple muscles across an entire limb to yield a singular, smooth, harmonized action. It seems likely that this function is enacted through interaction with motor planning areas, such as the premotor cortex. When the intermediate zone/interposed nuclei of the cerebellum are damaged, intended movements become decomposed into sequential actions at individual joints, leading to complex, convoluted pathways (like in Figure 4D). The other idea is that during complex movements involving multiple joints, small errors in motor commands to individual muscles (or as a consequence of unanticipated external perturbations) can quickly accumulate into large errors in the endpoint trajectory. Thus, the spinocerebellum uses sensory feedback from the limb to detect such errors and make corrections "on-the-fly" or to make longer-lasting, learned adjustments following repeated errors in the desired performance.

Interestingly, clinical or experimental evidence for the involvement of the spinocerebellum in adapting to new movement contingencies or learning new motor skills did not emerge until after theoreticians (Albus 1971; Marr 1969) hypothesized such a role for the cerebellum based on the characteristics of its neural circuitry (described below). For example, in studies involving cat reaching (like that shown in Figure 3), when experimenters placed a horizontal bar as an obstacle in the path taken by the forelimb to the target, intact cats readily learned after a trial or two to adjust the limb trajectory so as to avoid striking the obstacle on the way to the target (Martin *et al.* 2000). However, when the interposed nuclei were inactivated, cats seemed unable to learn the new contingencies of the task and continued to strike the obstacle on repeated trials. Such a disability did not occur with inactivation of the fastigial or dentate nuclei.

In a similar vein, some human cerebellar patients also exhibit a conspicuous inability to learn new motor tasks. Figure 5A depicts a subject throwing a ball at a target while wearing prism glasses (Martin *et al.* 1996).

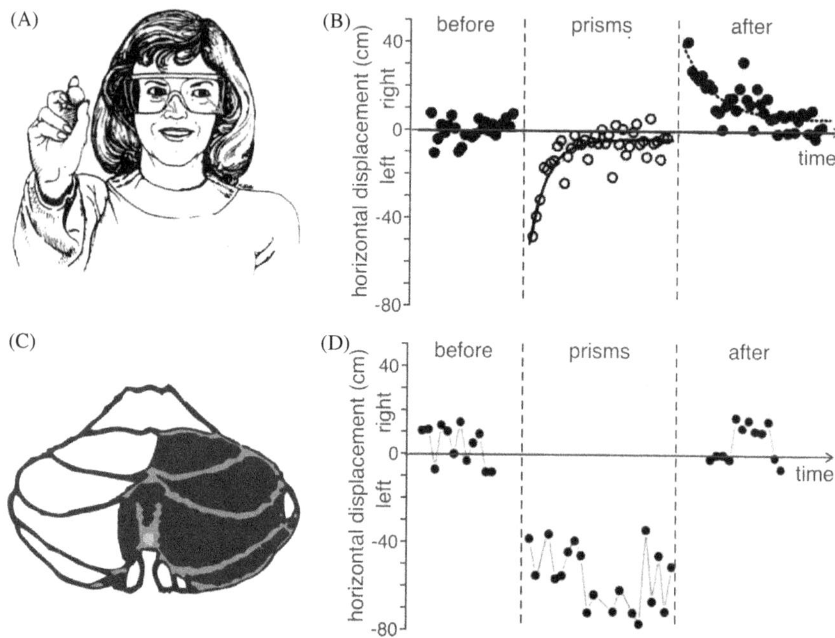

Figure 5.   Impaired learning of a new motor task with cerebellar damage. (A) A healthy subject throwing a ball at a vertical target while wearing prism glasses that required rotating the eyes about 20 degrees to the left (gray arrows) to see directly forward toward the target. (B) Before donning the prisms, the subject was reasonably accurate with throws mostly within 10 cm of the vertical target. However, when the prisms were first worn, the subject threw far off to the left. With repeated trials while wearing the prisms, the accuracy of the throws progressively improved. When the prisms were then removed, the subject initially threw the ball off to the right, an aftereffect of learning the new contingency to throw to the right of where one looks. (C) Darkened region indicates area of cerebellar damage in patient. (D) When the patient threw balls at the vertical target, accuracy was poorer (but not substantially) than that of the healthy subject. After donning the prisms, the patient persistently threw to the left, apparently unable to adjust to the new visual-motor situation. When removing the prisms, the patient immediately returned to pre-prism performance, showing no aftereffect of learning. (Adapted from Martin *et al.* [1996].)

In this case, the prism bent the light entering the eye so that in order to see what was straight ahead, the subject needed to look to the left about 20 degrees (Figure 5A). The experimenters quantified the accuracy of throwing by measuring the location that the ball hit to the left or right of a vertical target placed ~2 m in front of the subject. Before putting on the prisms, typical healthy subjects show reasonable accuracy, with the ball landing a few centimeters left or right of the target on repeated trials (dots, Figure 5B). Immediately after donning the prisms, however, healthy subjects invariably threw with large errors to the left of the target (Figure 5B). Such errors likely arise because of the well-learned association between direction of gaze and throwing direction. Consequently, because the eyes were rotated to the left (in order to see the target straight ahead), the throwing action was also to the left, that is, in the direction that the eyes pointed.

With repeated trials wearing the prisms, subjects gradually adjusted their throwing movements to improve accuracy. After ~10–15 trials, throws were back close to the target (Figure 5B). It was as though the subjects had now learned a new contingency: direct the throw made by your arm about 20 degrees to the right of where your eyes are looking to achieve success. This new learning was vividly revealed when the subjects removed the prisms. As shown in Figure 5B, immediately after removing the prisms, subjects now threw the ball far to the *right* of the target. In this case, the eyes were able to look straight ahead and at the target. However, the new learning impelled throwing to the right of where one looks. Again, with repeated trials with the prisms off, the subjects relearned to throw in the direction of eye gaze.

When the experiment was repeated with patients with cerebellar damage, a different result often occurred. Figure 5C shows the area of damaged cerebellum due to a stroke in a patient. As is most often the case, such damage was not isolated to a single part of the cerebellum. In this patient, damage included part of the vermis and much of the intermediate and lateral zones on one side of the cerebellum. Despite this expansive lesion, the patient's throwing accuracy before using the prisms was reasonable—just somewhat more variable than the healthy subject (Figure 5D). When the patient put on the prisms, he too threw off target to the left (Figure 5D, middle). However, the patient persisted in throwing to the left without any discernible adjustments despite seeing the errors after each throw. When the prisms were removed, the patient immediately returned to pre-prism performance, with no aftereffects as seen in the healthy subject. This result strongly indicated that the damage to the cerebellum prevented this individual from learning the "new rules" of this motor task.

This outcome is not unlike that in monkeys (described above) who could not change the trajectory of their limbs to avoid an obstacle when the interposed nuclei were inactivated.

Cerebrocerebellum Damage/Inactivation

Despite its relatively large size, damage or inactivation of the cerebrocerebellum/dentate nucleus is not associated with obvious deficits in motor function. The one subtle feature that does appear is a slowing in reaction time. For example, in a task involving pointing to targets, monkeys with the dentate nucleus temporarily inactivated initiated movements about 30–60 ms later than before inactivation (Trouche & Beaubaton 1980). Reaching movements otherwise seemed normal. In human patients with cerebellar damage involving the cerebrocerebellum (but other areas as well), reaction times have also been reported to be about 60 ms slower than in healthy controls (Inhoff *et al.* 1989). Therefore, one function of the cerebrocerebellum/dentate nucleus seems to be in the initiation of movement. However, as pointed out by Thatch *et al.* (1992): "*Unless the purpose of the dentate is to provide that little extra speed of reaction, the paucity of the observed deficit does not appear commensurate with the phylogenetically increasing size of the dentate nucleus.*"

Indeed, it may be that the large dentate nucleus and cerebrocerebellum in humans and other higher primates serve functions other than those involved in movement control (Schmahmann 1996; Strick *et al.* 2009). This idea has partly derived from detailed anatomical studies demonstrating connectivity between the dentate nucleus/cerebrocerebellum and non-motor association cortices (Bostan *et al.* 2013). Functional imaging studies have shown activation in the cerebrocerebellum or dentate nucleus during a variety of non-motor cognitive tasks, such as those involved in sensory perception (Gao *et al.* 1996), memory (Chen & Desmond 2005), and language (Leiner *et al.* 1988). Furthermore, a wide range of non-motor deficits associated with cerebellar damage have been described, including disorders of planning, attention, verbal communication, affect and mood, and visceral function (Benagiano *et al.* 2018). Nevertheless, some doubt still remains as to the actual significance of the cerebellum in regulating non-motor functions (Buckner 2013; Glickstein 2007; Manto 2008).

Cerebellectomy

Studies of damage (either experimentally induced or due to disease) to different parts of the cerebellum have provided important insights into function. However, the outcomes and interpretations can be uncertain. One might rightfully ask what deficits would be observed if the entire cerebellum was removed, rather than just inactivation of certain regions. Surprisingly, the long-term deficits of such a radical intervention can be quite modest.

Immediately following *surgical removal of the cerebellum* (**cerebellectomy**), monkeys were impaired in walking and running (Wirth & O'Leary 1974). Five months after the operation, however, the animals could walk and run but with a wider base of support than normal. The ability to climb ropes was modestly affected immediately following surgery. However, following 3 months of recovery, climbing was practically normal. The ability of the hand to pick up small pieces of food was good following the surgery. Furthermore, strength quickly recovered following cerebellectomy (Wirth & O'Leary 1974). Interestingly, the degree of impairment with cerebellectomy was less in monkeys than in raccoons or cats.

These findings in monkeys parallel those observed in a unique human patient in whom a complete absence of a cerebellum was discovered only when she was in her 20s (Yu *et al.* 2015). She was admitted to a hospital complaining of some unsteadiness of gait and dizziness. She was married and had children. Her speech and walking developed slowly as a child. Astonishingly, brain scans revealed no remnants of cerebellar tissue (Figure 6). Further testing showed mild ataxia on the finger-to-nose test, some irregularity and slowing during repeated pronation–supination of the wrist, and some slurring of speech. She was able to walk without support, while her gait was described as "moderately unsteady." At face value, these findings associated with a complete absence of the cerebellum are startling—more than half the neurons in the entire brain can be absent but

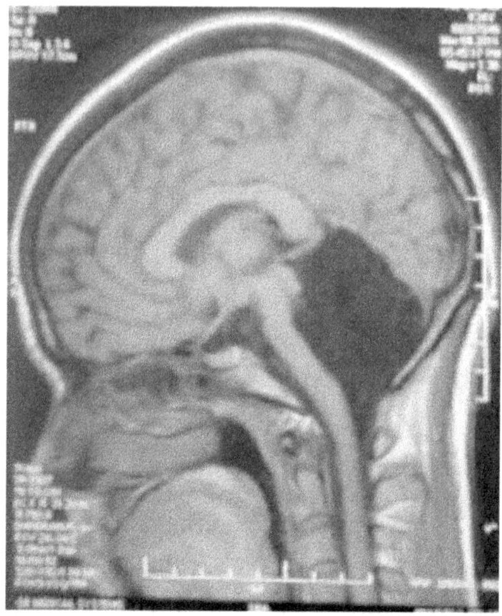

Figure 6.   Sagittal magnetic resonance image of a young woman with moderate motor symptoms reveals no recognizable cerebellar structure. The region normally occupied by the cerebellum is filled by cerebrospinal fluid (dark area). (Adapted from Yu *et al.* [2015].)

with relatively modest consequences. Some concerns, however, related to the interpretation of brain damage in humans or lesion/inactivation experiments in animals are warranted. These concerns are briefly considered in Appendix C.

Cerebellum as a Comparator

As discussed in previous chapters, movement plans are thought to be conveyed to the primary motor cortex from the premotor cortex. The motor cortex then issues motor commands that either directly or through brainstem or spinal cord circuits produce movements. It seems likely, however, that the transformation of descending commands (representing a desired movement) into an actual movement is not without errors. Keep in mind that even professional basketball players make only about 75% of their free throws despite tens of thousands of practice trials on this one task

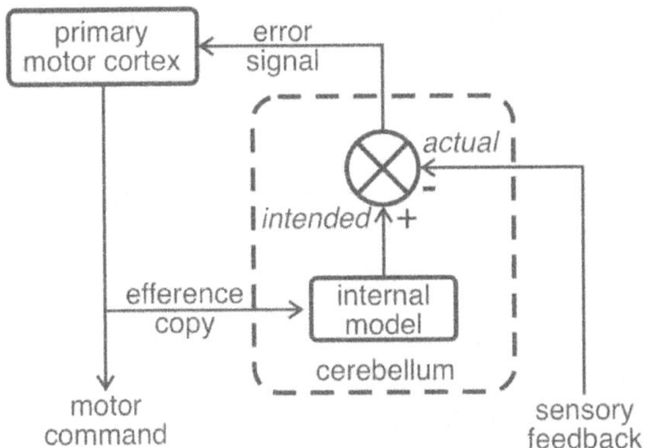

Figure 7.   Feedback control to correct movement errors. A copy of the motor command (efference copy) is delivered to an internal model that simulates the intended movement. The simulated intended movement is compared to the actual movement, signaled by sensory feedback arriving to the cerebellum from the moving body part. The outcome of the comparison (actual—intended) serves as a signal conveyed to the involved motor pathway to correct movement errors.

under highly standardized conditions. The cerebellum is thought to play an important role in helping to tidy up these errors (although not perfectly).

One way this may be accomplished is through online feedback by which desired actions are compared to that which actually occurs (Figure 7). In this scheme, a replica of the motor commands that drive the output machinery in the brainstem/spinal cord is conveyed to the cerebellum. This *facsimile of the motor command is referred to as an* **efference copy**. Such a representation of the motor command, presumably related to which muscles to engage, their intensities, and timing of activations, is then thought to be used by the cerebellum to "simulate," moment-by-moment, what the movement outcomes (e.g., limb displacements) should be. In order for the cerebellum to carry out such simulations, it needs a model (an "internal model," Figure 9) that accurately predicts movement outputs based on motor command inputs (Wolpert *et al.* 1998). This is not unlike a computer program that simulates movements of a system (an aircraft, an autonomous vehicle) given information on the inputs actuating the system. In this case, the "program" presumably is coded in the extensive and plastic interconnections among neurons in the cerebellum (discussed below).

The output of the internal model, therefore, is a representation of the desired action (i.e., the "intended" movement, Figure 7). The intended action is then compared to what is actually occurring, signaled by the massive sensory feedback to the cerebellum originating from somatosensory receptors in the limbs. The operation of this comparison can be thought of as a subtraction: the signal representing what is actually occurring is subtracted from that which was intended. This is shown schematically in Figure 7 as a summing junction (circle) with intended actions shown as positive and actual as negative.

Now, if the sensory feedback signal perfectly matched the intended signal, then there would be zero output from the summing junction. This means that the actual movements are taking place exactly as planned, and there is no need for any adjustments. If intended and actual movements are not in register, then the operation of this comparison is to make appropriate, quick adjustments to put the movement back on target. For a simple example, assume that at a particular moment in time, the intention was for the elbow joint angle to be at 90 degrees. However, sensory feedback indicates the actual joint angle was only 60 degrees. Subtracting the actual from the intended actions would yield 90 − 60 = +30 degrees. This positive outcome would then be forwarded as a proportionate magnitude excitatory input ("error signal," Figure 7) to the motor cortex to immediately boost drive to the limb in order to correct the lagging motion of the elbow. Alternatively, if sensory feedback indicated that the actual angle of the elbow was 120 degrees, then in this case subtraction would yield 90 − 120 = −30 degrees. As such, the forwarded error signal would be a proportionate negative signal representing inhibition of the motor cortex to throttle back drive to the limb that is too far forward of where it should be.

Some of the ataxia and associated movement errors observed in patients with cerebellar damage may be due to this disrupted comparator function of the cerebellum. It should be stated that the idea of an efference copy playing a role in comparing desired to actual movements has a long history. The more formalized and modern concept of efference copy was made by von Holst (1954). Yet, despite substantial efforts over the years, clear-cut demonstrations of the specific neural underpinnings associated with the comparator function of the cerebellum have been difficult to come by. Relatively recently, however, convincing evidence filling in some of the outlines of the scheme shown in Figure 7 has begun to emerge. For example, a specific class of spinal neurons that receive descending motor commands and then relay that information back up to the cerebellum has recently been identified as a likely source of efference copy (Azim *et al.* 2014). In addition, another study demonstrated that population activity across many cerebellar neurons (PCs, see below) collectively appears to encode the intended actions against which sensory signals can be compared (Herzfeld *et al.* 2015).

Cerebellar Circuitry

The cellular circuit within the cerebellum is striking for at least three reasons. One, the layout of the circuit has been clearly delineated and has been known for many decades. Two, the basic circuit is virtually the same everywhere in the cerebellum—repeated millions of times. And three, the circuit is fairly simple. Nevertheless, how this cellular system underlies the various functions of the cerebellum remains only partially understood.

Figure 8A shows a micrograph of a small section of the cerebellar cortex. Unlike the cerebral cortex, the *cerebellar* cortex has only three layers. The *innermost layer is called the* **granule cell layer** because it possesses billions of small cells that look grainy in histology (similar to layer 4 in some parts of the cerebral cortex). Indeed, **granule cells** *of the cerebellum are the smallest and most numerous neurons in the brain* (D'Angelo 2016). They typically have only four short dendrites. Consequently, they receive only a few synaptic contacts—indeed, cerebellar granule cells represent one of the smallest levels of synaptic convergence in the CNS.

Figure 8A also shows the cell bodies of a few **Purkinje cells** (named after their discoverer, the Czech anatomist Jan Purkinje in 1837). *These neurons have elaborate dendritic arbors (Figure 8B) and are highly unusual in that the dendrites are mostly confined to a single plane, like a handheld oriental fan* (see also the frontispiece). *The cell bodies of the PCs are large and comprise the middle layer of the cerebellar cortex,*

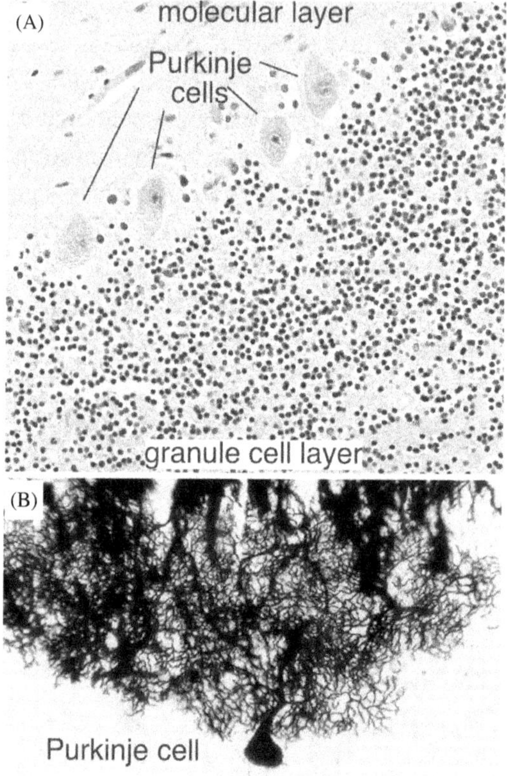

Figure 8.   (A) Small section of cerebellar cortex showing granule cells (small black dots) in the granule cell layer, the somas of a few Purkinje cells in the Purkinje cell layer, and the cell-sparse outer molecular layer. (B) Golgi-stained Purkinje cell showing extensive two-dimensional dendritic tree. (Adapted from University of Minnesota Veterinary Neurohistology Atlas, vanat.ahc.umn.edu/neurHistAtls/.)

called the **Purkinje cell layer**. The *outermost layer* is the **molecular layer** (Figure 8A), which *mostly possesses the dendrites of the PCs and the axons of the granule cells that make connections to the PCs* (described below).

Figure 9A is a basic schematic representing the connectivity among the neurons in the cerebellar cortex (a few cell types have been excluded for simplicity). The granule cells send axons up to the molecular layer, where they bifurcate and run in long stretches called parallel fibers (Figure 9A). In the molecular layer, the parallel fibers make repeated

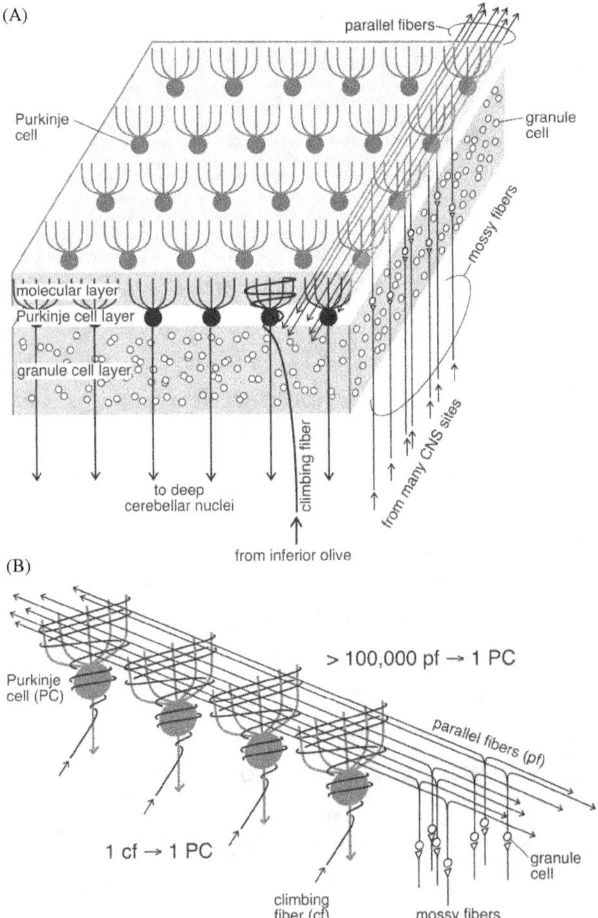

Figure 9. Cellular components of the cerebellar cortex. (A) The cerebellar cortex has three layers: the deep granule cell layer, the middle Purkinje cell layer, and the outer molecular layer. Inputs axons from many regions of the CNS, called mossy fibers, make excitatory contacts onto granule cells. Granule cell axons ascend into the molecular layer, where they bifurcate and run in long tracts with other axons called parallel fibers. Parallel fibers make excitatory synaptic contacts onto the dendrites of Purkinje cells. Purkinje cells also receive input from single climbing fibers that originate in the inferior olive of the brainstem. The only output from the cerebellar cortex is from Purkinje cells that make inhibitory connections to neurons in the deep cerebellar nuclei. (B) Schematic depicting connectivity pattern in cerebellar cortex. Massive numbers of parallel fibers make excitatory contacts onto long columns of Purkinje cells. As such, each Purkinje cell (PC) may receive greater than 100,000 parallel fiber (pf) inputs. On the other hand, each climbing fiber (cf) makes extensive contact with just one Purkinje cell.

synaptic contacts onto the dendritic arbors of successive PCs. PCs are laid out in a highly organized way in the cerebellar cortex, with long columns and rows, not unlike rows of vegetables planted in a garden. *A set of parallel fibers that pass through (and synapse upon) a column of PCs* is sometimes referred to as a "**beam**"—like a ray of information conveyed to a long array of cells (one such beam is depicted in Figure 9A). The plane of the PC dendrites is oriented perpendicular to the beam, acting like a large antenna to efficiently gather in large quantities of synaptic data carried on the beam.

There are two main sources of input to the cerebellar cortex. One is from **mossy fibers** *that arise from the massive set of axons that enter the cerebellum via the peduncles (see Figure 1B) from various locations in the CNS* (see Figure 2B). The mossy fibers make excitatory connections onto the granule cells (Figure 9A). The other source is the **climbing fibers**, *which arise from the inferior olive in the brainstem.* Climbing fibers are highly distinctive in that a single climbing fiber "climbs" all over a Purkinje cell, like a vine on a trellis (Figure 9A). In so doing, a single climbing fiber makes multiple synaptic contacts onto the dendrites of a single PC, forming an exceptionally potent excitatory synaptic connection. Interestingly, the only *output* from the cerebellar cortex is from the PCs that make inhibitory connections to neurons in the various DCN (Figure 9A).

Numerical features of connectivity among the elements of the cerebellar circuit are impressive. Figure 9B shows a schematic of a beam of parallel fibers coursing through the dendrites of a column of PCs—not unlike cables strung on the crossbeams of closely spaced electric poles. As parallel fibers pass by each PC, they give off excitatory synaptic contacts. The scale of this is enormous: a typical PC may receive in excess of 100,000 synaptic inputs from parallel fibers. At the other extreme, each PC receives input from only one climbing fiber (Figure 9B).

We can take this information and construct a basic representation of the cerebellar circuit (Figure 10). The region in Figure 10 above the dashed line represents the cerebellar cortex. The plane of the PC dendrites would be into and out of the page in Figure 10, and therefore, looks sparse in this depiction. Mossy fibers provide massive, continuous input indicating the somatosensory, vestibular, and movement planning states of the

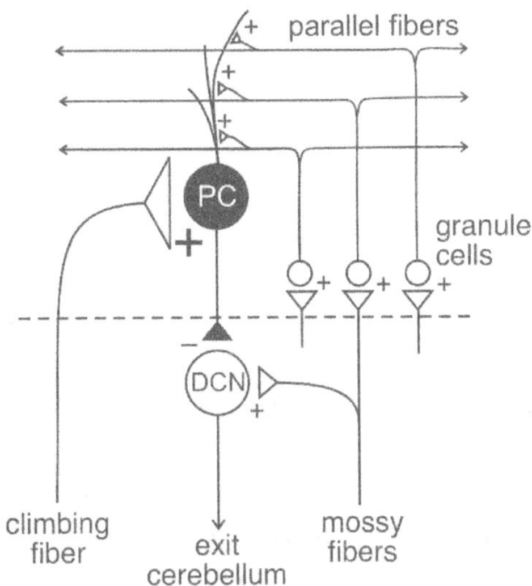

Figure 10. Simplified representation of cerebellar cellular circuit. Mossy fiber input provides excitatory input to granule cells and to neurons in the deep cerebellar nuclei (DCN). Granule cells, in turn, excite Purkinje cells (PCs) via the parallel fibers. PCs project back to neurons in the DCN with inhibitory input. Thus, DCN neurons, which provide the output of the cerebellum, receive converging excitatory and inhibitory inputs. Climbing fiber input provides brief massive depolarization of PCs. Cerebellar cortex is above the dashed horizontal line.

animal. Those inputs excite huge numbers of granule cells that, in turn, send excitatory projections via parallel fibers to lengthy columns of PCs. Prior to entering the cerebellar cortex, mossy fibers give off collaterals that provide excitatory input to the DCN (Figure 10). Climbing fibers, arising from the inferior olive in the brainstem, terminate in an elaborate plexus encompassing a PC. Because of the multifold glutamate release sites, this connection has been depicted as a large excitatory presynaptic terminal in Figure 10. Indeed, a *single* action potential in a climbing fiber leads to a large depolarization in a PC that, by itself, provokes a rapid burst of two to five action potentials. Such *climbing-fiber-induced bursts in a PC are referred to as a* **complex spike**. As will be discussed below, climbing fiber input and associated complex spikes are typically sparse and seem to occur significantly only under specific circumstances. While climbing fibers also send weak excitatory synaptic contacts to the DCN, their functional significance is uncertain (Lu *et al.* 2016) and are not shown in Figure 10.

Functions of Cerebellar Circuitry

Given the relative simplicity of the circuit depicted in Figure 10, it might be expected that some unifying theory as to how the operations of this circuit subserve the various functions of the cerebellum would have been set forth. No such theory, however, has yet been clearly articulated (or at least one that has been widely accepted). This is not to say that important ideas derived from extensive and rigorous experimental and theoretical work on the cerebellum have not been presented. Furthermore, there are aspects of the circuit that invite comparison to concepts discussed earlier. For example, converging excitatory inputs of mossy fibers and inhibitory inputs from PCs onto neurons of DCN (Figure 10) has some of the same flavor that the convergence of excitatory and inhibitory inputs had in the comparator representation of the cerebellum in Figure 7. In that representation, mismatches between those two sources of input are thought to lead to adjustments (up or down) in the output of the cerebellum that, in turn, serves to correct errors in movements.

In the cellular representation (Figure 10), neurons of the DCN would seem to serve a similar function as the "summing junction" (Figure 7) shown in the comparator circuit. Likewise, mossy fiber input would seem generally well suited to provide sensory feedback reporting on the actual circumstances taking place during a movement, as also depicted in Figure 7. Further, relatively recent work has shown that population activity in PCs provides a prediction of upcoming movements (Herzfeld *et al.* 2015). Such activity could represent intended actions driven by efference copy as laid out in the comparator circuit.

It could also be that some aspects of the comparator function depicted in Figure 7 may largely occur outside of the cerebellum, in the inferior olive (Oscarsson 1979). The inferior olive does receive substantial somatosensory input from ascending pathways (representing what is taking place) and converging descending inputs from the motor cortex via brainstem nuclei (perhaps representing the intended action) (Armstrong 1974). Furthermore, climbing fiber activity arising from the inferior olive is

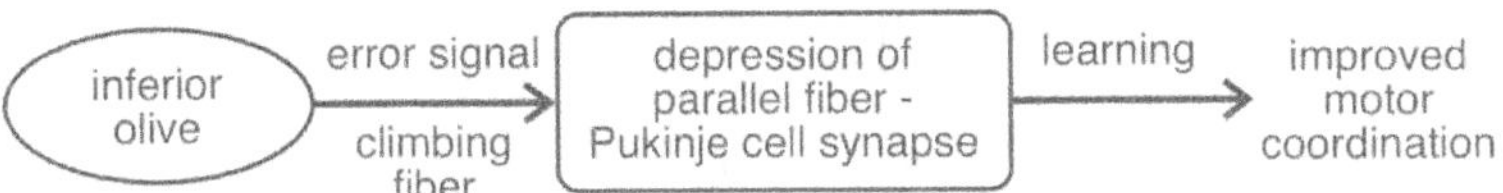

Figure 11.   Hypothesized mechanism by which mismatch between intended and actual movements leads to an error signal arising on climbing fibers from the inferior olive to reduce the strength of parallel fiber synaptic input onto Purkinje cells. This depression causes a long-term decrease in Purkinje cell output that is thought to underlie adjustments needed to reduce motor errors. This idea is attributed to Marr (1969), Albus (1971), and Ito (2001).

enhanced during movements when an unexpected perturbation (creating a mismatch between intended and actual movements) is applied to a limb (Gilbert & Thatch 1977). Such climbing fiber activity might serve as an error signal that, as proposed by theoreticians, could act as a "teaching" signal to selectively change the strength of synaptic connections between those parallel fibers and the PCs that are active at the moment of climbing fiber input (Figure 11). The change in synaptic strength is thought to modify the PC activity and leads to long-lasting adjustments in the output of the cerebellum that serves to overcome movement errors.

Long-Term Depression

Unlike the type of synaptic plasticity discussed in Chapter 7, where coincident activity in pre and postsynaptic neurons can lead to increases in synaptic strength, in the cerebellum, *coincident activity in climbing fibers and parallel fibers leads to a sustained reduction in the strength of parallel fiber synapses onto PCs*. This type of synaptic plasticity is called **long-term depression (LTD)** (see Figure 11). Figure 12A shows the type of experimental arrangement that was used to demonstrate LTD in isolated slices of the cerebellum (Daniel *et al.* 1998). An intracellular electrode was used to record PC responses to stimulation of a bundle of parallel fibers. In this situation, the PC electrode was used to record the net synaptic *current* associated with activating the parallel fibers. Recall from Chapter 5 (Figure 5) that inward current carrying positive (depolarizing) charges into a cell is conventionally represented as being in the "downward" direction. Figure 12B shows an example of such an inward current measured in a PC in response

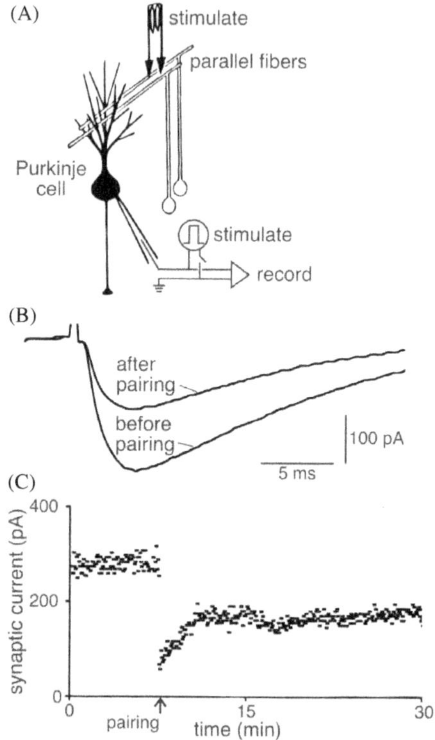

Figure 12.   Demonstration of long-term depression (LTD) in synapses between parallel fibers and Purkinje cells. (A) Experimental setup. An intracellular electrode was placed in a Purkinje cell that could be used to record net synaptic currents in response to stimulation of a set of parallel fibers or stimulate the Purkinje cell to mimic the depolarization caused by climbing fiber input. (B) Examples of inward synaptic current recorded in a Purkinje cell to stimulation of the same bundle of parallel fibers prior to ("before pairing") and following ("after pairing") concurrent climbing-fiber-like depolarization of the Purkinje cell with activation of parallel fibers. (C) Peak inward synaptic current measured over many minutes prior to and following paired (arrow) stimulation of parallel fibers and Purkinje cells. Synaptic efficacy is weakened for prolonged duration following the pairing—the signature of LTD. ([A] adapted from Daniel *et al.* [1998], [B] from Blond *et al.* [1997].)

to stimulating a set of parallel fibers (labeled "before pairing") (Blond *et al.* 1997). In this case, the peak inward current was ~300 pA.

The PC electrode was then connected to a stimulator (Figure 12A). Stimulation through this electrode was designed to elicit the same type of depolarization that occurs with climbing fiber input. The investigators then paired the stimulation of the parallel fibers (four stimuli/s for 1 minute) to coincide with repeated strong depolarizations of the PC (like that which would occur with climbing fiber input). Following this pairing protocol, the electrode in the PC was again used to record responses to stimulation of parallel fibers. After pairing, the inward current response in the PC to activation of the same parallel fibers was reduced by almost half (see the "after pairing" trace, Figure 12B). Moreover, this marked reduction in synaptic transmission was maintained over a long period of time, as shown in Figure 12C. Each dot in Figure 12C represents the peak inward current measured in the same PC to parallel fiber stimulation before and several minutes following the pairing protocol (Blond *et al.* 1997). Such an enduring reduction in synaptic efficacy is the hallmark of LTD.

Mechanism of Long-Term Depression

The strength of synapses can be *increased* between many types of neurons when presynaptic and postsynaptic neurons are active at the same time. Such Hebbian plasticity (see Chapter 7) comes about through activation of NMDA receptors in postsynaptic neurons that requires both binding of glutamate (provided by activity in presynaptic neurons) and strong membrane depolarization (reflective of activity in the postsynaptic neurons). This leads to Ca^{+2} influx through the NMDA-receptor channels that triggers synthesis and insertion of more glutamate AMPA receptors in the postsynaptic membrane, endowing the involved synapses with a long-lasting enhanced capability to depolarize the postsynaptic neuron. This type of plasticity is sometimes referred to as long-term potentiation (LTP).

Some of the same players associated with LTP are also involved in the long-lasting weakening of synapses at parallel fiber–PC synapses associated with LTD. These include the release of glutamate from presynaptic neurons (parallel fibers), strong depolarization of the postsynaptic neuron (in PCs caused by climbing fiber input), and an influx of Ca^{+2} triggering the changes that cause weakening of synaptic strength.

Figure 13 shows a schematic of some of the processes thought to be involved in LTD in the cerebellum. The presynaptic terminal is from a parallel fiber, and the postsynaptic side represents a dendrite of a PC.

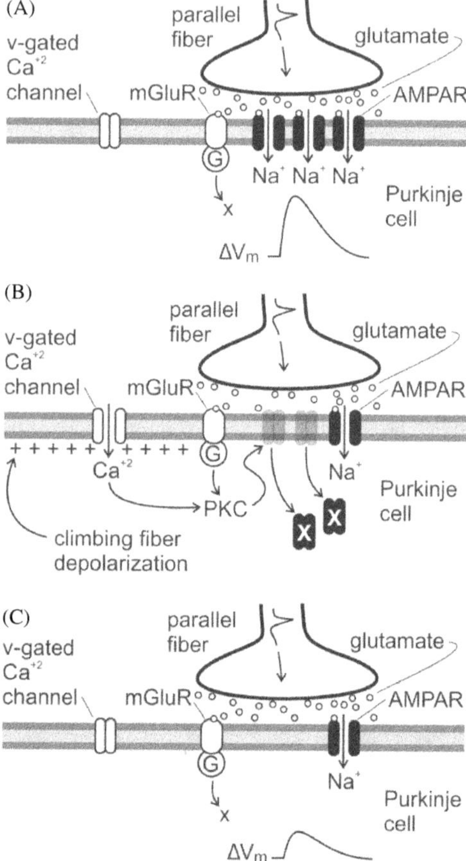

Figure 13.   Simplified representation of the cellular mechanisms underlying long-term depression in the cerebellum. (A) In an unmodified synapse, the release of glutamate from parallel fiber acts on both AMPA and mGluRs in the postsynaptic membrane of Purkinje cell dendrites. Several AMPA channels open together, leading to Na^+ influx and local depolarization (ΔV_m) of Purkinje cells. The activation of the mGluR has no downstream effect ("x") because the cascade requires the presence of Ca^{+2}. (B) Input from climbing fiber causes large depolarization of Purkinje cell, triggering influx of Ca^{+2} through voltage-gated Ca^{+2} channels. Parallel fibers that have released glutamate around the same time will engage mGluRs to instigate a cascade supported by the presence of Ca^{+2}. That metabolic pathway activates protein kinase C (PKC), which prompts the internalization of AMPA receptors in the vicinity of the synapse. (C) Following this process, the strength of the parallel fiber—Purkinje cells synapse is weakened because of fewer AMPA receptors and will be associated with a smaller depolarization (ΔV_m) after paired parallel and climbing fiber inputs.

Two types of receptors for glutamate are co-localized at the synapse in the postsynaptic membrane: AMPA receptors (ionotropic-receptor channel that leads to depolarization of the postsynaptic membrane—see Chapter 7) and metabotropic glutamate receptors (mGluR). Recall that such receptors do not directly open ion channels but instead often instigate a G-protein-coupled metabolic cascade that can influence a variety of processes in the postsynaptic cell.

In the non-modified state (Figure 13A), entry of an action potential into the presynaptic terminal of the parallel fiber triggers release of glutamate. Glutamate binds to both the AMPA and mGlu receptors in the postsynaptic membrane. Opening of the multiple AMPA receptor channels leads to an influx of Na^+ ions and localized membrane depolarization (ΔV_m) of the PC dendrite. Activation of the mGluR has minimal consequence ("x" in Figure 13A) because the effective metabolic cascade also requires the presence of Ca^{+2}.

When *climbing fiber* input causes a massive depolarization of the PC (Figure 13B), this leads to the opening of voltage-gated Ca^{+2} channels and the influx of Ca^{+2} into the PC dendrites. If the metabolic cascade initiated by the binding of glutamate to mGluRs occurs around the same time as the climbing fiber input and associated influx of Ca^{+2}, this will activate the intracellular substance protein kinase C (PKC, Figure 13B). PKC then provokes the internalization and removal of AMPA receptors at those synapses whose mGluR were just activated. The extent of this removal is greater with repeated pairings of the same parallel fibers with climbing fiber activation. Subsequent excitation of those parallel fibers (Figure 13C) will be associated with a smaller synaptic current and weaker level of depolarization because of the smaller number of AMPA receptors. The associated long-lasting reduction in synaptic strength is the manifestation of LTD in the cerebellum.

Functional Consequence of LTD at Parallel Fiber–Purkinje Cell Synapses

Although debated (e.g., see Schonewille *et al.* 2011; Welsh *et al.* 2005), LTD at synapses between parallel fibers and PCs has been considered to be critical for learning new motor skills (Ito 2001). But how might weakening those synapses be beneficial to motor learning? To help explain, let's consider a case involving adaptation to a new contingency that arises during simple movements. For example, Gilbert and Thatch (1977) trained monkeys to hold a lever at a particular position. On each trial, a motor attached to the lever would displace the lever away from the target position by abruptly increasing the force required to hold the lever in the target position. Monkeys were required to rapidly return the lever to the target position by increasing the force exerted on the lever to obtain a juice reward.

The monkeys were well trained on this task involving a fixed displacement force over a period of several months during which they performed the task with great skill. Then, while the monkeys were performing this well-trained behavior, the experimenters suddenly *changed* the displacement force applied to the lever. The monkey's ability to do the task immediately dropped under these novel circumstances. However, over several trials, the monkeys adapted to the new load and eventually were performing at the same level as before the change in the task.

Gilbert and Thatch recorded the activity of PCs in the monkeys during this period of learning new task requirements. The extracellular electrodes used allowed them to distinguish the occurrence of climbing fiber-mediated complex spikes (driven by input from climbing fibers) from regular spikes (called "simple" spikes), driven by activity received from parallel fibers. Figure 14A shows a recording from a PC over multiple trials (each row) of the task just prior to and then following the sudden change to a novel displacement force (horizontal arrow, Figure 14A). Prior to the change to the new load (top set of trials), complex spike activity (indicated by large dots, Figure 14A) was sporadic and was at a low rate, ~1.5 complex spikes/s on average. Simple spike activity (small dots) at the outset (initial ~0.15 s) of each trial (when the monkey was responding to the displacement force) was very high, on the order of 150 spikes/s. (It should be noted that even under resting conditions, PCs discharge at rates up to 100 spikes/s.) Immediately following the unexpected increase in displacement load, complex spikes were triggered near the onset of each trial. Such activity in climbing-fiber input (causing complex spikes) during this time would seem consistent with the idea that it might signal a mismatch between expected and actual movements. After multiple trials

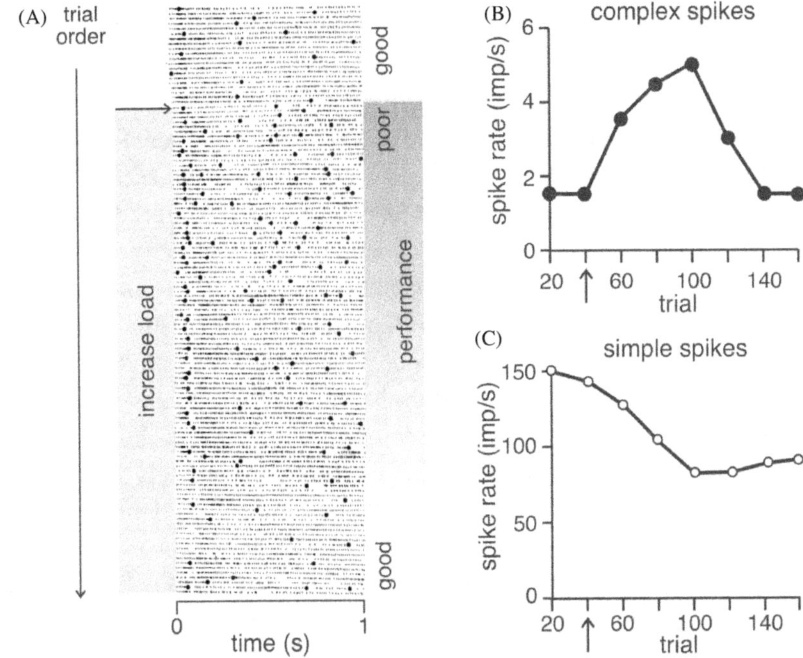

Figure 14.   Changes in complex spike and simple spike activities associated with learning a new task contingency. (A) Each row represents a complex spike (large dots) and a simple spike (small dots) recorded in a Purkinje cell of a monkey performing a task that involved rapidly moving a lever back to a target zone after a load was abruptly applied to the lever (at time 0 s). The first ~20 trials (top rows) were those for a load that the monkey had extensive experience, and his performance was good. On the trial indicated by the horizontal arrow, the magnitude of the load was unexpectedly increased. The monkey's performance with the new load was now poor. However, over the next ~60 trials, performance with the new load progressively improved until it was just about as good as before the imposition of the new load. (B) The incidence of complex spikes (measured over the initial 0.15 s of the task) increased when the new load was applied (vertical arrow). However, as the monkey gradually learned the new task and performance improved, the rate of complex spikes decreased back to the initial level. (C) Simple spike rate (measured just over the initial period of the task) was high. However, with the application of the novel load and increased complex spike activity, simple spike activity decreased. (Adapted from Gilbert and Thatch [1977].)

with the increased load, the monkey's performance progressively improved (right-hand side of Figure 14A). Importantly, complex spike activity associated with the onset of each movement gradually dissipated (see bottom of Figure 14A), returning to levels similar to that prior to the change in load. Presumably, movements were now occurring "according to plan," and there was no longer a mismatch between intended and actual movements. These findings are shown quantitatively in Figure 14B, depicting an initial increase in average complex spike activity following the increase in load applied to the lever (arrow, Figure 14B). After about 60 trials under this new situation, complex spike rate begins to fall, eventually returning to the initial level before the change in load.

More subtly, the rate of simple spikes can be seen to diminish over this period of learning. If one focuses on the density of small dots (the simple spikes) during the initial period of each trial, one can discern it to be relatively high in the set of trials before the new load was applied (Figure 14A). If one examines the same initial period of simple spike activity after the monkey had learned to respond accurately to the new load (bottom set of trials, Figure 14A), it appears to be less dense than that prior to the application of the new load. This impression is confirmed when simple spike activity (quantified over the initial 0.15 s) is plotted across the entire set of trials prior to and following the imposition of the new load (arrow) in Figure 14C. Simple spike rate decreased from ~150 spikes/s before the new load was added to about 100 spikes/s after learning to respond appropriately to the new load. In concept, the increased complex spike activity provoked by the new load situation (and when performance was poor) led to the weakening of the synapses of those parallel fibers activated during the task by LTD. LTD-mediated diminution of the depolarization caused by those parallel fibers, in turn, would cause simple spike output of the PCs to decrease.

But why would such a decrease in PC output serve to increase performance in this task? One possibility is outlined in Figure 15. Under nominal conditions (Figure 15A), like that associated with performing a well-learned task, neurons in the DCN receive converging excitatory input from the mossy fibers and inhibitory input from the PCs. The output of the DCN in response to these opposing inputs can be considered to represent an appropriate level of activity needed to perform the task accurately. When there is an unexpected change to the task (like increasing the load in Figure 14), climbing fiber activity signals the presence of an error (Figure 15B). This instigates LTD in the synapses of the granule cell—parallel fibers that were active during the error. When repeated over

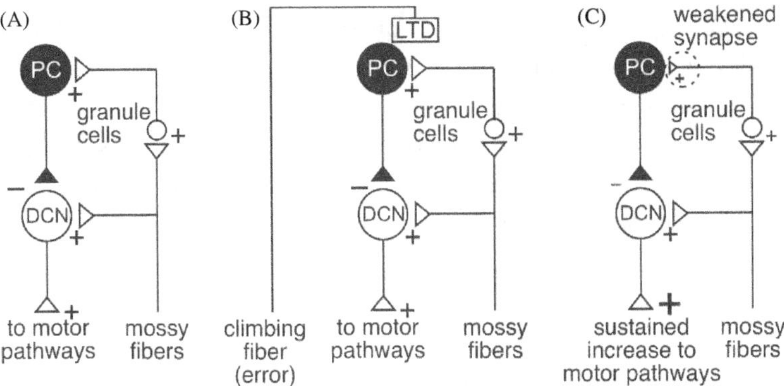

Figure 15.   Schematic depicting how long-term depression (LTD) of granule cell—parallel fiber synapses onto Purkinje cells (PCs) might improve responses to novel movement contingency. (A) Nominal state with consistent converging excitation from mossy fibers and inhibition from PCs leading to an appropriate output from the deep cerebellar nuclei (DCN) needed to perform a task. (B) If, for example, the load that must be overcome to perform a task unexpectedly increases, climbing fiber input from the inferior olive will signal a movement error and lead to LTD of the involved granule cell—parallel fiber synapses onto the PCs. (C) Weakening of parallel fiber excitation to PCs will lessen the inhibition delivered to the DCN and thereby enhance the output of the DCN to cope with the new increased load.

multiple trials, the weakening of the parallel fiber synapses (depicted as a smaller synapse in Figure 15C) lessens the inhibitory output of the PCs onto the DCN. Consequently, the degree of inhibition delivered to the DCN decreases, leading to an increased output of the DCN, providing an added surge of drive needed to cope with the increased load and restore movement accuracy.

Summary

The cerebellum is an enigmatic structure involved in coordination and learning of movements. It receives rich input from motor and somatosensory areas of the brain and spinal cord. Its output modifies and shapes commands that drive movements. Damage to the cerebellum can lead to dyscoordination and the inability to learn new movements. The cellular circuitry of the cerebellum is reasonably straightforward and has been well delineated. Features of the circuit seem to act as a feedback control system—comparing desired movements (efference copy) to what actually occurs (via sensory feedback from the periphery) to make appropriate adjustments when errors are detected. The circuit also possesses a form of synaptic plasticity called LTD that seems to facilitate the learning of new motor skills and adapting to new movement contingencies.

References

Albus JS (1971). A theory of cerebellar function. *Mathematical Biosciences* **10**, 25–61.

Armstrong DM (1974). Functional significance of connections of the inferior olive. *Physiological Reviews* **54**, 358–417.

Azim E, Jiang J, Alstermark B & Jessell TM (2014). Skilled reaching relies on a V2a propriospinal internal copy circuit. *Nature Publishing Group* **508**, 1–21.

Bastian AJ, Martin TA, Keating JG & Thach WT (1996). Cerebellar ataxia: Abnormal control of interaction torques across multiple joints. *Journal of Neurophysiology* **76**, 492–509.

Benagiano V, Rizzi A, Lorusso L, Flace P, Saccia M, Cagiano R, Ribatti D, Roncali L & Ambrosi G (2018). The functional anatomy of the cerebrocerebellar circuit: A review and new concepts. *The Journal of Comparative Neurology* **526**, 769–789.

Blond O, Daniel H, Otani S, Jaillard D & Crépel F (1997). Presynaptic and postsynaptic effects of nitric oxide donors at synapses between parallel fibres and Purkinje cells: Involvement in cerebellar long-term depression. *Neuroscience* **77**, 945–954.

Bostan AC, Dum RP & Strick PL (2013). Cerebellar networks with the cerebral cortex and basal ganglia. *Trends in Cognitive Sciences* **17**, 241–254.

Buckner RL (2013). The cerebellum and cognitive function: 25 years of insight from anatomy and neuroimaging. *Neuron* **80**, 807–815.

Chen SHA & Desmond JE (2005). Cerebrocerebellar networks during articulatory rehearsal and verbal working memory tasks. *NeuroImage* **24**, 332–338.

D'Angelo E (2016). Granule cells and parallel fibers. In: D.L. Gruol *et al.* (eds.), Essentials of Cerebellum and Cerebellar Disorders, Springer: Switzerland.

Daniel H, Levenes C & Crépel F (1998). Cellular mechanisms of cerebellar LTD. *Trends in Neurosciences* **21**, 401–407.

Filipek PA, Richelme C, Kennedy DN & Caviness VS (1994). The young adult human brain: An MRI-based morphometric analysis. *Cerebal Cortex* **4**, 344–360.

Gao J-H, Parsons LM, Bower JM, Xiong J, Li J & Fox PT (1996). Cerebellum Implicated in sensory acquisition and discrimination rather than motor control. *Science* **272**, 545–547.

Gilbert PFC & Thach WT (1977). Purkinje cell activity during motor learning. *Brain Research* **128**, 309–328.

Glickstein M (2007). What does the cerebellum really do? *Current Biology* **17**, R824–R827.

Herculano-Houzel S (2009). The human brain in numbers: A linearly scaled-up primate brain. *Front Human Neuroscience* **3**, 31, 11 pgs.

Herzfeld DJ, Kojima Y, Soetedjo R & Shadmehr R (2015). Encoding of action by the Purkinje cells of the cerebellum. *Nature* **526**, 439–442.

Inhoff AW, Diener HC, Rafal RD & Ivry R (1989). The role of cerebellar structures in the execution of serial movements. *Brain* **112**, 565–581.

Ito M (2001). Cerebellar long-term depression: Characterization, signal transduction, and functional roles. *Physiology Review* **81**, 1143–1195.

Kelly RM & Strick PL (2003). Cerebellar loops with motor cortex and prefrontal cortex of a nonhuman primate. *Journal of Neuroscience* **23**, 8432–8444.

Leiner HC, Leiner AL & Dow RS (1993). Cognitive and language functions of the human cerebellum. *Trends Neuroscience* **16**, 444–447.

Lu H, Yang B & Jaeger D (2016). Cerebellar nuclei neurons show only small excitatory responses to optogenetic olivary stimulation in transgenic mice: In vivo and in vitro studies. *Front Neural Circuits* **10**, 21.

Manto M (2008). The cerebellum, cerebellar disorders, and cerebellar research—Two centuries of discoveries. *Cerebellum* **7**, 505.

Marr D (1969). A theory of cerebellar cortex. *Journal of Physiology* **202**, 437–470.

Martin JH, Cooper SE, Hacking A & Ghez C (2000). Differential effects of deep cerebellar nuclei inactivation on reaching and adaptive control. *Journal of Neurophysiology* **83**, 1886–1899.

Martin TA, Keating JG, Goodkin HP, Bastian AJ & Thach WT (1996). Throwing while looking through prisms I. Focal olivocerebellar lesions impair adaptation. *Brain* **119**, 1183–1198.

Milak MS, Shimansky Y, Bracha V & Bloedel JR (1997). Effects of inactivating individual cerebellar nuclei on the performance and retention of an operantly conditioned forelimb movement. *Journal Neurophysiology* **78**, 939–959.

Nagao S, Kitamura T, Nakamura N, Hiramatsu T & Yamada J (1997). Differences of the primate flocculus and ventral paraflocculus in the mossy and climbing fiber input organization. *The Journal of Comparative Neurology* **382**, 480–498.

Oscarsson O (1965). Functional organization of the spino- and cuneocerebellar tracts. *Physiology Review* **45**, 495–522.

Oscarsson O (1979). Functional units of the cerebellum—sagittal zones and microzones. *Trends Neuroscience* **2**, 143–145.

Park H-K, Kim J-S, Strupp M & Zee DS (2013). Isolated floccular infarction: Impaired vestibular responses to horizontal head impulse. *Journal of Neurology* **260**, 1576–1582.

Phillips SC, Harper CG & Kril J (1987). A quantitative histological study of the cerebellar vermis in alcoholic patients. *Brain* **110**, 301–314.

Purves D, Augustine GJ, Fitzpatrick D, Katz LC, LaMantia A-S, McNamara JO & S Williams M. (2001). Neuroscience. Sinauer: Sunderland, MA.

Schmahmann JD (1996). From movement to thought: Anatomic substrates of the cerebellar contribution to cognitive processing. *Human Brain Mapped* **4**, 174–198.

Schonewille M, Gao Z, Boele H-J, Veloz MFV, Amerika WE, Šimek AAM, Jeu MTD, Steinberg JP, Takamiya K, Hoebeek FE, Linden DJ, Huganir RL & Zeeuw CID (2011). Reevaluating the Role of LTD in Cerebellar Motor Learning. *Neuron* **70**, 43–50.

Strick PL, Dum RP & Fiez JA (2009). Cerebellum and nonmotor function. *Annual Review of Neuroscience* **32**, 413–434.

Sullivan EV, Deshmukh A, Desmond JE, Lim KO & Pfefferbaum A (2000). Cerebellar volume decline in normal aging, alcoholism, and Korsakoff's syndrome: Relation to ataxia. *Neuropsychology* **14**, 341–352.

Thach WT, Goodkin HP & Keating JG (1992). The cerebellum and the adaptive coordination of movement. *Annual Review of Neuroscience* **15**, 403–442.

Trouche E & Beaubaton D (1980). Initiation of a goal-directed movement in the monkey. *Experimental Brain Research* **40**, 311–321.

von Holst E (1954). Relations between the central nervous system and the peripheral organs. *The British Journal of Animal Behaviour* **2**, 89–94.

Welsh JP, Yamaguchi H, Zeng X-H, Kojo M, Nakada Y, Takagi A, Sugimori M & Llinás RR (2005). Normal motor learning during pharmacological prevention of Purkinje cell long-term depression. *Proceedings of the National Academy of Sciences of the United States of America* **102**, 17166–17171.

Wiesendanger R, Wiesendanger M & Rüegg DG (1979). An anatomical investigation of the corticopontine projection in the primate (*Macaca fascicularis* and *Saimiri sciureus*)—II. The projection from frontal and parietal association areas. *Neuroscience* **4**, 747–765.

Wirth FP & O'Leary JL (1974). Locomotor behavior of decerebellated arboreal mammals—monkey and raccoon. *Journal of Comparative Neurology* **157**, 53–85.

Wolpert DM, Miall RC & Kawato M (1998). Internal models in the cerebellum. *Trends in Cognitive Sciences* **2**, 338–347.

Yu F, Jiang Q, Sun X & Zhang R (2015). A new case of complete primary cerebellar agenesis: Clinical and imaging findings in a living patient. *Brain* **138**, e353–e353.

Chapter 21

Basal Ganglia

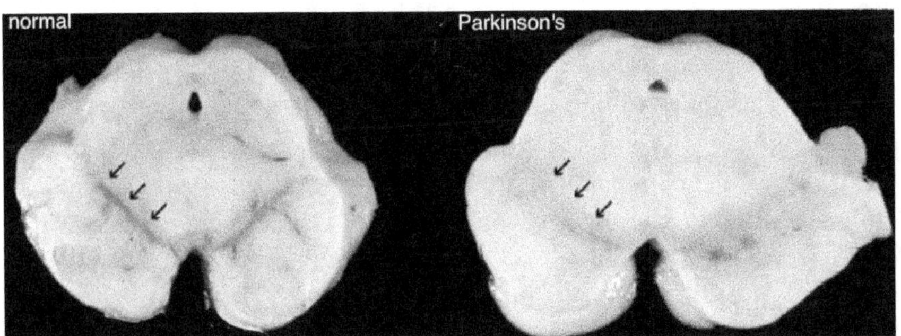

Post-mortem cross section through midbrain region of human brains. Left is from a normal healthy individual and the right is from an individual that suffered from Parkinson's disease. The arrows on the left point to the substantia nigra, a pigmented region that is a key source of the neurotransmitter dopamine. This region degenerates in Parkinson's disease and is barely detectable in the brain of the individual with Parkinson's disease. (Adapted from Halliday [2004].)

The basal ganglia (also referred to as the basal nuclei) are a collection of prominent brain structures found deep in the cerebrum and midbrain. Like parts of the cerebellum, the basal ganglia receive rich inputs from the cerebral cortex and project back to motor areas of the cerebral cortex. However, the extent of cerebral cortical input and the expanse of cortical regions targeted by the basal ganglia are much greater than for the cerebellum. As such, the basal ganglia are involved in a number of functions, not just those associated with motor control. Furthermore, the basal ganglia are implicated in a host of neurological disorders. Therefore, an understanding of the basic circuitry of the basal ganglia can provide important insights into the nature of these disorders and therapeutic approaches used to treat them, as will be discussed in this chapter.

Anatomy of the Basal Ganglia

The basal ganglia are a set of bilaterally paired structures that lie deep in the brain. Figure 1A is a lateral view of the brain with some of the entities that make up the basal ganglia made visible. The *outer (most lateral) structure is the oval-shaped* **putamen** (means nutshell in Latin). As shall be described, it is one of the entities of the basal ganglia that receives input from the cerebral cortex. *Extending from the dorsal region of the putamen is the long, curved, tail-like structure called the* **caudate nucleus** (meaning tail). The caudate, like the putamen, is a key structure that receives cortical input.

If part of the putamen were scraped away, *the more medially situated* **globus pallidus** (pale globe) would become visible (Figure 1A). It has complex functions, some of which are described below. Also seen in Figure 1A near the midline is the thalamus (not part of the basal ganglia). The remaining components of the basal ganglia are not readily visible in a lateral view. Therefore, a coronal section through the brain, taken at the level of the dashed line in Figure 1A, is useful for identifying the remainder of the basal ganglia.

In the coronal section of the half brain shown in Figure 1B, the prominent oval form of the thalamus is evident near the midline. Clustered dorsal (above), lateral, and ventral (below) to the thalamus, most of the components of the basal ganglia are visible and are highlighted in Figure 1B. The most lateral of these is the putamen. If one examines the dashed line in Figure 1A (representing the level of the section in Figure 1B), it can be seen to pass through the C-shaped caudate at two locations: one dorsal and one ventral. Those two sites are visible in cross-section in Figure 1B: dorsal and ventral to the thalamus. The putamen and the caudate serve similar functions as the structures receiving input from the cortex. They are *collectively referred to as the* **striatum** (Figure 1B), so called because where the caudate emerges from the dorsal putamen (see Figure 1A), there are gray matter bridges between bundles of white matter that give this region a striped (i.e. striate) appearance.

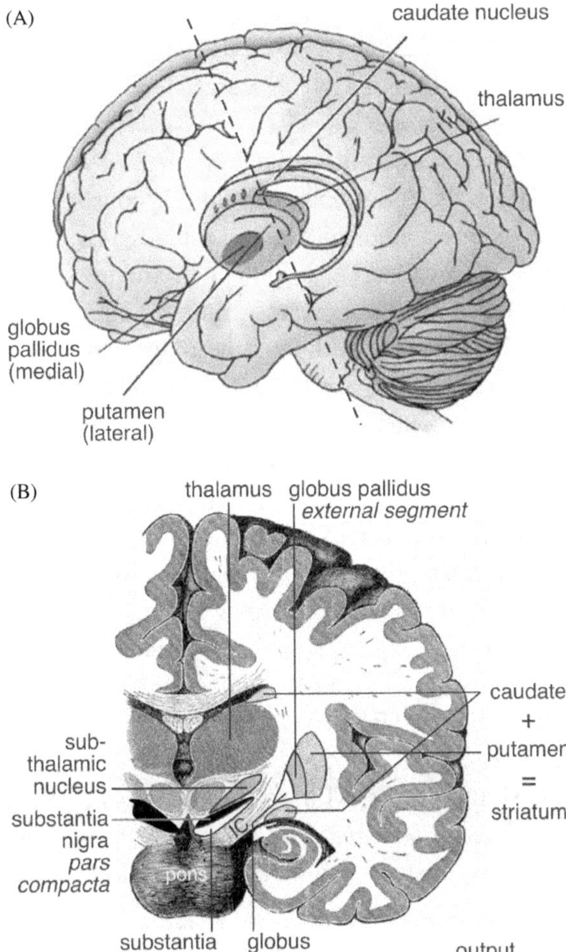

Figure 1.   (A) Lateral view of the brain showing some of the structures that make up the basal ganglia. Dashed line shows approximate level of section used in B. (B) Coronal section showing thalamus and components of the basal ganglia. ([B] adapted from Gray [1918].)

Situated immediately medial to the putamen is the wedge-shaped globus pallidus, which has two *functional* subdivisions. One (the most lateral) is called the **globus pallidus external (GPe) segment**, and the other more medial portion is called the **globus pallidus internal (GPi) segment** (Figure 1B). The **GPe** *is a processing station within the basal* *ganglia*, whereas the **GPi** *serves as an output structure* (as will be discussed). Situated *immediately ventral to the thalamus* is the aptly named **subthalamic nucleus** (Figure 1B)—*a stand-alone entity* whose function will also be discussed below.

Lastly, there is the **substantia nigra,** *a nucleus that sits in the mid-brain* (Figure 1B). Like the globus pallidus, it consists of two distinct functional subdivisions. One is the ventral-lateral **substantia nigra pars reticulata (SNpr)**—so called because the cell architecture is not clearly organized, like a loose meshwork or reticulum. The **SNpr** *functions similarly to the GPi.* Indeed, it is as though the SNpr was pulled away from the GPi early in development, like twins separated at birth, by the growth of the massive white matter tract called the **internal capsule** (IC, in Figure 1B). The IC is a *key conduit carrying axons between the cerebral cortex, brainstem, and spinal cord.* Collectively, the *GPi and SNpr comprise a single functional entity* (Nauta 1979) *that acts as the output station of the basal ganglia* (Figure 1B). Unfortunately, unlike the striatum, no single term has been articulated to designate this functional amalgam, so we are left referring to it as *GPi/SNpr.* Finally, there is the dorsal-medial region of the substantia nigra, called the **substantia nigra pars compacta (SNpc)** (Figure 1B). It has this designation because *it consists of densely packed cells that are darkly pigmented* by a substance similar to melanin—the skin pigment. As described below, the cells in the **SNpc** *release the neurotransmitter **dopamine** into the striatum.* Degeneration of the SNpc is the key histological feature of Parkinson's disease (see frontispiece).

Flow of Information through the Basal Ganglia

Like was done for the cerebellum, it is useful to first consider the general flow of information through the basal ganglia, including where inputs arrive from and where outputs project to (Figure 2). Inputs to the basal ganglia arise from a wide expanse of the cerebral cortex. The main outputs of the basal ganglia, on the other hand, are directed to nuclei in the thalamus. Those nuclei then project back to two main regions in the frontal lobe of the cerebral cortex: one is the supplementary motor area (SMA),

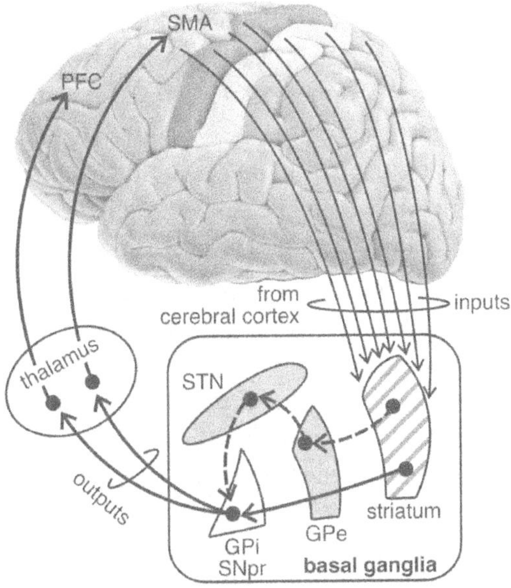

Figure 2.   Pathways through the basal ganglia (elements with the box). Inputs to the basal ganglia are from various regions of the cerebral cortex. Outputs from the basal ganglia project to the prefrontal cortex (PFC) and supplementary motor area (SMA) via nuclei in the thalamus. Cortical inputs to basal ganglia are received by the striatum. Outputs from the basal ganglia are from the globus pallidus internal (GPi) segment and substantia nigra pars reticulata (SNpr). Direct path (solid arrow) links striatum to GPi/SNpr. The indirect path involves projections from the striatum to the globus pallidus external (GPe) segment, GPe to the subthalamic nucleus (STN), and STN to GPi/SNpr.

and the other is a *broad rostral region of the frontal cortex* referred to as the **prefrontal cortex**. As discussed in Chapter 19, the SMA is thought to be involved in planning internally generated movements (i.e., those that don't necessarily include an overt external target). The prefrontal cortex, on the other hand, participates in a number of high-level cognitive processes, like reasoning, decision-making, and short-term memory. It also includes areas linked to personality, social behavior, speech control, and eye movements. The general operations of the basal ganglia associated with each of these disparate functions are thought to be similar but to occur across distinct, parallel pathways (Alexander *et al.* 1986).

Here we focus primarily on the motor pathway through the basal ganglia. In this case, the dominant cortical inputs are from the premotor, primary motor, and somatosensory cortex (Figure 2). The region of the basal ganglia that receives cortical input is the striatum. The entity that provides the output from the basal ganglia to nuclei in the thalamus is the composite structure GPi/SNPr. The thalamic nuclei in this case primarily project to the SMA (Schell & Strick 1984). There are two ways that information entering the input structure (striatum) gets passed to the output structure (GPi–SNpr). One is via *direct connections from the striatum to the GPi–SNpr* (solid arrow inside basal ganglia, Figure 2). As such, it is referred to as the **direct pathway**. In the other case, the flow of information from input to output structures within the basal ganglia takes a detour (dashed arrows, Figure 2). For this route (called the **indirect pathway**), *neurons in the striatum project to the GPe; the GPe then sends output to the subthalamic nucleus (STN), which in turn communicates with the output entity, GPi–SNpr.*

Functional Organization of Basal Ganglia

Figure 3 provides a simplified schematic of some of the main connections among the various elements of the basal ganglia (gray boxes) and their connections from and to other structures. This scheme is largely based on early reports from Albin *et al.* (1989), Alexander and Crutcher (1990), and Gerfen *et al.* (1990). Input to the striatum of the basal ganglia from the cerebral cortex is excitatory (glutamatergic). The output from the GPi–SNpr directed at nuclei within the thalamus is inhibitory (GABAergic). That output is persistently active and continuously acts to suppress the thalamus from engaging the SMA to promote internally generated movements. In a nutshell, the greater the output from the basal ganglia, the less likely that internally generated movements will be produced.

The neurons in the striatum that project directly to the GPi–SNpr (i.e., the direct pathway) are inhibitory (GABAergic) (Figure 3). As such, when this pathway is active, it will tend to suppress the GPi/SNpr. This, in turn, will lessen the inhibition of the thalamus directed at it from the GPi/SNpr, increasing the excitation of the SMA. In simple terms, one can think of this as "two negatives make a positive." In this case, the two negatives are

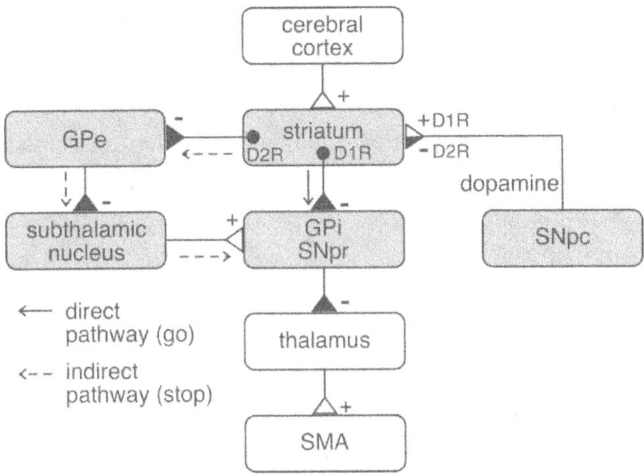

Figure 3.   Connections and pathways through the basal ganglia (gray boxes). Excitatory input from the cortex is delivered to the striatum. Output from the basal ganglia is from the globus pallidus internal (GPi) segment and substantia nigra pars reticulata (SNPr). That output is inhibitory and is directed to nuclei in the thalamus that, in turn, provide excitatory drive to the supplementary motor area (SMA). Inhibitory projections from the striatum directly to the GPi/SNpr reduce basal ganglia output. Such inhibition of a structure that tonically inhibits the thalamus (disinhibition) leads to increased thalamic activity. Increased excitation of the thalamus facilitates activity in the SMA and enhances the likelihood that a movement will be produced. As such, this direct pathway (solid arrow) is referred to as the "go" pathway. A different set of striatal neurons project to and inhibits the globus pallidus external (GPe) segment. The GPe sends inhibitory projections to the subthalamic nucleus (STN), which is the structure that provides tonic excitation of the GPi/SNpr. The net effect of activity in this indirect pathway (dashed arrows) will be to enhance excitation of the GPi/SNpr. Such increased activity will suppress thalamic drive of the SMA, reducing the likelihood of movement. Thus, the indirect pathway is referred to as the "stop" pathway. Dopamine release into the striatum by substantia nigra pars compacta (SNpc) excites neurons of the direct pathway that possess dopamine-1 receptors (D1R) and inhibits striatal neurons of the indirect pathway possessing D2R. Collectively, dopamine release into the striatum will potently promote movement by simultaneously facilitating the direct pathway and inhibiting the indirect pathway.

the inhibition by the striatum of the GPi/SNpr and the inhibition by the GPi/SNpr directed at the thalamus. Such *inhibition of inhibitory neurons* is sometimes referred to as **disinhibition,** leading to a next excitation of downstream targets. Collectively, therefore, engagement of the direct pathway will tend to promote movements. Thus, this pathway is sometimes referred to as the "go" pathway.

For the indirect pathway (dashed arrows, Figure 3), a different set of neurons in the striatum from those that make up the direct pathway also receive excitatory input from the cortex and project to the GPe. These projection neurons are inhibitory (also GABAergic). The GPe sends inhibitory inputs to the STN that tends to reduce activity in the continuously and intrinsically active STN. Lastly, the STN provides key excitatory input (glutamatergic) to the output structures of the basal ganglia, the GPi–SNpr. In some respects, the STN is the linchpin in the indirect pathway. Note that it is the only structure in the basal ganglia to provide direct excitation. When its activity increases, it further excites the GPi/SNpr to more strongly suppress the thalamus from exciting the SMA. When its activity diminishes, the output from the GPi/SNpr will also fall, reducing its inhibition of the thalamus and increasing drive to the SMA.

Inhibitory inputs to the STN from the GPe serve to temper the activity of the STN and thereby prevent excess activation of the GPi/SNpr (Figure 3). However, when neurons in the striatum that are part of the indirect pathway are activated, they suppress this tempering action of the GPe. This serves to remove some of the inhibition of the STN, increasing its excitatory drive to the GPi/SNpr. Again, one can think of the tandem inhibition of the striatum to the GPe and the GPe to the STN as two negatives making a positive. This disinhibition leads to increased activity in the STN and increased braking action by the GPi/SNpr of the thalamus. To put it briefly, increased activity in the neurons of the striatum at the headwaters of the indirect pathway will tend to suppress the production of movement. As such, the indirect pathway is sometimes called the "stop" pathway.

Role of the Substantia Nigra Pars Compacta

The direct and indirect pathways converge upon the output entity, the GPi/SNpr, with opposing influences. The direct pathway acts to restrain the GPi/SNpr, thereby lifting inhibition from the thalamus, enabling excitation of the SMA to promote movement. The indirect pathway enhances activation of the GPi/SNpr, increasing inhibition of the thalamus and impeding the production of movement. How is the standoff between these two pathways shifted in favor of one over the other? This turns out to be a key role of the other component of the basal ganglia, the SNpc.

This small structure is a main source of the neurotransmitter dopamine in the brain. **Dopamine** *typically acts as a neuromodulator (having a broad impact over a region of the brain) working through G-protein-coupled metabotropic receptors.* Another *important source of dopamine in the brain* is the **ventral tegmental area (VTA)**. The VTA is diffusely situated in the midbrain and supplies dopamine to a number of brain areas, including the prefrontal cortex. Dopamine release from the VTA is considered as a reward signal, underlying highly positive feelings associated with food, sex, and love. It is also critically implicated in the development of drug dependence because many addictive drugs act on the VTA.

In terms of dopamine's role in movement control, the release of dopamine into the striatum by neurons projecting from the SNpc has two parallel but differential effects (Figure 3). Neurons in the striatum that express the dopamine-1 receptor (D1R) become excited by the binding of dopamine. A different set of neurons in the striatum that express the dopamine-2 receptor (D2R) are inhibited by dopamine (Gerfen *et al.* 1990). These neurons are thoroughly intermingled within the striatum. Furthermore, dopamine release is widespread within a region of the striatum (Matsuda *et al.* 2009). This leads to concurrent binding of dopamine to both types of neurons (those expressing D1Rs and those possessing D2Rs).

The striatal neurons endowed with D1Rs and that become excited by dopamine are those that project to the GPi/SNpr, that is, those that underlie the direct pathway (Figure 3). On the other hand, neurons in the striatum that possess D2Rs and are inhibited by dopamine are mainly those that project to the GPe, namely, the neurons driving the indirect pathway. Consequently, the release of dopamine into the striatum from neurons in the SNpc will simultaneously boost activity in the direct pathway and suppress it in the indirect pathway. Because the direct pathway is considered as the "go" pathway and the indirect pathway the "stop" pathway, dopamine release into the striatum will strongly promote the production of movement. If we use a car as an analogy, dopamine release is like pressing on the gas pedal (facilitating the go pathway) while removing the foot from the brake (inhibiting the stop pathway) to actuate movement.

One reasonable question to ask is what inputs regulate the activity of the SNpc to deliver dopamine to the striatum? This question has not been completely answered. It is known that the SNpc receives excitatory, inhibitory, and neuromodulatory inputs from multiple structures in the brainstem, cerebrum, and even feedback from nuclei in the basal ganglia (Paladini & Tepper 2017). Of note, one intriguing source of input to the SNpc is from the amygdala (Fudge & Haber 2000). The **amygdala** *is a multinucleated structure found in the medial temporal lobe and is thought to identify the significance or emotional value of stimuli.* It receives converging input from most sensory association cortices and from the prefrontal cortex (Aggleton *et al.* 1981). The sensory inputs inform the amygdala as to "what" is occurring, while inputs from the prefrontal cortex may indicate the significance of a particular set of circumstances. Those inputs are processed, and if warranted, engage output neurons to set into motion behavioral and autonomic responses to a given situation. Such output from the amygdala, directed to the SNpc, could motivate action by enhancing the release of dopamine into the striatum, thereby facilitating the direct pathway and inhibiting the indirect pathway.

Activation of the Direct Pathway

Figure 4 shows neural responses recorded from different parts of the basal ganglia and thalamus to stimulation of the direct pathway (from Chevalier & Deniau 1990). In this case, a puff of glutamate was delivered to the striatum using a micropipette in an anesthetized rat to mimic the release of glutamate into the striatum from the cerebral cortex. A recording electrode in the striatum detected an abrupt increase in firing rate of a striatal neuron to the delivery of glutamate (arrow). The inhibition delivered to the GPi/SNpr from activated striatal neurons that are part of the direct pathway contributed to cessation of otherwise tonic activity in GPi/SNpr (right column, middle panel, Figure 4). The suppressed output of the GPi/SNpr then relieved the thalamus from its tonic inhibition, leading to a marked increase in its firing rate (right column, bottom panel, Figure 4). Such increased activity in thalamic nuclei would excite the

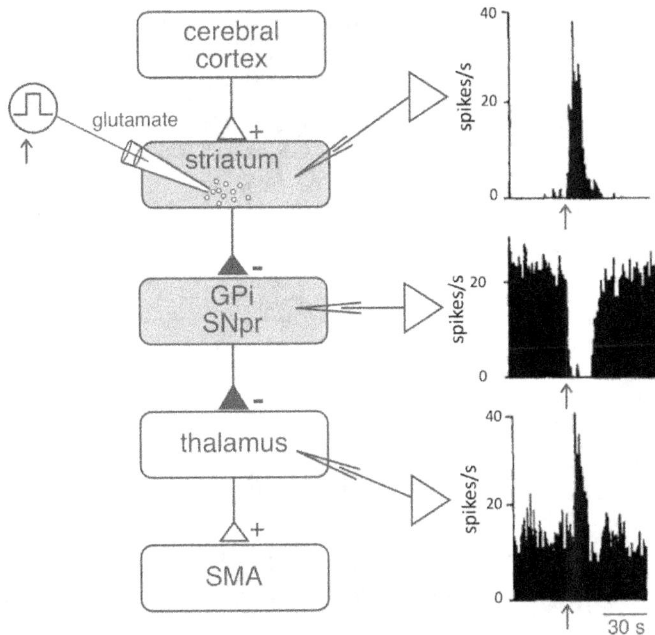

Figure 4.   Neural responses to excitation of the direct pathway. Left: Representation of direct pathway with micropipette that delivered the excitatory neurotransmitter glutamate into the rat striatum. Top right: increased spiking activity of a neuron in the striatum to a puff of glutamate (arrow). Middle right: reduction in spiking of neurons in the GPi/SNpr caused by increased activity in striatal neurons of the direct pathway. Bottom right: Increased firing in the thalamus caused by reduction in the inhibitory output of the GPi/SNpr. (Right panels adapted from Chevalier and Deniau [1990].)

SMA to increase the likelihood that the animal (if not anesthetized) to produce a movement.

Interruption of the Indirect Pathway

Figure 5 depicts the neural and behavioral changes associated with damage to the STN, a critical element of the indirect pathway. In this case, a toxic chemical was injected into the STN of monkeys that partially destroyed it (Figure 5A). The activities of individual neurons in the GPi were recorded before and following the lesion (Hamada & DeLong 1992a). The top panel in Figure 5B shows the activity of a typical GPi

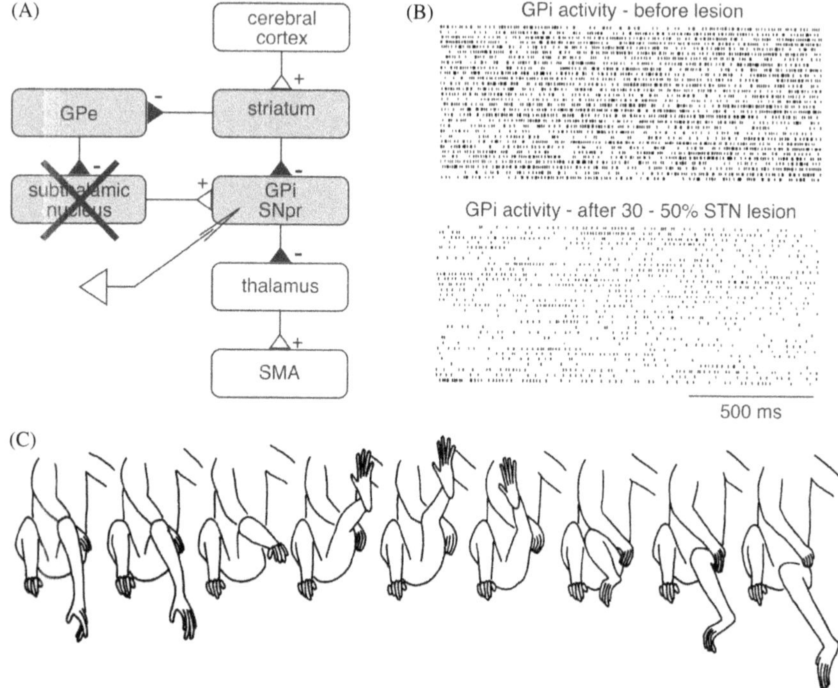

Figure 5. Interruption of the indirect pathway leads to uncontrolled movements. (A) Schematic indicating site of chemotoxic lesion placed in the subthalamic nucleus of monkeys. (B) Recording of neural activity (dots indicate spikes of a neuron) in the globus pallidus internal (GPi) segment before (above) and following the lesion (below). (C) Tracings made from video frames of a monkey following a lesion of the subthalamic nucleus showing uncontrolled flinging motions of the leg. ([B] adapted from Hamada and DeLong [1992a], [C] from Hamada and DeLong [1992b].)

neuron before the lesion. Each row of dots represents a 1.5 s-sample of spikes taken when the monkey was in a resting state. This high level of tonic activity, driven by excitatory input from the STN, continuously subdues the thalamus. The bottom panel in Figure 5B shows the distinctly reduced activity of a GPi neuron recorded after a lesion destroyed 30%–50% of the STN. Such reduced activity of the GPi would lessen the inhibition delivered to the thalamus. Indeed, soon after such lesions, monkeys developed pronounced *uncontrolled movements* (referred to as **dyskinesias**) that persisted for a few hours (Hamada & DeLong 1992b). For example, Figure 5C shows video frames of a monkey that had received an

STN lesion that prompted dyskinesia of the leg. These flinging motions of the leg occurred repetitively at a rate of almost one/s. These results highlight the role of the indirect pathway in preventing unwanted movements: indeed, when this pathway is impaired (i.e., the brake is disabled), uncontrollable movements emerge.

Optogenetics

While the experiments in Figures 4 and 5 illustrate how stimulation or lesions can elicit striking neurophysiological or behavioral responses, there are aspects of such experiments that make interpretation challenging. For example, chemical (or electrical) stimulation, as used in Figure 4, will tend to excite many neuron types in the vicinity of the micropipette. Typically, therefore, it is not known if the responses measured are due to activation of one type of neuron or others (e.g., those possessing D1R or D2R) or some combination. Likewise, as explained in Appendix C, the outcome of lesion experiments can be difficult to interpret because rapid plasticity may endow regions neighboring the lesions with compensatory functions, and small areas of a targeted structure that are undamaged by a lesion may take on an outsized role in continuing to perform the functions of that structure.

In the past 20 years, a powerful new methodology, largely developed and advanced by Karl Deisseroth and colleagues at Stanford University, can overcome some of the difficulties associated with using stimulation or lesions. This methodology, called **optogenetics**, *enables precise activation or suppression of specified cells with millisecond time resolution* (Deisseroth 2010). To accomplish this, genes from simple organisms (algae or bacteria) (Figure 6A) that express *light-sensitive ion channels* (called **channelrhodopsins [ChRs]**) are introduced into the DNA of mammalian neurons. This is done using non-toxic viruses (Figure 6B) that have been engineered to carry and insert the ChR producing genes into neurons. The viruses are then injected into the brain region of interest (Figure 6C). The virus then infects most neurons in the neighborhood of where the virus was injected. Also packaged with the virus is a genetic switch (a "promoter") that drives expression of the ChR protein only in cells that possess distinct genetic features associated with the particular functions of the cell, for example, that associated with the production of

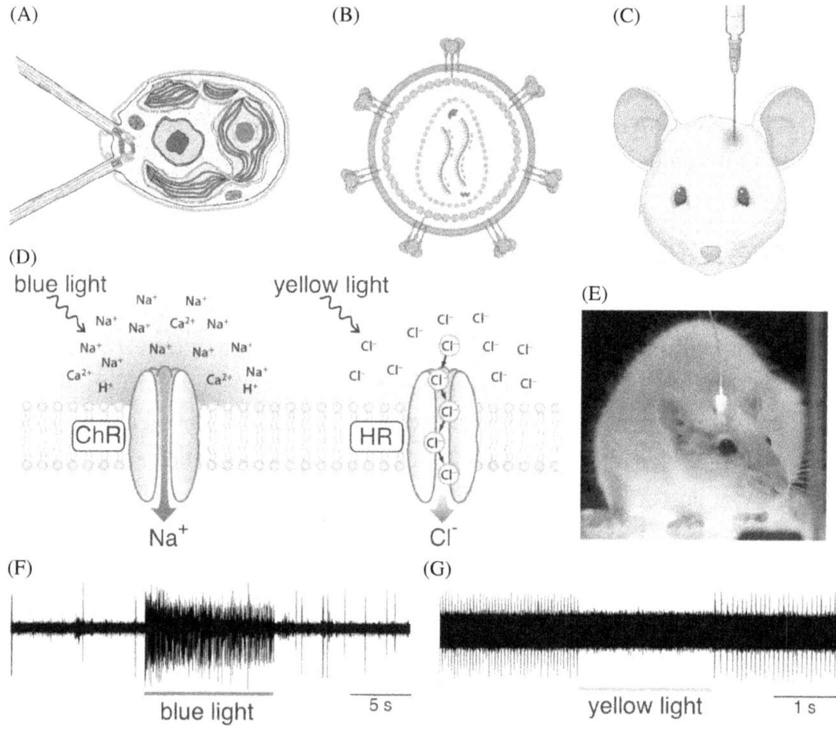

Figure 6.   Optogenetics. (A) Certain microbes possess ion channels that respond to light, such as the algae *Chlamydomonas reinhardtii*, which uses light to trigger motion of its flagella. (B) The genes that encode the light-sensitive channels (channelrhodopsins, ChRs) in microbes are introduced into the DNA of harmless viruses. (C) The viruses are injected to infect a target region of the brain. The viruses are packaged with a promoter that drives expression of the ChR genes only in specified neurons. (D) Some light-sensitive ion channels (ChR) respond to blue light, leading to Na^+ influx, whereas light-sensitive ion pumps respond to yellow light (halorhodopsin HR), leading to Cl^- influx. (E) Fiber optic cables are implanted into the infected brain region to deliver light of the appropriate wavelength to activate the light-sensitive channels or pumps. (F) A single neuron in the rat brain that expressed ChR was immediately excited by switching on blue light. (G) A neuron in the rat brain that expressed halorhodopsin was inhibited by delivery of yellow light. ([A] adapted from Merchant *et al.* [2007], [C] from Zhou *et al.* [2022], [D] from Fenno *et al.* [2011], [E] Gradinaru *et al.* [2009], [F & G] from Gradinaru *et al.* [2010].)

specific neurotransmitters. Thus, only neurons having the specified genetic identity will produce the ChR.

While optogenetics is a rapidly evolving field with many new light-sensitive systems being developed, there are two main types. One responds to blue light by opening a channel (i.e., ChR) that mostly leads to Na^+ influx and excitation of the neuron (Figure 6D) (Fenno *et al.* 2011). The other is actuated by yellow light and leads to Cl^- entry and inhibition of neurons. This latter type is not technically an ion channel but an ion pump and is called **halorhodopsin** (**HR**, Figure 6D). To deliver light of the appropriate wavelength (color) to a brain region genetically manipulated to have light sensitivity, thin fiber optic cables can be chronically implanted near the area (Figure 6E) to excite on or suppress targeted neurons in awake animals.

The fiber optic cables can be instrumented with recording electrodes to observe changes in neural activity associated with light delivery. Figure 6F shows such spiking activity recorded in an optogenetically manipulated neuron responding to blue light leading to sustained excitation (Gradinaru *et al.* 2010). Likewise, Figure 6G shows the marked suppression in the activity of a different neuron in response to yellow light in an animal engineered to express halorhodopsin (Gradinaru *et al.* 2010). Note that in both cases, activity changes almost immediately with the delivery of light and returns to the initial state upon cessation of the light stimulus. Therefore, with optogenetics, it is possible to excite or suppress activity (like flipping a switch) only in neurons of interest in awake animals and observe how those changes impact the behavior of an animal. This method has led to dramatic improvements in our understanding of basic operations of neural circuits (such as those in the basal ganglia, as discussed below) and insight into the nature of a number of neurological disorders (Steinberg *et al.* 2015).

Optogenetic Control of the Direct and Indirect Pathways

The notion that two parallel pathways (direct and indirect) exist in the basal ganglia and that these promote or suppress movement is based on convincing, yet circumstantial evidence. As such, questions have arisen as to the validity of this idea. To more rigorously evaluate the direct–indirect pathway hypothesis, mice were engineered to express ChR either in neurons of the striatum possessing dopamine-1 (D1) receptors or D2 receptors (Kravitz *et al.* 2010). As shown in Figure 7A, blue laser light was then delivered to the striatum in both types of mice, and the changes in neural

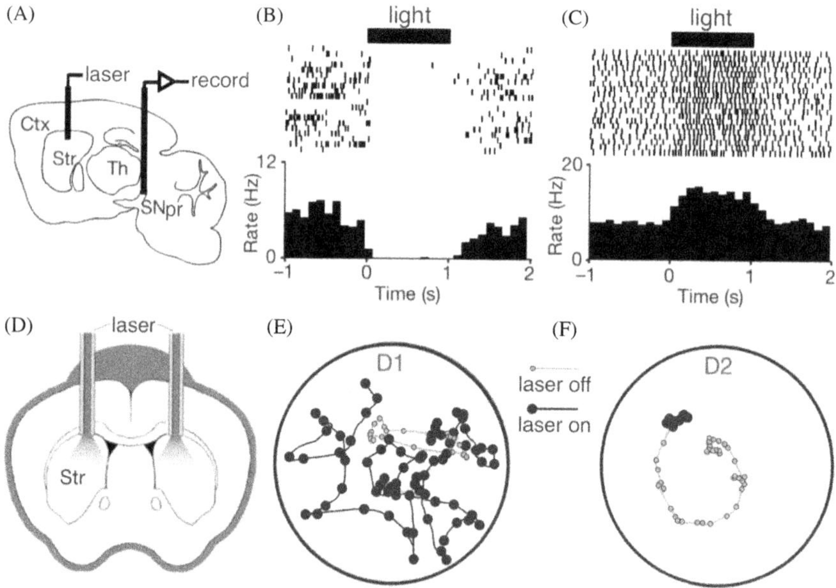

Figure 7.   Optogenetic demonstration of direct and indirect pathways in basal ganglia. (A) A blue laser was used to excite either neurons possessing dopamine 1 (D1) receptors or D2 receptors in the mouse striatum that had been targeted to express channelrhodopsin (ChR). Response to light excitation was recorded downstream in the output region of the basal ganglia, substantia nigra pars reticulata (SNpr). (B) Response of SNpr neuron in a mouse with ChR expressed in striatal neurons possessing D1 receptors ("D1 mice"). This represents the response to selective activation of the direct pathway. (C) Response in SNpr neuron in a different mouse with ChR expressed in striatal neurons possessing D2 receptors ("D2 mice"). This represents the response to selective activation of the indirect pathway. (D) Chronically implanted bilateral fiber optic cables used to deliver blue light to the striatum of freely moving D1 or D2 mice. (E) Top-down view of circular arena showing location of a D1 mouse every 1/3 of a second with laser off (light gray lines and dots) or on (black lines and dots). (F) Same as for E but for a D2 mouse. (Adapted from Kravitz *et al.* [2010].)

activity were recorded downstream in the output structure, SNpr. When the light was delivered to mice with ChR expressed in neurons possessing D1 receptors ("D1 mice"), activity in SNpr immediately decreased (Figure 7B). On the other hand, when blue light was delivered to the striatum of D2 mice, SNpr activity increased. These findings provide strong support for the direct–indirect pathway hypothesis. Selective activation of the direct pathway by engaging neurons expressing D1 receptors leads to inhibition of the output structure of the basal ganglia, whereas activation of the indirect pathway does the opposite (refer to Figure 3).

According to the hypothesis, activation of the direct pathway ("go" pathway) should promote movement, whereas excitation of the indirect pathway ("stop" pathway) should suppress movement. Kravitz and colleagues (2010) tested this idea in their D1 and D2 mice. Bilateral illumination of the striatum with fiber optic cables (Figure 7D) was performed in mice freely moving inside a circular arena. Figure 7E is a top-down view of the arena showing the movement of a D1 mouse. Each dot indicates the location of the mouse every 1/3 of a second. The small dots and gray lines show the movements of the mouse with the laser off, whereas the large dots and black lines show the trajectory of the animal when the laser was switched on. Compared to the laser-off period, activation of the D1 pathway with the laser caused a marked increase in locomotor activity in the mouse. Conversely, activation of the laser in a D2 mouse (Figure 7F) caused the animal to stop ambulating. Collectively, these findings strongly support the idea that there are two independent pathways through the basal ganglia that have opposing effects on the instigation of movement.

Hyperkinetic Disorders Associated with Dysfunction of the Indirect Pathway

There are a number of neurological disorders that may stem from damage or dysfunction of the indirect pathway. In a general sense, *when the stop pathway is disrupted (i.e., "the brake is broken"), unintended movements or behaviors occur.* Collectively, these conditions are referred to as **hyperkinetic disorders** (Albin *et al.* 1989). One such disorder is **hemiballism**, so-called because of unceasing ballistic or flinging motions of one of the limbs (typically an upper limb) in individuals with this disorder. Autopsies of individuals with this disorder invariably found damage to the STN contralateral to the limb exhibiting the hyperkinesia, typically caused by a stroke (Whittier 1947). This disorder is not unlike that described in monkeys with experimental lesions of the STN (see Figure 5). In human patients, the disorder usually resolves within a few months of onset (Posturna & Lang 2003).

Another disorder that gives rise to hyperkinesis is **Huntington's disease**. *Huntington's disease is a devastating genetic disorder that leads to degeneration of neurons in the striatum.* The most susceptible neurons appear to be those that express the D2 receptor and project to the GPe (Reiner *et al.* 1988). Those neurons are at the origin of the indirect pathway (Figure 3). The initial symptoms of Huntington's disease appear around age 40 years and include uncontrollable writhing movements of the limbs (called "chorea"—from the Greek word for dance), face, and tongue. Because the basal ganglia not only influence motor pathways but also the prefrontal cortex (Figure 2), individuals with Huntington's disease exhibit a wide range of personality and cognitive disorders, including impulsivity, irritability, aggression, anxiety, apathy, dementia, and memory deficits (Anderson & Marder 2001). As the disease progresses, neurons in the striatum that are part of the direct (go) pathway also degenerate, leading to a diminution in hyperkinetic behaviors and the emergence of hypokinetic symptoms (Reiner *et al.* 1988). Individuals with Huntington's disease eventually become bedridden, have difficulty swallowing, and die within ~15–20 years of diagnosis. At present there is no cure nor therapies that ameliorate the progression of Huntington's disease, although a number of gene-therapy-based treatments are being tested (Tabrizi *et al.* 2022).

Another hyperkinetic disorder with a clear genetic basis that affects almost 1% of the population is **Tourette's syndrome** (Robertson *et al.* 2017). *The symptoms of this disorder typically emerge around the age of five years and usually consist of various repetitive motor tics (such as eye blinking, head jerks, and facial muscle contractions) or vocal tics (such as throat clearing, sniffing, and coughing).* In more severe cases, the motor tics can be more intense, like repeated jumping, bending the trunk, and touching. The motor and vocal tics occur in bouts that wax and wane over a period of a day. Individuals with Tourette's have a growing awareness and sense of discomfort preceding a bout of tics that is temporarily relieved by producing the tic behavior. Because such motor and vocal tics lead to a sense of shame and embarrassment and are disruptive in social situations, Tourette's interferes with school participation, social relations, and companionship. As it happens, it is not uncommon for the vocal tics to include the uttering of obscenities. It is as though the "brake" that normally restrains us from expressing the various thoughts that pass through one's mind does not operate properly in Tourette's. Indeed, circumstantial evidence points to dysfunction of the indirect pathway in Tourette's syndrome, although the specific mechanisms underlying the disorder are not yet known. Interestingly, by the age of 20 years, many of the symptoms associated with Tourette's largely disappear.

And lastly, another example of a hyperkinetic disorder is **obsessive–compulsive disorders (OCD)**. *Individuals with OCD have invasive thoughts (obsessions) that increase anxiety and that can be partially relieved by repeatedly carrying out a stereotyped behavior (compulsions).* Typical examples of the obsession–compulsion pairings include worry about germs leading to excessive hand washing, concern about safety leading to repeating checking that doors are locked, distress about having sufficient food or other household items leading to hoarding behaviors, and worry about symmetry leading to excessive organizing and aligning of objects (Stein *et al.* 2019). OCD affects about 3% of the population and usually manifests in late childhood. Individuals with OCD typically recognize that the behaviors are excessive and unnecessary but can't halt them. It too has a clear genetic link and involves the basal ganglia (Burguière *et al.* 2015), but specific information about the causes of OCD is lacking. Like most hyperkinetic disorders described here, treatment for OCD often involves the use of dopamine *antagonists* (Roessel *et al.* 2023). This makes intuitive sense because hyperkinetic disorders involve unwanted movements or behaviors, and dopamine promotes movements. Dopamine antagonists, therefore, should dampen the incidence of such uncontrolled behaviors.

Parkinson's Disease

The prototypical *hypo*kinetic disorder is **Parkinson's disease**. *It is caused by degeneration of dopamine-producing cells in the* SNpc (see frontispiece).

The reason for this degeneration is not known. Some of the main symptoms of Parkinson's disease include paucity of movements (akinesia), slowed movements (bradykinesia), absence of facial expression (facial masking), and tremor. Because of the basal ganglia's influence on the prefrontal cortex, cognitive and personality disorders may also arise with Parkinson's disease. Eventually, Parkinson's patients typically become bedridden, have difficulty speaking and swallowing, and often develop pneumonia secondary to inhaling food or saliva into the lungs that ultimately contributes to their death.

Given dopamine's dual effect to facilitate activity in the direct pathway (promoting movement) and suppress activity in the indirect pathways (withdrawing restraints on movement production), its depletion from the striatum in Parkinson's disease potently undercuts the ability to move. However, Parkinson's does not cause explicit paralysis. Instead, it mainly impairs one type of movement, namely, that associated with internally generated movements. It is useful to recall that the main motor target of thalamic activity regulated by the basal ganglia is the supplemental motor area (SMA, Figure 2). The SMA is implicated in the planning and playout of *internally* generated motor behaviors (see Chapter 19). Indeed, individuals with Parkinson's disease may display surprisingly brisk, normal-looking movements to an external target. As pointed out in Chapter 19, such *externally* guided movements involve the lateral premotor cortex, a region less influenced by the basal ganglia, and therefore, not so severely affected by Parkinson's disease (Berardelli *et al.* 2001).

Oliver Sacks describes in his extraordinary book *Awakenings* (1973) practically immobile Parkinsonian patients adroitly reaching out to catch a ball thrown to them. Similarly, Sacks recounts the case of a Parkinson's patient who could readily climb stairs, with each step providing a distinct visual target. Yet, upon reaching the top of the stairs, the patient could not proceed—"freezing" with the absence of well-defined visual cues to aid further progression. Such anecdotes have been confirmed in experimental studies wherein Parkinson's patients and healthy subjects were asked, under their own internal drive, to reach out with maximal speed (Majsak *et al.* 1998). Movement speeds were substantially slower for Parkinson's patients compared to the healthy subjects. However, when the task involved reaching to grasp a moving ball, the Parkinson's patients moved just as quickly as the healthy subjects (and more quickly than their self-initiated "maximal" efforts). Such findings highlight Parkinson's disease as a profound impairment primarily in the ability to produce self-motivated behaviors.

Treatments for Parkinson's Disease

At present, there are no cures for Parkinson's disease. Nevertheless, a number of approaches have been used to mitigate symptoms of the disease. A treatment performed in the 1940s–1950s involved *surgical ablation of part of the globus pallidus* (**pallidotomy**). This surgical intervention was employed before the standard model of the pathways and connectivity among the elements of the basal ganglia (Figure 3) was described. As such, the surgical outcomes were highly variable. Death and complications of the surgery occurred in a relatively large proportion of patients (Guridi & Lozano 1997). Yet, a significant portion of Parkinsonian patients did show substantial and long-lasting improvement. With refinements in surgical methods and targeting of the GPi segment for lesioning, the success rate increased while mortality and adverse effects diminished (Svennilson *et al.* 1960). Because Parkinson's disease is associated with heightened activity in the GPi, ablating the GPi should dampen its inhibitory effect on the thalamic neurons that project to the SMA to promote movement.

The use of pallidotomy was greatly curtailed with the advent of a drug that potently reduced the symptoms associated with Parkinson's disease. That drug is levodopa (**L-DOPA**), *a precursor of dopamine that can pass through the blood–brain barrier and be synthesized into dopamine in the striatum.* Its utility in ameliorating the symptoms of Parkinson's was originally reported in experimental animals by the Nobel Prize winner Arvid Carlsson and colleagues (1957) and later in Parkinson's patients (Cotzias *et al.* 1967). It remains the key therapeutic in treating Parkinson's disease. While a crucial drug in the treatment of Parkinson's, its efficacy gradually diminishes over a period of years. Also, for reasons not completely understood, most patients on L-DOPA therapy eventually develop disabling *hyper*kinesias (also called dyskinesias)—not unlike that in Huntington's disease (Bezard *et al.* 2001). Therefore, L-DOPA treatment requires careful titration to maximize benefits while minimizing dyskinesias, plus combination with other drugs that attenuate dyskinesias.

Given some of the limitations of L-DOPA therapy, a number of other treatments have been attempted. For example, in the 1990s, dopamine-producing cells obtained from the substantia nigra of aborted human fetuses were transplanted directly into the striatum of Parkinson's patients (Freed *et al.* 1990; Lindvall *et al.* 1990). The procedures were safe, and the grafted cells survived and continued to produce dopamine several years after the transplant (Piccini *et al.* 1999). In some patients there was marked improvement in symptoms. In others, however, the transplant had little effect (Freed *et al.* 2001). There was also some evidence that transplanted cells eventually showed hallmarks of cell degeneration characteristic of that in Parkinson's disease (Li *et al.* 2008)—perhaps suggesting that the disease might "spread" from the host to the grafted cells. Furthermore, a large clinical trial using fetal tissue transplants failed to show clear-cut efficacy (Barker *et al.* 2024). For these reasons, plus logistical and ethical challenges, fetal tissue implants are unlikely to be used to treat Parkinson's disease in the future. However, recent advances in the use of **stem cells** (*cells that can be induced to proliferate into almost any form of cell*) obtained from adult human tissue and programmed into dopamine-producing cells (Parmar *et al.* 2020) overcome many limitations of fetal tissue grafts. Indeed, several clinical trials are ongoing to evaluate the efficacy of such stem-cell-derived dopamine cells when grafted into the brains of Parkinson's patients.

Deep Brain Stimulation

One of the most dramatic and effective treatments for the symptoms of Parkinson's disease involves **deep brain stimulation (DBS)**. *For Parkinson's disease, the targeted structure is the STN, into which an electrode is surgically placed (Figure 8). A stimulus generator (like a pacemaker) is implanted into the chest that delivers continuous, high-frequency stimulation to the electrode via a small subcutaneous cable (electrode lead).* When turned on by an external wand, symptoms such as tremor, bradykinesia, and difficulties with balance and walking almost instantly

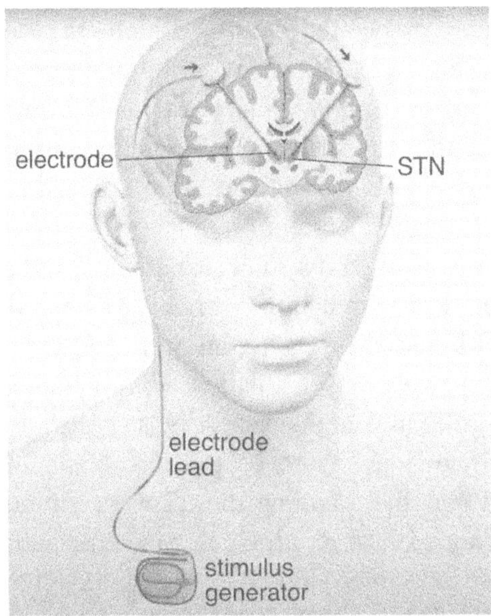

Figure 8.   Deep brain stimulation for treatment of Parkinson's disease symptoms. A stimulus generator implanted in the chest sends continuous, high-frequency stimulus pulses to electrodes implanted in the subthalamic nuclei (STN) via a small cable (electrode lead) that runs under the skin. (From Stanford Health Care, https://stanfordhealthcare.org/ stanford-health-care-now/videos/deep-brain-stimulation-dbs-for-parkinsons-disease-essential-tremor-epilepsy.html.)

fade away (see side-by-side videos of a Parkinson's patient recorded on the same day without and with DBS activated, https://www.youtube.com/ watch?v=_tkmSn2m0Ck). The improvements in motor function are retained up through at least 10 years, although the effectiveness of the stimulation wanes with the natural progression of the disease (Faggiani & Benazzouz 2017). Because the efficacy of DBS is more consistent and associated with fewer side effects than drug treatments, it has become the gold standard therapy for Parkinson's disease (Faggiani & Benazzouz 2017).

The discovery that DBS would be effective for treating parkinsonian symptoms was serendipitous (Hariz *et al.* 2010). Electrical stimulation was often used in neurosurgery to establish a location targeted for lesioning, like that associated with pallidotomy (described above). Because patients were typically awake during these procedures, surgeons could observe the effect stimulation had on disease symptoms. The site of stimulation that led to the most effective reduction in symptoms was then lesioned by passing high electrical current to damage brain tissue in the immediate vicinity of the electrode. It was eventually recognized, however, that the disease symptoms might be treated just as effectively by using chronic electrical stimulation, without the need for destruction of brain tissue. After a period of testing and refinement in non-human primates, the first human Parkinson's patient was implanted and effectively treated with DBS in France in the early 1990s (Pollak *et al.* 1993).

When considering the layout of the direct and indirect pathways through the basal ganglia, targeting the STN for stimulation with DBS (Figure 9) would not seem a very logical choice, perhaps even a counterproductive one. Keep in mind that excitation of the STN should enhance activity in the GPi/SNpr, which in turn would suppress the recipient

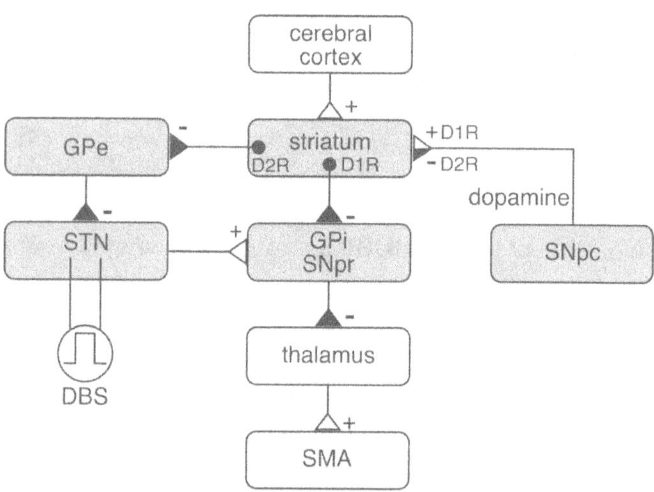

Figure 9.   Pathways and connections among structures making up the basal ganglia. Deep brain stimulation (DBS) electrodes are typically implanted in the subthalamic nucleus (STN) for treating Parkinson's disease. Such a placement might seem paradoxical given that STN excites the globus pallidus internal (GPi) segment and substantia nigra pars reticulata (SNpr) whose activities tend to suppress the production of movement.

thalamic nucleus, leading to less drive of the SMA. In other words, such stimulation, in theory, should suppress rather than promote movements. One of the major problems Parkinson's patients confront is not being able to effectively initiate internally generated movements. Therefore, DBS of the STN is in some ways a mysterious paradox.

Nevertheless, there are some ideas as to why DBS might work. One is that neural activity in the STN is suppressed (rather than increased) with the high-frequency stimulation (>100 pulses/s). Recall from Chapter 4 that there are brief refractory periods following each spike that hinder the production of a subsequent spike if a stimulus occurs within that period, as might happen with high-frequency stimulation. Furthermore, excessive and sustained depolarization by stimulation can cause neurons to stop firing altogether (see Figure 3D, Chapter 4). This is because spike-generating ion channels are maintained in persistently inactive states. Another possibility is that the stimulating electrodes excite the nerve endings of inhibitory inputs entering into the STN from the GPe. That would then effectively suppress output neurons of the STN projecting to the GPi/SNpr, ultimately lessening inhibition of the thalamus and SMA. It should be said, however, that none of these possibilities have yet been definitively proven to be the case (Gradinaru *et al.* 2009).

Summary

The basal ganglia are an assembly of subcortical structures that interact to promote movement and regulate cognitive functions. Inputs to the basal ganglia are from various regions of the cerebral cortex, and the outputs of the basal ganglia target the SMA and prefrontal cortex via relay nuclei in the thalamus. There are two main routes through which activity propagates through the motor basal ganglia: the direct path, which promotes movements, and the indirect path, which restrains movements. Dopamine, released into the striatum from the SNpc, potently facilitates the production of movement by promoting the direct pathway and inhibiting the indirect pathway. The basal ganglia are implicated in a number of neurological disorders. Disorders associated with impairment of the indirect pathway lead to excessive, unwanted movements. Parkinson's disease, on the other hand, is characterized by diminished voluntary movements caused by degeneration of dopaminergic neurons in the SNpc. A number of strategies have been used to treat symptoms of Parkinson's disease, including surgical ablation, dopamine replacement (with drugs or brain implants), or DBS. At present, however, no cure for Parkinson's disease has been developed.

References

Aggleton JP, Burton MF & Passingham RE (1980). Cortical and subcortical afferents to the amygdala of the rhesus monkey (*Macaca mulatta*). *Brain Research* **190**, 347–368.

Albin RL, Young AB & Penney JB (1989). The functional anatomy of basal ganglia disorders. *Trends Neuroscience* **12**, 1–10.

Alexander GE & Crutcher MD (1990). Functional architecture of basal ganglia circuits: Neural substrates of parallel processing. *Trends in Neurosciences* **13**, 266–271.

Alexander GE, DeLong MR & Strick PL (1986). Parallel organization of functionally segregated circuits linking basal ganglia and cortex. *Annual Review of Neuroscience* **9**, 357–381.

Anderson KE & Marder KS (2001). An overview of psychiatric symptoms in Huntington's disease. *Current Psychiatry Reports* **3**, 379–388.

Barker RA, Björklund A & Parmar M (2024). The history and status of dopamine cell therapies for Parkinson's disease. *BioEssayse*, 2400118.

Berardelli A, Rothwell JC, Thompson PD & Hallett M (2001). Pathophysiology of bradykinesia in Parkinson's disease. *Brain* **124**, 2131–2146.

Bezard E, Brotchie JM & Gross CE (2001). Pathophysiology of levodopa-induced dyskinesia: Potential for new therapies. *Nature Reviews Neuroscience* **2**, 577–588.

Burguière E, Monteiro P, Mallet L, Feng G & Graybiel AM (2015). Striatal circuits, habits, and implications for obsessive–compulsive disorder. *Current Opinion in Neurobiology* **30**, 59–65.

Carlsson A, Lindqvist M & Magnusson T (1957). 3,4-Dihydroxyphenylalanine and 5-hydroxytryptophan as reserpine antagonists. *Nature* **180**, 1200–1200.

Chevalier G & Deniau JM (1990). Disinhibition as a basic process in the expression of striatal functions. *Trends Neuroscience* **13**, 277–280.

Cotzias GC, Woert MHV & Schiffer LM (1967). Aromatic amino acids and modification of Parkinsonism. *The New England Journal of Medicine* **276**, 374–379.

Deisseroth K (2010). Controlling the brain with light. *Scientific American* **303**, 48–55.

Faggiani E & Benazzouz A (2017). Deep brain stimulation of the subthalamic nucleus in Parkinson's disease: From history to the interaction with the monoaminergic systems. *Progress in Neurobiology* **151**, 139–156.

Fenno L, Yizhar O & Deisseroth K (2011). The development and application of optogenetics. *Annual Review of Neuroscience* **34**, 389–412.

Freed CR, Breeze RE, Rosenberg NL, Schneck SA, Wells TH, Barrett JN, Grafton ST, Huang SC, Eidelberg D & Rottenberg DA (1990). Transplantation of human fetal dopamine cells for Parkinson's disease: Results at 1 year. *Archives of Neurology* **47**, 505–512.

Freed CR, Greene PE, Breeze RE, Tsai W-Y, DuMouchel W, Kao R, Dillon S, Winfield H, Culver S, Trojanowski JQ, Eidelberg D & Fahn S (2001). Transplantation of embryonic dopamine neurons for severe Parkinson's disease. *The New England Journal of Medicine* **344**, 710–719.

Fudge JL & Haber SN (2000). The central nucleus of the amygdala projection to dopamine subpopulations in primates. *Neuroscience* **97**, 479–494.

Gerfen CR, Engber TM, Mahan LC, Susel Z, Chase TN, Monsma FJ & Sibley DR (1990). D1 and D2 dopamine receptor-regulated gene expression of striatonigral and striatopallidal neurons. *Science* **250**, 1429–1432.

Gradinaru V, Mogri M, Thompson KR, Henderson JM & Deisseroth K (2009). Optical deconstruction of parkinsonian neural circuitry. *Science* **324**, 354–359.

Gradinaru V, Zhang F, Ramakrishnan C, Mattis J, Prakash R, Diester I, Goshen I, Thompson KR & Deisseroth K (2010). Molecular and cellular approaches for diversifying and extending optogenetics. *Cell* **141**, 154–165.

Gray H (1918). *Anatomy of the human body.* https://commons.wikimedia.org/wiki/File:Gray717.png

Guridi J & Lozano AM (1997). A brief history of pallidotomy. *Neurosurgery* **41**, 1169–1183.

Halliday G (2004). The human nervous system. Substantia Nigra and Locus Coeruleus (2nd Edition), Chapter 14, Academic Press, pp. 449–463.

Hamada I & DeLong MR (1992a). Excitotoxic acid lesions of the primate subthalamic nucleus result in reduced pallidal neuronal activity during active holding. *Journal of Neurophysiology* **68**, 1859–1866.

Hamada I & DeLong MR (1992b). Excitotoxic acid lesions of the primate subthalamic nucleus result in transient dyskinesias of the contralateral limbs. *Journal of Neurophysiology* **68**, 1850–1858.

Hariz MI, Blomstedt P & Zrinzo L (2010). Deep brain stimulation between 1947 and 1987: The untold story. *Neurosurg Focus* **29**, E1.

Kravitz AV, Freeze BS, Parker PRL, Kay K, Thwin MT, Deisseroth K & Kreitzer AC (2010). Regulation of Parkinsonian motor behaviours by optogenetic control of basal ganglia circuitry. *Nature* **466**, 622–626.

Li J-Y, Englund E, Holton JL, Soulet D, Hagell P, Lees AJ, Lashley T, Quinn NP, Rehncrona S, Björklund A, Widner H, Revesz T, Lindvall O & Brundin P (2008). Lewy bodies in grafted neurons in subjects with Parkinson's disease suggest host-to-graft disease propagation. *Nature Medicine* **14**, 501–503.

Lindvall O, Brundin P, Widner H, Rehncrona S, Gustavii B, Frackowiak R, Leenders KL, Sawle G, Rothwell JC, Marsden CD & Björklund M (1990). Grafts of fetal dopamine neurons survive and improve motor function in Parkinson's disease. *Science* **247**, 574–577.

Majsak MJ, Kaminski T, Gentile AM & Flanagan JR (1998). The reaching movements of patients with Parkinson's disease under self-determined maximal speed and visually cued conditions. *Brain* **121**, 755–766.

Matsuda W, Furuta T, Nakamura KC, Hioki H, Fujiyama F, Arai R & Kaneko T (2009). Single nigrostriatal dopaminergic neurons form widely spread and highly dense axonal arborizations in the neostriatum. *Journal of Neuroscience* **29**, 444–453.

Merchant SS *et al.* (2007). The *Chlamydomonas* genome reveals the evolution of key animal and plant functions. *Science* **318**, 245–250.

Nauta HJW (1979). A proposed conceptual reorganization of the basal ganglia and telencephalon. *Neuroscience* **4**, 1875–1881.

Paladini CA & Tepper JM (2017). Chapter 17 Neurophysiology of substantia nigra dopamine neurons: Modulation by GABA and glutamate. *Handbook of Behavioral Neuroscience* **24**, 335–359.

Parmar M, Grealish S & Henchcliffe C (2020). The future of stem cell therapies for Parkinson disease. *Nature Reviews Neuroscience* **21**, 103–115.

Piccini P, Brooks DJ, Björklund A, Gunn RN, Grasby PM, Rimoldi O, Brundin P, Hagell P, Rehncrona S, Widner H & Lindvall O (1999). Dopamine release from nigral transplants visualized in vivo in a Parkinson's patient. *Nature of Neuroscience* **2**, 1137–1140.

Pollak P, Benabid AL, Gross C, Gao DM, Laurent A, Benazzouz A, Hoffmann D, Gentil M. & Perret J (1993). Effects of the stimulation of the subthalamic nucleus in Parkinson disease. *Revue Neurologique* **149**, 175–176.

Posturna RB & Lang AE (2003). Hemiballism: revisiting a classic disorder. *Lancet Neurology* **2**, 661–668.

Reiner A, Albin RL, Anderson KD, D'Amato CJ, Penney JB & Young AB (1988). Differential loss of striatal projection neurons in Huntington disease. *Proceedings of the National Academy of Sciences* **85**, 5733–5737.

Robertson MM, Eapen V, Singer HS, Martino D, Scharf JM, Paschou P, Roessner V, Woods DW, Hariz M, Mathews CA, Črnčec R & Leckman JF (2017). Gilles de la Tourette syndrome. *Nature Reviews Disease Primers* **3**, 16097.

Roessel PJ van, Grassi G, Aboujaoude EN, Menchón JM, Ameringen MV & Rodríguez CI (2023). Treatment-resistant OCD: Pharmacotherapies in adults. *Comprehensive Psychiatry* **120**, 152352.

Sacks O (1973). *Awakenings*. New York: Summit.

Schell G & Strick P (1984). The origin of thalamic inputs to the arcuate premotor and supplementary motor areas. *Journal of Neuroscience* **4**, 539–560.

Stein DJ, Costa DLC, Lochner C, Miguel EC, Reddy YCJ, Shavitt RG, Heuvel OA van den & Simpson HB (2019). Obsessive–compulsive disorder. *Nature Reviews Disease Primers* **5**, 52.

Steinberg EE, Christoffel DJ, Deisseroth K & Malenka RC (2015). Illuminating circuitry relevant to psychiatric disorders with optogenetics. *Current Opinion in Neurobiology* **30**, 9–16.

Svennilson E, Torvik A, Lowe R & Leksell L (1960). Treatment of parkinsonism by stereotactic thermolesions in the pallidal region. A clinical evaluation of 81 cases. *Acta Physiologica Scandinavica* **35**, 358–377.

Tabrizi SJ, Estevez-Fraga C, van Roon-Mom WMC, Flower MD, Scahill RI, Wild EJ, Muñoz-Sanjuan I, Sampaio C, Rosser AE & Leavitt BR (2022). Potential disease-modifying therapies for Huntington's disease: Lessons learned and future opportunities. *The Lancet Neurology* **21**, 645–658.

Whittier JR (1947). Ballism and the subthalamic nucleus (nucleus hypothalamicus; Corpus luysi): Review of the literature and study of thirty cases. *Archives of Neurology & Psychiatry* **58**, 672–692.

Zhou K, Han J, Wang Y, Zhang Y & Zhu C (2022). Routes of administration for adeno-associated viruses carrying gene therapies for brain diseases. *Frontiers in Molecular Neuroscience* **15**, 988914.

Appendix A

Review of Electricity and Electrical Circuits

In order to understand the operations of the nervous system, which largely functions through electrical signaling, it is imperative to have a good grasp of electricity and electrical circuits. What follows is a conceptual, rather than a rigorous analytical overview of these topics needed to have a reasonably firm footing for understanding electrophysiology relevant for the nervous system and other physiological systems.

Charge

Like gravity, electricity is one of the fundamental forces of nature. Whereas gravitational forces depend on the <u>mass</u> of the objects, electrical forces depend on the <u>charge</u>. The symbol for charge is q. **Charge** *is a basic property of the elementary particles (electrons and protons) that make up matter.* Like the kilogram as the unit of measure for mass, the *unit of measure for charge is the* **coulomb,** C (named for Charles-Augustin de Coulomb). And how much charge is in one coulomb? **Plus one coulomb** (+1 C) of charge is equivalent to the charge carried by 6.25×10^{18} *protons,* while **minus one coulomb** (−1 C) of charge is equal to the charge carried by 6.25×10^{18} electrons. The **total charge** possessed by an object is *the algebraic sum of the individual charges.* Therefore, if we poured a bucket containing +1 C of charge into a bucket containing −1 C of charge,

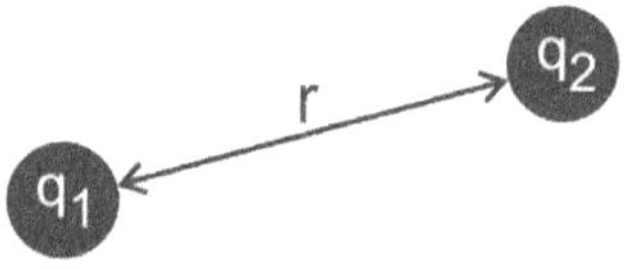

Figure 1.   Two charges separated by a distance *r*.

we would have a bucket with 0 C of charge (even though there would be 12.5×10^{18} charged particles in the bucket).

Electrical Force

The **electrical force** (i.e., the push or pull) set up between two objects (Figure 1) is given by an equation that is remarkably similar to that for gravitational forces:

$$F_E = K \cdot \frac{q_1 \cdot q_2}{r^2}$$

where **K is the universal electric constant** ($K = 9 \times 10^9 \ N \cdot m^2/C^2$), q_1 is the charge (in *C*) on one object, q_2 is the charge (in *C*) on the other object, and *r* is the distance (in meters, *m*) between the two objects. The unit *N* in the universal electric constant indicates newtons of force. And while gravitational forces are always attractive, electrical forces can either attract or repel the two objects, depending on the sign of the charges on the two objects. Like in many human relationships, opposites (i.e., oppositely charged objects) attract, whereas alike (i.e., same sign of charge on both objects) repel.

As a simple example, let's calculate the electrical force set up between two objects; object 1 has +1 C of charge, and object 2 has −1 C of charge, and the two objects are 1 m apart. Therefore, using the equation for electrical force, we have:

$$F_E = K \cdot \frac{q_1 \cdot q_2}{r^2} = 9 \times 10^9 \, N \cdot m^2/C^2 \cdot \frac{(+1C) \cdot (-1C)}{1m^2}$$

$$F_E = -9 \times 10^9 \, N \cdot m^2/C^2 \cdot \frac{C^2}{m^2}$$

Both the C^2 and the m^2 terms cancel out, leaving an electrical force of:

$$F_E = -9 \times 10^9 \; N$$

The units for F_E are in newtons (N), as appropriate for a force. When the electric force has a negative value (as in this case), the direction of the force is to pull the two objects toward one another (to attract), whereas if the electrical force is positive (as would occur when both objects have positive charge or both objects have negative charge), then the direction of the force is to push the two objects away from one another (to repel). The magnitude of this force is enormous: 9×10^9 N is roughly equivalent to one million metric tons of force. This outcome highlights an important point: *electrical forces are extremely potent.* As such, only tiny amounts of charge on two objects can give rise to significant electrical forces. This is a point addressed in Chapter 2 when discussing the factors that underlie the membrane potential in neurons.

Potential

The somewhat inconvenient aspect of electrical force is that the strength of the push or pull depends on the charges on the *two* objects. But what if you possessed an object and simply wanted to be able to express its capability (its "potential") to push or pull on other objects? Well, we can "derive" a term that represents such electrical potential from the equation for electrical force. First, let's rewrite the equation for electrical force in an equivalent form, but let's give one r in the denominator to each q in the numerator:

$$F_E = K \cdot \left(\frac{q_1}{r} \right) \cdot \left(\frac{q_2}{r} \right)$$

Then, we sharpen a knife and slice off the rightmost term associated with q_2 (the object we don't care about). What we are left with is indeed an expression for **electrical potential (Pot)**:

$$Pot = K \cdot \left(\frac{q_1}{r} \right)$$

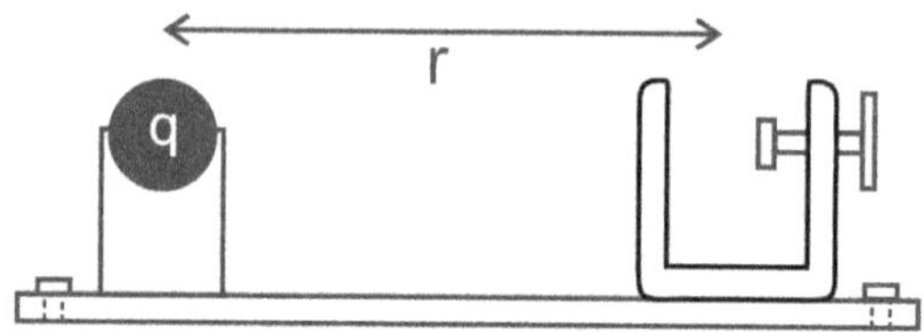

Figure 2.   Apparatus for holding charged objects a fixed distance away from the apparatus charge. The electrical potential of this apparatus is given by $K\,q/r$.

that represents the capability (*potential*) of an object to push or pull on other objects that are placed a certain distance away from the object.

For example, let's calculate the electrical potential for an apparatus that is bolted to the floor and that has an object with charge $q = 2$ C welded to it (Figure 2). A vise, at a distance $r = 0.5$ m away, is used to hold objects of different charges. The electrical potential of this apparatus is given by:

$$Pot = K \cdot \left(\frac{q}{r}\right) = 9 \cdot 10^9\, N \cdot m^2 / C^2 \cdot \frac{2C}{0.5\,m}$$

$$Pot = 36 \times 10^9 N \times m/C$$

Note that in this case only one m and one C canceled out in the units. As such, we are left with $N \cdot m/C$ as the units for electrical potential. This gets clunky to write out all the time, so we refer to one $N \cdot m/C$ as a **volt** (named to honor Alessandro Volta, the inventor of the battery). The most important concept to keep in mind related to electrical potential is simply that the electrical potential is directly proportional to the amount of charge on the object:

$$\boldsymbol{Pot\ \alpha\ q}$$

Therefore, the capacity of an object to push or pull on other objects with charge depends on how much charge the object itself possesses. If we double the amount of charge on the object, we double its electrical strength (its potential).

Current

Another important concept in electricity is that: *if allowed to, charge will move from a place of high potential toward a site of low potential.* But first, what do we mean by "if allowed to"? A medium that enables the movement of charge is referred to as a *conductor*. Typical conductors include ions in solution and metals. Conversely, a medium that tends to prevent the movement of charge is called an *insulator*. Typical insulators include air, oil (lipids), glass, and plastic. Therefore, if we connect two objects together with a conductor, charge will flow from the object with higher potential toward the object with lower potential.

Let's think about these concepts in mechanical terms. Let's say that we lift and hold a bowling ball 2 m above the earth surface (left part of Figure 3). The bowling ball is now at a site of high potential energy. If we release it, it will move to a site of lower potential energy (just as charges will do), namely to the earth surface (a site with zero mechanical potential). If we imbed the bowling ball in a column of concrete (middle part of Figure 3), it still has high mechanical potential with respect to the earth surface but is in a medium that resists the movement of bowling balls (just like an insulator resists the movement of charge). Finally, if we dig a hole

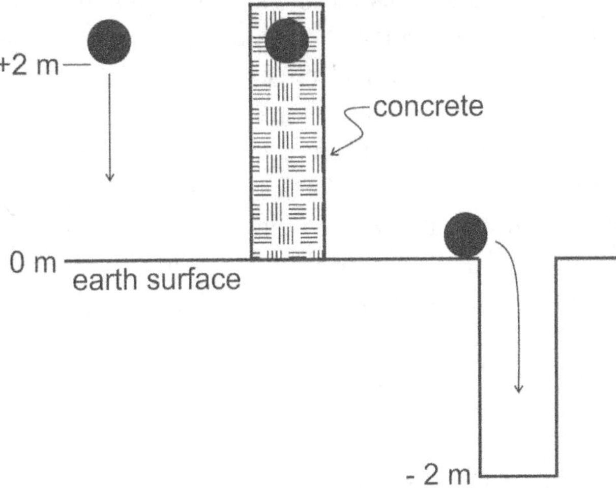

Figure 3.   Mechanical analogy of objects moving from high to low potential and insulators.

in the earth that is 2 m deep, and we nudge the bowling ball from its resting position on the earth surface (with zero mechanical potential) over the hole (right side of Figure 3), it will move to a new site that has negative potential, namely to −2 m below the earth surface. This highlights an important point, namely, that zero potential is *higher* than negative potential. Likewise, an object sitting at −1 m has higher potential than an object sitting at −2 m.

These concepts hold true for electrical potential. An object with zero electrical potential has higher potential than an object with negative potential. As such, if the two objects are connected with a conductor, charges will move from the object with zero potential to the object with negative potential. Similarly, an object with −1 coulomb of charge has higher potential than an object with −2 coulombs of charge. If these two objects are connected with a conductor, then charge will move from the object with −1 C to the object with −2 C. One crucial point (and something that we will return to) is that the *movement of charge* is always considered to be in the *direction that positive charges would move.*

Another essential concept for understanding electrical circuits is that of electrical current. **Current** *(I) is a measure of the <u>movement</u> of charge.* As such, it is a measure of flow, just like the flow of water in a pipe. We can quantify flow in a pipe as the amount of water (the stuff) passing through the pipe in a given amount of time, for example, *Flow = 100 L/minute*. Likewise, in an electrical circuit, current is a measure of the amount of charge (the stuff) passing through a part of a circuit in a given amount of time, and as such is expressed as $I = q/t$. The unit of measure of current, therefore, is *coulombs/s*. For brevity, a *coulomb/s is called an ampere, A* (named for the French physicist André-Marie Ampère). Therefore, 1 ampere of current means that exactly 1 coulomb of charge (i.e., 6.25×10^{18} protons) would pass through a particular location in a circuit in 1 second. In a nutshell, current represents *how fast* charges are moving through a circuit or part of a circuit.

To gain a conceptual understanding of current and the factors that influence it, let's begin with some simple examples. First, let's consider charge movement and associated current between two objects (Figure 4), one that has 4 units of charge (could be coulombs, micro-coulombs, pico-coulombs ... it doesn't matter) and the other has no net charge (remember,

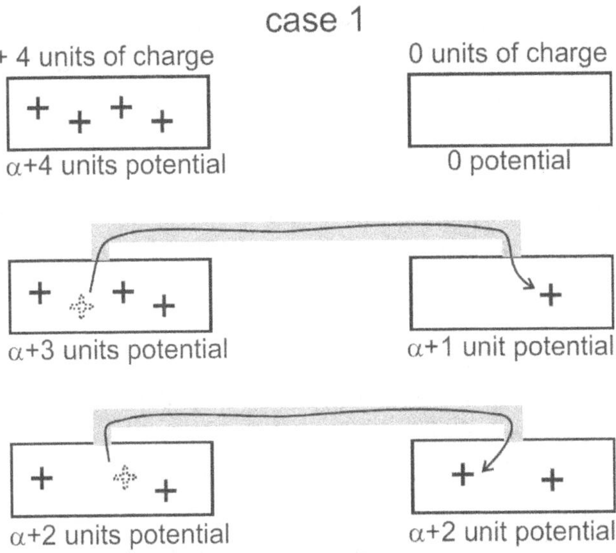

Figure 4.   Movement of charge from object with high potential to object with low potential.

this simply means that there are equal numbers of positive and negative charges on this object). Also, keep in mind that potential is directly proportional to the amount of charge, *Pot α q*. Therefore, the object on the left has 4 units of potential, whereas the object on the right has zero potential. At first, the two objects are not connected together (top row, Figure 4), and therefore, there is no medium to enable movement of charge. If we now connect the two objects with a conductor, let's say a tube filled with electrolyte solution, then charge can move. Charge will move from the high-potential object on the left toward the low-potential object on the right. After the movement of one unit of charge from the left to the right object, the object on the left will now have 3 units of potential, whereas the object on the right will now possess one unit of potential (middle row, Figure 4). The object on the left still has higher potential than the object on the right, so again charge will move from the left object to the right one. After another unit of charge has moved from left to right (bottom row, Figure 4), we now end up with 2 units of potential on the left object and 2 units of potential on the right. At this point, there is no site of lower potential, and therefore, movement of charge halts.

Before moving on, it is a good time to address one of those confusing bits of information picked up in physics classes. Students are often informed that electrons, not positively charged particles, carry the movement of charge in circuits. This, however, is not generally true. It is true in the specific case where metals serve as the conductor but is not necessarily true when ions in solution serve as the conductor (as in biological systems). Furthermore, it doesn't matter—the effects are identical. To illustrate this, let's reconsider the case shown in Figure 4 but where electrons are the charge carriers (Figure 5). Once the two objects are connected (let's say by a copper wire), negative charge is pulled off the object on the right, leaving behind its companion and now exposed positive charge (middle row, Figure 5). The arrival of the negative charge on the left object joins with and cancels out one of the excess positive charges on the left, leaving three positive charges (and 3 units of potential on the left object). Because there remains a difference in potential between the two objects (and a medium to conduct charge), charge will continue to move. Another negative charge is pulled off the object on the right (bottom row,

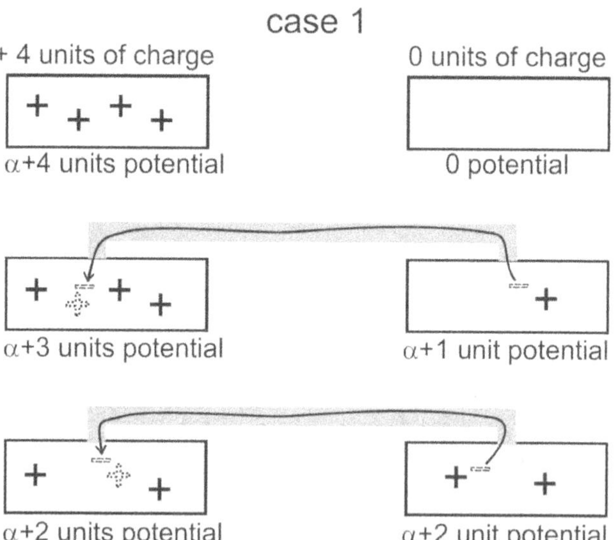

Figure 5.   Equivalence of negative charge movement with positive charge movement (see Figure 4).

Figure 5), leaving behind and exposing its companion positive charge. When the negative charge arrives on the left object, it combines with an excess positive charge, and they cancel one another out. Now, we end up in exactly the same situation as we did for the case involving the movement of positive charge (Figure 4), namely, with two units of potential on both the left and right objects and no further movement of charge. As mentioned above, by convention, *current is always considered to be in the direction that positive charges would flow*. As such, when dealing with electrical circuits, it is (for the most part) helpful to forget that electrons carry charge in metal-based circuits and just think about positive charges moving around. It will make your life simpler.

Now that we have that out of our hair, we can return to the important matter of what factors determine electrical current. Let's do a cartoon-like calculation of the average current associated with the case depicted in Figure 4. In that case, 2 units of charge (let's call it 2 C) were moved in a certain amount of time, let's say 1 second. Therefore, the average current over the one-second time period can be crudely calculated as: $I = q/t = 2$ $C/1s = 2$ $C/s = 2$ *amperes (A)*.

Now, let's examine a second case (Figure 6) for which at the outset there are +2 units of charge (and +2 units of potential) on the left object and −6 units of charge (and −6 units of potential) on the right object. Keeping in mind the very important concept that *if allowed (by the presence of a conductor), charge moves from high to low potential*, then when connected with a conductor, charge will move from the site of high potential (+2 on the left) toward the site of low potential (−6 on the right). The first movement of charge (second row, Figure 6) will leave +1 unit of potential on the left and −5 units of potential on the right. Another movement of charge from left to right will leave zero potential on the left and −4 units of potential on the right (third row, Figure 6). Remembering that zero potential is *higher* than negative potential (see the right part of Figure 3), charge will again move from the object on the left to the object on the right. After this movement (fourth row, Figure 6), there will be −1 unit of potential on the left object and −3 on the right. As in the case of the bowling ball, where 1 m down in a hole (−1 m) is *higher* than 3 m deep in a hole (−3 m), −1 unit of electrical potential is higher than −3 units of potential. Therefore, again, charge will move from the left object to the

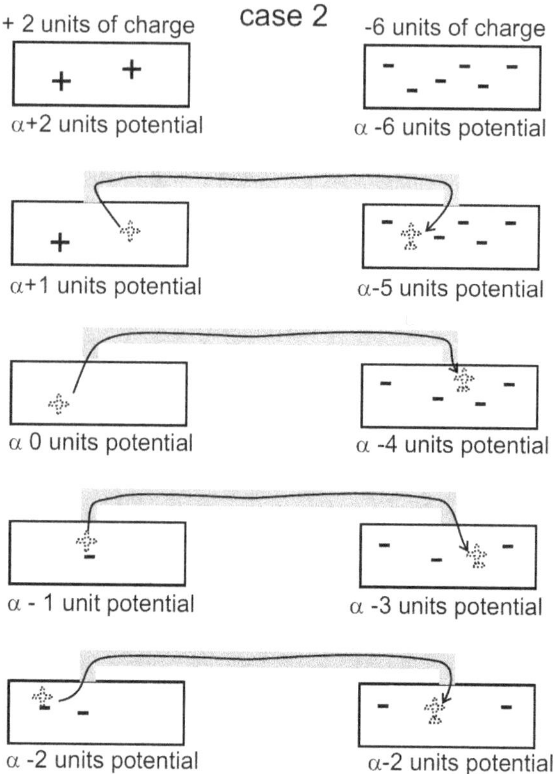

Figure 6.   Movement of charge from site of high potential to low potential. The difference in potential here is greater than that in Figure 4.

right. After this move, there will be −2 units of potential on both the left and right objects (fifth row, Figure 6). At this point, there is no site of higher or lower potential, and therefore all movement of charges ceases.

Let's do our simple calculation of average current for this second case (Figure 6). If we count up the number of unit-charge movements from left to right, there were four. Let's again assume that all charge movement is complete within one second. When we do our calculation, this yields: $I = q/t = 4\ C/1\ s = 4\ A$.

There are three key points to highlight at this stage: (1) *charge moves from high to low potential*, (2) *the total charge in the system does not change*, and (3) the magnitude of the *current is directly proportional to the difference in potential between the two ends*. Point 1 has already been discussed. With regard to the second point, note that for Case 1 (Figure 4), the total charge at the start was +4 units (all on the left object). After the two objects were connected and current eventually came to a halt, there were still +4 units of charge (+2 on the left and +2 on the right). Likewise, for Case 2, the total charge in the system at the outset was +2 + (−6) = −4 units of charge. After connecting the two objects together and allowing charges to move, there ended up with −2 units on the left and −2 units on the right for again a total of −4 units of charge.

With regard to the third point, note that for Case 1 (Figure 4), the *difference in potential* between the two objects at the outset was +4 − 0 = +4 units of potential. We estimated the current for this situation to be *2 A*. For Case 2 (Figure 6), the difference in potential between object 1 and object 2 at the outset was +2 − (−6) = +8 units of potential. This is twice that for Case 1. The current for Case 2 was calculated to be *4 A*, exactly twice that of Case 1. As such, the magnitude of the current is directly related to the difference in potential between the two ends of a circuit.

Now, let's change the property of the conductor (e.g., a tube filled with electrolyte solution) that connects the two objects. Let's reduce the diameter of the tube so it is more difficult for charges to squeeze through (i.e., we've increased its resistance). Figure 7 shows the start and end states for Case 1 (on the left) and for our new situation (Case 3, on the right), which is exactly like Case 1 except for the thinner tube. For both cases, two units of charge are moved, but because of the thinner conductor that more strongly impedes movement of charge, it takes longer to reach the end state in Case 3. Let's say it takes 2 seconds. Therefore, our average

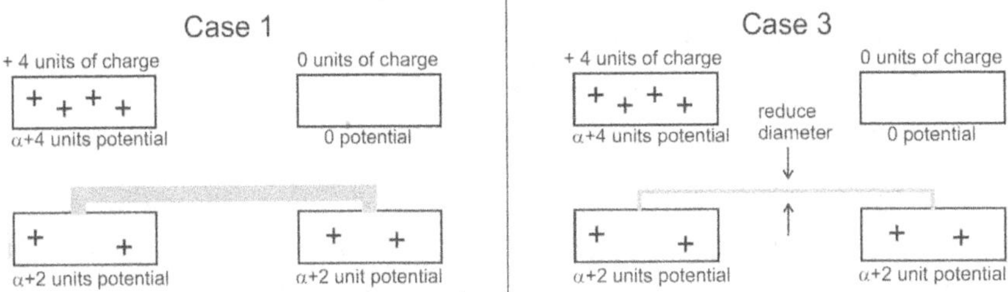

Figure 7.   Movement of charge with low-resistance path (Case 1) and high-resistance path (Case 3).

current for Case 3 is $I = q/t = 2$ $C/2$ $s = 1$ $C/s = 1$ A, half that associated with Case 1.

Ohm's Law

Without even knowing it, we've just (more or less) derived **Ohm's Law**. First, we showed that current is proportional to the difference in potential between the two ends of our system, namely: $I \propto V_1 - V_2$, where V_1 and V_2 are the potentials measured in volts at each end. For simplicity, we write this as $I \propto \Delta V$. Second, we suggested that the current is inversely proportional to the resistance (R) in the pathway connecting the two ends, namely: $I \propto 1/R$. When we combine these two observations, we get Ohm's Law: $I = \Delta V/R$, which indicates that the current set up along a path is precisely equal to the difference in potential between the two ends of the path divided by the resistance offered by the path. Ohm's law is also sometimes written as $\Delta V = I \cdot R$, from which one can deduce the difference in potential that must exist across a path by knowing the current and the resistance in the path.

But what precisely do we mean by the term resistance, R? Resistance is a function of both the physical geometry of the pathway through which charges move and an intrinsic property of the material making up the pathway called **resistivity** (r). Resistivity, in turn, is a function of the molecular structure of the material such that conductors (like ions in solution, metals) have low values of resistivity, whereas insulators (like lipids, glass, and air) have high resistivities. The unit of measure for resistivity is ohm · meter ($\Omega \cdot$ m). For example, to calculate the resistance of a cylindrically shaped object (like a wire, tube, axon, dendrite, and muscle fiber), we use the following equation:

$$R = \frac{\rho \cdot L}{A}$$

where L is the length of the cylinder and A is the cross-sectional area of the cylinder. Therefore, the longer the object, the higher will be its resistance. Conversely, the larger the cross-sectional area, the lower the resistance. The units associated with this equation are:

$$R = \frac{(\Omega \cdot m) \cdot m}{m^2} = \Omega$$

But what is an ohm (Ω)? The ohm (named for the German physicist Georg Simon Ohm) is a derived unit based on the following kind of experiment. You have a little circuit with a *difference* in potential between the two ends of precisely 1 V. You also have a device to measure the current in the circuit. Then you keep tweaking the properties of the conductor (e.g., by repeatedly changing the diameter) until you measure a current of precisely 1.0 A. By definition, then, the conductor in your circuit has exactly 1 Ω of resistance. In other words, a 1-Ω resistor is that resistance that gives rise to exactly 1 A of current in a path that has a difference of potential across the path of 1 V. From Ohm's law ($I = \Delta V/R$), therefore, we have 1 $A = 1V/1\Omega$. If we rearrange this expression to solve for ohms, we get $\Omega = V/A$. As such, the base unit of measure for Ωs is V/A. Remember that Ohm's law, $I = \Delta V/R$, indicates that the current (measured in amperes) is equal to the difference in potential divided by the resistance. Therefore, the units on the right side of the equation must have units of amperes (A). If we substitute in V/A for Ω, then indeed we get $I = \Delta V/R = V/\Omega = V/(V/A) = A$.

Battery

Up till now, we've discussed the movement of charge between two objects connected with a conductor (i.e., Figures 4–7). But current only exists when there is a difference in potential, and in each of these cases, charge movement quickly leads to equal potential on both objects, causing current to halt. From a practical sense, this is not very useful. Let's create an apparatus that continuously maintains a difference in potential and thereby maintains current moving through the circuit. To do this, we begin with the same two objects used previously, let's say with +4 V of potential on the left object and −4 V of potential on the right (Figure 8A). These two objects (let's say they are small metal bars) are connected by a tube of a certain length and diameter, filled with an electrolyte solution, thereby defining the overall resistance of this pathway. Next, we simply bend the

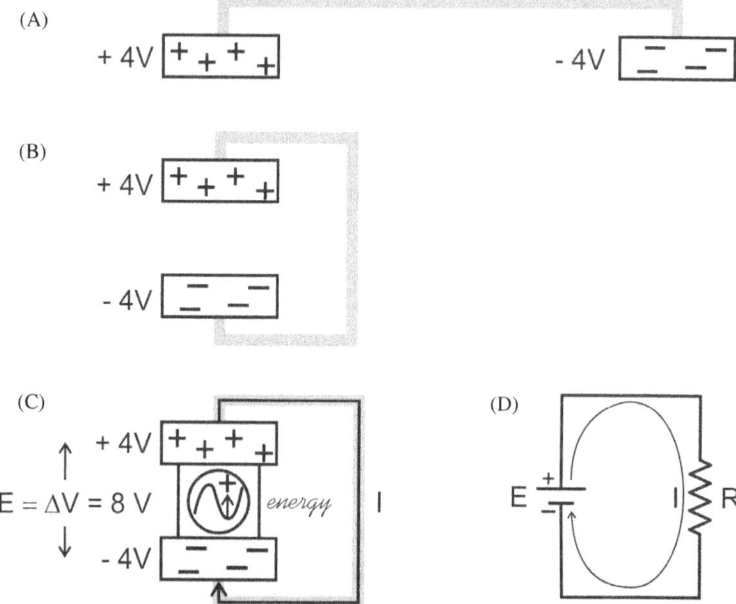

Figure 8.   (A) Two objects with different potentials connected by a resistive path. (B) Same two objects but with path bent. (C) "Pump" requiring energy inserted between high-potential and low-potential bars that moves positive charges onto high-potential bar to maintain a constant difference in potential. This device is a battery. The constant difference in potential maintained by the battery is the electromotive force, E. (D) symbolic representation of battery and resistor.

tube around such that the bar with the negative charge is situated below the bar with the positive charge (Figure 8B). The length and diameter of the tube are the same, so the resistance is the same. Now, we insert a device between the two bars (Figure 8C). This device works like a pump such that as soon as any positive charge arrives on the bottom bar (that has been delivered from the top bar), it is scooped up by the pump and pushed back onto the top bar. The process of pushing a positive charge onto a bar with positive charges requires energy that is fueled by chemical processes within the device. The beauty of this system is that it keeps the amount of charge, and therefore the potential, constant on the top and bottom bars. As such, the *difference* in potential between one end of the circuit (i.e., the top bar with +4 V) and the other (i.e., the bottom bar with −4 V) is also maintained constant (i.e., at 8 V). From Ohm's law we know that the current is directly proportional to the difference in potential. Therefore, if the difference in potential is not changing (and the resistance is constant), then this system will set up a steady flow of charge (i.e., a steady current) that will persist indefinitely until the chemical fuel is expended. This device is a **battery**. The *difference in potential between one end and the other of a battery* is referred to as the **electromotive force** (i.e., how pushy the battery is in driving current in a circuit) and as such, is abbreviated as **E**. And while an actual battery doesn't quite work in the way described in Figure 8, the concepts are similar.

Of course, it gets cumbersome to draw circuits using pumps, bars, and tubes of given lengths and diameters. Therefore, we use symbols for different electrical elements in order to facilitate the representation of complex circuits. Figure 8D shows the same circuit as in Figure 8C but using symbols. The symbol for the battery is two lines: a long top line labeled with a "+" representing the high potential bar and a short bottom line labeled with a "−" representing the low potential bar. The whole thing is labeled with an E indicating the potential difference between the top and bottom bars.

In the real world, resistance depends critically on the geometry of the conductor. This presents a challenge for representing resistance diagrammatically. The clever solution was to consolidate all of the resistance associated with some conductor (such as the electrolyte-filled tube in Figure 8C) into a single location (the zigzag in Figure 8D). All the elements of a circuit are then interconnected with lines (like superconducting wires) that offer no resistance. As such, one can change the length and bends of these lines as much as desired without having any effect on the circuit. Lastly, arrows are sometimes drawn to indicate the direction that positive charges would flow (i.e., the current) in the circuit.

Analysis of Circuits

Often an electrical circuit consists of a network of interconnected elements like the one shown in Figure 9A. An equivalent hydraulic circuit is shown in Figure 9B. In the hydraulic circuit, the pump produces high positive pressure on the exit side, driving fluid toward the negative

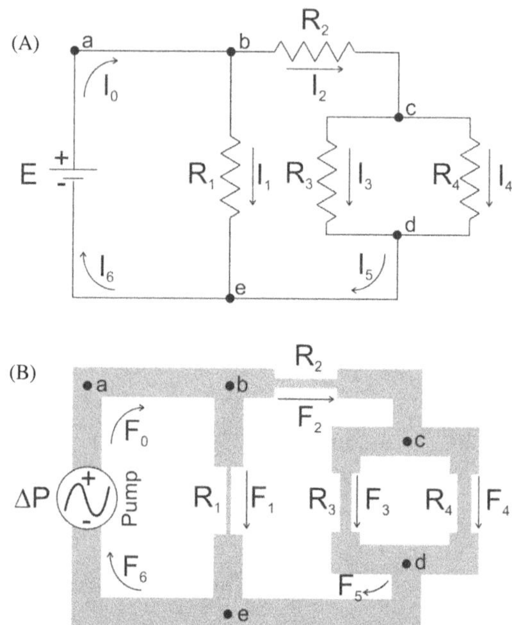

Figure 9.   (A) Electrical circuit and (B) a hydraulic equivalent to the electrical circuit.

pressure (suction) side through a network of pipes of varying diameters that offer different amounts of resistance to fluid flow (F). Typically, a goal of circuit analysis is to determine the amount of current (Figure 9A) or flow (Figure 9B) in each branch of the circuit given the resistances and difference in potential (E) across the battery (Figure 9A) or difference in pressure (ΔP) across the pump (Figure 9B).

The analysis of electrical circuits, like the one shown in Figure 9A, involves the use of Ohm's law and a couple of other principles known as Kirchhoff's laws (named for the German physicist Gustav Kirchhoff). **Kirchhoff's first law** states that *the total current entering a point in a circuit must equal the total current exiting the point.* Note that this law has to do with *current* at a single *point* in a circuit. In a nutshell, Kirchhoff's first law simply tells us: *what goes in = what comes out.*

For example, in Figure 9A, the total current entering node *a* is I_0, and therefore, the total current exiting *a* is also I_0. At node *b*, the total current entering is I_0, but the path then splits into two branches that carry currents

I_1 and I_2 out of node b. Kirchhoff's first law, therefore, tells us that at node b: $I_0 = I_1 + I_2$. Likewise, at node c, what enters is I_2 and what exits is I_3 and I_4, therefore, $I_2 = I_3 + I_4$. At node d, two paths carrying current converge, and only one path emerges. As such, at d, what goes in (I_3 and I_4) must equal what comes out (I_5): $I_3 + I_4 = I_5$. The part of the circuit involving the branches through R_3 and R_4 operates just like a river splitting into two branches to go around an island (Figure 10). Let's say the flow of water F_2 entering into c is 10,000 L/s. That flow splits into two branches, F_3 and F_4, say 4,000 and 6,000 L/s, respectively, such that their sum equals what was entered. The flows F_3 and F_4 are then carried around the island, where they merge at point d. According to Kirchhoff's first law, the flow that enters d must equal what exits, namely, $F_3 + F_4 = F_5$, in other words, $4,000 + 6,000 = 10,000$ L/s. Note also that the total flow into this system, F_2, is equal to the total flow that exits, F_5. All the water must be accounted for ... it is not sneaking away through some unknown pathway.

Kirchhoff's second law states that *the change in potential (voltage) between two points in a circuit is the same for any path that connects those two points.* In contrast to Kirchhoff's first law, this law refers to change in potential and two points in a circuit. While perhaps less intuitive than Kirchhoff's first law, we can get a conceptual idea about the second

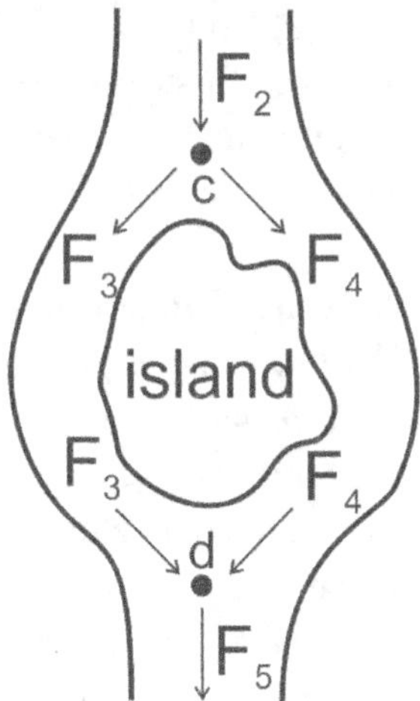

Figure 10.   Flow in a river splitting into two branches to go around an island.

law by considering the following. Imagine a little stick figure of a human standing on the "wire" connecting point *a* and *b* in the circuit drawn in Figure 9A. In this mechanical analogy, assume that that wire represents a long hallway on the second floor of a building. At node *b* there is a stairway (R_1) that runs all the way from the second floor down to the basement at point *e*. If the person takes that stairway, then their mechanical potential will change from being one floor above the earth surface to one floor below. Now, further along the hallway on the second floor is another stairway (R_2) that runs from the second floor down to the ground floor (point *c*). From there, the person could then take the hallway to the left and descend stairway R_3 or take the hallway to the right and descend down stairway R_4. Both of those stairways would bring the person to the same location in the basement at point *d*. The person could then walk around the corner and along the basement hallway to arrive at point *e*. And there is another path by which the person could descend from the second floor to the basement. The person could walk to the left on the second floor, go around the corner at position *a*, and take the elevator (E) directly down to the basement. Once exiting the elevator, the person could walk along the hallway, take a turn, and also arrive at position *e*.

For all these paths that connect point *b* on the second floor to point *e* on the bottom floor, the *change* in the person's mechanical potential is exactly the same; namely, it went from a mechanical potential associated with being one floor above the earth surface to one floor below. This is exactly the same principle for Kirchhoff's second law—the change in electrical potential is the same for any path in a circuit that connects two points.

Related to this principle is the **Voltage Law**, which simply indicates that the *total change in potential along a path is equal to the algebraic sum of the individual changes in potential.* For example, in Figure 9A, taking a path from point *b* to *c* through R_2, then from point *c* to *d* through R_3, and then from point *d* along the connector to point *e*, the total change in potential from *b* to *e* is given as $\Delta V_{b \to e} = \Delta V_{b \to c} + \Delta V_{c \to d} + \Delta V_{d \to e}$. You should note that $\Delta V_{d \to e}$ is zero because this path has no resistance associated with it. Recall from Ohm's Law, $\Delta V = I \times R$, and if the resistance is zero, then there will be no change in potential. This is no different than walking along a hallway in the basement; there is no change in mechanical potential because your vertical position is not changing.

Application to a Simple Circuit

Kirchhoff's laws, Ohm's law, and the Voltage law are like tools in your toolbox that you can pull out at different times to help solve a circuit problem. Let's begin by applying these principles in a very simple circuit (Figure 11) for which we want to know the magnitude of the current, I, given the difference in potential across the battery, E, and the resistance, R. First, from *Kirchhoff's first law*, you should recognize that the current is the same everywhere in this circuit. This is because there are no branches where the current can be split up into different parts (like in the river example in Figure 10). Now, let's use *Kirchhoff's second law* in a strategic way. Let's consider two pathways that connect point a to point d. One pathway connects a to d moving clockwise through b, R, and c. The other pathway connects a to d directly through the battery, E. Kirchhoff's second law tells us that the change in potential must be identical for both pathways. In other words, the total change in potential from a to d through the path including the resistor ($\Delta V_{a,d \to R}$) must equal the total change in potential from a to d through the path that includes the battery ($\Delta V_{a,d \to E}$), that is, $\Delta V_{a,d \to R} = \Delta V_{a,d \to E}$. The left side of the equation includes components associated with three separate segments: a to b, b to c, and c to d.

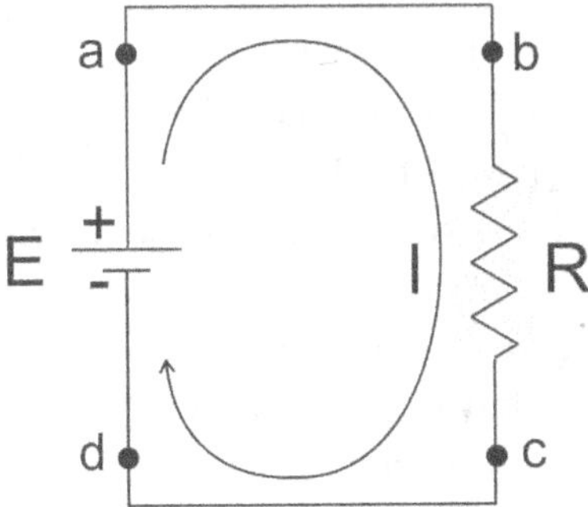

Figure 11.   Simple circuit with battery and resistor.

These different contributions can be accounted for using the *Voltage law*, as: $\Delta V_{a,b} + \Delta V_{b,c} + \Delta V_{c,d} = \Delta V_{a,d \to E}$. We now can pull out our *Ohm's law* tool that tells us that the change in potential across a part of the circuit is equal to the product of the current in that part of the circuit and the resistance offered by that part of the circuit. Keeping in mind that Kirchhoff's first law tells us that the current is the same for each part of this circuit and that the connectors offer no resistance, we can write: $(I \times 0) + (I \times R) + (I \times 0) = \Delta V_{a,d \to E}$. Now, on the right side of the equation, the difference in potential across a battery is simply E, and therefore we end up with $I \times R = E$. This can be rearranged to solve for the current, $I = E/R$. Finally, we can solve for I given a battery voltage E, say of 12 V, and a resistor R, say of 6 Ω: I = 12 V/6 Ω = 2 V/Ω. Remembering that an Ω is equivalent to V/A, we have $I = 2$ V/V/A = **2 A**.

The point of this exercise was not to just extract a value of current for this simple circuit but to demonstrate the method by which one deploys Kirchhoff's, Ohm's, and the Voltage laws in just about any circuit. Furthermore, while the circuit in Figure 11 may seem trivial, there are some subtle aspects to it that may not be so obvious when pondered carefully. For example, one may legitimately ask: why is the current in the segment *a* to *b* with no resistance the same as that through *b* to *c* with resistance? Doesn't Ohm's law tell us that current is inversely proportional to the resistance, and clearly, in these two segments, we have different resistances? Good questions! Perhaps an unsatisfactory explanation to these questions is that charges move along a given pathway (with no branches) at the same pace because they are tightly packed, one behind the other, with no "space" to move at different rates. Maybe a better way to conceptualize this is to consider the cafeteria from hell (Figure 12). In this situation, the only resistance for the poor souls moving through the lunch line is at the cash register, R. And while the cashier is only dealing with (and resisting flow for) the customer in front of her, it nevertheless affects everyone in the line in the same way. Indeed, one can only move in the line as fast as the slowest person moving past the cash register. And since this is the cafeteria from hell, as soon as you pay for your food, you must stay in line, pick up your food, and pay again (... forever more).

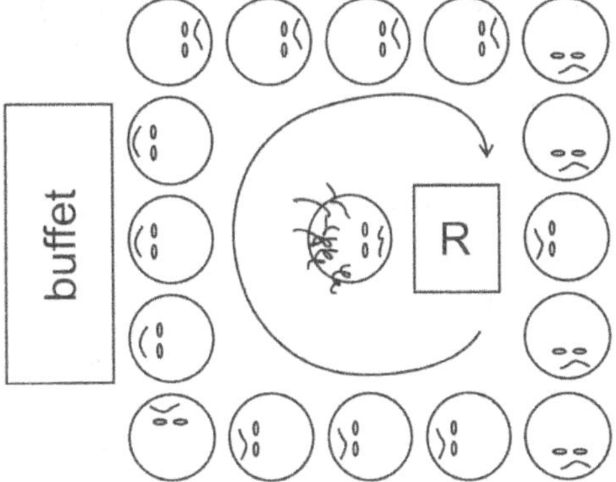

Figure 12.   Cafeteria from hell. Everyone in line moves at the same pace even though resistance for movement occurs only at a single location, R.

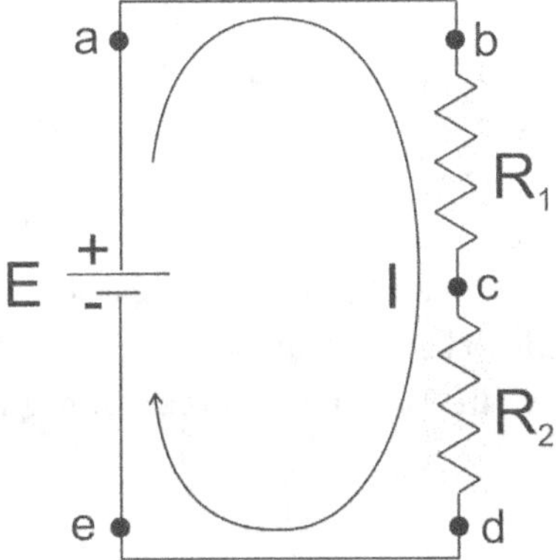

Figure 13.   Circuit with two resistors in series.

Resistors in Series

Let's make the circuit slightly more challenging and calculate the current in a circuit that has two resistors, R_1 and R_2 (Figure 13). In this case, the resistors are arranged in series. Now, the term "in series" simply means that the current that goes through one element is the same as goes through the other; there are no intervening branches or junctions. Indeed, in this circuit configuration, *Kirchhoff's first law* tells us that the current that goes through R_1 and R_2 (as well as through the battery, E, and any other point in the circuit) is the same. Now, let's use *Kirchhoff's second law* and consider the change in potential for two paths that connect point a to e; one through the resistors and one across the battery. We know that the total change in potential across these two pathways must be equal to one another. Furthermore, the total change in potential along a path is equal to the sum of the individual changes in potential (*Voltage law*). Therefore, we can write: $\Delta V_{a,b} + \Delta V_{b,c} + \Delta V_{c,d} + \Delta V_{d,e} = \Delta V_{a,e \to E}$. From *Ohm's law* we know that the change in potential across a segment of a circuit is equal to the product of the current and the segment resistance, and we also know that the change in potential across a battery is simply E. As such, we can write: $I \times 0 + I \times R_1 + I \times R_2 + I \times 0 = E$, which reduces to $I \times (R_1 + R_2) = E$. Now, oftentimes when dealing with circuit problems, one ends up with an equation that looks like Ohm's law except that there are a bunch of resistance terms inside a set of brackets (in our case, just R_1 and R_2). It can be convenient to represent those resistance terms as a single equivalent resistance, R_{eq}. In this simple case, for two resistors in series, we have $R_{eq} = R_1 + R_2$, so we can rewrite our equation as $I \times R_{eq} = E$ yielding $I = E/R_{eq}$.

In general, for a set of n resistors in *series*, the equivalent resistance is simply the algebraic sum of the individual resistors: $R_{eq} = R_1 + R_2 + R_3 + \cdots R_n$. However, one needs to be mindful as to what constitutes resistors in series. Take, for example, the set of resistors shown in Figure 14. Although

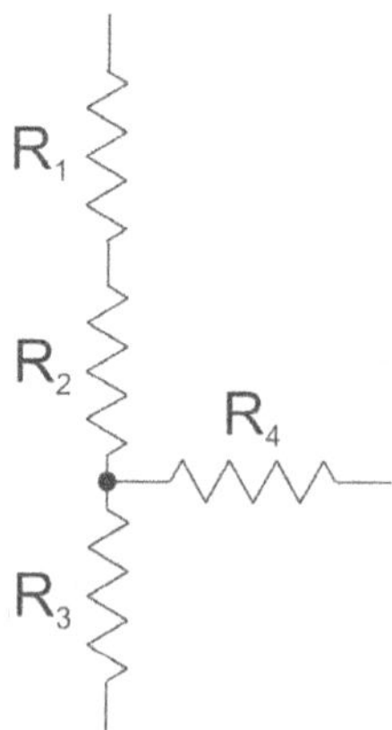

Figure 14.   Resistors R_2 and R_3 are not in series. Resistors R_3 and R_4 are in parallel.

arranged in a line, resistors R_1, R_2, and R_3 are <u>not</u> in series. This is because the current that passes through R_1 and R_2 (which are in series) is not the same current that passes through R_3. At the node, some of the current exiting R_2 goes toward R_4, and some of the current goes through R_3. Indeed, resistors R_3 and R_4 are in parallel (meaning different currents pass through each of those elements), even though they are not drawn as physically parallel elements.

Let's briefly return to the two-resistors-in-series circuit (Figure 13) and plug in some numbers. The values we calculate here will be compared to those calculated for a different circuit later. Let's say $E = 12$ V, $R_1 = 2$ Ω, and $R_2 = 4$ Ω. Therefore, the equivalent resistance is given as $R_{eq} = 2$ $\Omega + 4$ $\Omega = 6$ Ω. The current in the circuit can then be calculated as: $I = E/R_{eq} = 12$ V$/6$ $\Omega = 2$ V$/\Omega = 2$ V$/$V$/$A $= \underline{2 \text{ A}}$.

Resistors in Parallel

Now let's examine a circuit that has two resistors in parallel (Figure 15). From *Kirchhoff's first law*, we know that the current that enters node a must equal that what exits, namely $I = I_1 + I_2$. Likewise, at node b, what enters is $I_1 + I_2$, and what exits must be I. From *Kirchhoff's second law*, we know that the change in potential along the path from point a to b through R_1 must be equal to the change in potential from a to b through R_2. Furthermore, that change in potential must also be equal to the change in potential along the path on the left that just includes the battery, E. Therefore, we can write: $\Delta V_{a,b \to R1} = \Delta V_{a,b \to R2} = \Delta V_{a,b \to E}$. Handling the change in potential separately for each resistor, setting them equal to E (i.e.,

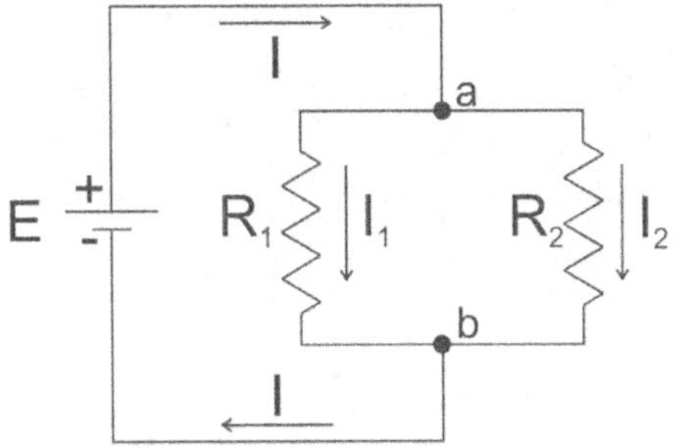

Figure 15.   Circuit with two resistors in parallel.

$\Delta V_{a,d\to E}$), and applying Ohm's law to calculate the change in potential across a resistor, we get: $I_1 \times R_1 = E$ and $I_2 \times R_2 = E$. Rearranging to calculate the current in each branch, we obtain: $I_1 = E/R_1$ and $I_2 = E/R_2$. Now, we can substitute the values I_1 and I_2 into the equation we derived above from *Kirchhoff's first law* to obtain: $I = I_1 + I_2 = E/R_1 + E/R_2 = E\,(1/R_1 + 1/R_2)$.

As mentioned earlier, it is often convenient to express such equations as Ohm's law involving a single equivalent resistor, such as $I = E/R_{eq}$. This equation and the one we just derived are both equal to the current I; therefore, we can set them equal to one another, namely, $E/R_{eq} = E\,(1/R_1 + 1/R_2)$. If we divide both sides by E, we end up with $1/R_{eq} = 1/R_1 + 1/R_2$. We have just derived the general form for the equivalent resistance for n resistors in parallel: $1/R_{eq} = 1/R_1 + 1/R_2 + 1/R_3 + \cdots + 1/R_n$. It is difficult (for most of us), however, to estimate equivalent resistances with such an inverted equation form. Let's perform a little algebra trick and get a form that is much easier to deal with. First, multiply both sides of the above equation for the equivalent resistance with two resistors in parallel by $R_1 \times R_2$ to get: $R_1 \times R_2 \times 1/R_{eq} = R_1 \times R_2 \times (1/R_1 + 1/R_2)$. This gives $R_1 \times R_2/R_{eq} = R_1 \times R_2/R_1 + R_1 \times R_2/R_2$. The right-hand side of the equation reduces to $R_2 + R_1$, so we now have $R_1 \times R_2/R_{eq} = R_2 + R_1$. This rearranges to yield: $R_{eq} = R_1 \times R_2/(R_1 + R_2)$. As such, the equivalent resistance for two resistors in parallel is simply equal to their *product* over their *sum* (now this is something one can do in their head!). However, be forewarned, this form of equation doesn't work for more than two resistors in parallel.

Now let's plug in the values that we used previously for the circuit with resistors in series, namely, $E = 12$ V, $R_1 = 2\ \Omega$, and $R_2 = 4\ \Omega$. In this case, the equivalent resistance is given by $R_{eq} = R_1 \times R_2/(R_1 + R_2) = 2\ \Omega \times 4\ \Omega/(2\ \Omega + 4\ \Omega) = 4/3\ \Omega$. The total current that leaves the battery is given as $I = E/R_{eq} = 12$ V$/4/3\ \Omega = 9$ A. The current through R_1 is $I_1 = E/R_1 = 12$ V$/2\ \Omega = 6$ A, and the current through R_2 is $I_2 = E/R_2 = 12$ V$/4\ \Omega = 3$ A. As a confirmation, we check that indeed $I = I_1 + I_2$, that is, 9 A $= 6$ A $+ 3$ A.

Three Key Observations

Based on our simple analyses of circuits with resistors in series and parallel, we can make the following three observations. *One*, the current, I, that exited ("was drawn") from the battery was substantially larger for the case where the resistors were arranged in parallel compared to in series. Why is that? ... we used the same battery and the same two resistors. The reason is that **when resistors are arranged in parallel, the equivalent resistance is smaller than when arranged in series**. For the parallel case, $Req = 4/3\ \Omega = 1.3\ \Omega$, whereas for the series case, $Req = 6\ \Omega$. Ohm's law tells us that the current in a circuit is inversely proportional to the resistance ($I = \Delta V/R$), and since ΔV is the same in both cases (E), then the current will be higher for the case with the parallel resistors having a small net resistance.

Two, in the parallel resistor circuit, the current through R_1 (6 A) was higher than that through R_2 (3 A). This relates to an important rule of thumb: **current tends to follow the path of least resistance**. As such, more current is directed through the low-resistance path ($R_1 = 2\ \Omega$) and less through the high-resistance path ($R_2 = 4\ \Omega$).

And *three*, when **resistors are arranged in parallel, the equivalent resistance is <u>less</u> than the smallest of the original resistors**. In our case, $R_1 = 2\ \Omega$ and $R_2 = 4\ \Omega$, yet the equivalent resistance was 1.3 Ω. Indeed, the more resistors one "adds" in parallel, the lower the effective resistance. Now how could this be—adding more gives you less? To help understand this, let's take a look at a hydraulic example in Figure 16. In hydraulic circuits, narrow pipes act as the resistors to fluid flow. In Figure 16A, there is just one such resistor. If we now add three of these resistors in parallel (Figure 16B), the effective resistance will diminish. This is because the net cross-sectional area across the three pipe resistances is increased, and resistance decreases as area increases. Indeed, an equivalent pipe resistance would have a cross-sectional area 3× larger than the original pipe. This idea is the same for *parallel resistors* in an electrical circuit—*more is less*.

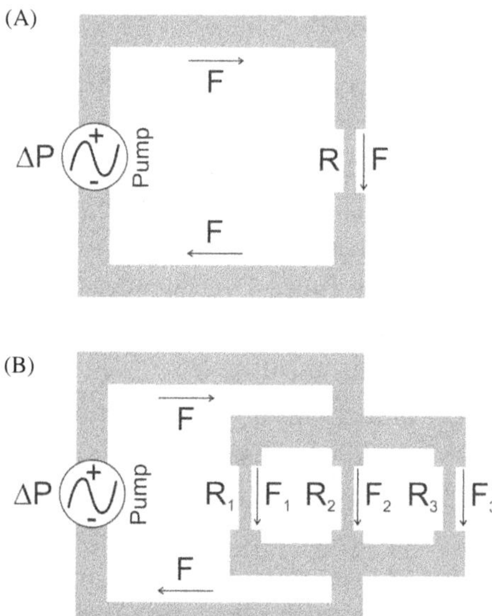

Figure 16.   Hydraulic analogy of circuit with single resistor (A) and with three resistors "added" in parallel (B).

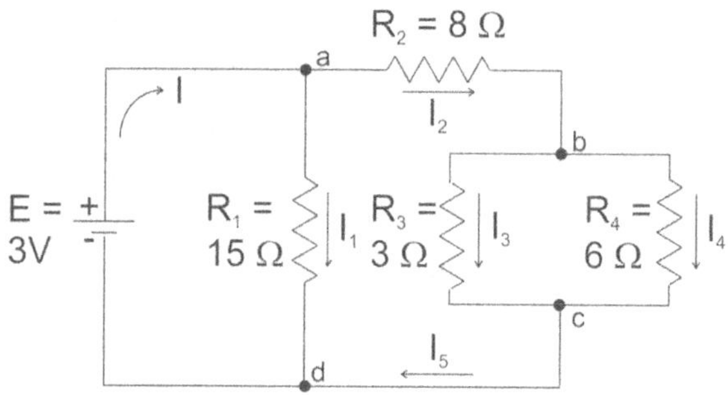

Figure 17.   Complex circuit.

Complex Circuit

Now we should be ready to tackle a more complicated circuit. Let's use our tools (Ohm's, Kirchhoff's, and Voltage laws) to determine the currents I, I_1, I_2, I_3, I_4, and I_5 in the circuit depicted in Figure 17. To begin, let's use our rules for combining resistors in parallel and series step-by-step until we have only a single equivalent resistor in the circuit. First, the single

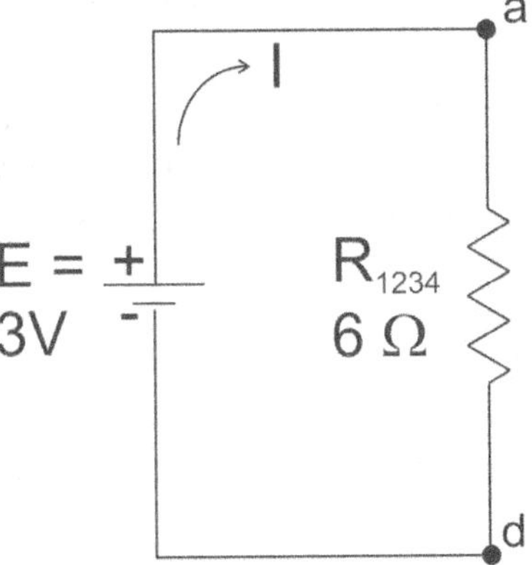

Figure 18.   The complex circuit shown in Figure 17 resolved to one with a single equivalent resistance, R_{1234}.

equivalent resistance (R_{34}) for resistors R_3 and R_4 in *parallel* can be found as (product over the sum):

$$R_{34} = \frac{R_3 \cdot R_4}{R_3 + R_4} = \frac{3\Omega \cdot 6\Omega}{3\Omega + 6\Omega} = \frac{18\Omega^2}{9\Omega} = 2\Omega.$$

Note that the equivalent resistance is less than either of the original resistances. Now the equivalent resistance R_{34} is in *series* with R_2. We can calculate the equivalent resistance R_{234} simply as the sum of these resistances:

$$R_{234} = R_2 + R_{34} = 8\ \Omega + 2\ \Omega = 10\ \Omega.$$

Finally, resistor R_1 is in *parallel* with the equivalent resistance R_{234}. Therefore, we can obtain the overall equivalent resistance, R_{1234}, again using the product over the sum rule:

$$R_{1234} = \frac{R_1 \cdot R_{234}}{R_1 + R_{234}} = \frac{15\Omega \cdot 10\Omega}{15\Omega + 10\Omega} = \frac{150\Omega^2}{25\Omega} = 6\Omega$$

where 6 Ω is less than either 15 Ω or 10 Ω.

We can now redraw our circuit as a simple one with just one resistor and a battery as (Figure 18).

We should recognize that in this representation, the current, I, is the same everywhere in this single path circuit (according to *Kirchhoff's first law*). From *Kirchhoff's second law* we know that:

$$\Delta V_{a,d \rightarrow R1234} = \Delta V_{a,d \rightarrow E}$$

We know that the change in potential across a battery is just E, and that change in potential through a resistor (left side of equation) is given from *Ohm's law*, so we obtain:

$$I \cdot R_{1234} = E$$

$$I = \frac{E}{R_{1234}} = \frac{3V}{6\Omega} = \textbf{0.5 A}$$

This value represents the total current drawn out of the battery. Now, let's determine how much of that current ends up in each of the different branches of the circuit.

If we return to the full representation of the circuit in Figure 17, we can calculate the current going through R_1 using *Kirchhoff's second law,* which tells us that the change in potential is the same for any path connecting two points. Let's consider points a and d. One path that connects a to d is through the R_1, and another convenient path connecting a to d just includes the battery, E. Therefore, we can write:

$$\Delta V_{a,d \rightarrow R1} = \Delta V_{a,d \rightarrow E}$$

Again, from *Ohm's law*, we know the change in potential through a resistor is the product of the current and the resistance, and the change in potential across the battery is E:

$$I_1 \cdot R_1 = E$$

$$I_1 = \frac{E}{R_1} = \frac{3V}{15\Omega} = \textbf{0.2 A}$$

Now let's consider what happens to the current at point *a* in the circuit (Figure 17). What enters is *I*, but what exits is I_1 and I_2. Thus, according to *Kirchhoff's first law*, we know that:

$$I = I_1 + I_2$$

and therefore:

$$I_2 = I - I_1 = 0.5 \, A - 0.2 \, A = \mathbf{0.3 \, A}$$

Now, let's tackle the current going through R_3 and R_4. It is important to note that, for example, the change in potential from *b* to *c* through R_3 is **not** equal to the change in potential across the battery, *E*. This is because the path from *b* to *c* that includes the battery also includes a change in potential through R_2. A more strategic use of *Kirchhoff's second law* is to consider the total change in potential from *a* to *d* through both R_2 and R_3. That total change in potential is equal to the change in potential from *a* to *d* just through the battery. Therefore, we have

$$\Delta V_{a,d \to R2,R3} = \Delta V_{a,d \to E}$$

From the *Voltage law*, we obtain

$$\Delta V_{a,b \to R2} + \Delta V_{b,c \to R3} + \Delta V_{c,d} = \Delta V_{a,d \to E}$$

Using *Ohm's law* for the expressions on the left side of the equation and setting the right side of the equation to *E*, we get:

$$I_2 \cdot R_2 + I_3 \cdot R_3 + I_5 \cdot 0 = E.$$

This rearranges to

$$I_3 = \frac{E - I_2 \cdot R_2}{R_3} = \frac{3V - 0.3A \cdot 8\Omega}{3\Omega} = \frac{3V - 2.4\,A\Omega}{3\Omega} = \frac{3V - 2.4A \cdot V/A}{3\Omega}$$

$$= \frac{0.6V}{3\Omega} = 0.2 \, A$$

Now, we could calculate the current I_4 using the same strategy we just applied to I_3. However, there is an even easier way: let's use *Kirchhoff's first law*. At point *b*, what enters is I_2, and what exits are I_3 and I_4. Therefore, we have

$$I_2 = I_3 + I_4$$

$$I_4 = I_2 - I_3 = 0.3\ A - 0.2\ A = \textbf{0.1 A}.$$

Likewise, we can use *Kirchhoff's first law* to calculate I_5 at point *c*, where what enters is I_3 and I_4 and what exits is I_5, giving:

$$I_3 + I_4 = I_5;\ I_5 = 0.2\ A + 0.1\ A = \textbf{0.3 A}.$$

And lastly, we can apply *Kirchhoff's first law* again, but now at point *d* to double-check that the current that exits from *d* and then enters the battery is equal to what comes out of the battery, *I*. As such, at point *d*, what enters is I_1 and I_5, and what exits should be *I*:

$$I_1 + I_5 = 0.2\ A + 0.3\ A = 0.5\ A = \textbf{\textit{I}}.$$

It is important to point out that the approach just illustrated to calculate the current in each branch of the example circuit in Figure 17 is just one of several equally valid sets of steps that can be used to solve this

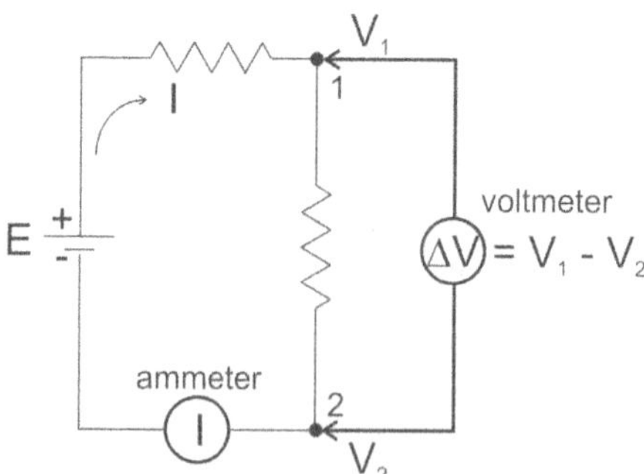

Figure 19.   Voltmeter measuring difference in potential between two locations (1 and 2) in the circuit and ammeter inserted into circuit to measure current at one location.

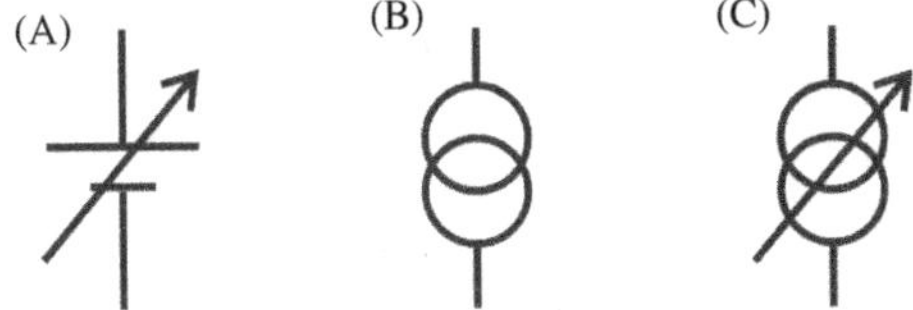

Figure 20.   Symbols for (A) voltage generator, (B) constant current device, (C) current generator.

problem. As long as one appropriately applies Ohm's, Kirchhoff's, and Voltage laws, the specific order of the steps is not crucial.

Measuring Voltage and Current and Other Devices

Specialized devices have been developed to measure the difference in potential across a section of a circuit or the current flowing at a particular site within a circuit. The device for measuring difference in potential is simply called a **voltmeter**. As shown in Figure 19, a voltmeter has two probes that "taste" the potential at two different locations in the circuit. The voltmeter takes the potential sampled on probe 1 (V_1) and subtracts from it the potential sampled on probe 2 (V_2) to obtain the difference in potential (ΔV) across the two locations in the circuit. To measure current, we need a device that is actually inserted into the circuit at a specific location such that it detects the rate at which charges pass through it. This device is called an **ammeter**.

There are a few other devices that are widely used by electrophysiologists to assist them in understanding electrical signaling in excitable cells. One is like a battery, except that it allows the experimenter to set the difference in potential to any desired level. This device is called a **voltage generator** and is drawn as a battery with an arrow (dial) passing through it (Figure 20A). Another important piece of apparatus is the **constant current device**, drawn as two interlocking circles (Figure 20B). Whereas a battery maintains a constant difference in potential, a constant current device (as its name implies) maintains a steady level of current in a circuit regardless of the resistance in the circuit. Like the voltage generator, a **current generator** (drawn as two interlocking circles with an arrow

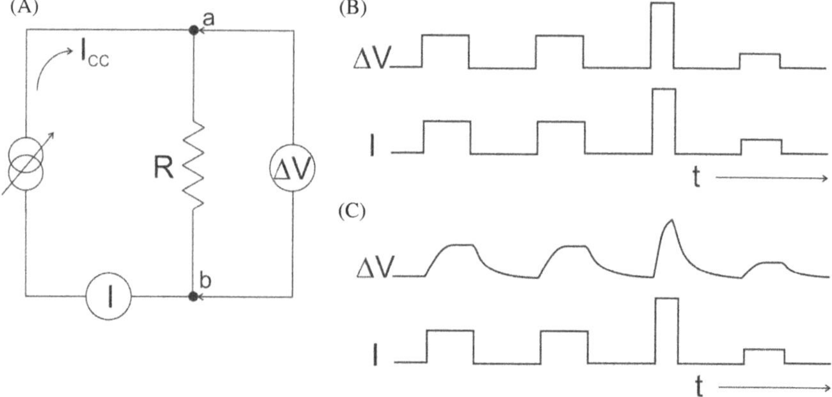

Figure 21.   (A) Circuit in which differences in potential and current are measured in response to changes in constant current (I_{CC}) delivered by a current generator. (B) Changes in potential and current measure in a purely resistive circuit. (C) Changes in potential and resistance measured in a circuit with resistance and capacitance.

passing through it, Figure 20C) enables the experimenter to set any desired level of constant current to be delivered to a circuit.

Capacitors

Resistors, batteries, voltage generators, and current generators are only a few of a number of elements used in electrical circuits. Another important element, particularly with regard to bioelectricity, is a *capacitor*. One important aspect of a circuit that has capacitors is that signals in the circuit vary as a *function of time*. To get an initial feel for this idea, consider a circuit with a resistor that is connected to a current generator rather than a battery (Figure 21A). We've also added a voltmeter so that we can measure the difference in potential between points *a* and *b* and an ammeter to measure the current.

Because there is a current generator in the circuit, the experimenter can vary the magnitude of the constant current (I_{cc}) delivered to the circuit as a function of time. Since we only have one path in this circuit, the ammeter inserted into the circuit detects those changes in current. As shown in the lower trace in Figure 21B, assume the experimenter first switches the current generator to deliver a particular level of current (e.g., 1 A) and then turns it off, then repeats that again, then switches the current to a higher level (e.g., 2 A) for a briefer time, and lastly switches the current to a lower level (e.g., 0.5 A). During this time, the readout of the difference in potential (upper trace, Figure 21B) will always be in direct proportion to the magnitude of the current. This is because Ohm's law tells us that $\Delta V = I \times R$, and since the resistance doesn't change, then ΔV will be directly proportional to I; if I doubles, then ΔV will also double. Also note that there are no time delays—as soon as current changes, the measured ΔV occurs instantaneously.

Now let's add a capacitor into the circuit somewhere between point a and b (we'll get to the details about how capacitors work in a moment). For the same pattern of current delivered to the circuit as in Figure 21B, we now get a different ΔV response when a capacitor is included in the circuit (Figure 21C). The key difference is that the voltage changes as a function of time. Note that when the current is abruptly increased, the voltage increases gradually before leveling out at a steady level. When the current is abruptly switched off, the voltage gradually, rather than instantaneously, returns to zero. It is as though the capacitor tends to "round off" the sharp corners in the voltage response and extend the time that the voltage response hangs around even when the driving current has been shut off. If a circuit with a light bulb possesses a capacitor, when the light switch is first turned "on," the light bulb wouldn't immediately glow brightly. Instead, the intensity of the light would gradually increase over time to a steady level and then stays at that level indefinitely. When the light is switched "off," instead of instantly turning dark, the light bulb would gradually dim until going completely dark.

To get a conceptual understanding of how a capacitor works, let's return to our original description of a battery (Figure 22A). A "pump" is situated between the two bars of the battery, and the entire pathway connecting the top to the bottom bar provides resistance to current flow. Recall that as charge "lands" on the bottom (low potential) bar, it is moved to the upper (high potential) bar through a process requiring energy. In this way, the difference in potential (say 16 V) is held constant, and therefore, the current is maintained constant.

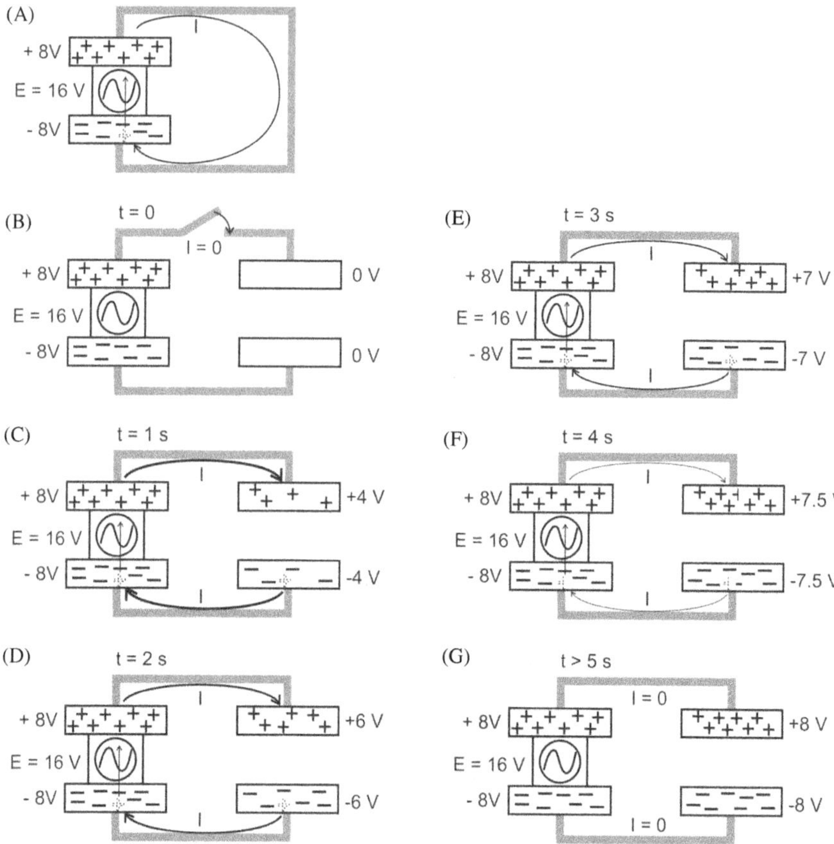

Figure 22.   (A) Cartoon circuit with battery and resistive path. (B) Circuit with battery, resistive path, capacitor, and switch. (C–G) Time course of charge movement, potential changes, and current in a resistor–capacitor circuit.

Now, let's insert another device into the circuit that looks very similar to a battery (Figure 22B). This device too consists of two conductive bars, however, in this case the two bars are not connected to one another. This weird device is a capacitor. Initially, a switch is disengaged in the circuit so that no current can flow. (No current flows because the disconnected end of the conductor at the switch offers near-infinite resistance, and Ohm's law, $I = \Delta V/R$, indicates that as resistance goes to infinity, the current goes to zero.) It is important to note that the top bar of the battery is now connected (or will be when the switch is engaged) to the top bar of the capacitor while the bottom bar of the battery is connected to the bottom bar of the capacitor.

At the moment the switch is engaged (at $t = 0$ s), what is going to happen? As we know, charge will move from a place of high potential to low potential. In this case, charge will move from the top bar of the battery (at +8 V of potential) toward the top bar of the capacitor (at 0 V of potential). Remember also that the rate at which charge moves (i.e., the current) is proportional to the difference in potential between the two ends. In this case, the difference in potential is +8 V − 0 V = +8 V. Likewise, and at the same time, charge will move from the bottom bar of the capacitor (at 0 V of potential) toward the bottom bar of the battery (at −8 V of potential ... remember zero volts is higher than any negative potential). The difference in potential on the bottom side of the circuit is 0 V − (−8 V) = +8 V. Because the difference in potential (+8 V) is the same for the top and bottom halves of the circuit, the current flowing along the top segment of the circuit will be identical to that flowing along the bottom. Perhaps surprisingly, this state of affairs is exactly what Kirchhoff's first law predicts (current in = current out): the current flowing into the top of the capacitor is exactly what flows out from the capacitor on the bottom. However, no charges actually directly pass from one bar to the other in the capacitor.

After one time step (say 1 s), let's "freeze" the circuit and examine what has taken place (Figure 22C). During the initial time period, the top bar of the capacitor has gained 4 units of positive charge from the top bar of the battery, whereas the bottom bar of the capacitor has given away 4 units of positive charge to the bottom bar of the battery, leaving behind 4 units of exposed negative charge. All those excess positive charges that were delivered to the bottom bar of the battery were pushed up onto the top bar of the battery, maintaining the difference in potential of 16 V across the battery. However, the difference in potential between the top bar of the battery and the top bar of the capacitor has changed; it is now reduced to +8 V − (+4 V) = +4 V. Similarly, the difference in potential across the bottom part of the circuit has also been reduced by the same amount to −4 V − (−8 V) = +4 V. Because the difference in potential has decreased, this means that the rate at which charge moves (current) will now also decrease.

Therefore, in the next time step (t = 2 s, Figure 22D), only two additional units of charge will move from the top bar of the battery to the top bar of the capacitor and from the bottom bar of the capacitor to the bottom bar of the battery. This means that the difference in potential across the top half of the circuit is now +8 V − (+6 V) = +2 V, and across the bottom half is −6 V − (−8 V) = + 2 V. As such, the current will again slow down. Therefore, in the next time step (t = 3 s, Figure 22E), only 1 unit of charge will move across the top and bottom parts of the circuit, leaving a potential difference across both parts of +1 V. The current again reduces even further, so that at the next time point (t = 4 s, Figure 22F), perhaps only a half unit of charge will move across the top and bottom parts of the circuit. In this situation, the difference in potential across the top and bottom halves of the circuit will become quite small (0.5 V), meaning that the current flowing slows down to just a trickle. At some time point, let's say somewhat greater than 5 s (Figure 22G), just enough charge will move across the top part and bottom parts of the circuit such that the difference in potential across those two parts of the circuit is zero. If there is no difference in potential, then no charge will move, and all current in the circuit will halt.

Time-Dependent Changes in Current and Potential in a Capacitive Circuit

To approach a more quantitative understanding of time-dependent movement of charge, current, and potential in a capacitive circuit, let's first plot the cumulative amount of charge moved in the circuit shown in Figure 22. As shown in Figure 23A, over the first-time step (1 s), a total of 4 units of charge (coulombs) was moved. Then, in the next time step, an additional 2 coulombs were moved for a cumulative total of 6. Then 1 additional coulomb was moved for a cumulative total of 7 coulombs, then a half coulomb was moved for a total of 7.5 coulombs, and finally, after more than 5 s, an additional half coulomb was moved to reach the final total of 8 coulombs of charge moved from one site in the circuit to another.

From these movements in charge, we can calculate the average current over each time step from the basic equation for current, $I = \Delta q/\Delta t$.

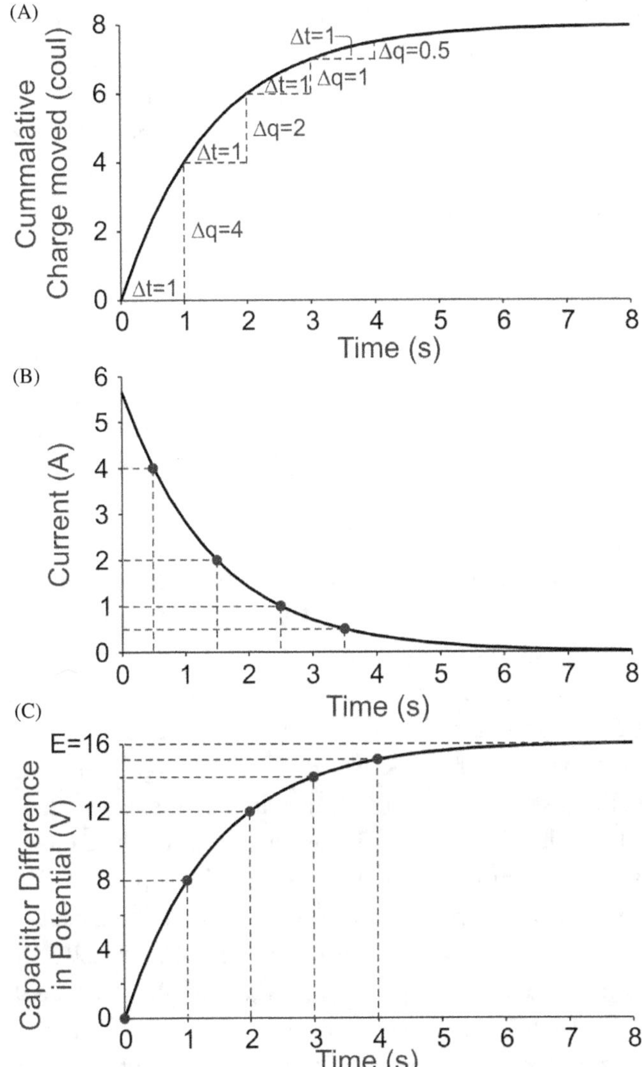

Figure 23.   (A) charge movement, (B) current, and (C) change in potential for the circuit shown in Figure 22.

Therefore, the average current over the first-time step is $I = 4$ $C/1$ $s = 4$ A. You should note that this is equivalent to taking the average slope of the charge movement curve over each time increment. When calculating the slope in this way, the value calculated is represented as occurring at a time halfway through the time interval. Therefore, in this case, we would indicate a current of 4 A at a time of 0.5 s, as shown in Figure 23B. Likewise, for the next 1-s interval, the amount of charge moved was 2 C, and therefore, the current is 2 A at a time of 1.5 s. Similarly, the current then drops to 1 A at 2.5 s, and then to 0.5 A at 3.5 s. Eventually (some time beyond 5 s), the current halts altogether.

During this process, let's say that we used a voltmeter to measure the difference in potential across the two bars of the capacitor. One probe (V_1) is placed on the top bar of the capacitor in Figure 22, and the second probe (V_2) is placed on the bottom bar of the capacitor. As such, the difference in potential will be measured as: $\Delta V = V_1 - V_2$. At time $t = 0$ s (Figure 22B), there is zero net charge on both the top and bottom bars of the capacitor, and therefore the difference in potential is zero (Figure 23C). At $t = 1$ s, the potential on the top bar is +4 V, and the potential on the bottom bar is −4 V (Figure 22C) for a ΔV of +8 V (Figure 23C). At 2 s, the top bar is at +6 V and the bottom bar at −6 V (Figure 22D) for a ΔV of 12 V (Figure 23C). Likewise, at 3 s, $\Delta V = 14$ V, at 4 s $\Delta V = 15.5$ V, and eventually (> 5 s), the difference in potential is at 16 V (Figure 23C).

When examining the plots of charge movement, current, and difference in potential (in Figure 23), one sees that after about 5 s, there are no further time-dependent changes. No additional charge is moved, the current in the circuit stops, and the difference in potential across the capacitor reaches a steady level. Interestingly, in this state, the difference in potential across the capacitor is exactly equal to the difference in potential across the battery, E. We refer to this state of affairs as the capacitor being "fully charged." When looking at this situation in Figure 22G, the capacitor looks almost like a battery—it has two bars or plates with a difference in potential across the plates. Indeed (as we shall see), if a charged capacitor is connected to another circuit or part of a circuit, it can act like a temporary battery, driving charge from its high potential bar toward its low potential bar (just as a battery does). The only difference is that there is no pump in the capacitor to keep the potential difference constant. As such, the difference in potential across the capacitor progressively runs down and eventually stops driving current in the circuit.

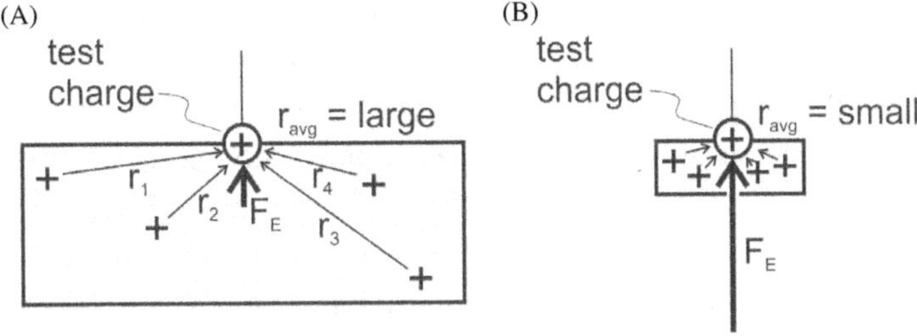

Figure 24.   Influence of capacitor size on electrical force (F_E) and potential possessing the same amount of charge. (A) distances (r) between capacitor charges and test charge on large capacitor and (B) small capacitor.

Time to Charge Capacitor

Before we consider the actions of capacitors in a circuit, let's first consider how long it takes for a capacitor to get charged in the first place. To do this, we need to return to our original definition for electrical potential, namely,

$$Pot = \frac{k \cdot q}{r}$$

If you recall, this equation indicates the capacity (i.e., the potential) of an object with charge to push or pull on other objects. We emphasized that potential is directly proportional to the charge on the object. But now we need to confront the other variable in this equation, r, representing the distance between charges on our object and that of a test object.

To do this, let's consider two conductive bars, each with four units of charge on them, but one bar is large (Figure 24A) and the other is small (Figure 24B). When we try to push a test charge onto each bar by sliding it along a wire fixed to the top of the bars, the charges on the bars tend to repel this addition. However, in the case of the large bar (Figure 24A), the charges are distributed across the bar such that the average distance, r_{avg}, of the charges to the site where the test charge is being added is relatively large. Because of this, the push back (i.e., the electric force, F_E) of the bar onto the test charge is relatively weak (remembering that F_E is *inversely* related to r^2). It is as though we have diluted the pushiness of the bar by distributing its charges over a large surface area. Conversely, the charges on the small bar are more physically concentrated (Figure 24B). Their small average distance to where the test charge is being added to the bar will greatly increase the overall force that repels the addition of the test charge.

As such, the large bar in Figure 24 will have a low electrical potential, whereas the small bar will have a high potential even though they both have the same amount of charge. This is in accordance with the equation for potential (*Pot = k·q/r*) with *r* being large for the large bar and small for the small bar. This issue is important in order to understand the time required to charge a capacitor. Recall from our example circuit (Figure 22) that the current comes to a halt when the potential on a bar of the capacitor is equal to that on the bar of the battery to which it is connected (see Figure 22G). If the capacitor bar were large (like in Figure 24A), then much more charge would need to be deposited on it in order to build up a potential equal to that of the battery. The process of delivering the additional charge onto the capacitor bar takes more time. Conversely, if the capacitor bar were small (like in Figure 24B), then relatively little charge would need to be delivered in order for its potential to equal that of the battery, and as such, it occurs quickly. Therefore, the *time to charge* (i.e., the time needed for the capacitor to build up sufficient charge to exert a potential equal to the battery to which it is connected) *is directly related to the physical size of the capacitor.*

This idea is similar to that of filling up a container with water. The height of the water in the container determines the pressure (i.e., the potential) exerted at the bottom of the container. For example, the time to fill an Olympic-sized swimming pool to a depth of 2 meters with a water pump will take markedly longer than to fill a small backyard pool to the same depth. Yet the pressure felt by someone at the bottom of either pool will be the same.

Capacitance

We refer to this notion of capacitor size as **capacitance**. In the case of the swimming pools, the Olympic-sized pool has a much bigger *capacity* to hold or store water than the small backyard pool even though the water depth (pressure or potential) is the same for both. Likewise, a physically larger electrical capacitor has a larger capacitance. The volume of water (the stuff) stored in a container (e.g., swimming pool) is equal to its height multiplied times its cross-sectional area (i.e., its size):

$$Volume = Height \times area$$

The height of water in the container is directly related to the pressure exerted at the bottom of the container. Likewise, for a capacitor, the amount of charge (the stuff) stored on a capacitor bar is equivalent to the potential set up on the bar (like the height or pressure) multiplied times a measure related to the surface area of the bar, namely, its capacitance:

$$Charge = potential \times capacitance$$

If we rearrange this equation, we get:

$$Potential = \frac{Charge}{Capacitance}$$

indicating that the potential on a capacitor bar is inversely related to capacitor size (capacitance), just as we illustrated in Figure 24. If we further rearrange the equation to solve for capacitance, we can get the units for capacitance as:

$$Capacitance = \frac{Charge}{Potential} = \frac{Coulombs}{V} = Farad$$

As a simple example, let's calculate the amount of charge stored on a capacitor bar when connected to a 10 V bar of a battery and the capacitor is fully charged. Let's do this for two capacitors, one with 1 farad of capacitance and one with 2 farads of capacitance. As such, we have for the first capacitor:

$$Charge = Potential \times capacitance = 10\,V \times 1\,farad = 10\,V \times 1\frac{Coulomb}{V}$$

$$= 10\;\boldsymbol{coulombs}$$

For the other second capacitor, we have:

$$Charge = Potential \times capacitance = 10\,V \times 2\,farad = 10\,V \times 2\frac{Coulomb}{V}$$

$$= 20\;\boldsymbol{coulombs.}$$

Therefore, the amount of charge that is stored on the second capacitor for the same potential exerted by the capacitors is twice as large as the first capacitor because of its larger capacitance (size).

Distance between Capacitor Plates Affects Capacitance

Not to confuse the matter even further (!) but there is another factor that also affects the capacitance—so we should address it here. This has to do

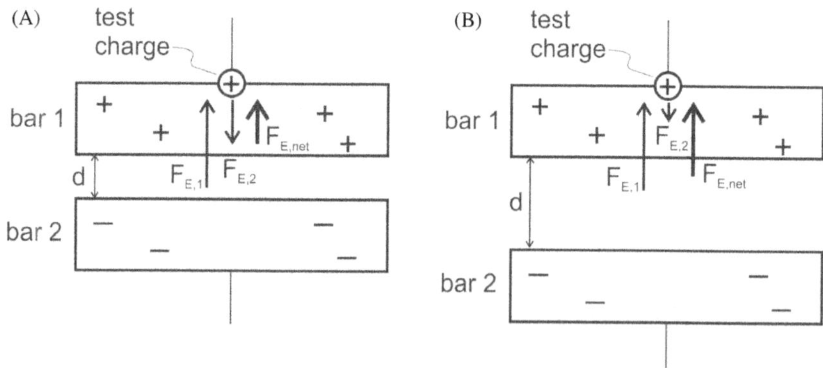

Figure 25.   Effect of distance (d) between capacitor bars and net electric force ($F_{E,net}$) for two bars close to another (A) and two bars far apart (B).

with how physically close together the two plates or bars of the capacitor are to one another. For simplicity, we began our discussion of capacitance by only considering what takes place on one of the bars of the capacitor ... it was as though the other bar was far away and therefore had little effect on the bar under consideration. In reality, however, the two bars or plates of capacitors are usually quite close to one another. As such, the charge built up on one bar will affect (push or pull on) charges being deposited on the other bar. The *net* push or pull (i.e., the potential) of a capacitor, therefore, will depend on the charges built up on both bars and the distance their charges are from the site where charges are delivered to the capacitor. To understand this, let's consider two capacitors, one in which the distance (d) between the two bars is relatively small (Figure 25A) and another where d is relatively large (Figure 25B). In both cases, the amount of charge on the capacitors is the same.

Note that in Figure 25A, the negative charges on bar 2 will tend to pull (rather than repel) on the test charge delivered to bar 1. However, because the average distance from the negative charges on bar 2 to the test charge is larger than that of the positive charges on bar 1 to the test charge, the magnitude of the electrical force set up by bar 2 ($F_{E,2}$) will be smaller than that of bar 1 ($F_{E,1}$). The net force ($F_{E,net}$), therefore, will be to moderately repel the addition of the test charge; the associated electrical potential of the capacitor system in this case will also be moderate. Now if we move the bars farther apart (Figure 25B), then the average distance of the negative charges on bar 2 to the test charge will be large. This large distance will weaken the electrical force of bar 2 onto the test charge ($F_{E,2}$). Therefore, the net force ($F_{E,net}$) in this case will remain relatively large to repel the addition of the test charge. The overall electrical potential (i.e., the ability of an apparatus to push or pull on other objects) of the capacitor in Figure 25B, therefore, will be relatively strong.

One should note (even though it is not shown on Figure 25) that there is an equal magnitude but oppositely directed effect on bar 2. Regardless, *the closer together* the two bars are to one another, the *weaker the net force*. It is as though the negative charges on bar 2 "cancel out" some of the effects of the positive charges on bar 1, and the closer bar 2 is to bar 1, the greater the effect of the "canceling out." As a consequence, to build up a certain level of potential in a capacitor in order to equal that of a

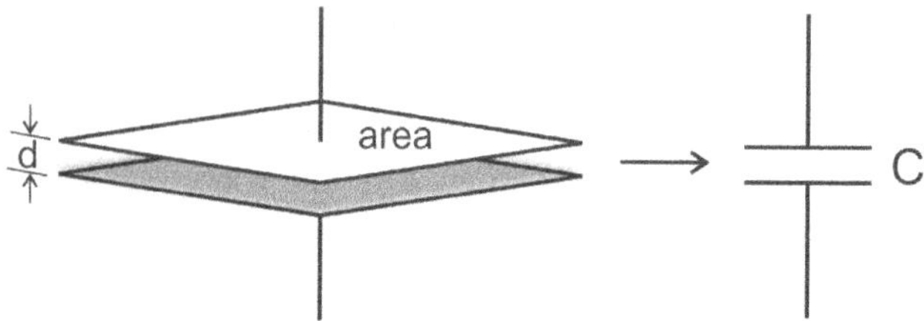

Figure 26.   An actual capacitor consists of two conductive plates separated by an insulator of thickness d. The symbol for a capacitor (C) is two parallel lines with a gap between them.

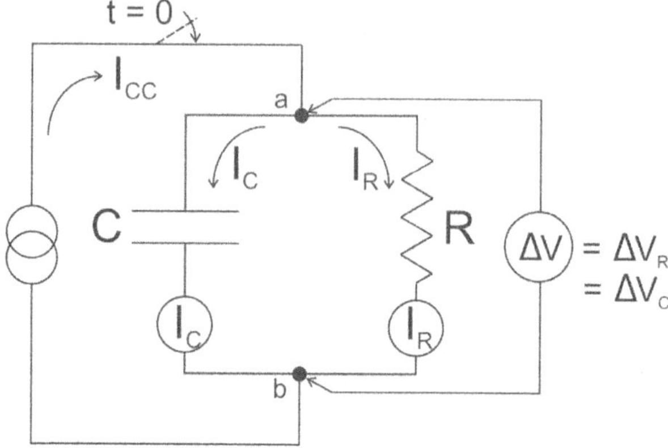

Figure 27.   RC circuit with the resistor and capacitor in parallel. Current is driven by a constant current device. At time $t = 0$, the switch is engaged. Some of the current is directed to the capacitor (I_C) and some through the resistor (I_R). The change in potential across the capacitor is identical to that across the resistor.

battery attached to it (i.e., to fully charge the capacitor), much more charge needs to be delivered and stored on the capacitor when the capacitor bars are close to one another. Collectively, therefore, the capacitance of a capacitor (i.e., ability to store charge) is proportional to the surface area of the capacitor and inversely proportional to the distance (d) between the capacitor bars:

$$\textit{Capacitance} \propto \textit{area}/d$$

Resistor–Capacitor (RC) Circuits

As for other circuit elements, we need a simple symbol to represent a capacitor. Typically, a real capacitor consists of two thin conductive plates separated by an insulator with small wires extending from the plates to connect to other parts of a circuit (Figure 26). The *capacitance* of a capacitor, that is, its ability to store up charge, depends on the surface area of the plates and the distance (d) between the plates. The symbol for a capacitor (C) is two parallel lines with a gap between them and with connecting wires emerging from each line.

Let's consider a diagrammatic circuit that includes both resistors and capacitors (Figure 27). In this case, the resistor and capacitor are arranged in parallel and are connected to a constant current device. When the switch is engaged at time t = 0, a steady level of current, I_{CC}, will be delivered to the circuit. At point a, the current divides into two parts, one going toward the capacitor (I_C) and one going to the resistor (I_R). As Kirchhoff's first law tells us, the sum of I_C and I_R must always equal the constant value of I_{CC}. As a consequence, if current diminishes in one of the branches, then current must increase by the same amount in the other branch so that their sum is always a constant value. Ammeters are placed in each branch to measure the currents in these two pathways.

At time $t = 0$ (Figure 27), a steady level of current, I_{CC}, is delivered to point a. Some of that current will go to the capacitor and some will go to the resistor—but how much to each path and how will that change over time? One way to consider this is to think of a big queue of ice skaters backed up at position a who are eagerly awaiting the chance to skate. The top plate of the capacitor represents a smooth ice-skating pond that presently has no skaters on it. The resistor represents a gravely path. Now, at the time the switch is engaged and the skaters are allowed to start moving, the skaters at the front of the line naturally all head toward the capacitor (the ice-skating pond). Indeed, the first skater in line is able to slide out onto the pond with absolutely no interference or resistance; she has the pond to herself for a moment. Now as other skaters go out onto the pond, skaters must be more cautious so as to not run into other skaters, and therefore movement on the pond becomes more restricted. Some people in the line may decide to forgo this increasingly crowded pond and instead take the gravely path (through the resistor) in search of other less crowded skating opportunities. Eventually, the ice-skating pond will become so crowded that there is barely any room to maneuver, and it is not possible to add further skaters. When that happens, everyone in line will now be forced to take the gravely path.

The same principles apply to our electrical circuit (Figure 27). At time $t = 0$, there is no charge on the top plate of the capacitor and therefore no charge to push back onto charges we might want to add to the plate. Furthermore, the capacitor plate has a large surface area. Therefore, moving charge onto the plate at this moment is like sliding charge along a very low-resistance wire or connector. Furthermore, from our rule of thumb that *current tends to follow the path of least resistance*, when there is *no* effective resistance along one path, then *all* of the current will take that path. Therefore, in the very first moment, all the current that enters point a will be directed toward the capacitor (at $t = 0$, $I_C = I_{CC}$), and none will go toward the resistor (at $t = 0$, $I_R = 0$). After a moment, positive charge will start to build up on the top capacitor plate. This charge will start to oppose the addition of other charges, that is, it starts to resist the deposition of charges onto the capacitor. Therefore, some of the charge will start to pass through the resistor. Eventually, with more charge added to the capacitor, the push back provided by those charges on the capacitor will equal the push forward provided by the constant current device. When that happens, no further charge is deposited on the capacitor, and the current toward the capacitor drops to zero. We refer to this situation as the capacitor being fully charged. When this happens, then all of the current entering point a is directed toward the resistor.

The time required to reach this fully charged state is partially dependent on the capacitance (size) of the capacitor. By analogy, if one has a very large ice-skating pond, then many more skaters will need to go out on the ice before it becomes so crowded that no new skaters can be added compared to a tiny pond. The same holds for a capacitor (as we discussed previously related to Figure 24). The larger the surface area, the lower the pushback (potential) that the capacitor plate exerts on charge attempting to enter the plate. As such, more charge needs to be added (requiring more time) to reach a certain level of potential for a large capacitor compared to a small capacitor.

The time courses of current to the capacitor (I_C) and to the resistor (I_R) are shown graphically in Figures 28A and B, respectively. Initially (at

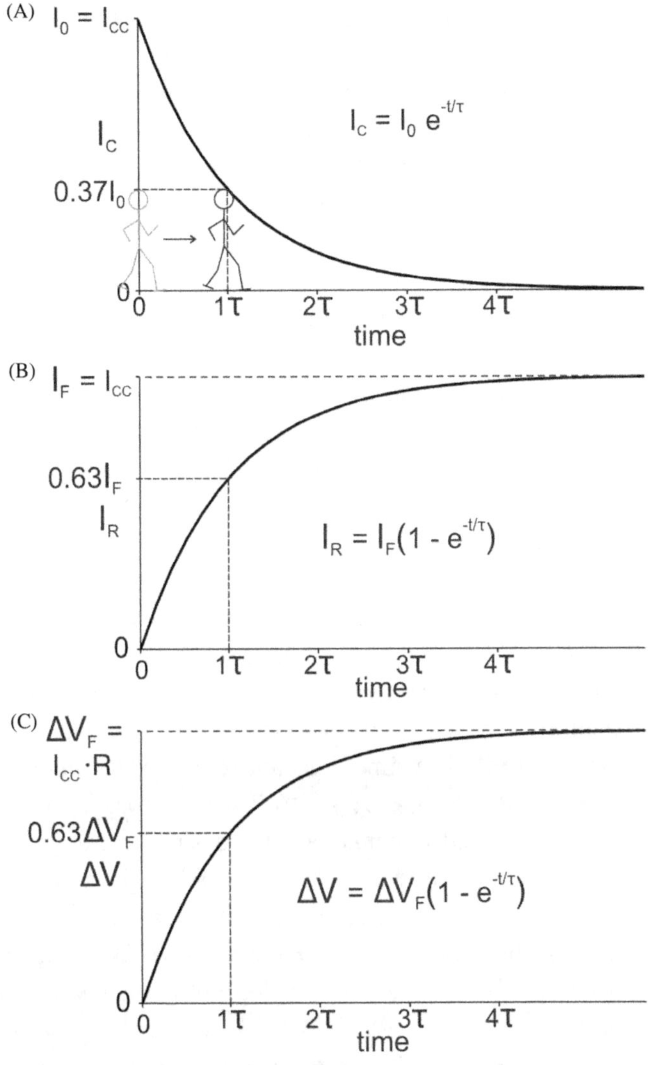

Figure 28.   Time courses of change in current through the capacitor (A), through the resistor (B), and change in potential across both the capacitor and resistor (C) for the parallel RC circuit shown in Figure 27.

time = 0), all the current pushed out by the constant current device (I_{CC}) goes to the capacitor (Figure 28A, $I_0 = I_{CC}$) and none goes to the resistor (Figure 28B, $I_0 = 0$). As mentioned above, as time progresses, charges build up on the plates of the capacitor, slowing down and eventually stopping current directed to the capacitor (Figure 28A). On the other hand, current directed to the resistor progressively increases (Figure 28B). Eventually, the final level of current (I_F) going to the resistor will be equal to the total current delivered by the constant current device (i.e., $I_F = I_{CC}$). This state of affairs will persist indefinitely unless the switch in the circuit (Figure 27) is disengaged. One should note that the current going to the capacitor (I_C, Figure 28A) and that to the resistor (I_R, Figure 28B) are exact mirror images of one another. As such, at any time, the sum of I_C and I_R will always be a constant value, namely, I_{CC}.

The types of curves shown in Figure 28 are ubiquitous in nature, and there are standardized equations to represent them. Let's first take a look at the equation for the curve depicting the fall in current directed to the capacitor over time, $I(t)$, as shown in Figure 28A:

$$I(t) = I_0 \cdot e^{-t/\tau}$$

This type of equation is referred to as a **falling exponential**. I_0 is the initial value of the current and, in this case, is the total current delivered by the constant current device (I_{CC}). e is Euler's constant (2.72) and is the base of the natural logarithms, t is the variable for time, and τ is referred to as the **time constant**. The time constant refers to the *amount of time required for the signal to change by ~63%*. The time constant is a standard way to indicate how rapidly signals are increasing or decaying. In this case, because we are dealing with a decaying signal, it is the amount of time for the signal to fall to a value that is 37% of the initial value, or to $0.37 I_0$ (we'll get to the reason why the number is 37% momentarily). A simple way to think about this is to consider a little man whose height is 37% of the initial value (Figure 28A). When he walks along the x-axis and bumps his head on the curve, his feet are at a position equivalent to one time constant, 1τ.

Let's put some time values into this falling exponential equation and see what we get. To use some actual numbers, let's say from the graph in Figure 28A we determine that 37-percentile man bumps his head into the curve at time $t = 5$ s. As such, $t = 5$ s. Therefore, at time $\tau = 0$ we get:

$$I(t=0)=I_0 \cdot e^{-\frac{0s}{5s}}=I_0 \cdot e^0=I_0 \cdot 1=I_0$$

Now, let's calculate the value of the current at a time equal to one time constant, that is, at $t = 1\tau = 5$ s:

$$I(t)=I_0 \cdot e^{-t/\tau}$$

$$I(t=1\tau=5s)=I_0 \cdot e^{-\frac{5s}{5s}}=I_0 \cdot e^{-\frac{1\tau}{\tau}}=I_0 \cdot e^{-1}=I_0 \cdot \frac{1}{e}=I_0 \cdot \frac{1}{2.72}=\mathbf{0.37 \cdot I_0}$$

As you can see, the 0.37 associated with one time constant derives from the value that is the inverse of e (2.72). Now, let's repeat this calculation but for a time = two time constants, namely, $t = 2\tau = 10$ s:

$$I(t=2\tau=10s)=I_0 \cdot e^{-\frac{10s}{5s}}=I_0 \cdot e^{-\frac{2\tau}{\tau}}=I_0 \cdot e^{-2}=I_0 \cdot \frac{1}{e^2}=I_0 \cdot \frac{1}{7.39}=\mathbf{0.135 \cdot I_0}$$

If we repeated this calculation for times $t = 3\tau = 15$ s and $t = 4\tau = 20$ s, we would get values of $\mathbf{0.05 \cdot I_0}$ and $\mathbf{0.02 \cdot I_0}$, respectively. Therefore, after about four time constants, the current has practically come to a halt, and the capacitor is fully charged.

While we could empirically measure the time constant, it would be nice to be able to calculate it from first principles. As we argued in relation to Figure 24, the *time to fully charge a capacitor is directly related to its capacitance*. We also know that the larger the resistance in a circuit, the slower charges move. Therefore, the *time to charge* will also be *directly proportional to the resistance in the circuit*. As such, it turns out that the time constant is precisely equal to the product of the resistance (R) and the capacitance (C):

$$\tau = R \cdot C$$

But how could the product of resistance with units of ohms and capacitance with units of farads yield a time value? Let's plug in the units and see what we get:

$$\tau = R \cdot C = \Omega \cdot Farads = \frac{V}{A} \cdot \frac{Coulombs}{V} = \frac{Coulombs}{\frac{Coulombs}{s}} = s$$

Therefore, in the circuit shown in Figure 27, if the resistor was 500 Ω and the capacitor had a capacitance of 1 microfarad (1×10^{-3} farads), then the time constant would be 0.5 s and it would take about 2 s (i.e., four time constants) for the capacitor to fully charge.

As mentioned above, the current to the resistor (Figure 28B) is a mirror image of the current to the capacitor. This type of function is referred to as a **rising exponential** and has the form:

$$I(t) = I_F \cdot \left(1 - e^{-t/\tau}\right)$$

where I_F represents the final value of current directed to the resistor if given sufficient time. In this case, it is I_{cc}. If one plugs in different values of time t into this equation, say 0, 1τ, 2τ, 3τ, and 4τ (where τ is calculated as the product of the resistance and capacitance), the calculated values of I_R would be 0, $0.63I_{cc}$, $0.86I_{cc}$, $0.95I_{cc}$, and $0.98I_{cc}$. As such, after four time constants, the current directed to the resistor is practically equivalent to the total current exiting the constant current device.

It is important to note that just because we now have capacitors involved, Kirchhoff's laws do not go out the window. According to Kirchhoff's second law, the difference in potential across the two plates of the capacitor (one path connecting point *a* to *b*, see Figure 27) must always be equal to the change in potential across the resistor (another path connecting point *a* to *b*). Therefore, in Figure 28C, only one voltage-time graph is shown, as it is identical for both ΔV_C and ΔV_R. There are two ways to conceptualize how the change in potential varies as a function of time. First, we know from Ohm's law that $\Delta V_R = I_R \times R$. Therefore, the ΔV time graph must look exactly like the I_R time graph (Figure 28B). It starts low and eventually reaches a level equivalent to $I_{cc} \times R$. The other way to think about the change in potential as a function of time is to consider what happens to the capacitor. At time zero, there

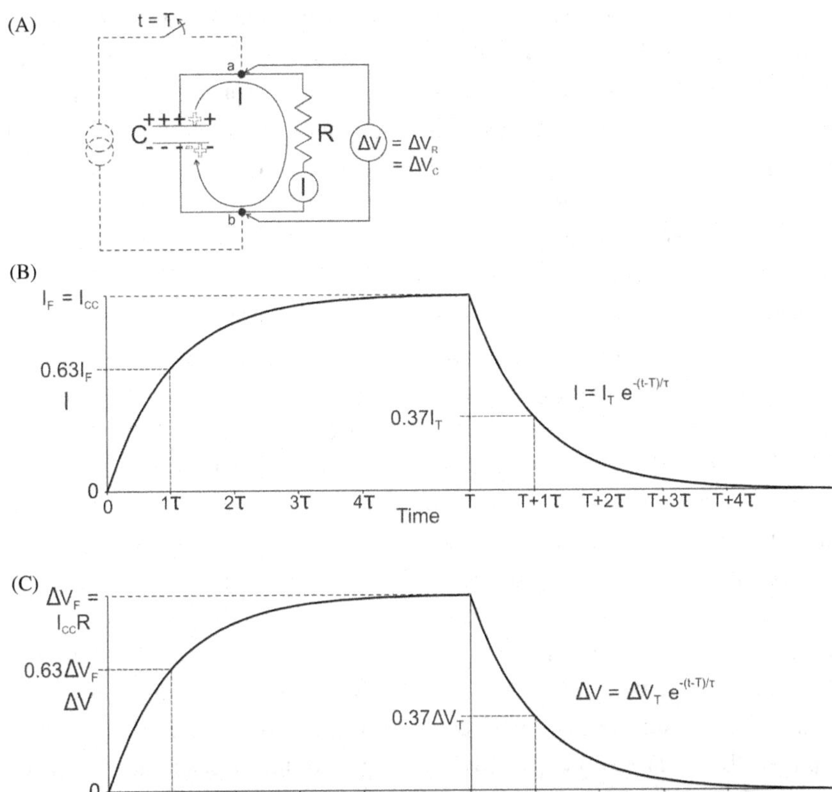

Figure 29.   After the capacitor is fully charged in the RC circuit, the switch is disengaged at time $t = T$. Following that time, just the inner loop containing the capacitor and resistor is operational (solid lines). (B) and (C) show time courses of change in current (I) and potential (DV) following disengagement of the switch at time T. The plots to the left of time T are identical to those shown in Figures 28B and C during the time the circuit was charging.

is no charge on either plate of the capacitor, and therefore, the difference in potential at this time is zero. As positive charges are deposited on the top plate and removed from the bottom plate, the difference in potential will grow. Eventually, the potential on the capacitor reaches a value equal to $I_{CC} \times R$.

Once the capacitor is fully charged and we keep the switch engaged, all the current is directed through the resistor. As such, all the action takes place through the resistor. Consequently, the capacitor does nothing from this point forward until the switch is disengaged. Indeed, the behavior of the circuit during this time when the capacitor is fully charged is no different from a circuit that has no capacitor but only a resistor. However, when the switch is disengaged (say at time $t = T$), then the charge stored on the capacitor comes back into play (Figure 29A). Note that the part of the circuit that contains the opened pathway, including the constant current device, essentially drops out of operation. The top plate of the capacitor (having high potential) is now connected to the bottom plate (with negative potential) through a pathway that has resistance (Figure 29A). Therefore, charge will move (current) from the top to the bottom plate. Also, there is now only one path, not two separate branches, so only one ammeter is needed to measure current. At the moment the switch is opened (at time t = T, Figure 29B), the current starts at a high level because the difference in potential across the capacitor is large. As the charges move from the top to the bottom plate, lost charges are not replenished as they are in a battery. The arrival of positive charges on the bottom plate joins with negative charges and cancels out one another (Figure 29A). Therefore, the potential difference across the capacitor progressively decreases, and the current follows suit. Eventually, all the excess charge from the top plate of the capacitor is delivered to the bottom plate and, at that point, there is zero potential difference across the capacitor and current stops. The capacitor has been discharged. The time courses of these changes are falling exponentials with a time constant $\tau = R \times C$ (Figure 29B, C). Note again that the change in potential across the resistor (ΔV, Figure 29C), from Ohm's law, must be proportional to the current flowing through the resistor. Thus, the change in potential over time has the identical shape as the current-time plot in Figure 29B. Interestingly, the circuit shown in Figure 27 (and its properties described in Figures 28 and 29) is often used to model the electrical properties of neurons and other excitable cells (see Chapter 5).

Appendix B

Nernst Equation

The Nernst equation is used to calculate the membrane potential at which the *electrical* force acting on a particular ion perfectly counteracts the *chemical* driving force. The *electrical force* between two objects is proportional to the magnitude of the charges possessed by the two objects. In the case of a cell, the relevant objects are the cell membrane and an ion. The charge on the membrane is directly proportional to its membrane potential. The charge on the ion is given by its valence, Z ($+1, -1, +2$). The *chemical force* acting on an ion X is related to the difference in concentrations of the ion outside $[X]_o$ and inside $[X]_i$ the cell.

In brief, the Nernst equation determines the membrane potential, E_X (and the associated electrical force acting on ion X of valence Z) that counteracts the chemical force. As such, it is given by:

$$E_X = \frac{R \cdot T}{Z \cdot F} \cdot \ln\left(\frac{[X]_o}{[X]_i}\right)$$

where R and F are constants, T is the temperature in degrees Kelvin, and *ln* is the natural logarithm. R is the gas constant and has a value of 8.3 (J K^{-1}mol^{-1}) and represents the energy (J = joules) per temperature increment (K = degrees Kelvin) per amount of substance (mol = moles). F is Faraday's constant (96,485 C/mol), representing the amount of charge (in coulombs, C) per unit amount (mol) of substance.

The natural logarithm indicates the power (i.e., exponent) that Euler's constant, e (2.718) must be raised to obtain the particular number that follows *ln*. For example, if $e^3 = 2.718^3 = 20.1$, then *ln* (20.1) = 3. Because it is somewhat easier to think in terms of log_{10} (i.e., the power 10 must be raised to obtain a particular number), let's convert *ln* to log_{10} (or simply *log*). This can be done empirically as follows. Take the natural log of some number, say 10,000: *ln* 10,000 = 9.21 (need to raise e to the 9.21 power to get 10,000). Now take the logarithm of the same number: *log* 10,000 = 4 (i.e., need to raise 10 to the power 4 to get 10,000). Therefore, the *ln* of some number X is the same as the *log* of that number multiplied by (9.21/4) = 2.3. In other words, *ln* X = 2.3 *log* X.

Therefore, we can rewrite the Nernst equation as

$$E_X = 2.3 \frac{R \cdot T}{Z \cdot F} \cdot log \left(\frac{[X]_o}{[X]_i} \right).$$

Let's now convert the typical lab temperature of 25°C (at which many experiments are performed) to degrees Kelvin (K) using K = 273 + degrees C = 273 + 25 = 298 K. When we substitute that temperature along with the constant values, we obtain:

$$E_X = \frac{2.3}{Z} \cdot \frac{8.3 \left(\frac{J}{K \cdot mol} \right) \cdot 298 \ K}{96,485 \ C/mol} \cdot log \left(\frac{[X]_o}{[X]_i} \right).$$

Keeping in mind that $1 \ J = 1 \ \text{N·m}$ (newton-meter), we obtain

$$E_X = \frac{2.3}{Z} \cdot \frac{8.3 \left(\frac{N \cdot m}{K \cdot mol} \right) \cdot 298 \ K}{96,485 \ C/mol} \cdot log \left(\frac{[X]_o}{[X]_i} \right).$$

The units K and *mol* cancel out of the equation as shown below:

$$E_X = \frac{2.3}{Z} \cdot \frac{8.315 \left(\frac{N \cdot m}{\cancel{K} \cdot \cancel{mol}} \right) \cdot 298.16 \ \cancel{K}}{96,485 \ C/\cancel{mol}} \cdot log \left(\frac{[X]_o}{[X]_i} \right).$$

to leave:

$$E_X = \frac{2.3}{Z} \cdot 0.025 \frac{N \cdot m}{C} \cdot \log\left(\frac{[X]_o}{[X]_i}\right).$$

From Appendix A, we know that 1 N·m/C = 1 volt. Therefore, we end up with

$$E_X = \frac{0.0575\,V}{Z} \cdot \log\left(\frac{[X]_o}{[X]_i}\right)$$

$$E_X = \frac{57.5\,mV}{Z} \cdot \log\left(\frac{[X]_o}{[X]_i}\right).$$

As a quick way to estimate the equilibrium potential, one can use the following table for different concentration ratios outside and inside a cell and for a valence of $Z = +1$. For other valances, divide the values in the right column by Z.

$[X]_{out}/[X]_{in}$	log	E_X (for $Z = +1$)
100	2	115 mV
10	1	57.5 mV
1	0	0 mV
0.1	−1	−57.5 mV
0.01	−2	−115 mV

Appendix C

Challenges in Interpreting Brain Lesions, Inactivation, and Damage

Despite its widespread use, there are a number of interrelated challenges associated with the interpretation of behavioral changes caused by lesions or inactivation in experimental animals or caused by brain damage in humans. One has to do with recovery of function following lesions. The brain has a fecund capacity to recover with sufficient time after damage. In clinical terms, this is clearly revealed in extensive recovery following a stroke. Stroke most often comes about due to occlusion of blood flow (an ischemic stroke) to a part of the brain, leading to permanent, and in many cases, extensive tissue **necrosis** (*cell death*). Nevertheless, about 75% of individuals who survive a stroke, and initially present with some form of paralysis, exhibit only mild or no motor symptoms six months following the stroke (Bonita & Beaglehole 1988).

This recovery may be due to neighboring, nondamaged areas being "repurposed" via neuroplasticity to carry out operations previously performed by the damaged region (see Chapter 13). Indeed, some evidence of such repurposing following stroke was demonstrated in monkeys (Nudo *et al.* 1996). The experimenters induced ischemic strokes that led to necrosis of a region of the motor cortex that when stimulated before the stroke caused movements of the fingers. Following about a month of recovery that included rehabilitation exercises of the hand, the experimenters retested the responses to stimulation in the area surrounding the lesion. These neighboring areas, which prior to the stroke responded to stimulation with movements of the shoulder and elbow, now evoked movements of the fingers.

Given the challenges associated with the characterization of the function of a brain area following accident or stroke-related damage because of recovery, it would therefore seem advantageous to carry out experiments in animals involving lesions or inactivation, and then evaluate behavior as soon as practical thereafter to minimize the chance of recovery. Indeed, there is a long history of such work. In some cases, however, the outcomes of this approach seem bewildering and difficult to reconcile with accepted views of the function of various brain areas.

An illustrative example is the remarkable experiments carried out by Leyton and Sherrington (1917) in which they surgically removed different portions of the cerebral cortex in apes and then documented behavioral deficits immediately upon recovery and then for several weeks thereafter. In one chimpanzee, for example, the region of the left motor cortex that most readily evoked movements of the fingers, wrist, elbow, and shoulder of the right arm upon electrical stimulation was excised. Immediately upon recovery from surgery, the chimp exhibited wrist-drop, clear paralysis of the thumb and index finger, but no obvious paralysis of the elbow of the right arm. The day following the surgery, the animal was able to climb on its cage, with good use of its right shoulder and elbow, and use of the fingers to grasp the bars of the cage. Two weeks following the surgery, virtually no deficits could be observed in the use of the right arm or hand.

A few months after the original surgery, regions adjacent to the lesion were stimulated to determine whether those areas now evoked movements of the right arm or hand. Figure 1 shows the outcome of that experiment. The symbols indicate what movements were evoked upon stimulation. A "0" indicates that no movement was elicited. Stimulation of areas immediately ventral to (below) the lesion evoked movements of the mouth and ears. Stimulation of the area bounding the lesion dorsally (above) caused contraction of chest muscles. Neither stimulation of the primary somatosensory cortex, caudal to (to the right) nor stimulation of the premotor cortex, rostral to (to the left) the lesion, evoked any movements.

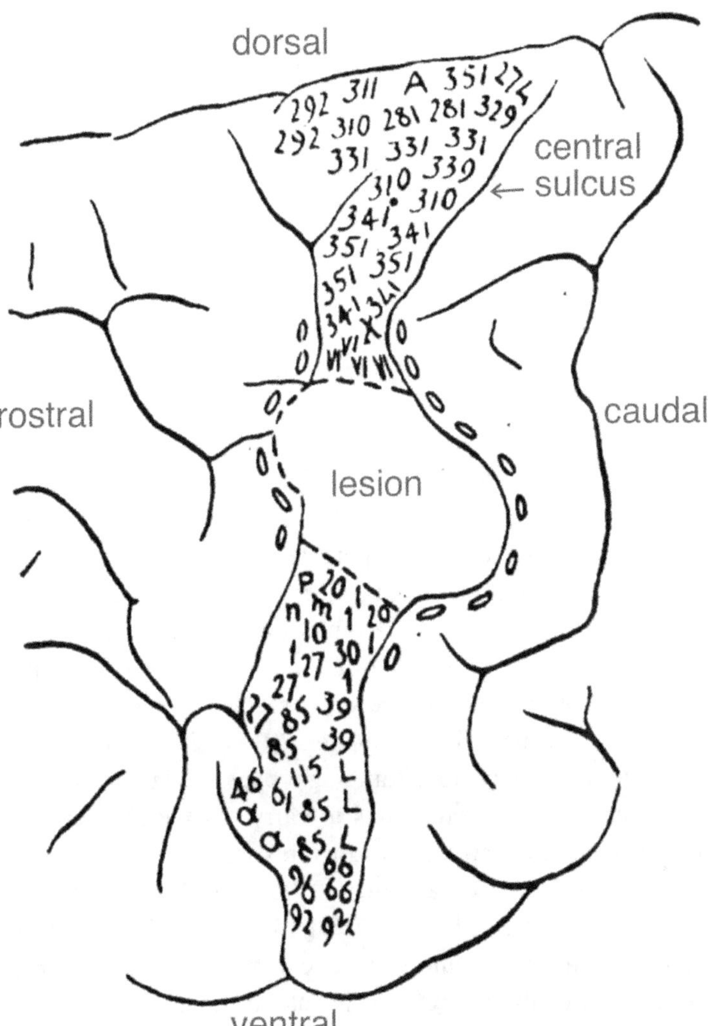

Figure 1.   Drawing of a portion of the cerebral cortex in a chimpanzee that had the finger/
wrist/elbow/shoulder region of the primary motor cortex surgically excised ("lesion") a
few months prior to testing. The numbers and symbols surrounding the lesion indicate the
types of movements evoked with electrical stimulation at various sites. "0" indicates no
movement elicited. "VI" the contralateral chest muscles, "P" the contralateral ear, "20" the
upper lip, "1" the mouth. No regions evoked arm/hand movements, yet the animal exhibited little impairment in use of the limb. (Adapted from Leyton and Sherrington [1917].)

Therefore, unlike the work of Nudo *et al.* (1996) described above, no evidence was found of neighboring regions "taking over" the function of the lesioned area in the Leyton and Sherrington study. To test the possibility that the motor cortex contralateral to the lesion (i.e., on the right side of the brain) might have undergone plastic changes to enable control of the right arm via ipsilateral connections to the spinal cord, Leyton and Sherrington then also lesioned the right motor cortex. Immediately upon recovery from this surgery, as described in the typical ornate language of Sherrington: *"Not the slightest recrudescence of symptoms of paresis and clumsiness in the right arm was detected."* It should be noted that a similar outcome to the Leyton and Sherrington (1917) study was more recently described in rats (Kawai *et al.* 2015).

What is one to make of such findings? If a large portion of the cerebellum or the motor cortex is removed, the behavior is little impaired, and there is little evidence that regions neighboring the lesion are repurposed to carry out operations of the damaged area, then what part of the brain is used to control the movements? One possibility is that the computations and production of neural signals needed to carry out such movements are actually performed by the "low-level" structures, such as those in the brainstem or the spinal cord (Kawai *et al.* 2015). "High-level" input from the cerebral cortex or the cerebellum might play more of an enabling role, exciting those lower-level structures to carry out the elaboration of the desired movement. If the high-level structures are disabled, time-dependent changes in the intrinsic excitabilities of the lower-level structures might enable them to be activated with minimal high-level input (Otchy *et al.* 2015). The consequence would be recovery of function in the absence of the areas conventionally thought to mediate the behavior.

It is also possible that if a small portion of a targeted structure remains intact following inactivation or lesion, it could take on an outsized role in continuing to perform the functions of that structure. For example, in cats with 85% to 98% of their optic tract (connection between retina and visual thalamus) severed bilaterally, virtually no gross visual impairments could be detected a week after the surgery (Galambos *et al.* 1967). The animals also performed normally on tests of visual discrimination. It is important to point out that it is very difficult to ensure that the entirety of a targeted brain structure is lesioned or inactivated in such experiments. Indeed, the original goal of the Galambos *et al.* (1967) study was to observe adaptive changes that occur in response to complete elimination of the optic tract.

In a similar vein, and as discussed in Chapter 16, Mott and Sherrington (1895) showed that when all the dorsal roots supplying the arm and hand in monkeys were severed, the arm was more or less permanently paralyzed. However, if they left just one dorsal root intact, few deficits were detectable. Those results were fully confirmed in a later study by Twitchell (1954). Therefore, it appears as though retention of even a modicum of a neural structure can largely prevent the development of overt impairments. This possibility markedly complicates the interpretation of lesion or inactivation experiments.

References

Bonita R & Beaglehole R (1988). Recovery of motor function after stroke. *Stroke* **19**, 1497–1500.

Galambos R, Norton TT & Frommer GP (1967). Optic tract lesions sparing pattern vision in cats. *Experimental Neurology* **18**, 8–25.

Kawai R, Markman T, Poddar R, Ko R, Fantana AL, Dhawale AK, Kampff AR & Ölveczky BP (2015). Motor cortex is required for learning but not for executing a motor skill. *Neuron* **86**, 800–812.

Leyton ASF & Sherrington CS (1917). Observations on the excitable cortex of the chimpanzee, orangutan, and gorilla. *Quarterly Journal of Experimental Physiology* **11**, 135–222.

Mott FW & Sherrington CS (1895). Experiments upon the influence of sensory nerves upon movement and nutrition of the limbs. Preliminary communication. *Proceedings of the Royal Society of London* **57**, 481–488.

Nudo RJ, Wise BM, Si Fuentes F & Milliken GW (1996). Neural substrates for the effects of rehabilitative training on motor recovery after ischemic infarct. *Science* **272**, 1791–1794.

Otchy TM, Wolff SBE, Rhee JY, Pehlevan C, Kawai R, Kempf A, Gobes SMH & Ölveczky BP (2015). Acute off-target effects of neural circuit manipulations. *Nature* **528**, 358–363.

Twitchell TE (1954). Sensory factors in purposive movement. *Journal of Neurophysiology* **17**, 239–252.

Index